Principles of Polymer Science and Technology in Cosmetics and Personal Care

COSMETIC SCIENCE AND TECHNOLOGY

Series Editor

ERIC JUNGERMANN

Jungermann Associates, Inc.
Phoenix, Arizona

1. Cosmetic and Drug Preservation: Principles and Practice, *edited by Jon J. Kabara*
2. The Cosmetic Industry: Scientific and Regulatory Foundations, *edited by Norman F. Estrin*
3. Cosmetic Product Testing: A Modern Psychophysical Approach, *Howard R. Moskowitz*
4. Cosmetic Analysis: Selective Methods and Techniques, *edited by P. Boré*
5. Cosmetic Safety: A Primer for Cosmetic Scientists, *edited by James H. Whittam*
6. Oral Hygiene Products and Practice, *Morton Pader*
7. Antiperspirants and Deodorants, *edited by Karl Laden and Carl B. Felger*
8. Clinical Safety and Efficacy Testing of Cosmetics, *edited by William C. Waggoner*
9. Methods for Cutaneous Investigation, *edited by Robert L. Rietschel and Thomas S. Spencer*
10. Sunscreens: Development, Evaluation, and Regulatory Aspects, *edited by Nicholas J. Lowe and Nadim A. Shaath*
11. Glycerine: A Key Cosmetic Ingredient, *edited by Eric Jungermann and Norman O. V. Sonntag*
12. Handbook of Cosmetic Microbiology, *Donald S. Orth*
13. Rheological Properties of Cosmetics and Toiletries, *edited by Dennis Laba*
14. Consumer Testing and Evaluation of Personal Care Products, *Howard R. Moskowitz*
15. Sunscreens: Development, Evaluation, and Regulatory Aspects. Second Edition, Revised and Expanded, *edited by Nicholas J. Lowe, Nadim A. Shaath, and Madhu A. Pathak*
16. Preservative-Free and Self-Preserving Cosmetics and Drugs: Principles and Practice, *edited by Jon J. Kabara and Donald S. Orth*
17. Hair and Hair Care, *edited by Dale H. Johnson*
18. Cosmetic Claims Substantiation, *edited by Louise B. Aust*
19. Novel Cosmetic Delivery Systems, *edited by Shlomo Magdassi and Elka Touitou*
20. Antiperspirants and Deodorants: Second Edition, Revised and Expanded, *edited by Karl Laden*
21. Conditioning Agents for Hair and Skin, *edited by Randy Schueller and Perry Romanowski*
22. Principles of Polymer Science and Technology in Cosmetics and Personal Care, *edited by E. Desmond Goddard and James V. Gruber*

ADDITIONAL VOLUMES IN PREPARATION

Botanicals in Cosmetics, *edited by Larry Smith*

Principles of Polymer Science and Technology in Cosmetics and Personal Care

edited by

E. Desmond Goddard

Former Corporate Research Fellow
Union Carbide Corporation
Tarrytown, New York

James V. Gruber

Amerchol Corporation
Edison, New Jersey

MARCEL DEKKER, INC. NEW YORK • BASEL

Library of Congress Cataloging-in-Publication Data

Principles of polymer science and technology in cosmetics and personal care / edited by E. Desmond Goddard and James V. Gruber.
p. cm.—(Cosmetic science and technology : v. 22)
Includes bibliographical references and index.
ISBN 0-8247-1923-9 (alk. paper)
1. Cosmetics. 2. Toilet preparations. 3. Polymers. I. Goddard, E. D. (Errol Desmond). II. Gruber, James V.
III. Series: Cosmetic science and technology series : v. 22.
TP983.P8924 1999
668′.5—dc21 99-17274
CIP

This book is printed on acid-free paper.

Headquarters
Marcel Dekker, Inc.
270 Madison Avenue, New York, NY 10016
tel: 212-696-9000; fax: 212-685-4540

Eastern Hemisphere Distribution
Marcel Dekker AG
Hutgasse 4, Postfach 812, CH-4001 Basel, Switzerland
tel: 41-61-261-8482; fax: 41-61-261-8896

World Wide Web
http://www.dekker.com

The publisher offers discounts on this book when ordered in bulk quantities. For more information, write to Special Sales/Professional Marketing at the headquarters address above.

Current printing (last digit):
10 9 8 7 6 5 4 3 2 1

PRINTED IN THE UNITED STATES OF AMERICA

Series Introduction

The Cosmetic Science and Technology series was conceived to permit discussion of a broad range of current knowledge and theories of cosmetic science and technology. The series is made up of books either written by a single author or edited with a number of contributors. Authorities from industry, academia, and the government are participating in writing these books.

The aim of this series is to cover the many facets of cosmetic science and technology. Topics are drawn from a wide spectrum of disciplines ranging from chemistry, physics, biochemistry, analytical and consumer evaluations to safety, efficacy, toxicity, and regulatory questions. Organic, inorganic, physical, and polymer chemistry, as well as emulsion technology, microbiology, dermatology and toxicology all play a role in cosmetic science.

There is little commonality in the scientific methods, processes, or formulations required for the wide variety of cosmetics and toiletries manufactured. Products range from hair care, oral care, and skin care preparations to lipsticks, nail polishes and extenders, deodorants, body powders and aerosols, to over-the-counter products, such as antiperspirants, dandruff treatments, antimicrobial soaps, and acne and sunscreen products.

Cosmetics and toiletries represent a highly diversified field with many subsections of science and ''art.'' Indeed, even in these days of high technology, ''art'' and intuition continue to play an important part in the development of formulations, their evaluation, and the selection of raw materials. There is a move toward more sophisticated scientific methodologies in the fields of preservative efficacy testing, claim substantiation, safety testing, product evaluation, and chemical analyses.

Emphasis in the Cosmetic Science and Technology series is placed on reporting the current status of cosmetic technology and science in addition to historical reviews. Several of the books have found an international audience and have been translated into Japanese or Chinese. Contributions range from highly sophisticated and scientific treatises to primers, practical applications, and pragmatic presentations. Authors are encouraged to present their own concepts, as well as established theories. Contributors have been asked not to shy away from fields that are still in a state of transition, or to hesitate to present detailed discussions of their own work. Altogether, we intend to develop in this series a collection of critical surveys and ideas covering diverse phases of the cosmetic industry.

Principles of Polymer Science and Technology in Cosmetics and Personal Care is the twenty-second volume published in this series. Polymers are important components in a broad range of cosmetic and personal care products. They fill a multitude of functions too numerous to list. This book covers the many classes of polymers used in almost every type of cosmetic formulation and their wide range of applications, special properties, and sometimes specialized requirements.

I want to thank the editors, E. Desmond Goddard and James V. Gruber, and all the contributors for collaborating in the editing and writing of this book. Special recognition is also due to Sandra Beberman and the editorial staff at Marcel Dekker, Inc. In addition, I would like to thank my wife Eva, without whose constant support and editorial help I would never have undertaken this project.

Eric Jungermann, Ph.D.

Preface

Although synthetic polymers first appeared in the last century, it has been the twentieth century, especially the second half, which has witnessed an explosive growth in the development and use of this category of material. Indeed, it is difficult to think of many industries today that do not employ polymers in some form or another. Such employment, of course, includes that by the cosmetic and personal care industry in which the use of polymeric materials continues to develop rapidly. This trend will continue in the next century.

Polymer science—already starting from a solid foundation with the early recognition that many natural products, including proteins and polysaccharides, are polymeric—has grown apace with these developments. Today some would aver that it has been difficult for many scientists, including those actually involved in research and development work involving polymers, to keep abreast of recent theoretical developments, let alone to retain a working familiarity with what has evolved today as basic polymer science. Be this as it may, a need was identified for a book that could be used not only as a reference source for the polymers currently used in the cosmetics industry, but also as a source of information on the basic physical chemistry of polymers as it applies to the functions they serve in the formulation and use properties of cosmetics. Furthermore, because of both the latter features and the overlapping of technology, it seems that such a text might also be found useful by investigators in related fields such as detergent formulation, pharmaceuticals, textiles, and even the latex paint industry. Bearing in mind the breadth of the field, we invited the participation of several other authors, all recognized as experts in their area(s) of polymer science. We believe the result is a comprehensive coverage of the field designated by the title of the book.

The body of the text consists of 12 self-standing chapters comprising a mix of the fundamental science of polymers, their solution and interfacial properties, their interactions with surfactants, the intrinsic properties of polymers employed in cosmetic formulations, and the properties they confer to treated surfaces. There is also an appendix which lists and groups the polymers used in cosmetics.

Chapter 1 is an introduction to polymer science, covering its history, fundamentals, and recent developments. The reader is introduced to the different types of polymers, their classification and synthesis, molecular weight definitions, and properties in the solid and semisolid state. There follows an overview of the properties of polymers in solution starting with their thermodynamics, considerations of molecular size and shape, and finally their rheology. It concludes with a list of about 50 definitions used in polymer science, potentially useful to newcomers and seasoned practitioners alike.

Many uses of polymers are concerned with the properties of polymers at interfaces. Chapter 2 presents a summary of theories of polymer adsorption and discusses the properties and state of polymers at interfaces and methods for determining the details of their structure, conformations, and so on. The basic theory of colloid-interaction forces in terms of DLVO theory is presented, together with a discussion of the different basic stabilization mechanisms of colloids.

In Chapter 3, the solution and surface properties of a relatively new class of material, namely, polymeric surfactants, are illustrated in some detail using Flory-Huggins theory and current polymer-adsorption theory. This is followed by a discussion of the phenomenon of steric stabilization of suspended particles and how it is affected by the detailed structure of the stabilizing polymeric species. It concludes with a discussion of the stabilization of emulsions by interfacial and bulk rheological effects, and presents closing comments on ''multiple'' emulsions.

When polymers are employed in personal care formulations, in many (if not most) cases they occur as cocomponents with surfactants. Recognizing a widespread tendency of such components to interact and affect each other's properties (sometimes in dramatic ways), Chapter 4 outlines a number of methods to investigate and analyze such interaction for the main types of polymers—nonionic, ionic, ''hydrophobic,'' and proteinaceous. Chapter 5 presents an illustrative selection of polymer/surfactant interactions in applied systems that demonstrates how they can be selected to achieve beneficial performance effects.

Realizing that many practicing formulation chemists and research scientists are seeking more immediate and nontheoretical discussion of the polymers used so frequently in cosmetics and personal care, the next four chapters were written to address, in a more nuts-and-bolts fashion, the most popular and widely used polymers employed in the industry, including synthetic polymers, silicone polymers, polysaccharides, and proteins. However, the intent of the authors of these four chapters was not simply to describe lists of formulations, but instead to try and discuss the basic knowledge of these four polymer groups and to develop insights into 1) how one might better formulate with these materials and 2) what behavioral aspects one might expect in using a particular polymer.

Synthetic polymers are ubiquitous in the personal care industry. Chapter 6 strives to address this rather broad topic in a straightforward and easily readable fashion. The chapter starts with a brief discussion of how synthetic polymers are made and the nomenclature used to describe some of the more basic structural principles of synthetic polymers. It expands to address many of the synthetic polymers used in personal care formulations based principally on their primary mode of operation, including thickening polymers, fixative polymers, conditioning polymers, and encapsulating polymers, the last subject becoming more important as formulators develop more sophisticated topical systems to deliver active materials.

Chapter 7 discusses the phenomenal range and use of silicone polymers that can be found in nearly every branch of personal care and cosmetic development. The chapter discusses how the polymers are made, essentially from sand, and the nomenclature used to describe the many different types of silicone-based polymers found in the industry.

A lengthy discussion follows, covering how the polymers behave in use, the spreading characteristics, and the many beneficial properties silicone polymers offer when delivered to keratinous surfaces. The chapter concludes with a thorough discussion of the safety and environmental impact of silicone-based polymers.

Chapter 8 is a review of the use of polysaccharides, perhaps some of the oldest and most well-known ingredients used in personal care. Because polysaccharides are derived from natural sources, the nature of the monosaccharides that comprise these sugar-based polymers and how nature designs the polysaccharides are addressed first. This discussion is followed by greater details of individual cosmetically important polysaccharides based primarily on the ionic nature of the polysaccharide, that is, anionic, cationic, nonionic, or amphoteric, which can be either naturally developed by the polysaccharide source or manipulated by human intervention and invention. The effects of hydrophobic modification of polysaccharides are also discussed. The chapter concludes with a brief discussion of certain polysaccharides that appear to have physiological effects on the human body when applied topically.

Chapter 9 addresses the important issues and chemistry surrounding the use of proteins in personal care. The chapter begins with a thorough review of the structural properties of proteins, including the basic amino acids of which they are composed, the various sources (both plant and animal) of the beneficial proteins, and how these amino-acid-based polymers develop secondary, tertiary, and quaternary structures as they form. The chapter then addresses how proteins behave in formulations and how their functionality can be interrupted or changed by formulations or modification of the proteins that affect these unique protein-folding structures. It concludes with a timely discussion covering protein contaminants, particularly bovine spongiphorm encephalopathy (BSE), a human contagion the nature of which has appeared to grip the industry somewhat emotionally.

Polycationic materials are well known and have long been used as conditioning agents for hair and skin. Chapters 10 and 11 discuss methods employed, and results obtained, in measurements of their sorption by these substrates. These model studies show that uptake of polymer can be substantial, vastly exceeding that required for simple ''monolayer'' coverage. Presumably what is involved is the substantial swelling, and the development of diffusion channels, in these substrates on immersion in water. Although some ionic surfactants, that is, anionic, or especially cationic surfactants, can substantially reduce the uptake, they do not eliminate it.

The last chapter (12) is concerned with evaluation methods of polymer-conditioned hair. The first part deals with single-fiber evaluation and includes contact angle, electrokinetic, fluorimetry, friction, and cuticle-cohesion measurements. The second part deals with hair assemblies and includes measurements of combing, ''body,'' optical properties, and static electrification.

Finally, in the appendix, there is a comprehensive listing—an ''encyclopedia''—of the polymers used in the cosmetic industry, together with their INCI designations and a brief description of the polymers. We believe that inclusion of this updated compendium adds substantially to the general utility of the book.

On a personal note, Dr. Goddard wishes to express his appreciation to Union Carbide and Amerchol Corporation for sustained support of his own research work on many of the subjects dealt with in this volume. This work would not have been possible without the cooperation and contributions of many of his former colleagues, including, especially, J. A. Faucher, R. B. Hannan, P. S. Leung, and K. P. Ananthapadmanabhan. In particular he wishes to thank the last-mentioned (''Ananth'') for many fruitful discussions during compilation of Chapter 5. Lastly, he wishes also to express his appreciation to J. V. Gruber who, as coeditor of this book and author of two chapters and in many other ways, played a key role in making this undertaking a reality.

Dr. Gruber would like to recognize the friendship and professional relationship which has developed with E. D. Goddard as a result of this undertaking, and to express his appreciation for being invited to become a part of this project. In addition, he wishes to recognize the help that Freida DeBaro provided in completing the chapters he worked on. Her assistance was invaluable. He would also like to thank Frank J. Freiler and the Amerchol Corporation for giving him the opportunity to work on this volume. Both editors thank Sandra Beberman for her help in making the project move along quickly and professionally. Dr. Gruber is indebted to Lori Riday for her patience and understanding as this project borrowed many weekends of personal quality time. He would like to dedicate his efforts on this book to his family and especially to his brother Steve Gruber.

E. Desmond Goddard
James V. Gruber

Contents

Contributors

Marianne D. Berthiaume, M.Sc. Personal Care–Worldwide, Wacker Silicones Corporation, Adrian, Michigan

E. Desmond Goddard, Ph.D. Former Corporate Research Fellow, Union Carbide Corporation, Tarrytown, New York

Peter C. Griffiths, Ph.D. Department of Chemistry, Cardiff University, Cardiff, Wales

James V. Gruber, Ph.D. Amerchol Corporation, Edison, New Jersey

Yashavanth Kamath, Ph.D. TRI/Princeton, Princeton, New Jersey

Robert Y. Lochhead, Ph.D. Department of Polymer Science, University of Southern Mississippi, Hattiesburg, Mississippi

Timothy M. Obey, Ph.D. School of Chemistry, University of Bristol, Bristol, England

Gianfranco Secchi Kelisema Italy, Tavernerio, Italy

Th. F. Tadros, Ph.D. Department of Chemical Engineering, Imperial College, London, England

Alessandro Teglia, Ph.D. Kelisema Italy, Tavernerio, Italy

Hans-Dietrich Weigmann, Ph.D. TRI/Princeton, Princeton, New Jersey

Françoise M. Winnik, Ph.D. Department of Chemistry, McMaster University, Hamilton, Ontario, Canada

Principles of Polymer Science and Technology in Cosmetics and Personal Care

1

Elements of Polymer Science

Françoise M. Winnik
McMaster University, Hamilton, Ontario, Canada

I. INTRODUCTION

Polymers are molecules consisting of a large number of identical low molar mass units, named repeat units, that are connected covalently. If -A- is the base unit, then a polymer molecule or macromolecule is represented by:

$$——\text{-A-A-A-A-A-A}———— \text{ or } —(\text{A})_n—$$

where n is an integer, called degree of polymerization of this macromolecule. Before 1930, polymer molecules were generally considered as physical aggregates of unchanged monomer molecules $(A)_n$, so-called association colloids. However, already in 1920, Staudinger had postulated that these colloidal particles were composed of a single, very long molecule, a macromolecule. This revolutionary concept paved the way for synthetic organic chemists, in particular Carothers, to start building such macromolecules in a systematic way from known monomers. Since the 1930s, many thousands of polymers have been prepared, but less than 100 of them have reached the phase of large-scale industrial production. For accounts of the history of polymer science and technology, see, for example, Refs. 1 and 1a.

Polymers represent a significant share of raw materials used in the cosmetics industry. They are usually classified according to their use, such as thickening agents, film formers, resinous powders, and humectants. Thickening agents are used to adjust the viscosity of products to make them easy to use and to maintain the product stability. For example, they are used to ensure the stability of milky lotions and liquid foundations by preventing the separation of emulsified particles and powders. Thickening agents polymers are in widespread use for this specific purpose. Natural polymers, gums and resins, have been used in the industry since the early 1940s as water-soluble binders, thickeners, and film-forming agents. In today's products they are added to many cosmetics formulations to fulfill these various functions, but often they are used simply because of the growing consumer demand for "natural products." There are drawbacks, however, to the use of polymers isolated from natural sources: they vary in purity and physical appearance, and they are relatively expensive, compared to common synthetic polymers. Problems securing stable supplies coupled with variations in viscosity and microbial contamination led to a change to synthetic or semisynthetic substitutes. Synthetic or semisynthetic polymers, which are chemically modified natural polymers, have been developed to match the properties of gums and resins. Today, the industry is driven by a need of improved formulations, attainable through the use of current synthetic methodology and through the understanding of the molecular interactions between the polymers and the other components of a care product.

This chapter covers the chemistry, physical properties, and thermodynamics of polymers. First are discussed various methods of macromolecule preparation. Next are discussed the physical properties of polymers in the bulk, with emphasis on the morphology and rheology of polymeric materials. Finally, several aspects of polymer solutions are discussed, including their thermodynamics and rheological properties, which will be related to molecular parameters such as chain conformation. Current theories that account for the properties of macromolecules in the bulk and in solution are presented briefly. The reader is encouraged to seek further information in specialized texts (2–7), dictionaries (8), and encyclopedia (9–11).

A. Natural and Synthetic Polymers

1. Biopolymers

Proteins, polysaccharides, natural rubber, and gums are all natural polymers. The repeat units in proteins are amino acids. Nucleic acids are composed of nucleotides and polysaccharides consist of sugar units.

a. Proteins and Polypeptides. Amino acids in proteins are linked by an amide linkage between the amino group of one molecule and the carboxyl group of another. This amide bond is often called peptide bond (Fig. 1). There are simple proteins composed only of amino acids, such as albumin, gelatin, casein, collagen, or keratin. Other proteins contain not only amino acid residues, but also other groups such as carbohydrates in glycoproteins, or lipids in lipoproteins. Proteins that possess catalytic activity are known as enzymes.

b. Polysaccharides. The repeat units of polysaccharides are simple carbohydrates (sugars) linked to each other by acetal bonds (Fig. 1). Among the important polysaccharides are homopolymers of glucose (starch, glycogen, and cellulose), mannose (guar), or amino-sugars, such as chitosan and hyaluronan. Polysaccharides are important materials of the cosmetics industry. Their chemistry and physical properties are presented in Chapter 8.

2. Synthetic Polymers

Carothers, in 1929, classified synthetic polymers into two classes, according to the method of their preparation, i.e., condensation polymers and addition polymers. In polycondensation, or step-growth polymerization, polymers are obtained by reaction between two polyfunctional molecules and elimination of a small molecule, for example water. Typical condensation polymers are shown in Figure 2. Addition (or chain reaction) polymers are formed from unsaturated monomers in a chain reaction. Examples of addition polymers are shown in Figure 2.

We will conform to Carothers' classification in the sections devoted to the preparation of synthetic polymers. However, when considering the application of polymers it is more useful to consider the following three categories: (1) *plastics*, which include thermosetting resins, such as urea resins, polyesters, or epoxies, and thermoplastic resins, such as poly-

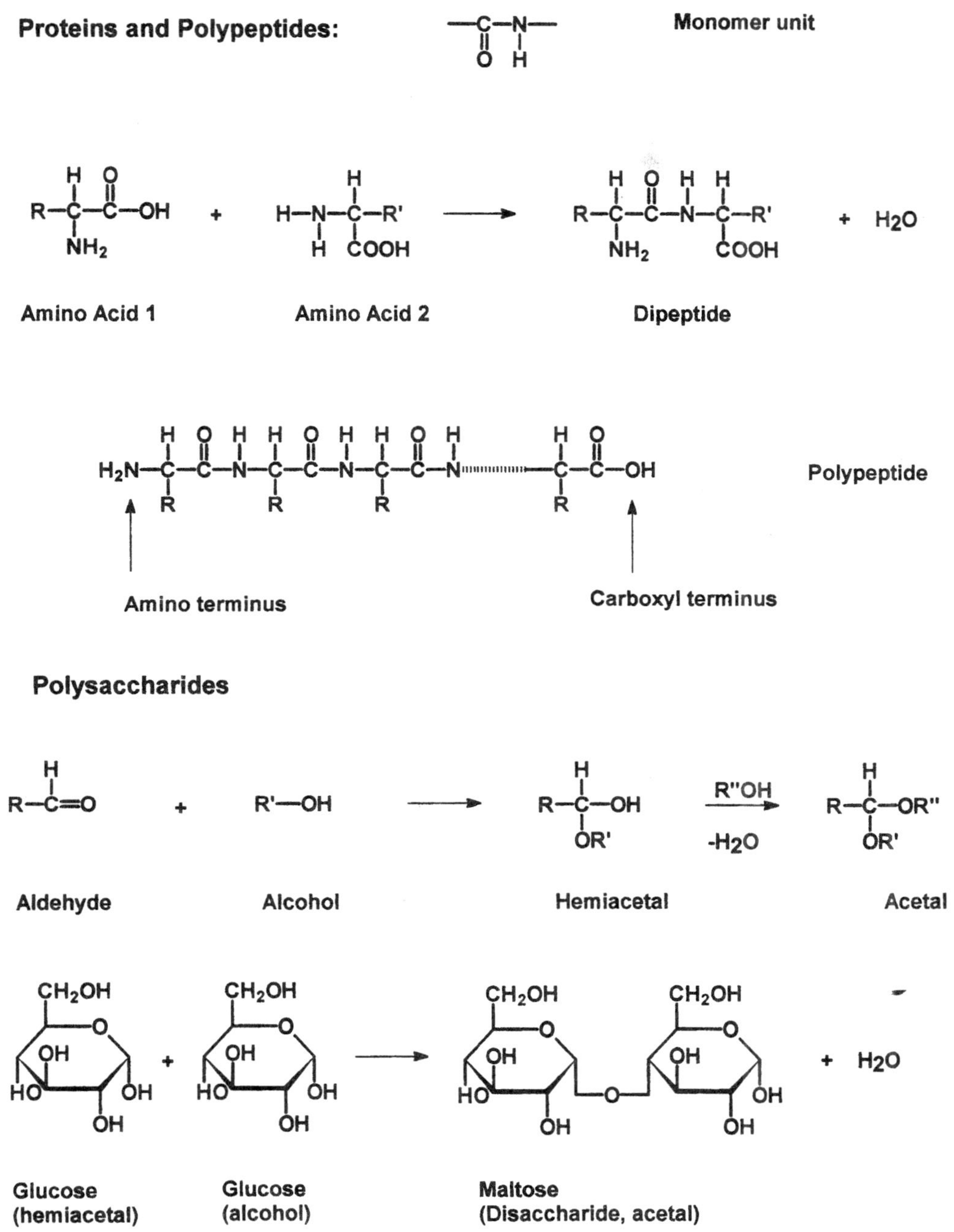

Figure 1 Chemical structures of natural polymers.

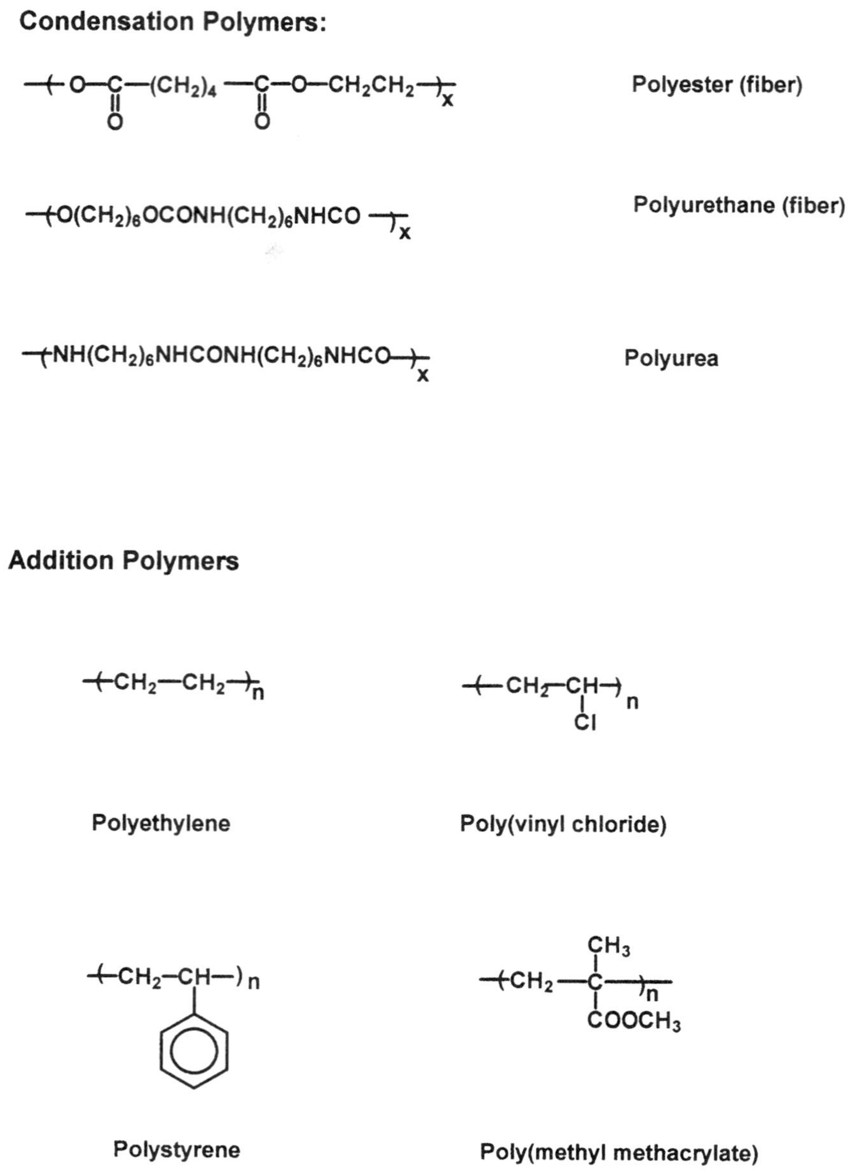

Figure 2 Chemical structures of synthetic polymers.

ethylene, polystyrene, or poly(propylene); (2) *fibers*, which include cellulosics, such as rayon and acetate, and noncellulosic polymers, such as polyester and nylon; and (3) *rubbers*, for example styrene-butadiene copolymer.

B. Definitions and Nomenclature

Homopolymers are derived from one type of monomer, whereas copolymers require two or more species of monomers. Copolymers are distinguished according to the sequence

Table 1 Sequence of Monomer Units in Various Copolymers

Copolymer type	Schematic composition
Statistical or random	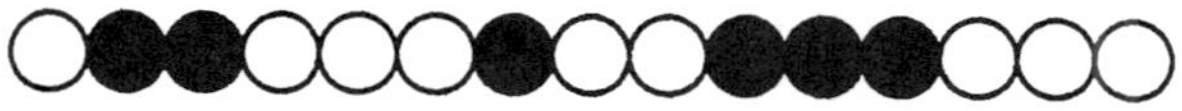
Alternating	
Diblock	
Triblock	
Graft	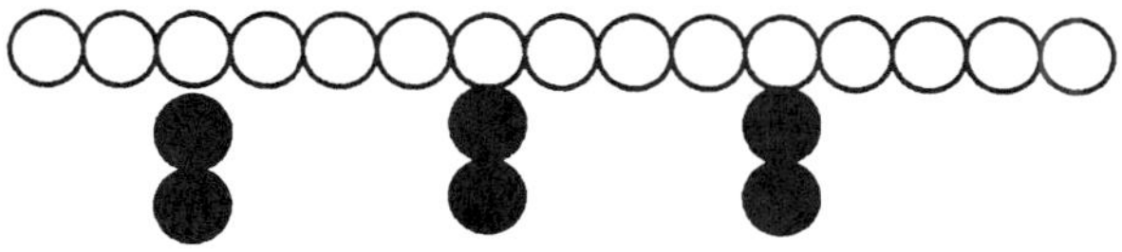

of the various monomer units. They are subdivided into the major classes listed in Table 1. The simplest polymers consist of regular macromolecules, with only one repeat unit in a single sequential arrangement. Examples are poly(acrylic acid), polystyrene, and polyethylene (Fig. 2). The constitutional units form a linear chain. Cyclic polymer molecules result if the two ends of a linear macromolecule are connected. They are called ‘‘macrocycles’’ (12). Small amounts of cyclic molecules are often formed as by-products during the synthesis of linear chains. Combinations of linear molecules, of linear molecules with cyclic molecules, and of cyclic macromolecules themselves lead to a great variety of molecular architectures (Fig. 3).

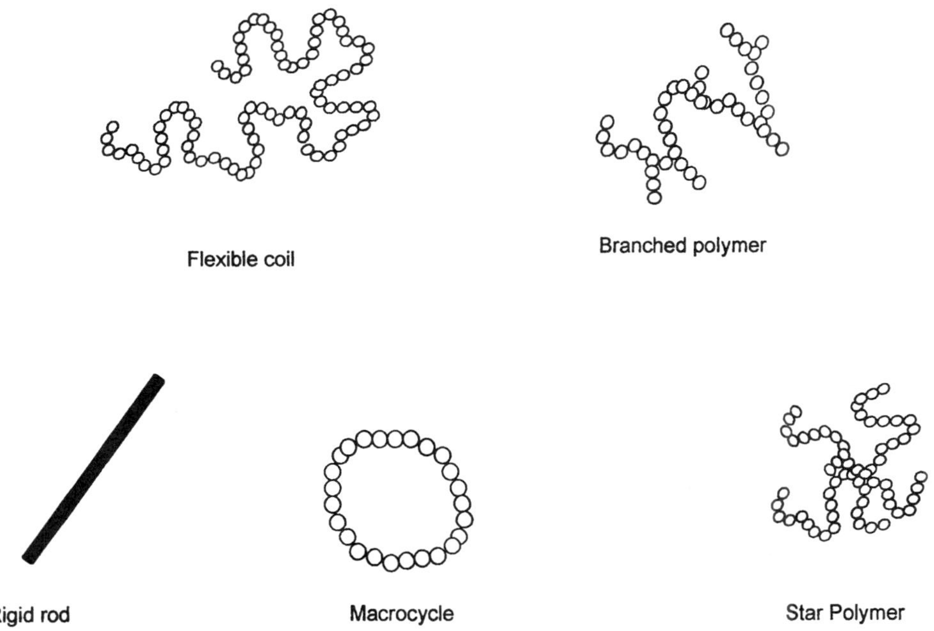

Figure 3 Major macromolecular architectures.

Linear chains may also be arranged at short intervals along a single main chain via trifunctional branch points. These ''comb'' polymers can be synthesized by polymerization of macromers (a monomer consisting of a polymerizable group linked to a short polymer chain) or by grafting (13). Branched polymers contain branch points (junctions) that connect three or four subchains, which may be side chains or parts of a main chain. Polymers are statistically branched if side chains of different lengths are irregularly distributed along the main chain. These polymers resemble trees. In star polymers (14) three or more branches sprout from a common core. Star polymers with multifunctional ends on the arms can add additional monomers. The resulting polymers, known as dendrimers (15), can be considered as tree polymers with regular sequences of branches or star polymers with subsequent secondary branches.

In cross-linked polymers, all molecules of a sample are interconnected by many bonds, resulting in a single, ''infinitely large'' molecule. Networks can be generated by intermolecular covalent bond or by physical junctions, such as ion clusters, crystallites, or microphases. Physical (noncovalently bound) networks can *in principle* be dissolved by a solvent, whereas chemical (covalently bound) networks are insoluble in all solvents. The chemical properties of polymer networks depend strongly on the chemical structure of the chemical chain and the type of junction. The mechanical properties are primarily dictated by the cross-link density and by the mobility of the chain segments. Networks may thus be soft, elastic, brittle, or hard. Two independent networks may interpenetrate to form interpenetrating networks (IPN) (16). Nail enamels are examples of physical networks formed upon solvent evaporation, with no chemical cross-linking during drying but only physical interactions among their polymer constituents, primarily nitrocellulose and synthetic resins.

A classification of polymers especially useful in the case of water-soluble polymers is based on the electric charge born by the macromolecule. Electrically neutral water-soluble polymers include various polysaccharides, mostly cellulose ethers, polyacrylamides, and certain polyethers, such as poly(ethylene glycols). Polyelectrolytes are water-soluble polymers with many electrically charged groups per molecule. They form polyions on dissociation. These polyions may be polyanions with negative charges as in dissociated poly(acrylic acid) $—[CH_2—CH(COO^-)]_n—$ or polycations as in protonated poly(vinylamine), $—[CH_2—CH(NH_3)^+]_n—$. They may also be polysalts, as in the sodium salt of poly(acrylic acid), $—[CH_2—CH(COONa)]_n—$. Polyions should be distinguished from macroions, which carry only one ionic group, usually at one chain end. Water-insoluble polymers with relatively few ionic groups in the chain are known as ionomers.

II. PREPARATIONS OF MACROMOLECULAR COMPOUNDS

Synthetic polymers are prepared by one of two fundamentally different approaches: (a) polymerization of monomer molecules or (b) modification of existent macromolecules into macromolecules of different constitution, a process known as polymer analog reaction (17–19). Both methods are described briefly in this section, starting with the polymerization reactions, which can proceed via two different processes, condensation reactions in step-growth polymerizations and addition reactions in chain-growth polymerizations.

A. Step-Growth Polymerization

The term ''step-growth polymerization'' refers to the process in which the polymer molecular weight increases in a slow, step-like manner as reaction time increases. This polymerization depends entirely on individual reactions of the functional groups of monomers. Random reactions of two molecules occur between any combination of a monomer, oligomer, or a longer-chain molecule. High-molecular-weight polymers are formed only near the end of the polymerization, when most of the monomer has been depleted. Polyesters, polyamides, polyurethanes, and polycarbonates are prepared by step-growth polymerization (Fig. 4).

The polycondensation technique can also be applied to prepare organic-inorganic polymers. The most important such polymers are the polysiloxanes, also known as silicone polymers such as dimethicone, based on the —Si—O— linkage present in glass or sand (see Chapter 7). They are made by polymerization of a low-molecular-weight cyclic analog, such as octamethylcyclotetrasiloxane. When this compound is heated above 100°C with a trace of an acid or base, it polymerizes to form a highly viscous liquid. Although the dimethylsiloxane structure forms the basis of most silicone polymers, other substituents have also been introduced as cosubstituents. These include vinyl, ethyl, phenyl, and *n*-alkyl groups. Polysiloxanes are among the most flexible macromolecules known. They also repel water. Partly because of this property, they are used in protective hand-and-body lotions and creams. They are incorporated also in hair-care formulations to improve luster and sheen.

Condensation polymers can be prepared by several techniques:

The melt technique, where an equimolar mixture of two monomers is heated, possibly in the presence of a catalyst. It is an equilibrium process in which the polymer is formed by driving the reaction to completion by removal of the by-products, such as water or hydrochloric acid.

The solution condensation, where equimolar amounts of the two monomers are dis-

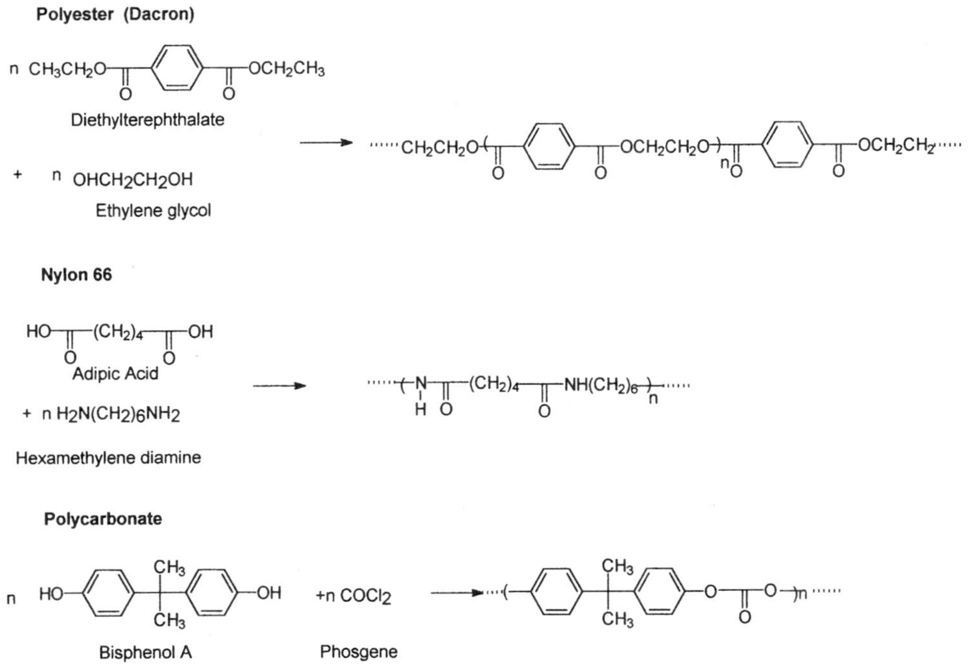

Figure 4 Synthetic scheme for the preparation of condensation polymers.

solved in a solvent, which should also be a solvent for the polymer. It is an equilibrium reaction, driven to completion by removal of the by-products, but it has to be carried out at temperatures lower than melt polycondensations.

The interfacial technique (20), which is a heterophase process where two fast-reacting reactants are dissolved in a pair of immiscible solvents, one of which is usually water. The aqueous phase contains a diol or a diamine; the organic phase contains a diacid chloride dissolved in a solvent such as dichloromethane, toluene, or diethyl ether. Condensation occurs at the water/organic solvent interface often in the presence of a phase transfer catalyst.

B. Chain-Growth Polymerization

In this process, the only chain-extension reaction is that of attachment of a monomer to a growing ''active'' chain. The active end group may be a free radical, an anion, or a cation. In contrast to step-growth polymerization, some high-molecular-weight polymer is formed in the early stage of the addition polymerization.

1. *Free-Radical Polymerization (21)*

The general scheme for free-radical polymerization can be expressed as follows:

$\text{Initiator} \rightarrow R^{\bullet}$	Initiation
$R^{\bullet} + M \rightarrow MR^{\bullet}$	Chain propagation
$MR^{\bullet} + M \rightarrow M_2R^{\bullet}$	
. . .	
$M_nR^{\bullet} + M_mR^{\bullet} \rightarrow M_{n+m}$	Chain termination

where M represents the monomer molecule and $R^{\bullet}$ a free radical produced in the initial step. Commonly used initiators are peroxides, such as potassium persulfate (soluble in water) or benzoyl peroxide (soluble in organic solvents), and aliphatic azo compounds, such as azobisisobutyronitrile (AIBN).

Various experimental techniques may be used to carry out free radical polymerizations. The choice of method is guided on the one hand by the solubility of the monomers and polymers and on the other hand by the preferred isolation method for the polymer. Common techniques are:

1. Bulk polymerization, where the reaction is carried out without solvent.
2. Solution polymerization, which is done in an inert liquid that dissolves both the monomer and the polymer.
3. Precipitation polymerization, which takes place in an inert liquid that dissolves the monomer, but not the polymer. The polymer is isolated by filtration or decantation.
4. Suspension polymerization, which is used with water-insoluble monomers suspended in water as droplets. Coalescing of the droplets is prevented by use of small amounts of a stabilizer, usually a water-soluble polymer, such as poly(vinyl alcohol). The polymer is isolated in the form of discrete particles 10–1000 nm in diameter.
5. Emulsion polymerization (22), which takes place in a suspension in water of a

water-insoluble monomer in the presence of a surfactant and a water-soluble initiator. Unlike suspension polymerization, this technique produces polymer in the form of a latex, or stable dispersion in water of polymer particles ranging in size from 0.05 to 5 nm.

2. *Ionic Polymerization*

Ionic polymerizations are initiated by ionic species. The active chain end is an ion, either a carbanion, C^-, in the case of anionic polymerizations (23,24) or a carbocation, C^+, in the case of cationic polymerizations (25,26). They have to be carried out in organic solvents under strictly anhydrous and oxygen-free conditions. Anionic polymerizations are performed with monomers that contain a double bond substituted with an electron-withdrawing group, such as styrene and various acrylic monomers, and also with oxiranes, such as ethylene oxide, which polymerize by a ring-opening mechanism. Macroanions in solution continue to grow until all initially present monomer molecules are consumed. Addition of new monomer leads to further polymerization. Such polymerizations without internal or external termination reaction are called living polymerizations. They are useful to synthesize homopolymers with narrow-molecular-weight distribution and star or block copolymers.

Cationic polymerizations are started by reaction of electrophilic initiator cations with electron-donating monomer molecules. Catalysts are Lewis acids and Friedel-Crafts catalysts, such as aluminum trichloride ($AlCl_3$), and strong acids, such as sulfuric acid (H_2SO_4). Monomer molecules able to undergo cationic polymerization include electron-rich olefins, such as vinyl aromatics and vinyl ethers, and ring compounds, such as ethylene oxide and tetrahydrofuran.

Other types of chain-growth polymerizations include: (a) insertion polymerizations, such as the Ziegler-Natta process used in the preparation of polyethylene and metathesis polymerizations (27,28), and (b) group transfer polymerizations, a process in which an initiator molecule transfers its active group to a monomer molecule under the action of a catalyst.

C. Polymerization Kinetics

Condensation reactions follow kinetic schemes similar to those of small molecule reactions. They are simple first-order, second-order, etc. reactions. In contrast, the kinetics of chain reactions, such as free-radical polymerization or ionic polymerization, are much more complicated.

1. *Condensation Reactions (29)*

We will discuss the case of polyesterifications, typical condensation reactions that take place by reaction of a diol (A, HO—R—OH) and a diacid (B, HOOC—R′—COOH):

$$n\ \mathrm{HO{-}R{-}OH} + n\ \mathrm{HOOC{-}R'{-}COOH} \rightarrow \mathrm{H{-}[O{-}R{-}OCO{-}R'{-}COO]_n^-}$$

The experimental rate of polycondensation polymerization is given by the following expression (Eq. 1), where k is the rate constant:

$$\frac{-d[B]}{dt} = k[B]^2[A] \quad (1)$$

If $[B] = [A] = c$, where c is the monomer concentration at time t, then the rate expression can be written as Eq. 2. Upon integration of the rearranged form (Eq. 3), we obtain Eq.

4, which is conveniently expressed in terms of P, the extent of reaction, defined as the fraction of functional groups that has reacted at time t. The concentration c can be expressed as a function of $1 - P$, the fraction of unreacted A and c_0, the initial concentration. Substituting c into Eq. 4, we obtain Eq. 5. A plot $1/(1 - P)^2$ versus time should be linear, with a slope of $2c_0^2\,k$, from which k can be determined.

$$\frac{-dc}{dt} = kc^3 \tag{2}$$

$$\frac{-dc}{c^3} = kdt \tag{3}$$

$$2\,kt = \frac{1}{c^2} + \text{constant} \tag{4}$$

$$2c_0^2\,kt = \frac{1}{(1 - P)^2} + \text{constant} \tag{5}$$

The number average degree of polymerization, DP_N, for condensation reactions can be expressed as:

$$DP_N = \frac{\text{number of original molecules}}{\text{number of molecules at time } t} = \frac{N_0}{N} = \frac{c_0}{c} = \frac{c_0}{c_0\,(1 - P)} = \frac{1}{1 - P} \tag{6}$$

For an essentially quantitative synthesis of polyesters, where $P = 0.9999$, the DP_N value calculated from Eq. 6 is equal to 10,000.

2. Free-Radical polymerizations

Free-radical polymerizations involve the simultaneous generation and disappearance of initiator radicals, monomer radicals, and macroradicals. After a few seconds the total concentration of all radicals becomes constant. This steady state or stationary state is obtained at very small monomer conversions. In terms of kinetics, the total free-radical concentration becomes stationary when the rate of radical formation equals the rate of radical disappearance (Eq. 7).

$$R_d = \frac{-\,d[I^\bullet]}{dt} = k_d\,[I] \tag{7}$$

Initiators I dissociate with a rate R_d giving two initiator radicals $I^\bullet$; therefore, the rate of radical formation R_r is double the rate of initiator decomposition:

$$R_r = \frac{d[I^\bullet]}{dt} = 2k_d[I] = 2R_d \tag{8}$$

However, since the initiator molecule dissociates in a ''cage'' surrounding monomer and solvent molecules, some of the newly formed radicals recombine immediately. Due to this cage effect, only a fraction f of initiator radicals $I^\bullet$ react with monomer in the start reaction: $I^\bullet + M \rightarrow IM^\bullet$ (st). The rate of radical formation is thus $R_r = 2\,f\,k_d\,[I]$. Monomer radicals are generated with a rate R_{st}, which is much greater than the rate R_d of initiator decomposition:

$$R_{st} = \frac{-\,d[I^\bullet]}{dt} = k_{st}[I^\bullet][M] \tag{9}$$

Initiator radicals are consumed as fast as they are generated. The rate-determining step is thus the initiator decomposition. Overall, the instantaneous concentration of initiator radicals and the rate of the start reaction are given by Eq. 10 and 11, respectively:

$$\frac{d[I^{\cdot}]}{dt} = 2fk_d[I] - k_{st}[I^{\cdot}][M] = 0 \quad (10)$$

$$R_{st} = k_{st}[I^{\cdot}][M] = 2fk_d\,[I] \quad (11)$$

Per initiator radical, only one monomer is consumed in the start of the reaction, but many hundreds in the subsequent propagation reaction. Monomers are thus practically only consumed by propagation. Their consumption by start, termination, and transfer to monomer is negligible. For irreversible reactions, the gross rate of polymerization, R_{gross}, thus approximates R_p (Eq. 12):

$$R_{gross} = \frac{-d[M]}{dt} \approx R_p = k_p[P^{\cdot}][M] \quad (12)$$

The following assumptions underlie the ideal polymerization kinetics:

1. Only initiator decomposition and start, propagation and termination reactions are considered.
2. All reactions are irreversible.
3. The effective concentration of initiator radicals is steady.
4. The concentration of macroradicals is stationary.
5. Termination occurs only by mutual deactivation of two macroradicals; hence:

$$R_{gross} \approx \frac{-d[M]}{dt} = k_p\left(\frac{2fk_d}{k_t}\right)^{1/2}[M][I]^{1/2} \quad (13)$$

The rate of polymerization $R_{\text{gross}} \approx R_p$ is thus directly proportional to the monomer concentration, under ideal kinetics conditions. Larger initiator concentrations lead to higher polymerization rates and to lower kinetic chain length, ν, defined as the number of monomer molecules that are added to an initiator radical before the resulting macroradical is terminated. The kinetic chain length is given by the ratio of the rate of propagation, R_p, to the sum of the rates of all terminations; the type of termination does not matter (Eq. 14).

$$\nu = \frac{R_p}{\sum_i R_{t,i}} \quad (14)$$

The ideal polymerization kinetics are rarely followed in practical polymerizations. One complication is related to the ‘‘gel effect’’: toward the end of a polymerization, the reaction mixture becomes extremely viscous, resulting in a rapid increase in the rate of polymerization, R_p, as a result of the decrease in k_t. Another complication results from undesired chain transfer reactions, which terminate the polymerization prematurely, and consequently, polymers of molecular weights lower than predicted will be formed. There are several mechanisms for chain transfer, for example:

Chain transfer to monomer:

$M_n^{\cdot} + M \rightarrow \text{polymer} + M^{\cdot}$

Chain transfer to solvent:

$M_n^{\cdot} + S \rightarrow \text{polymer} + S^{\cdot}$
$S^{\cdot} + M \rightarrow SM^{\cdot} \rightarrow \ldots$

Chain transfer to initiator

$M_n^{\cdot} + \text{I} \rightarrow \text{polymer} + R^{\cdot}$

Chain transfer agents may be added intentionally to a polymerization mixture as a way of controlling the (low) molecular weight of a polymer. Such compounds are known as ''regulators.'' When used in large amounts, they are called telogens, since they produce low-molecular-weight polymers, or telomers. Examples of chain transfer agents are mercaptans, alkyl halides, phenols, and alcohols. The chain transfer reaction decreases the average chain length in accordance with the concentration of chain transfer agent [*S*]. The deMayo equation (Eq. 15) can be used to predict the molecular weight of a polymer upon addition of a chain transfer agent:

$$\frac{1}{DP} = \frac{1}{DP_0} + C_s \frac{[S]}{[M]} \tag{15}$$

In this equation, DP and DP_0 are the degrees of polymerization of the polymer with and without chain transfer agent, respectively, [*S*] is the concentration of chain transfer agent, [*M*] is the monomer concentration, and C_s is the chain transfer constant or the ratio of the rate of termination by transfer to the rate of propagation. This constant is related to relative bond strengths in the chain transfer agent and the stability of the new free radical produced.

D. Polymer Analog Reactions (30,31)

In polymer analog modifications, a reaction takes place along the polymer chain to convert certain chemical functionalities into different functions, without altering the degree of polymerization of the starting polymer. This approach is particularly useful for the transformation of naturally occurring polymers, but it is applied also to modify synthetic polymers. For example, saturated polymers, such as polyethylene, can be chlorinated or oxidized. Polyenes, such as rubber, can be hydrogenated, halogenated, or epoxidized. Pendant groups, such as the ester groups in poly(vinyl acetate), can be hydrolyzed by transesterification with butanol or methanol to yield poly(vinyl alcohol). The latter can be modified further by reactions typical of alcohols, such as ether formation, esterification, or formation of acetal by treatment with butyraldehyde to form poly(vinyl butyral). The hydroxyl groups in polysaccharides are converted to corresponding ethers and esters. Cellulose ethers, for example, result from the reaction of cellulose with ethylene oxide or propylene oxide (see Chapter 8). Hydrophobically modified polymers such as the cationic cellulose ether derivative, Quatrisoft LM-200 (Amerchol), are obtained via polymer analog reactions (see later chapters).

Esters, amides, or nitriles pendant groups can be converted to the corresponding carboxylic acids. Poly(carboxylic acids) may be dehydrated upon heating to poly(carboxylic acid anhydrides). Phenyl pendant groups, such as those in polystyrene, undergo the characteristic reactions of aromatic rings, such as alkylation, halogenation, or sulfonation. In all cases, competing polymer degradation may take place. It is important to assess whether the molecular weight of the polymer is affected by the chemical transformation.

III. DISTRIBUTION OF MOLECULAR WEIGHTS

With the exception of naturally occurring proteins, all polymers are mixtures of many molecular weights. They are polydisperse: in any polymer sample, the individual polymer chains do not all have the same size. The distribution of molecular weights has been shown to be important in many applications, including the flow of melts or solutions, adhesion, flocculation, or aging behavior. Because of the difficulties involved in measuring a distribution of molecular weights in detail, several mathematical forms are used and related to the averages measured experimentally. As described below, the type of average determined will depend on the experimental method used to measure it.

A. Types of Molecular Weight (32,33)

The simplest average is the number-average molecular weight, M_n, where n_i is the number of species with molecular weight M_i (Eq. 16) Physically, the number-average molecular weight can be determined by any technique that ''counts'' molecules based on the colligative properties of solutions (34), such as freezing point depression, boiling point elevation, and osmometry.

The weight-average molecular weight, M_w, is given by Eq. 17, where wt_i is the weight of all species with molecular weight M_i. Weight-average molecular weights are determined from techniques such as size-exclusion chromatography, in which each macromolecule makes a contribution to the measured value relative to its size. The weight average is more dependent on the number of heavier molecules than is M_n, which depends simply on the total number of polymers. The z-average molecular weight M_z, obtained, for instance, by ultracentrifugation techniques, is defined by Eq. 18:

$$M_n = \frac{\sum_i n_i M_i}{\sum_i M_i} \tag{16}$$

$$M_w = \frac{\sum_i wt_i M_i}{\sum_i wt_i} = \frac{\sum_i n_i M_i^2}{\sum_i n_i M_i} \tag{17}$$

$$M_z = \frac{\sum_i wt_i M_i^2}{\sum_i wt_i M_i} = \frac{\sum_i n_i M_i^3}{\sum_i n_i M_i^2} \tag{18}$$

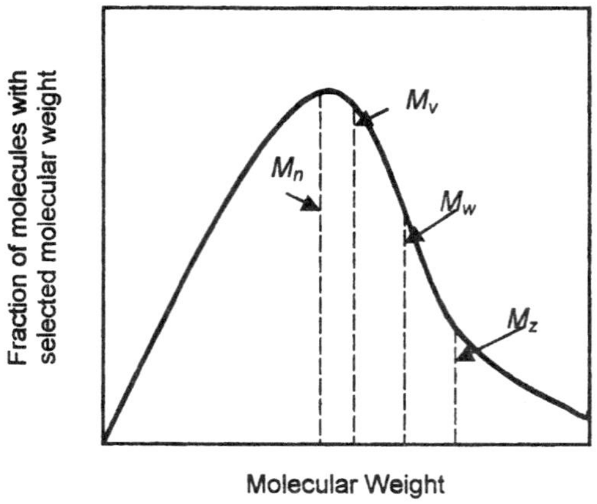

Figure 5 Molecular weights of polymers.

For systems heterogeneous in size, the three average molecular weights are such that $M_n < M_w < M_z$ (Fig. 5). The ratio M_w/M_n, called the polydispersity, is a useful measure of the spread of a polymer distribution. Larger values of M_w/M_n (>2) indicate a very wide spread with substantial amounts of material at both extremes. When $M_w/M_n \sim 1$, all polymer molecules have the same molecular weight.

Viscosity measurements yield yet another average molecular weight, M_v. Its value is usually intermediate between M_n and M_w. It is obtained from the Mark-Houwink-Sakurada equation (see below).

B. Experimental Methods for Determining Molecular Weight and Molecular Weight Distribution (35)

Absolute methods yield experimental data that can be used to determine molecular weights without any assumption about the polymer structure. Listed below are some of the well-known experimental techniques for determining absolute molecular weights of polymers:

1. Methods yielding number-average molecular weights: osmotic pressure, melting point depression, boiling point elevation
2. Methods yielding weight-average molecular weights: diffusion, light scattering
3. Methods yielding z-average molecular weights: ultracentrifugation

Relative methods for determining molecular weights require calibrations with standards of known molecular weight and molecular weight distribution. They are influenced by the chemical and physical nature of the polymer and its interactions with solvent molecules. Gel permeation chromatography, fractional precipitation, and electrophoresis are used most frequently, with electrophoresis particularly useful to determine the molecular weight of proteins.

Gel permeation chromatography (GPC) (36–38) is a type of liquid-solid elution chromatography that separates polydisperse samples into fractions by means of the sieving action of a cross-linked gel. Such gels, which serve as the stationary phase, are commercially available with a wide distribution of pore sizes (1–10^6 nm). Since the smaller molecules permeate the gels preferentially, the larger molecules elute faster than the smaller ones. Therefore, molecules are separated on the basis of their size. The separation can be carried out with polymers soluble in organic solvent, with calibration against polystyrene standard samples, or with water-soluble polymers, using poly(ethylene oxides) or dextrans standards.

Equivalent methods require information about the chemical structure of a polymer. End-group determinations allow the calculation of relative molar masses if the constitution of end groups is known (39). The sensitivity of end-group determinations depends on the experimental methods. ^{13}C NMR spectrometry can yield information on polymers of molecular weight up to ~8000. Titrations are applicable if the end group is either an acid or a base. They yield molecular weights up to ~40,000.

Mass spectrometry is the only method that delivers the mass of a molecule, as the ratio of molecular mass to the number z of charges per molecule. Until recently mass spectrometry was of little use for the analysis of polymers, since polymers could not be vaporized in the spectrometer without thermal decomposition. However, newer techniques, such as matrix-assisted laser desorption ionization mass spectrometry (MALDI-MS), which uses a volatile carrier, "the matrix," to transport nonvolatile polymers to the magnetic field of the spectrometer, allow the determination of molecular masses of polymers up to 200,000.

IV. PHYSICAL PROPERTIES OF POLYMERS IN THE BULK

A. Polymer Morphology (40–42)

When polymers are irradiated by a beam of X-rays, scattering produces diffuse halos on the screen for some polymers, whereas for others a series of sharply defined rings superimposed on a diffuse background is recorded. The former pattern is characteristic of amorphous polymers and illustrates the fact that a limited amount of short-range order exists in all polymer solids. The latter pattern indicates considerable three-dimensional order and is typical of polycrystalline samples containing a large number of unoriented crystallites associated with amorphous regions. No bulk polymer is completely crystalline. Some commercial polymers, for example polyethylenes, are highly crystalline materials with well-defined crystalline morphology consisting of chain-folded lamellae joined in supramolecular structures called "spherulites." Another important polymer, poly(vinylchloride), has a very low level of crystallinity. Many other polymers, such as atactic polystyrene or poly(methyl methacrylate), are totally amorphous. In each case the presence of crystalline structure controls to a significant level the physical, thermal, and mechanical properties of the material. Polymer microstructure depends first on molecular parameters, such as the chemical structure of the base unit and the molecular weight of the polymer, but it is influenced also by the processing techniques employed to manufacture a specific material.

To appreciate how polymers attain their morphology, let us consider what may happen when an initially molten polymer is cooled down gradually. In the melt, a polymer can be viewed as made up of highly entangled chains that have a considerable segmental motion and conformational freedom. The polymer melt behaves like a liquid. As the temperature decreases, the viscosity of the molten polymer increases. When the temperature has come down far enough, individual chains undergoing the strongest attraction start to solidify. These chains separate from the molten polymer as crystallites. Then, as the temperature decreases further, the remaining polymer chains solidify as amorphous unorganized domains outside the domains of crystallinity (Fig. 6). The difference between flexible and rubbery polymeric materials arises from the significant degree of crystallinity of the former, as opposed to an almost totally amorphous state in the latter.

1. The Amorphous State

Polystyrene and poly(methyl methacrylate) are typical glassy polymers (43) at ambient temperature. They are rigid and optically transparent materials. As thin samples, they become slightly flexible. They have moderate strength and some impact resistance, but can be shattered quite easily. If a small stress is applied, the glass exhibits a rapid elastic response resulting from local deformations. However, the sample has no means of dissipating large stresses other than by rupture. A polymer glass is therefore brittle and prone to fractures.

Elastomers (44) exhibit many of the properties of liquids: they change shape and flow readily when subjected to weak forces. But unlike liquids they reassume their original shape once the distorting force has been removed. This unique behavior is a consequence of the large size of polymer chains, compared to typical low-molecular-weight liquids, coupled with a high mobility of backbone bonds, compared to glassy polymers. The ability of an elastomer to reassume its original shape after deformation can be attributed to en-

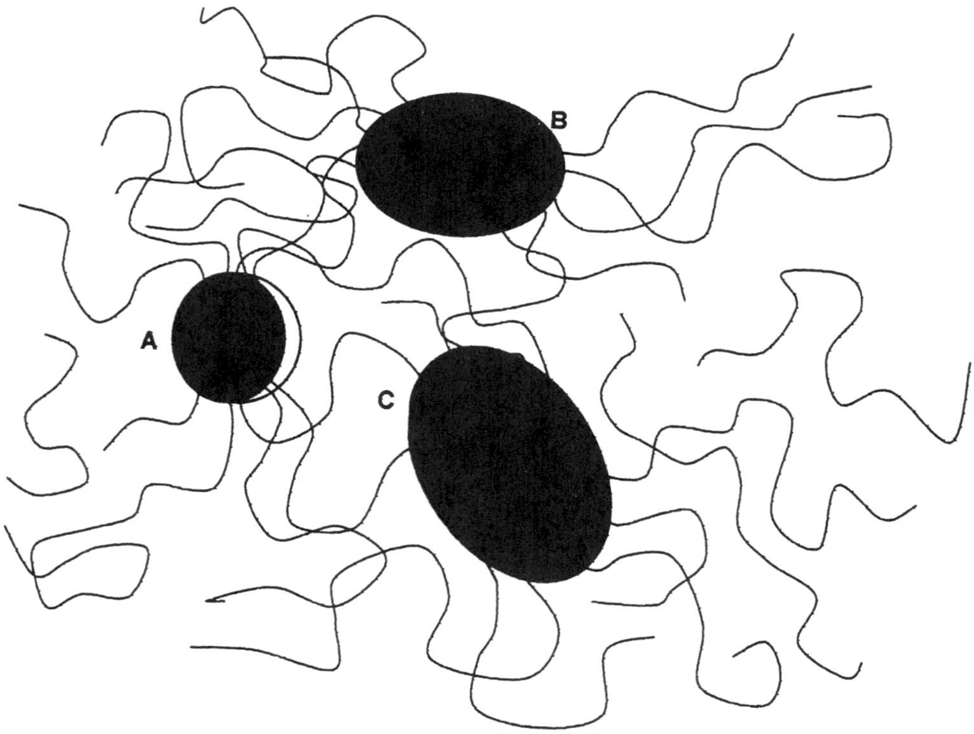

Figure 6 Schematic representation of a thermoplastic polymer (semicrystalline state). Each line corresponds to the backbone of polymer chain. The encircled zones A, B, and C represent zones of crystallinity.

tropic features: a stretched chain will tend to contract to allow maximization of the entropy, once the tension is released.

At low enough temperatures, all amorphous polymers are stiff and glassy. On warming, polymers soften in a characteristic temperature range, known as the glass transition temperature (T_g) range (45–47). The transition from the glass to the rubber-like state is an important characteristic of amorphous polymers, because it marks the region of dramatic changes in their physical properties, such as stiffness and elasticity. For most common polymers this temperature ranges between −120°C and +200°C. Structural factors influencing the magnitude of T_g include: (1) the molecular structure in particular possible steric effects, (2) the chain flexibility, (3) the molecular weight, and (4) the degree of branching and cross-linking. The relative importance of each of these factors is illustrated by the examples listed in Table 2.

a. Measurement of the Glass Transition Temperature. The glass temperature of a polymer can be observed experimentally by measuring basic thermodynamic, physical, mechanical, or electrical properties as a function of temperature. Thermal methods are

Table 2 Relationships Between the Structure of Polymers and Their Glass Transition Temperature (T_g)

Polymer structure	Main chain unit	T_g(°C)
Chain flexibility		
Polyethylene	$-(CH_2CH_2)_n-$	−125
Polydimethylsiloxane	$-[O-Si(CH_3)_2]_n-$	−123
Polyethylene oxide	$-(CH_2CH_2O)_n-$	−47
Steric restrictions and substituent sizes		
Polyethylene	$-(CH_2CH_2)_n-$	−125
Polystyrene	$-[CH_2CH(C_6H_5)]_n-$	+100
Poly(4-methylstyrene)	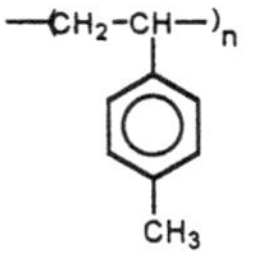	+115
Poly(α-vinylnaphthalene)	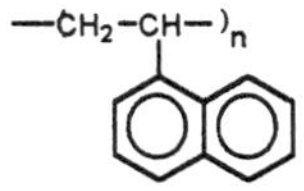	+135
Size of the substituent group		
Poly(methyl methacrylate)	$-[CH_2CH(COOCH_3)]_n-$	+105
Poly(ethyl methacrylate)	$-[CH_2CH(COOCH_2CH_3)]_n-$	+65
Poly(propyl methacrylate)	$-[CH_2CH(COOCH_2CH_2CH_3)]_n-$	+35
Interchain forces (H-bonds, dipole-dipole interactions)		
Polyethylene	$-(CH_2CH_2)_n-$	−125
Polyoxymethylene	$-(OCH_2)_n-$	−85
Polypropylene	$-[CH_2CH(CH_3)]_n-$	−15
Polyvinylchloride	$-(CH_2CHCl)_n-$	+80
Polyacrylonitrile	$-[CH_2CH(CN)]_n-$	+105
Polycaprolactone	$-[(CH_2)_5-COO]_n-$	−60
Polycaprolactam (nylon 6)	$-[(CH_2)_5-CONH]_n-$	+60

used routinely (48,49). Two closely related thermal methods dominate, an older method, differential thermal analysis (DTA), and a newer method, differential scanning calorimetry (DSC) (50). In making DTA measurements, the temperature of a sample is compared with a reference material, such as powdered alumina. Both the sample and the reference are heated at a uniform rate, typically 10–20°C/min. Since the two materials have different heat capacities, each maintains slightly different temperatures throughout the scan. The difference in temperature, ΔT, is monitored as a function of the temperature T. The glass transition temperature will be marked by a significant deviation in the otherwise smooth profile of ΔT versus temperature (or time) (Fig. 7). The DSC method uses a servo system to supply energy at a varying rate to the sample and the reference, so that the two stay at equal temperature (50). A DSC trace plots energy supplied against average temperature. The area under the peaks corresponding to the glass transition temperature can be related directly to the enthalpy change associated with the transition. Melting temperatures of crystalline polymers (see below) are also measured by DSC.

b. Molecular Interpretation of the Glass Transition (48). In the amorphous state the distribution of polymer chains in the matrix is completely random. At sufficiently high molecular weight interpenetrating chains form flow-restricting entanglements. The minimum polymer chain length, or critical molecular weight (M_c), for the formation of stable entanglements is an important characteristic of a polymer. Relatively flexible chains, such as polystyrene, have high M_c, while stiffer chains, such as polycarbonates, have relatively lower M_c. A second parameter of importance is M_e, the molecular weight between entanglements. Typically the molecular weight of commercial polymers (100,000–500,000) is much larger than M_e (10,000–30,000). Therefore, in most commercial polymers the individual chains are highly entangled. The question then arises: how can long-range motion of the chains take place as the polymer is heated through its glass transition temperature?

Several models have been proposed to describe the motion of a single polymer chain in an entangled network of chains. In the reptation model, proposed by De Gennes (51),

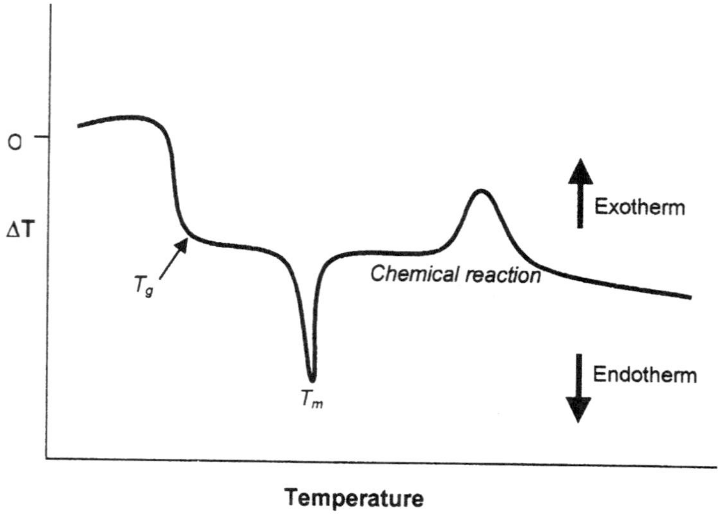

Figure 7 Schematic differential thermal analysis plot (DTA).

the chain is assumed to be contained in a hypothetical tube placed in the network. The ''knots'' in the network are seen as obstacles around which the chain must ''wriggle'' during translation. Two types of motions can be envisaged: (1) conformational changes within the confines of the tube; and (2) reptation, a snake-like motion that translates the chain within the tube until it finally escapes at the tube end (Fig. 8). The theory of reptation has been applied with large success to develop theories describing the dynamics and viscoelastic properties of entangled polymers.

The most severe mechanism for decreasing molecular freedom in a polymeric material is by chemical cross-linking: linking polymer chains through chemical bonds. This can be made either during the polymerization process, by use of polyfunctional monomers, or in a separate process, often described as a curing step (52). A number of extreme changes accompany cross-linking. If previously soluble, the polymer will no longer dissolve. In the presence of a solvent, a cross-linked polymer swells as the solvent molecules penetrate the network. A solvent-swollen polymer forms a gel. If the gel particles are very small these are called microgels, which can be viewed as tightly packed spheres suspended in solvents (53). These materials have found many applications, as support for solid-phase reactions and delivery systems (54).

2. *The Crystalline and Semicrystalline States* (55–58)

The formation of stable crystalline regions in a polymer requires that a closely packed arrangement of chains can be achieved in three dimensions and that a favorable change in internal energy is obtained during the crystallization process. This imposes restrictions on the type of chains that can be crystallized with ease. Polyesters, polyamides, and polyethylene, which have a high degree of symmetry, are expected to crystallize readily. General factors influencing the crystallinity of a polymer include: (1) the symmetry of the chain, (2) the occurrence of intermolecular bonding (van der Waals forces, hydrogen bonding, dipole-dipole interactions), (3) the tacticity, (4) the branching (if the chain is substantially branched the packing efficiency deteriorates), and (5) the molecular weight of the polymer.

Crystalline polymers are generally tougher, stiffer, more opaque, more resistant to solvents, and of higher density than their amorphous counterparts. The higher the degree of crystallinity, the more pronounced are these properties. The superior mechanical properties are a reflection of the greater cohesive strength arising from more effective intermolecular secondary forces among the closely packed chains. Examples of highly crystalline

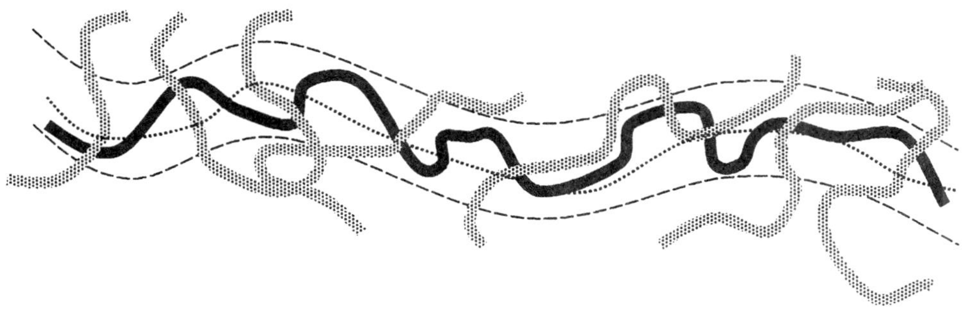

Figure 8 Reptation of a chain within a tube. (A test chain [black] reptates through a tube with ''walls'' formed by segments of the chains [gray]).

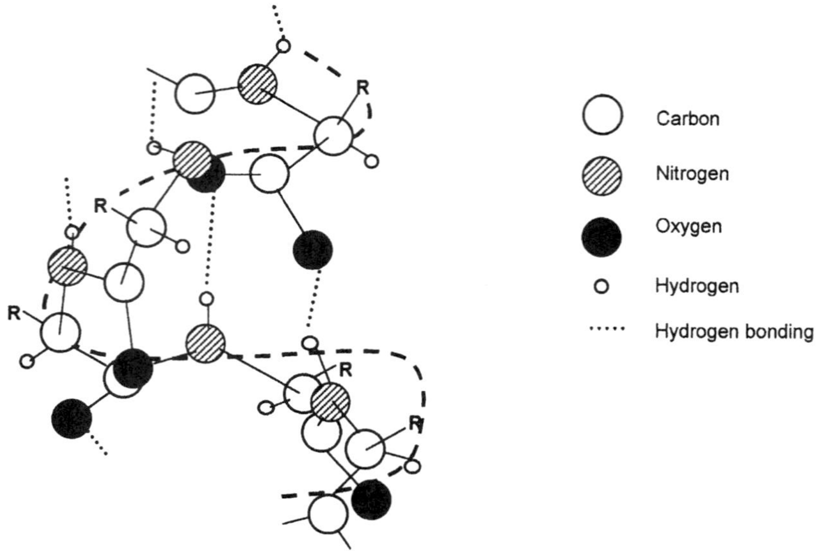

Figure 9 Section of α-helix of α-keratin.

polymers include proteins, polysaccharides, such as cellulose, and synthetic polymers, such as certain forms of polyethylene.

Proteins tend to form stable geometries, generally those that allow the greatest degree of hydrogen bonding. The conformation of a protein chain is referred to as its secondary structure. X-ray analysis, notably by Linus Pauling, has shown that a right-handed helical arrangement, called the α-helix, is probably the most important secondary structure. Such an arrangement allows room for bulky substituents present in most amino acids. It is stabilized by intramolecular hydrogen bonding between the amide nitrogen atoms and the carbonyl oxygens. A short section of the peptide chain of α-keratin, the main constituent of hair and nails, is shown in Figure 9 (59). Proteins that have predominantly small substituents, for example silk fibroin (60), can assume a configuration that is essentially an extended chain, but with some contraction so that crowding between substituents of one chain and those of a neighboring chain is minimized. The chains can lie side by side in a sheet-like arrangement, referred to as a pleated sheet or beta-arrangement (Fig. 10).

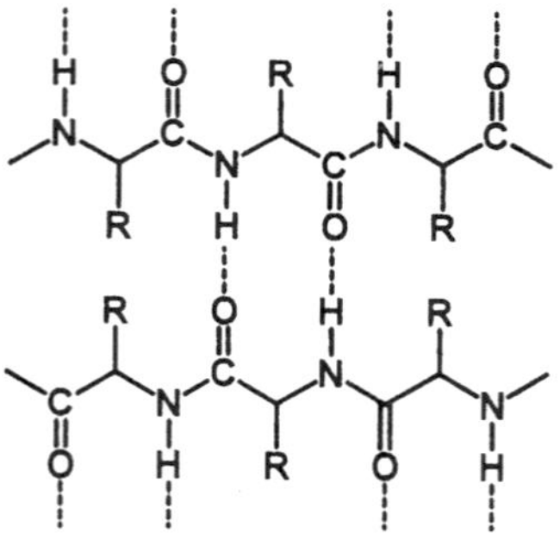

Figure 10 Pleated sheet structure (β-arrangement) of silk fibroin.

The shape of protein molecules is not given completely by their secondary structure. Sections of peptide chains may be linked chemically through sulfur bonds of cystein groups, as in the case of keratins, or by salt bridges between carboxyl groups and ammonium groups, such as the glutamic acid-lysine links present in α-keratin (59). This overall three-dimensional structure of a protein molecule is known as its tertiary structure. In addition to tertiary structure, a protein may exhibit a quaternary structure that originates from associations of several proteins or of proteins and nonprotein sustances.

B. Rheology and Mechanical Properties of Polymers (61,62)

In the course of their use, polymers are subjected to various physical treatments, first during product manufacture and then during use in their intended applications. Therefore, the mechanical properties of polymeric materials need to be controlled and tested rigorously. Mechanical properties of polymers include their resistance to deformation and their ultimate failure as static or dynamic loads are applied. Deformations can be generated by drawing, shearing, pressurizing, compressing, bending, or torsion.

1. *Deformation Under Tension* (63)

The simplest mechanical test method is tensile testing, where a rectangular or dumbbell-shaped specimen is placed between two clamps and then uniaxially drawn with constant speed (64,65). In the case of pure elastic deformation, the stress σ and the resulting deformation are proportional to each other. The original dimensions of the test specimen are completely and immediately restored after removal of the stress. The proportionality constant E is called the modulus. It is given by Hooke's law (Eq. 19), where σ is the tensile stress ($N\ m^{-2}$), γ the strain, and E Young's modulus ($N\ m^{-2}$):

$$\sigma = E\gamma \tag{19}$$

Polymers behave very differently upon drawing. They can be subdivided into six classes (Table 3) according to moduli and stress-strain behavior. The changes of Young's modulus E with temperature give a good insight into the properties and applicability of a polymer over a given temperature range. For an amorphous non-cross-linked polymer five regions exist, as shown in Figure 11. It is clear that amorphous polymers below T_g have high E values that remain reasonably constant below T_g (region 1). At the glass transition temperature the polymer does not immediately become a viscous liquid ($E = 0$), as would be observed for low-mass compounds, but rather it undergoes a series of changes in mechanical behavior. In region 2, the modulus drops by a factor of 10^3 over a 20–30°C range. The behavior of the polymer in this region is described as leathery. Region 3 is

Table 3 Classification of Polymers According to Their Tensile Behavior

Class	E	σ	ε	Example
Rigid-brittle	Large	—	Small	Polystyrene
Rigid-strong	Large	Large	Small	Poly(methyl methacrylate)
Rigid-ductile	Large	Large	Large	Polycarbonate
Soft-ductile	Small	Small	Large	Low-density polyethylene
Soft-strong	Small	Small	Small	Poly(tetrafluoroethylene) (teflon)
Soft-elastic	Small	Large	Large	Styrene/butadiene/styrene copolymer

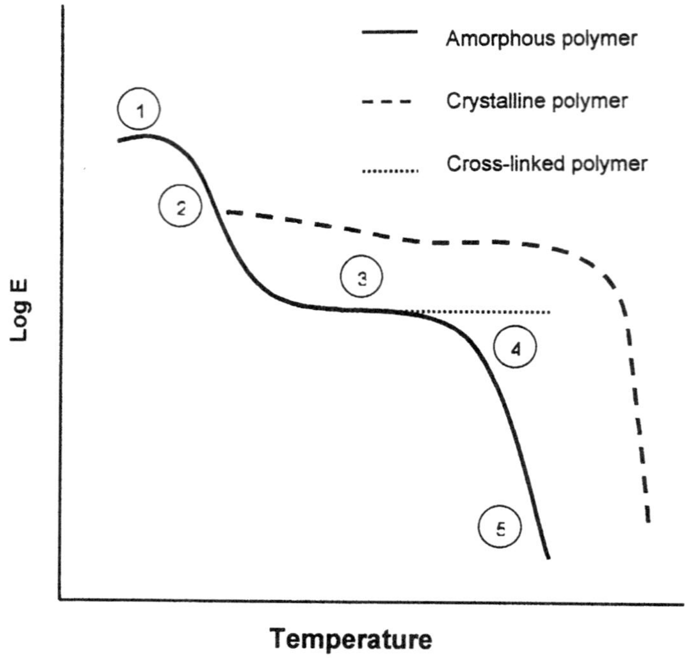

Figure 11 Five regions of viscoelastic behavior for a linear, amorphous polymer.

the rubbery plateau region. After a sharp drop, the modulus reaches a value that remains constant over a large temperature range. In the rubbery plateau, polymers exhibit long-range rubber elasticity, which means that they can be stretched maybe several hundred percent and snap back to nearly their original length. As the temperature is raised past the rubbery plateau, the polymer reaches the rubbery flow region (4), and finally the liquid flow region (5) at still higher temperatures.

A typical stress-strain curve of keratin, a crystalline polymer, is shown in Figure 12. If a keratin fiber is extended progressively under constant temperature and humidity conditions, once it is straightened, the stress-strain curve exhibits a nearly linear region. With further extension an increase in stress occurs with small increases in strain (yield region). Then the stress increases more rapidly with increasing strain. This region of increase in fiber stiffness is called the postyield region. The longitudinal stress-strain curves of α-keratin vary markedly with temperature, humidity, and time.

2. Deformations Under Shear

Instead of elongating or compressing a solid, we can subject it to various shearing or twisting motions. The ratio of the shear stress, σ, to the shear strain, γ, defines the shear modulus G (Eq. 20):

$$\sigma = G\gamma \tag{20}$$

Normally a body shrinks in volume upon exposure to increasing external pressure. The bulk modulus B is defined by Eq. 21, where P is the pressure and V the volume of the body. The inverse of the bulk modulus is the compressibility β.

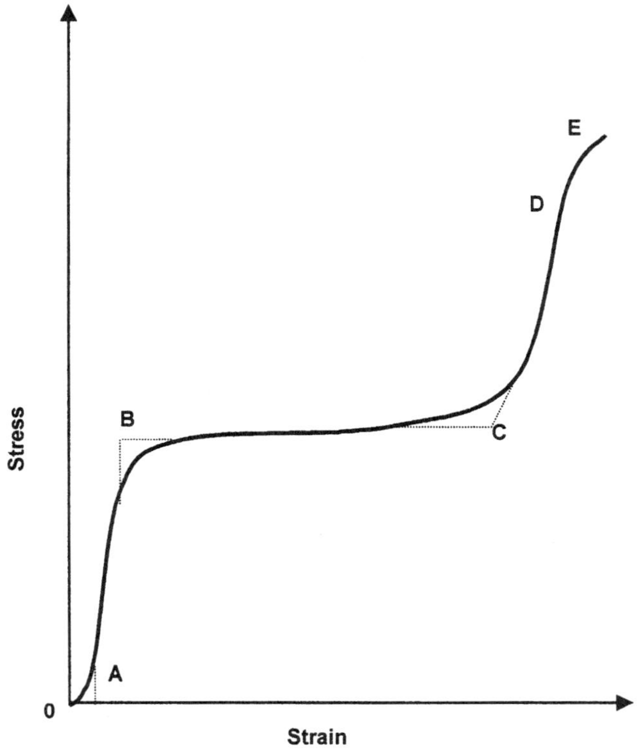

Figure 12 Typical stress-strain curve of an α-keratin fiber showing the Hookean region (AB), the yield region (BC), and the postyield region (CDE).

$$B = -V\left(\frac{\partial P}{\partial V}\right)_T \tag{21}$$

The modulus B is a measure of stiffness or hardness of an object. The compliance J is a measure of its softness. In regions far from transitions, the elongation compliance J is defined as in Eq. 22:

$$J \cong \frac{1}{E} \tag{22}$$

In a creep experiment the dimensions of a specimen are observed as a function of time under constant load. Usually a constant stress is applied to a sample and the dimensions are recorded as a function of time. The experiments can be generalized to include shear motions, compressions, etc. Creep experiments are usually reported as time-dependent compliance $J(t)$.

The quantities E and G refer to quasi-static measurements. When cyclic motions of stress and strain are involved, it is more convenient to use dynamical mechanical moduli. The complex Young's modulus is then defined as $E^* = E' + iE''$, where E' is the storage modulus and E'' the loss modulus. The storage modulus is a measure of the energy stored elastically during deformation; the loss modulus is a measure of the energy converted to heat. Similar definitions hold for G^*, J^*, and other mechanical properties.

3. *Models for Analyzing Stress Relaxation and Creep*

When dealing with very small deformations of materials with both elastic and viscous nature (viscoelastic materials) it is usual to combine a linear, Hookean stress-strain relationship with a linear Newtonian viscous relationship to illustrate the behavior of real materials. In these models, spring and dashpot elements are frequently used to model creep and relaxation measurements. A spring behaves like a purely elastic material, such as a metallic spring, stretching instantly under stress and holding the stress indefinitely. A dashpot is full of a purely viscous fluid. Under stress the plunger moves through the fluid at a rate proportional to the stress. On removal of stress there is no recovery. Springs and dashpots can be put together to model the viscoelastic behavior of polymers. Two simple arrangements are the Maxwell and Kelvin (or Voigt) elements (Fig. 13). In the Maxwell element, the spring and dashpot are in series; in the Kelvin element, they are in parallel. In the Maxwell element both the spring and the dashpot are subjected to the same stress but are permitted to have independent strains. The inverse is true for the Kelvin element. On application of stress to the Maxwell element, the spring instantly responds, as illustrated by the vertical line in Figure 14. The spring then remains extended as the dashpot gradually pulls out, yielding a line slanted upward. The spring and dashpot undergo concerted motions. On the other hand, in the Kelvin element the dashpot responds slowly to the stress and gradually transfers it to the spring as it becomes extended, resulting in the asymptotic behavior as a function of time depicted in Figure 14.

A few viscoelastic behaviors can be modeled adequately by a two-element model, but usually it is necessary to combine Maxwell and Kelvin elements. A series arrangement of the two elements, known as the four-element model, is the simplest model that exhibits all the features of viscoelasticity (Fig. 15). It is beyond the scope of this introductory chapter to derive the mathematical equations that describe the various models. Several excellent texts exist and can be consulted (66–68).

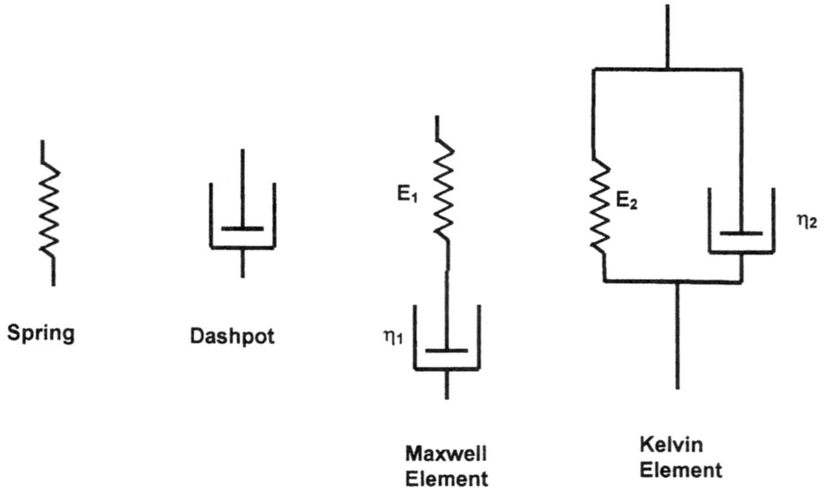

Figure 13 The Maxwell and Kelvin elements, representing simple series and parallel arrays of springs and dashpots.

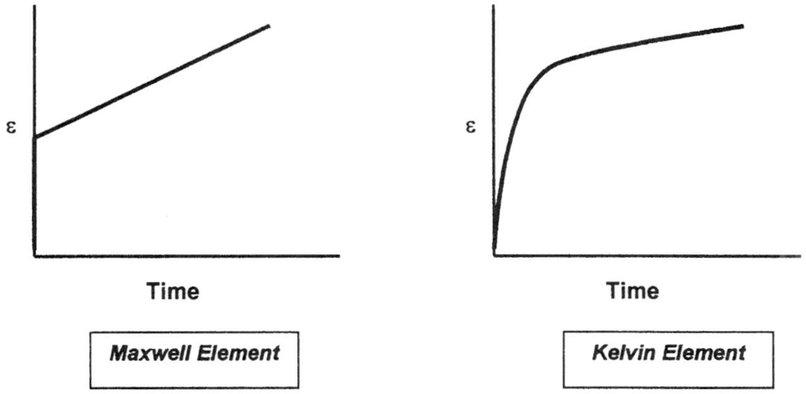

Figure 14 Creep behavior of the Maxwell and Kelvin elements. The Maxwell element exhibits viscous flow throughout the deformation, whereas the Kelvin element reaches an asymptotic limit to deformation.

V. POLYMER SOLUTIONS

Polymers are probably best known for their use as bulk materials, as discussed in the previous section. However, they also play an important role in the control of solution and dispersion rheology. This application includes fields as diverse as fuels, lubricants, water treatment chemicals, foodstuffs, and cosmetic formulations. In these areas polymers affect the flow behavior, and thereby the performance, of a fluid during and after application.

When one attempts to dissolve a polymer in solvents selected at random, many, per-

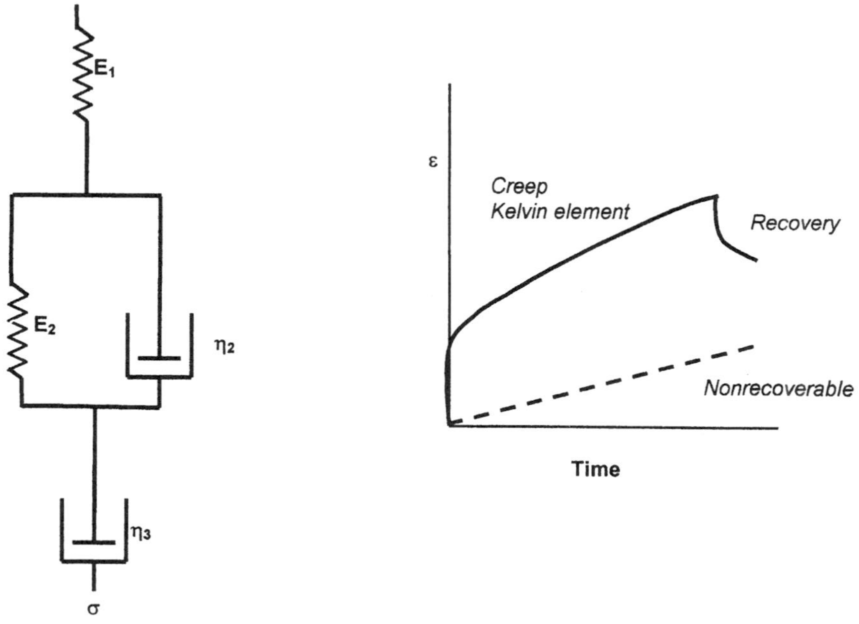

Figure 15 The four-element model and the creep behavior predicted by this model.

haps most, will not work. The experimentalist rapidly finds out that the higher the molecular weight of the polymer, the more difficult it is to select a good solvent. Attempts to understand polymer-solvent and polymer-polymer mutual interactions in a solvent, especially by Flory in the 1950s (69) and De Gennes in the 1970s, have led to many new theoretical developments in the thermodynamics of polymers in solution.

A. Thermodynamics of Polymers in Solution

One of the simplest notions in chemistry is that ''like dissolves like.'' Qualitatively, ''like'' can be defined in terms of similar chemical groups or similar polarities. Quantitatively, solubility of one component in another is governed by the free energy of mixing, ΔG_M (Eq. 23), where T is the absolute temperature, ΔS_M is the entropy of mixing, and ΔH_M is the enthalpy of mixing.

$$\Delta G_M = \Delta H_M - T\Delta S_M \tag{23}$$

A negative value of ΔG_M indicates that the dissolution process will occur spontaneously. The term $T\Delta S_M$ is generally positive, as there is usually an increase in entropy (disorder) on mixing. Hence the sign of ΔG_M depends primarily on the sign of the enthalpy of mixing. Surprisingly, the enthalpy of mixing is usually positive, opposing mixing. This is true for most small molecules and polymers alike. Exceptions occur when the solute and solvent attract each other in some way, for example through hydrogen bonding as is often the case during the dissolution process in water.

Historically, the theoretical understanding of how polymers interact with solvent molecules is credited to the pioneering work of Flory and Huggins (69). They introduced the idea of contact energy as the cause of the heat of mixing of polymer solutions. In this treatment, the energy change on mixing is assumed to arise from the formation of new solvent-polymer contacts, which replace some of the solvent-solvent and polymer-polymer contacts present in pure solvent and in the pure polymer, respectively (Fig. 16). By assuming that the size of polymer units, or segments, is similar to that of a solvent molecule, Flory and Huggins derived an expression for the partial molar Gibbs free energy, which included a dimensionless parameter, known as the Flory-Huggins interaction parameter, χ_i. This parameter is defined in Eq. 24, where the term ΔH_M is the contact energy, k is Boltzmann constant, T the absolute temperature, n_1 the number of solvent molecules, and V_2 the polymer volume fraction. The interaction parameter can be used as a measure of solvent power. It has a value of at least 0.5 for poor solvents and decreases for good solvents.

$$\chi_i = \frac{\Delta H_M}{k n_1 V_2} \tag{24}$$

To overcome some of the limitations of his early model, Flory, together with Krieg-baum (70), made a second assumption. They postulated the presence of the excluded volume, the volume occupied by a polymer chain that exhibits long-range intramolecular interactions. These interactions were introduced as an enthalpic term (K_1) and an entropic term ω_1, as described later. The two terms are equal if $\Delta G_M = 0$. The temperature at which these conditions prevail in a given solvent is the θ temperature. At this temperature the effects of the excluded volume are eliminated and the polymer chain adopts its unperturbed conformation in dilute solution. In other words, the θ temperature is the lowest temperature at which a polymer of infinite molecular weight is completely soluble in a given solvent.

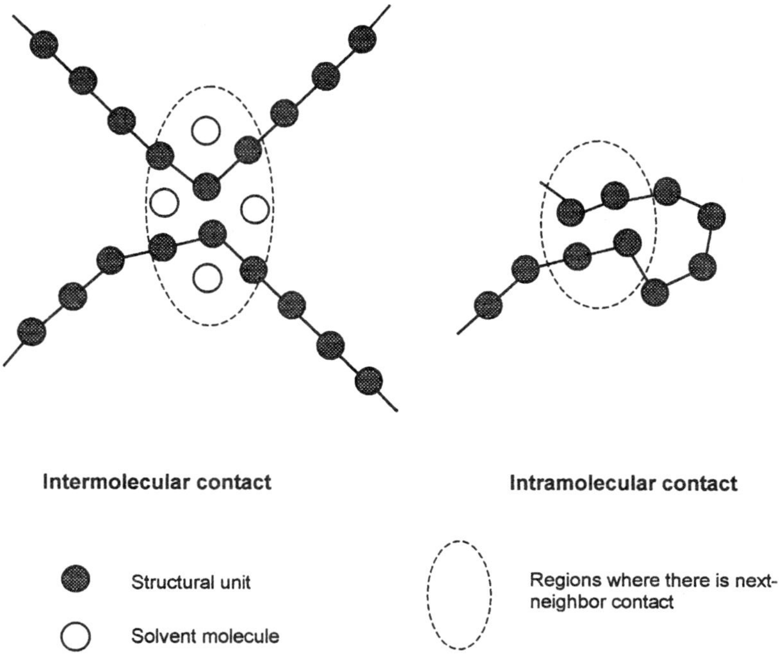

Figure 16 Schematic representation of polymer/polymer and polymer/solvent contacts in solution.

Above this temperature the coil expands and below this temperature the coil collapses with concomitant macroscopic phase separation.

1. Solubility Parameters and Cohesive Energy Density (71)

As there is no simple rule for predicting the solubility of a polymer in a specific solvent, polymer chemists and technologists use empirical relationships to guide solvent selection. In the early 1930s, both Scatchard and Hildebrand independently suggested that the enthalpy of mixing, ΔH_M, involved in the mixing of solute and solvent could be derived using the heat of vaporization of a liquid in binary mixtures. The cohesive energy density (CED) was introduced as a measure of the strength of the internal forces between polymer chains in the bulk. In this approach the enthalpy of mixing is obtained from Eq. 25:

$$\Delta \mathrm{H}_M = V_M \left[\left(\frac{\Delta E_1^v}{V_1} \right)^{1/2} - \left(\frac{\Delta E_2^v}{V_2} \right)^{1/2} \right]^2 \chi_1 \chi_2 \tag{25}$$

where ΔE_i^v is the energy of vaporization of the two species ($i = 1$: solvent, $i = 2$: polymer), $V_M = V_1 n_1 + V_2 n_2$ is the total volume of the solution with V_i and n_i, the molar volume and the number of moles of each component, respectively, and x_i is the molar fraction of each component. The quantity $\Delta E^v/V$ is taken as a measure of "internal pressure" or cohesive energy density. The square root of $\Delta E^v/V$ is defined as the solubility parameter, δ. Thus, we can write the following relations:

$$\Delta H_M = \mathrm{V}_M(\delta_1 - \delta_2)^2 \chi_1 \chi_2 \tag{26}$$

$$\text{or } \delta = \left(\frac{\Delta H_M - RT}{V_M} \right)^{1/2} \tag{27}$$

Therefore knowing the values of V_M and ΔH_M at a given temperature, T, it is possible to determine the value of δ for any solvent and polymer.

It is reasonably easy to use Eq. 26 to determine the solubility parameter of a solvent, but since the heat of vaporization of polymers is usually not known, other methods are needed to determine the solubility parameters of polymers. There are several experimental methods, based on polymer swelling measurements or on the determination of the intrinsic viscosity of polymer solutions. Alternatively, solubility parameters can be predicted from knowledge of the chemical structure of each component. The latter method is due to Small (72) and Hoy (73), who supplied values for molar attraction constants (G) of a large number of functional groups (Table 4). The constants G are additive. With these values it is possible to estimate the solubility parameter of any polymer using Eq. 28, where ρ represents the density and M the molecular weight of the polymer.

$$\delta = \frac{\rho \sum G}{M} \tag{28}$$

Solubility parameters of common solvents and polymers are given in Table 5 and Table 6, respectively. (For a comprehensive list of solubility parameters, see Ref. 74.) These tables provide a strong basis to predict the solubility of a polymer in a given solvent. It is usually found that polymers will dissolve in solvents having solubility parameters within about one unit of their own. Referring to Tables 5 and 6, it is easy to understand why polyethylene (δ 7.9) is not soluble in water (δ 23.4 or methanol (δ 14.5) but dissolves readily in *n*-hexane (δ 7.28).

2. *Statistical Thermodynamics of Mixing*

In the previous section the solubility of a polymer in a solvent was described in terms of the respective solubility parameters, which are controlled only by the heat of mixing. However, it is the free energy of mixing, $\Delta G_M = \Delta H_M - T\Delta S_M$, that ultimately controls polymer solubility in a given solvent. Therefore, the entropy of mixing needs to be taken into account as well. An expression of the entropy of mixing of a polymer in a solvent was derived by Flory and Huggins, using a simple lattice model. A representation of a lattice model in the case of mixing of two low-molecular-weight components is given in Figure 17a. The lattice sites are chosen to be the size of a solvent molecule. The solute

Table 4 Representative Group Molar Attraction Constants G [$(\text{cal/cm}^3)^{1/2}$ mol^{-1}] at 25°C

Group	G	Group	G
—CH_3	214	—CO— (ketone)	275
—CH_2	133	—COO— (ester)	310
>CH—	28	—CN	310
>C<	−93	—SH—	315
Six-membered ring	95–105	—S—	225
—CH=CH—	111	—Cl (primary)	270
>C=CH—	19	—Si—	−38
Phenyl	735	—CF_3	274
—O— (ether)	70		

Table 5 Solubility Parameters of Common Solvents

Solvent	δ (cal cm^{-3})$^{1/2}$
n-Hexane	7.28
Carbon tetrachloride	8.70
Toluene	8.90
Benzene	9.09
Chloroform	9.29
Tetrahydrofuran	9.48
Chlorobenzene	9.58
Acetone	9.82
Methylene chloride	9.92
1,4-Dioxane	10.0
N-Methyl-2-pyrrolidone	11.2
Dimethylformamide	12.1
Methanol	14.5
Water	23.4

molecule (component 2) is assumed to have the same size as the solvent molecule (component 1). The increase in entropy due to mixing of solvent and solute, ΔS_M, is obtained from Boltzmann's relation (Eq. 29), where Ω gives the total number of ways of arranging n_1 molecules of solvent and n_2 solute molecules in a lattice with $N = n_1 + n_2$ number of sites. The probability function is given by Eq. 30:

$$\Delta S_M = k \ln \Omega \tag{29}$$

$$\Omega = \frac{N!}{n_1!\, n_2!} \tag{30}$$

Using Stirling's approximation ($\ln n! = n \ln n - n$) leads to the expression for the entropy of mixing (Eq. 31), where R is the ideal gas constant, $x_1 = n_1/(n_1 + n_2)$ the molar fraction of the solvent, and $x_2 = n_2/(n_1 + n_2)$ the molar fraction of the solute.

$$\Delta S_M = -k\,(n_1 \ln x_1 + n_2 \ln x_2) = -R\,(x_1 \ln x_1 + x_2 \ln x_2) \tag{31}$$

Table 6 Solubility Parameters of Polymers

Polymer	δ (cal cm^{-3})$^{1/2}$
Polybutadiene	8.4
Polyethylene	7.9
Poly(methyl methacrylate)	9.45
Polytetrafluorethylene	6.2
Polyisobutene	7.85
Polystyrene	9.10
Cellulose triacetate	13.60
Nylon 66	13.6
Polysulfone	9.92
Poly(vinyl chloride)	10.5
Polyacrylonitrile	12.4

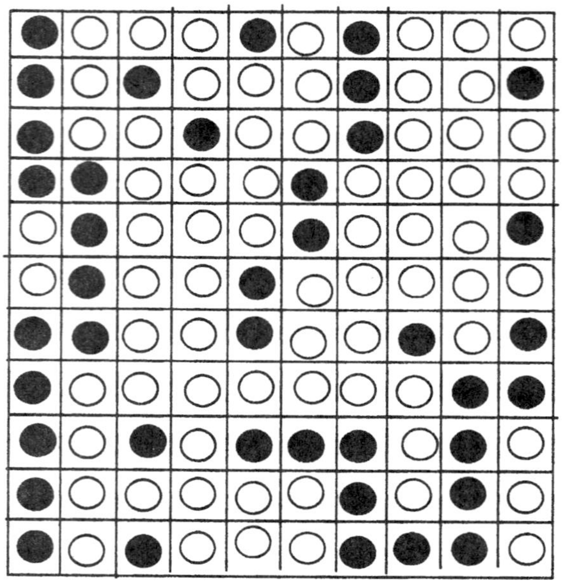

(a)

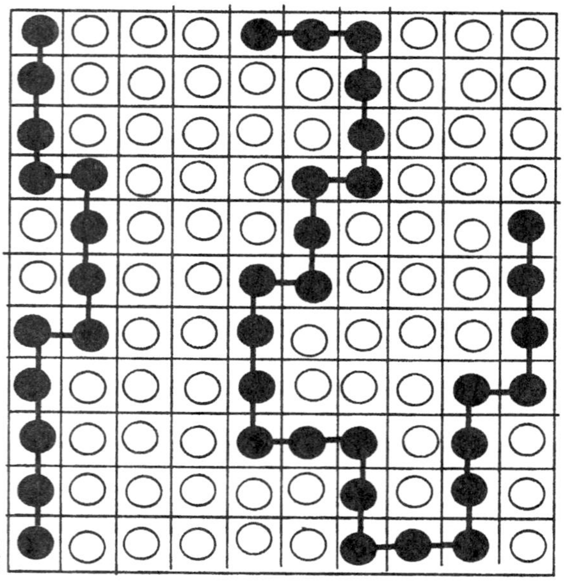

(b)

Figure 17 Lattice model for (a) a low- molecular-weight solute in solution (filled circle: solute; open circle: solvent molecule); (b) a polymer solution (filled circle: monomer segment; open circle: solvent molecule).

Flory derived general equations to describe the changes in molecular configuration of the polymer in the presence of a solvent using the lattice theory, which had been applied previously to describe solutions of small molecules. The central point is the filling of lattice sites in a three-dimensional space by polymer segments and solvent molecules (see Fig. 17b), neglecting the interaction potentials existing between polymer segments. A segment was defined by Flory as "that portion of a polymer molecule requiring the same space as a molecule of solvent." Thus, we assume that the polymer segment and the solvent molecule are of equal volume and that a lattice site is filled with either a solvent molecule or a polymer segment. Solvent molecules can be placed in any unoccupied site available. The possibilities for placing polymer segments are limited, since adjacent segments have to occupy adjacent sites (see Fig. 17b). Let y be the number of segments in a chain, n_1 the number of solvent molecules, n_2 the number of polymer chains, and N the total number of lattice sites; hence $N = n_1 + yn_2$. The derivations, described very clearly by Flory (75), lead to the expression of ΔS_M represented by Eq. 32, where ϕ_1 and ϕ_2 are the lattice *volume* fractions of solvent and polymer, respectively.

$$(32) \quad \Delta S_M = -k\,(n_1 \ln \phi_1 + n_2 \ln \phi_2)$$

$$\phi_2 = \frac{yn_2}{n_1 + yn_2} \tag{33}$$

$$\phi_1 = \frac{n_1}{n_1 + yn_2} \tag{34}$$

Combining the expressions for the entropy (Eq. 32) and the enthalpy of mixing (derived from Eq. 24) gives the Gibbs free energy of mixing of a polymer in a solvent (Eq. 35):

$$\Delta G_M = -kT(n_1 \ln \phi_1 + n_2 \ln \phi_2 + \chi_i \phi_2^2) \tag{35}$$

The Flory-Huggins theory in its simplest form considers all lattice sites to be occupied by one component or the other, in other words, incompressible solutions. It can be applied only to solutions sufficiently concentrated to have uniform segment density. It also assumes that there are no energetically preferred arrangements of polymer segments and solvent molecules in the lattice. Newer theories have extended the treatment to lattices with empty sites.

3. *Miscibility and Phase Equilibria* (76)

The mutual solubility, or miscibility, of a polymer and a solvent, or of two polymers, is governed by the sign of ΔG_M, the free energy of mixing of the two components. Three different cases can be envisaged. If ΔG_M is positive over the entire composition range (case I) the polymer and solvent are totally immiscible. They will coexist at equilibrium as two distinct phases. For total miscibility of polymer and solvent, two conditions have to be met: (1) the free energy of mixing must be negative for all compositions, and (2) the second derivative of ΔG_M with respect to the volume fraction of solvent or polymer must be positive over the entire composition range (Eq. 36):

$$\left(\frac{\partial^2 \Delta G_M}{\partial \phi_2^2}\right)_{P,T} > 0 \tag{36}$$

If condition (2) is not satisfied, the solution will phase-separate at equilibrium into two phases containing different concentrations of each component.

Phase equilibria are strongly affected by temperature: raising the temperature of a solution may increase the miscibility of the two components or, less frequently, may result in a decrease of their miscibility. In the first case, as depicted in the phase diagram in Figure 18, the two components are totally miscible above a point known as the upper critical solution temperature (UCST). At any temperature below the UCST, compositions lying outside the curve constitute homogeneous phases, while compositions inside the curve are thermodynamically unstable and will phase-separate. When the miscibility of a polymer in a solvent decreases as the temperature increases, the mixture possesses a lower critical solution temperature (LCST; Fig. 18). For temperatures below this point, the two components are totally miscible.

Phase diagrams presenting a UCST are often reported for polymers in nonpolar solvents. In these systems. ΔS_M is normally positive but weighted heavily by T, so the solubility depends mainly on the magnitude of ΔH_M, which is normally positive (endothermic dissolution process). Consequently when T decreases, $\Delta G_M = \Delta H_M - T\,\Delta S_M$, eventually becomes positive and phase separation takes place. Miscibility curves featuring an LCST are often observed in solutions of polymers in polar solvents, in particular in water. The occurrence of an LCST in water is a result of hydrogen-bond formation between the polymer and solvent, which enhances the solubility of the polymer at low temperature. As hydrogen bonds are thermally labile, a rise in temperature reduces the number of hydrogen bonds and causes eventual phase separation. Phase diagrams of polymer solutions may also present a miscibility gap between the two types of curves, as in the case of polystyrene in acetone.

B. Size and Shape of Polymers in Solution

One of the classic problems in polymer science has been the conformation of polymer chains in space. Over the years, several models have been proposed, based on theory and backed up by experimental determinations of the macromolecules' dimensions by scatter-

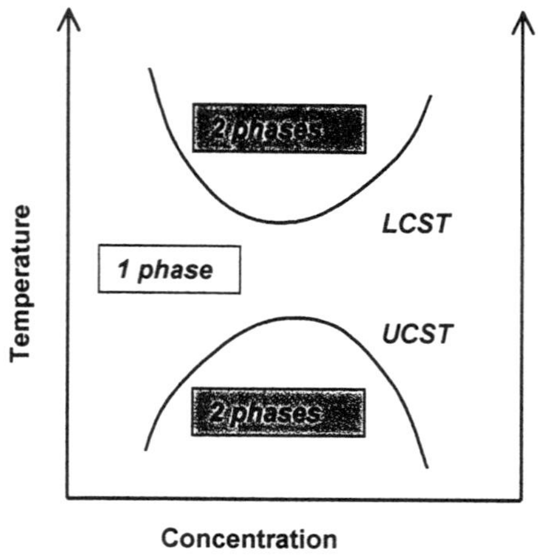

Figure 18 Phase diagram of a polymer solution with UCST (upper-critical-solution temperature) and LCST (lower-critical-solution temperature)

ing of light (77,78), X-rays (79), or neutrons (80). Polymer chain dimensions can also be obtained indirectly from size exclusion chromatography data, the viscosity of dilute solutions, and other hydrodynamic properties. The size and shape of single macromolecules can only be studied in solution, unlike small molecules that can be vaporized and observed in the gas phase, in the absence of solvent molecules. In solutions, solvent/polymer interactions cannot be ignored. In melts, macromolecules surrounding a single chain may be viewed as a type of solvent. The shape of a macromolecule will depend on inherent structural factors, such as the chemical structure of the base unit and the level of branching. It will also vary with solvent, temperature, and flow. The influence of the shape of macromolecules on their physical properties and performances cannot be overlooked. It may be as strong as the effect of chain constitution and configuration.

1. *Dilute Solutions* (81,82)

Once a polymer-solvent pair has been selected, the physical properties of the resulting solution are controlled by how the polymer behaves among the solvent molecules. Particularly important is the resultant size, or hydrodynamic volume, of the macromolecule. A polymer in solution can be pictured as a coil, continuously changing its shape, and hence its size, under the action of thermal fluctuations. Therefore, the only meaningful chain dimensions are those averaged over many conformations and chain lengths. If the polymer were fully extended, its size could easily be determined from the knowledge of bond lengths and bond angles. This is not the case with most common polymers. Two average dimensions are particularly useful:

The average root mean square distance between chain ends, $\langle r^2 \rangle^{1/2}$
The average root mean square radius of gyration, $\langle s^2 \rangle^{1/2}$, which is a measure of the average distance of a chain segment from the center of gravity of the coil (Fig. 19)

For simple linear chains, the two quantities are related, in the absence of excluded volume effects, by:

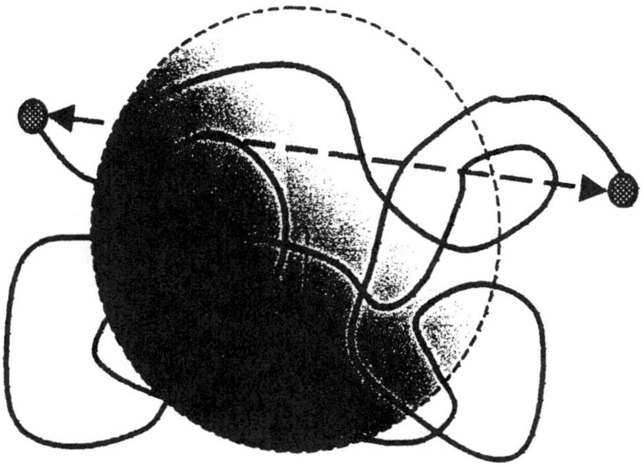

Figure 19 Coil conformation of a macromolecule in solution. The distance between chain ends and the radius of gyration are indicated.

$$\langle r^2 \rangle^{1/2} = \langle 6s^2 \rangle^{1/2} \tag{37}$$

Various models have been proposed to calculate the end-to-end distances of single linear chains. In simple cases only short-range interactions need to be considered. These involve two to five neighboring segments of the polymer chain. Long-range interactions are defined as those between spatially proximate groups that are separated along the chain by many segments. Both interaction types are intramolecular. The various models for random coils with short-range interactions are all nonspecific with respect to the type of interactions (Van der Waals, dipole-dipole, etc.). They differ in the number of interacting chain atoms and the restrictions applied to valence angles and torsion angles.

It is convenient to express r and s in terms of two factors, an unperturbed dimension (r_0 or s_0) and an expansion factor (α). Thus:

$$\bar{r}^2 = r_0^2\alpha^2 \tag{38}$$

$$\bar{s}^2 = s_0^2\alpha^2 \tag{39}$$

The unperturbed dimension refers to the size of the molecule, exclusive of solvent effects. It arises from a combination of free rotations and intermolecular steric and polar interactions. The expansion factor arises from interactions between the polymer and the solvent. In a ''good solvent'' α will be greater than 1 and the actual (perturbed) dimensions of the polymer will exceed its unperturbed dimensions. The greater the value of α, the better the solvent. For the special case where $\alpha = 1$, the polymer adopts its unperturbed dimensions and behaves as an ''ideal statistical coil''.

2. *Semidilute and Concentrated Solutions*

Random coils of polymer molecules are very loose entities. They occupy a large volume per mass. At very low polymer concentrations, they are separated from each other by many solvent molecules. With increasing polymer concentration, less and less space is available between the coils and finally a concentration is reached where they start to touch each other and then overlap. This critical concentration is known as the overlap concentration, c^*. If the concentration is increased to a point slightly higher than c^*, the coils become entangled and a network of mesh size ξ is formed. The parameter ξ refers to the distance between two entanglement points or two intersection points. The chain interactions and entanglements in the three concentration regimes are represented in Figure 20.

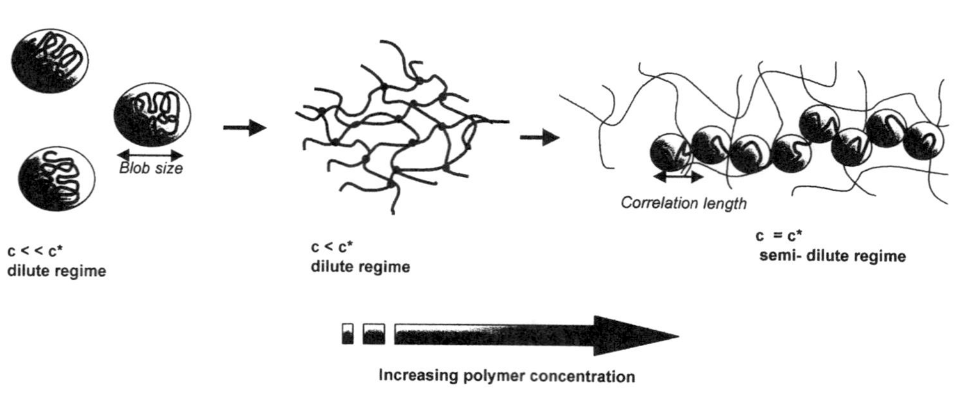

Figure 20 Chain entanglement.

In the dilute region an individual polymer chain can be conceived as confined in a blob of radius r or ξ. In the semidilute regime many chains interpenetrate into each other to form a mesh of size ξ. Still in the semidilute region, but with a concentration slightly higher than c^*, the same individual chain is in the form of a succession of blobs of radius ξ. The parameter ξ is known as the correlation length. In the concentrated region c'', the length ξ becomes smaller than the coil size. When the concentration is very high, ξ becomes similar to the monomer unit size. The chain exists in the collapsed state.

The phase diagram of a typical polymer solution is shown in Figure 21, where $\tau = (T - \theta)/\theta$ is the reduced temperature. Region I is the dilute region. Region II is the semidilute region, bound by the lines corresponding to the c^* and c''. An interesting quantity in region II is the screening length, ξ, which represents the average distance between nearest chain contacts. At c*, ξ can be identified as the radius of gyration. If the polymer is cross-linked it corresponds to the mesh size. Region III consists of the semidilute and concentrated θ state. Region IV occurs in the negative τ range. It is bound by the coexistence phase diagram curve (dashed line). Phase I′ represents the θ state.

3. *Polymer Association*

Coil overlap, described in the previous section, is a nonspecific event that is due only to the increased competition for space of segments of macromolecules as the polymer concentration increases. In many cases an increase in concentration induces *specific* interactions between certain groups or segments. These lead to polymer association and gelation. Specific interactions tend to begin at polymer concentrations well below c^*. Polymer association is a reversible process under thermodynamic control. This process should not be confused with polymer aggregation, an irreversible process. Association may occur within a single macromolecule, or intrapolymeric association. Alternatively, it may involve several chains (interpolymeric association). Intramolecular association leads to the contraction of the polymer coils. The coils become more compact and overall viscosity of the solution decreases. Intramolecular association shows no concentration dependence. On the contrary, interpolymeric associations increase with increasing polymer concentra-

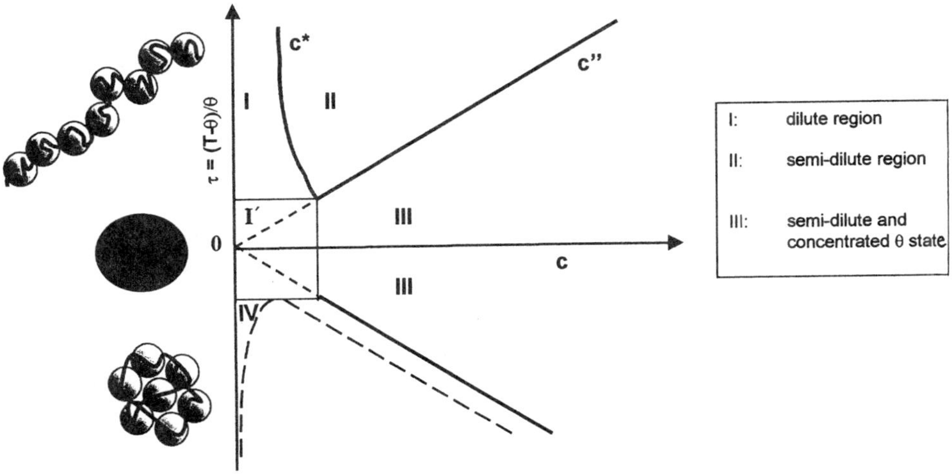

Figure 21 Phase diagram of a typical polymer solution. The quantity τ represents the reduced temperature, $(T - \tau)/\theta$ where θ is the Flory θ-temperature.

tion. They tend to induce an increase in the viscosity of the solution. Important advances have been made in the last two decades in unraveling the structure and dynamics of polymer association, especially in the case of aqueous polymers (83,84).

C. Rheology of Polymer Solutions

The simplest rheological properties are viscosity and elasticity. Liquids such as water or liquid paraffin have viscosity but no elasticity. They flow under even the smallest force, spending all the force in flowing. By contrast, materials such as rubber have elasticity but no viscosity. When they are subjected to a force, they change shape and the energy applied is stored, instead of being consumed. In cosmetics, the liquid state is usually handled as a purely viscous fluid, but disperse systems, such as milky lotions and creams, demonstrate complex rheological properties, displaying both viscosity and elasticity. Polymers strongly influence the rheological properties of these fluids as described in the following sections.

1. The Viscosity of Polymer Solutions

It is a common observation that, usually, polymer solutions flow more slowly through a tube than do pure solvents, under the same pressure. Viscosity is a measure of the energy dissipated by a fluid in motion as it resists an applied shearing force. Solution viscosity is a measure of the resistance to flow and thus, for polymer solutions, it is directly related to the size of the macromolecules and can be used to characterize the molecular weight of polymers. Practically, the flow of a polymer solution is measured and compared to the flow of the solvent alone. The ratio of the viscosity of a polymer solution, η, to that of the solvent, η_o, or relative viscosity, η_r, is used to define an important parameter of a polymer in a given solvent, the intrinsic viscosity $[\eta]$ (Eq. 40).

$$[\eta] = \lim_{c \to 0} \frac{\eta - \eta_0}{c\,\eta_0} = \lim_{c \to 0} \frac{\eta_{sp}}{c} \tag{40}$$

The extrapolation to zero concentration is performed to eliminate the effects of molecular interferences likely to occur even in dilute solutions and obtain the influence of an isolated polymer coil on the viscosity of the solution. Only η and η_o have the dimensions of viscosity (Poise or Pa. s). Specific viscosity and relative viscosity are dimensionless. Intrinsic viscosity, reduced viscosity, and inherent viscosity all have the dimension of inverse concentration. The nomenclature of viscosity parameters is given in Table 7.

A relationship between molecular weight and intrinsic viscosity was derived independently by Mark and Houwink in the late 1930s (Eq. 41):

$$[\eta] = KM^a \tag{41}$$

where K and a are constants (the Mark-Houwink constants) that vary with solvent and polymer. The exponent a is a function of the shape of the molecule in solution and a measure of the interaction of solvent and polymer, increasing in value as the polymer expands in a good solvent. For most polymer/solvent pairs, the coefficient a ranges between 0.5 and 0.8. In a θ-solvent, it takes a value of 0.5, characteristic of the ideal random coil. An extensive compilation of a and K values can be found, for example, in the *Polymer Handbook* for a large number of solvent/polymer pairs (85). Measurements of viscosity for the determination of molecular weight are usually done using a glass capillary viscometer, such as the Ostwald-Fenske or the Ubbelohde viscometer. Precise experimental conditions are described in various textbooks (86).

Table 7 Commonly Used Viscometry Terms

Common name	IUPAC name	Definition	Symbol	Common Units
Solution viscosity		η	η	Poise or Pa s
Solvent viscosity		η_0	η_0	Poise or Pa s
Relative viscosity	Viscosity ratio	η/η_0	$\eta_{rel} = \eta_r$	Dimensionless
Specific viscosity		$(\eta/\eta_0) - 1$ or $\eta_\rho - 1$	η_{sp}	Dimensionless
Reduced viscosity	Viscosity number	η_{sp}/c	η_{red}	dl/g
Inherent viscosity	Logarithmic viscosity number	$In\ (\eta_r)/c$	η_{ink}	dl/g
Intrinsic viscosity	Limiting viscosity number	$lim(\eta_{sp}/c)_{c \to 0}$	$[\eta]$ or LVN	dl/g

When dealing with solutions of charged water-soluble polymers, the linear Huggins relationship no longer holds as a result of the strong ionic interactions between polymer chains and solvent molecules. Charged polymers have been shown to follow the empirical relationship proposed by Fuoss and Strauss (Eq. 42) (87). The reciprocal of Eq. 42 yields a linear relationship between (c/η_{sp}) and $c^{1/2}$, with the slope given by B/A and the intercept by $(1/A)$. Physically, the value of A corresponds to the intrinsic viscosity.

$$\frac{\eta_{sp}}{c} = \frac{A}{1 + Bc^{1/2}} \tag{42}$$

2. *Rheological Properties of Polymer Solutions* (38)

In many practical systems, polymers are added to solutions to control their flow characteristics. The attractive feature of polymeric additives is that even in rather low concentrations they can dramatically affect the rheology of a fluid, imparting to a solution properties intermediate between those of elastic solids and those of viscous fluids. The elastic behavior is dominant in solids. It is described by Hooke's law ($\sigma = E\gamma$, Eq. 19, see above). Viscous behavior is dominant in simple liquids. It is described by Newton's law (Eq. 43), which states that the applied stress σ is proportional to the rate of strain $d\gamma/dt$, with a proportionality constant η, the viscosity.

$$\sigma = \eta \frac{d\gamma}{dt} = \eta\dot{\gamma} \tag{43}$$

Therefore, a liquid is said to exhibit Newtonian flow, if η is independent of $\dot{\gamma}$. Substances that show deviations from this flow pattern are termed non-Newtonian. There are two broad classes of non-Newtonian fluids:

1. Fluids with shear stresses that at any point depend on the shear rates only, and are independent of time. These include Bingham plastics, or materials that require a minimum amount of stress (yield stress) before deformation, pseudo-plastics or shear-thinning fluids, which exhibit a decrease of shear stress with shear rate, and dilatants, or shear-thickening fluids, for which the stress increases with the shear rate.
2. Fluids in which the ratio of shear stress to shear rate depends on time. They fall into two categories: thixotropic fluids, in which the microstructure of the fluid progressively breaks down and the viscosity decreases, and rheopectic fluids, where the applied shear promotes gradual formation of structure, and the viscosity increases with shear.

Most polymer solutions fall into one (or several) of these categories in certain concentration ranges. The nature and shape of the viscosity curves depend on a series of additional factors, such as polymer molecular weight and weight distribution, polymer molecular structure, and solvent power. A typical flow curve exhibits two Newtonian plateaus, one at low shear, or "zero-shear condition," and one at high shear, or "infinite shear condition." A shear-thinning region lies between the two limiting conditions. It may extend over several orders of magnitudes of shear rates (Fig. 22).

To understand the complex effect of shear on the flow of polymer solutions, one needs to consider its influence on the molecular interactions at play in solution. Shear-thinning behavior, for instance, reflects the effect of shear on entanglements, as illustrated

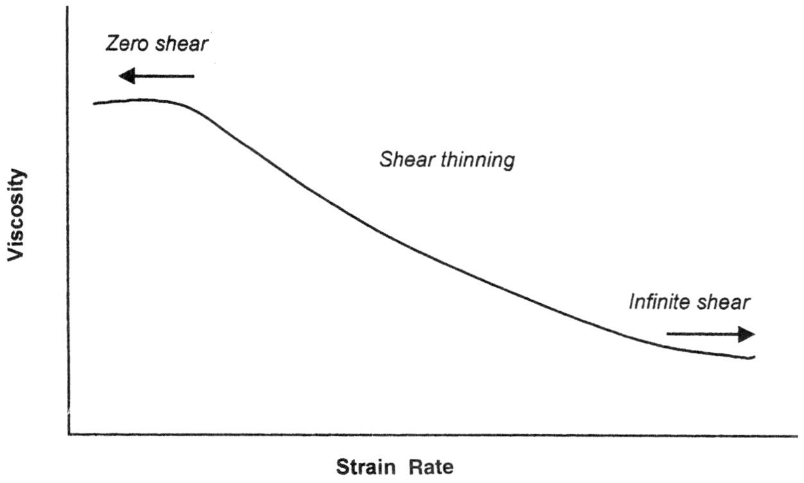

Figure 22 Typical viscosity curve of a polymer solution.

in Figure 23. At low shear rates, the entanglements impede shear flow, and therefore viscosity is high. As the shear rate increases, chains begin to orient in the flow direction and disentangle from one another, and the viscosity begins to drop. Finally the macromolecules become fully oriented in the flow direction at very high shear rates. At this point stable entanglements are no longer possible and the viscosity reaches a low level that is again independent of shear rate.

In some cases the viscosity of a fluid increases with increasing shear rate. This behavior is uncommon for polymers in organic solvents, where it was observed for the first time in ionomer solutions (89). Ionomers are hydrophobic polymers that carry a charged group at each chain end. When dissolved in organic solvents, the charged polymers associate via their ionic groups. The observed shear thickening of the solution is interpreted in terms of an increase in temporary associations among chains made possible by elongation under flow of the charged polymers. The phenomenon is highly dependent on chemical composition and is maximized with only a few associating groups per chain. Shear-thickening effect is observed also with certain water-soluble polymers, especially various new types of hydrophobically modified polymers, such as hydrophobically-modified ethylene oxide urethanes (HEUR) and hydrophobically-modified alkali-swellable emulsions (HASE) (90). In these solutions shear thickening is brought about by formation of polymer networks via hydrophobic interactions (91). The addition of small amounts of surfactant to these polymeric solutions may also result in exceptionally intense shear thickening.

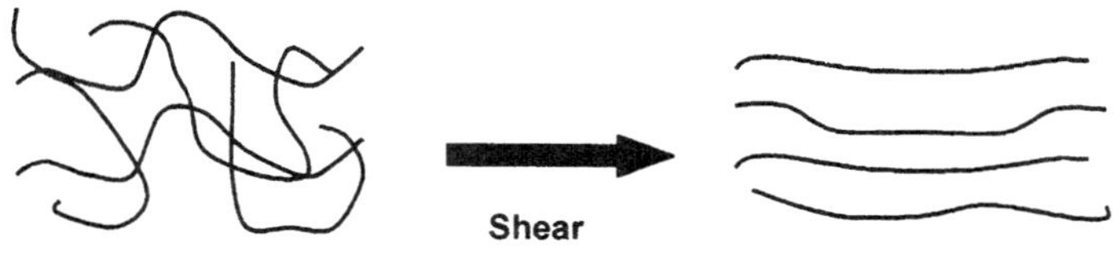

Figure 23 Idealized view of the effect of shear on the entanglements of concentrated polymer solutions and polymer melts.

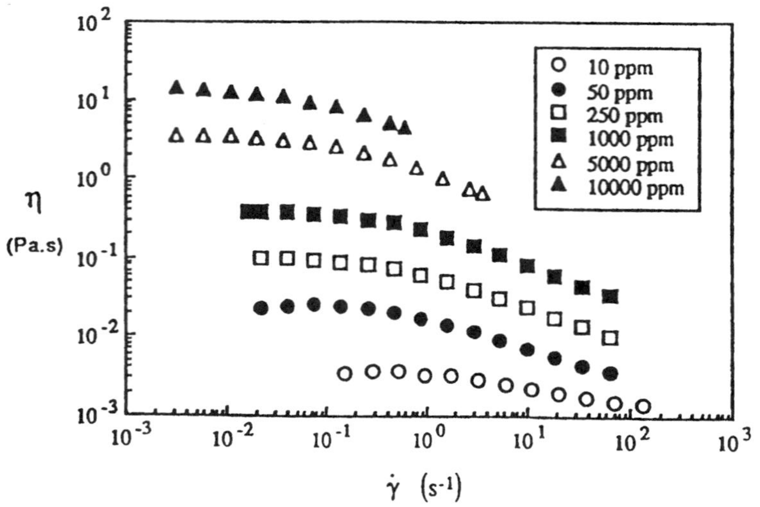

Figure 24 Shear-dependent viscosity of polyacrylamide solutions. (From KC Tam and C Tiu, Water-soluble polymers (rheological properties) in Polymeric Materials Encyclopedia, JC Salamone, ed. Boca Raton, FL: CRC Press, 1996, p. 8655.)

a. Effect of Polymer Concentration. Figures 24 and 25 show typical viscosity curves for two classes of polymers, the flexible poly(acrylamide) and the semirigid xanthan gum, in aqueous solutions. Shear-thinning behavior is observed in both cases, starting at a very low concentration in the case of the xanthan gum. The curves are identical for the two polymers at low concentration, despite considerable structural differences between the two. In the semidilute and concentrated regions ($c > 2$ g/L) the xanthan solutions are much more viscous than the polyacrylamide solutions and shear thinning starts at much lower shear rates, compared to the poly(acrylamide). The viscosity at low shear (η_0) is

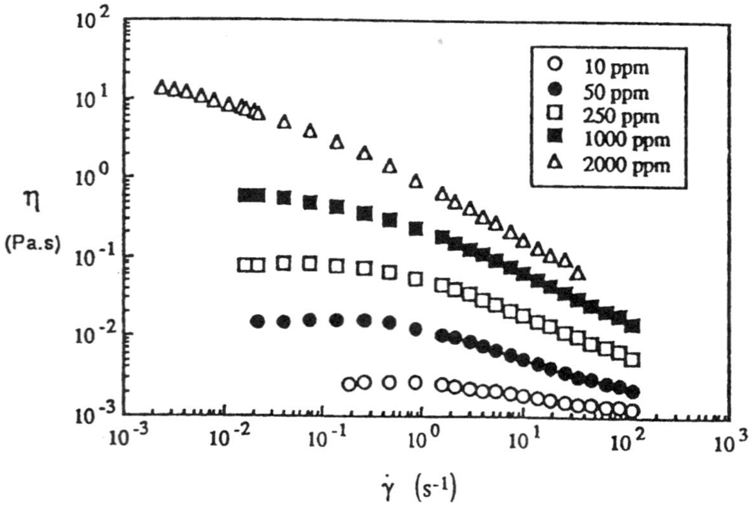

Figure 25 Shear-dependent viscosity of xanthan gum solutions. (From KC Tam and C Tiu, Water-soluble polymers (rheological properties) in Polymeric Materials Encyclopedia, JC Salamone, ed. Boca Raton, FL: CRC Press, 1996, p. 8655.)

often correlated as a function of $c[\eta]$ and the result is used as an approximate guide to identify various concentration regimes of a polymer solution. For many polymers, the dilute solution regime occurs up to $c[\eta]$ of 1.0, where the slope of η_0 versus $c[\eta]$ is about 1.0. This regime is followed by a transition zone between $1 < c[\eta] < 10$ with a varying slope, corresponding to the semidilute regime. Finally, when $c[\eta]$ exceeds about 10, the curve reaches a second linear region with a slope of about 3.4, corresponding to the concentrated solution regime. In the case of polyelectrolytes the interactions between charges on the polymer chains greatly affect the shape and size of the polymer coil, and hence the solution viscosity. In general, the values of zero-shear viscosity vary greatly among polymers for solutions of identical concentrations, even in the case of neutral polymers.

b. Temperature Effects. Temperature changes can dramatically affect the rheology of polymer solutions. Thus, the ability to predict the variations of the steady shear and dynamic properties with respect to temperature is critical in many applications. Newtonian fluids usually obey an Arrhenius-type exponential dependence on temperature (Eq. 44) where the constant B_T can be estimated from thermodynamic properties (92).

$$\eta(T) = A \exp\left(\frac{B_T}{T}\right) \tag{44}$$

Solutions of high-molecular-weight polymers exhibit similar temperature dependence, but the coefficient B_T cannot be predicted from thermodynamic properties. It depends on the structural and thermal properties of the polymer. Data are analyzed in terms of mathematical representations of viscosity in which appropriate coefficients are related to structural considerations.

c. Effects of Electrolytes. Polyelectrolytes in water are highly charged species producing a strong electrical field that attracts counterions. The electrical field is screened out when the concentration of small ions is large enough. This may be achieved by addition of simple electrolyte, such as sodium chloride. The effects of mono- and divalent salts on the zero shear viscosity and onset of shear thinning are illustrated in the case of polyacrylamide (Fig. 26).

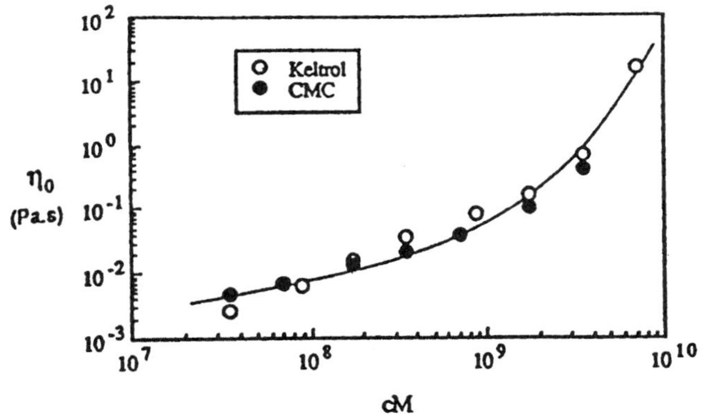

Figure 26 Dependence of zero-shear viscosity and critical shear rate concentration on salt concentration for polyacrylamide aqueous solutions. (From KC Tam and C Tiu, Water-soluble polymers (rheological properties) in Polymeric Materials Encyclopedia, JC Salamone, ed. Boca Raton, FL: CRC Press, 1996, p. 8655.)

d. Oscillatory Properties. When polymer solutions are subjected to oscillatory stresses of high frequency, their characterization as fluids with a viscosity η is no longer adequate, since their response to the applied stress also contains an elastic component (93). If the shearing strain in the $x - y$ plane is $\gamma_{xy} = \gamma_{xy}^{\circ}\sin(\omega t)$, where $\omega/2\pi$ is the frequency of the oscillations, the shearing stress s_{xy} has an elastic component in phase with γ_{xy} and a viscous component proportional to $d\gamma_{xy}/dt$, such that Eq. 45 is obeyed, where the shear storage modulus G' and the shear loss modulus G'' are functions of ω.

$$\sigma_{xy} = \gamma_{xy}^{0}\,[G' \sin(\omega t) + G'' \cos(\omega t)] \tag{45}$$

The shapes of G' and G'' versus ω curves for polymer solutions have been described by Ferry (93). At low frequency, G' and G'' are proportional to ω^2 and ω, respectively. As the frequency increases, the slope of these curves decreases. On a molecular basis this suggests that as the polymer concentration increases, the number density of macromolecules in solution increases, resulting in larger G' and G'' values. The effects of temperature on dynamic properties are similar to those on the steady shear behavior of polymer solutions. Also, similar to the steady shear properties, the presence of electrolytes significantly alters the elastic properties of polyelectrolyte solutions. Divalent salts have a much greater effect on the relaxation time, as the shielding effect is much stronger than in the case of monovalent salts. Therefore, addition of divalent salts to a polyelectrolyte solution will induce coiling of the chain in a more compact polymer coil. Such behavior results in a reduction in the effectiveness of a polymer as a drag-reducing agent when high salt concentrations are encountered.

e. Treatment of Viscosity Data: Master Curves. We have seen that the viscosity–shear rate curves for polymer solutions are dependent on a number of factors. It is possible to evaluate the effects of molecular structure on $\eta(\gamma)$ in terms of reduced variables. Graessley showed that such dependence can be represented by the characteristic relaxation time in spring-bead models, where β is given by Eq. 46 (94).

$$\frac{\eta - \eta_s}{\eta_0 - \eta_s} = fn\,(\beta) \tag{46}$$

$$\beta = \frac{(\eta_0 - \eta_s)M}{cRT}\,\dot{\gamma} = \lambda\,\dot{\gamma}$$

A classic example is the master curve obtained for concentrated polystyrene solutions in *n*-butylbenzene (94). The method is also applicable for dilute aqueous solutions of poly(acrylamide), xanthan gum and poly(ethylene oxide). In the case of polyelectrolytes, the method gives satisfactory results only in limited concentration ranges. Further refinements have to be added to the general method (95).

f. Correlation Between Steady-Shear and Oscillatory Data. The viscosity function is by far the most widely used and the easiest viscometric function determined experimentally. For dilute polymer solutions dynamic measurements are often preferred over steady-shear normal stress measurements for the determination of fluid elasticity at low deformation rates. The relationship between viscous and elastic properties of polymer liquids is of great interest to polymer rheologists. In recent years, several models have been proposed to predict fluid elasticity from shear viscosity data.

VI. CONCLUSION

Polymers are important components of most cosmetics and their role can be critical. Understanding the physical chemistry of polymer solutions is essential in designing cosmetic formulations and ensuring their stability. The rheological properties of cosmetics, controlled to a great extent by the incorporation of polymers, are of prime importance, not only from the standpoint of their final use and acceptance by the customer, but also in the design of manufacture processes. The dramatic effects that are often triggered by small modifications of polymer-containing fluids cannot be overlooked, as demonstrated in the following chapters.

ACKNOWLEDGMENTS

I thank Dr. E. D. Goddard for his constant support, his enthusiasm, and his excellent advice. Thanks are due also to Dr. V. Gruber for providing an early version of the chapters he wrote in this book and to Dr. K. Szczubialka (Jagiellonian University, Krakow, Poland) for his careful proofreading of the manuscript.

REFERENCES

1. Morawetz H. Polymers: The Origins and Growth of a Science. New York: Wiley, 1985.
1a. Meikle JL. American Plastic: A Cultural History. New Brunswick, NJ: Rutgers University Press, 1995.
2. Carraher CE Jr. Polymer Chemistry, an Introduction, 4th ed. New York: Marcel Dekker, 1996.
3. Allcock HR, Lampe FW. Contemporary Polymer Chemistry, 2nd ed. Englewood Cliffs, NJ: Prentice-Hall, 1990.
4. Fried JR. Polymer Science and Technology. Englewood Cliffs, NJ: Prentice-Hall, 1995.
5. Elias H-G. An Introduction to Polymer Science. Weinheim, Germany: VCH, 1997.
6. Campbell IM. Introduction to Synthetic Polymers. Oxford, UK: Oxford Science Publications, Oxford University Press, 1994.
7. Cowie JMG. Polymers, Chemistry and Physics of Modern Materials, 2nd ed. London: Blackie Academic & Professional, Chapman Hall, 1991.
8. Brandrup J, Immergut EH, eds. Polymer Handbook, 3rd ed. New York: Wiley, 1989.
9. Mark H, Overberger C, Menges G, Bikales NM, eds. Encyclopedia of Polymer Science and Engineering, 2nd ed. New York: Wiley, 1985 ff, 18 vols, and supplements.
10. Salamone JC, ed. Polymeric Materials Encyclopedia. Boca Raton, FL: CRC Press, 1986.
11. Allen G, Bevington JC, eds. Comprehensive Polymer Science. Oxford, UK: Pergamon Press, 1989.
12. Semlyen JA, ed. Cyclic Polymers. New York: Elsevier, 1986.
13. Ikeda Y. Characterization of graft copolymers. Adv Polym Sci 1978; 29:47.
14. Bywater S. Preparation and properties of star-branched polymers. Adv Polym Sci 1979; 30: 89.
15. Tomalia DA. Naylor AM. Goddard WA III. Starburst dendrimers. Angew Chem Int Ed Engl 1990; 29:138.
16. Sperling LH. Interpenetrating Networks and Related Materials. New York: Plenum Press, 1981.
17. Rempp P, Merrill EW. Polymer Synthesis, 2nd ed. Basel: Hüthig and Wepf, 1992.
18. Odian G. Principles of Polymerization, 3rd ed. New York: Wiley, 1992.

19. Kricheldorf HR, ed. Handbook of Polymer Synthesis. New York: Marcel Dekker, 1992. 2 vols.
20. Millich F, Carraher CE, eds. Interfacial Synthesis. New York: Marcel Dekker, 1977. 2 vols.
21. Free-Radical Polymerization, Comprehensive Chemical Kinetics, 14A. Amsterdam: Elsevier, 1976
22. Piirma I. Emulsion Polymerization. New York: Academic Press, 1982.
23. Morton M. Anionic Polymerization: Principle and Practice. New York: Academic Press, 1983.
24. Hsieh HL, Quirk RP. Anionic Polymerization. New York: Marcel Dekker, 1996.
25. Kennedy JP, Iván B. Designed Polymers by Carbocationic Macromolecular Engineering: Theory and Practice. Munich: Hanser, 1992.
26. Matyajaszewski K, ed. Cationic Polymerizations. New York: Marcel Dekker, 1996.
27. Kissin YV. Isospecific Polymerization of Olefins. Berlin: Springer-Verlag, 1986.
28. Fink G, Mülhaupt R, Brintzinger HH, eds. Ziegler Catalysts. Berlin: Springer-Verlag, 1995.
29. Kucera M. Mechanism and Kinetics of Addition Polymerizations. Amsterdam: Elsevier, 1992.
30. Carraher CE, Moore JA. Modification of Polymers. New York: Plenum Press, 1983.
31. Moore JA. Reactions of Polymers. Boston: D. Reidel, 1974.
32. Peebles LH. Molecular Weight Distribution in Polymers. New York: Interscience, 1971.
33. Slade PE Jr. Polymer Molecular Weights. New York: Marcel Dekker, 1975. 2 vols.
34. Laidler KJ, Meiser JH. Physical Chemistry, 2nd ed. Boston: Houghton Mifflin, 1995, Chapter 5.
35. Billingham NC. Molar Mass Measurements in Polymer Science. New York: Wiley, 1977.
36. Yau WW, Kirkland IJ, Bly DD. Modern Size Exclusion Liquid Chromatography. New York: Wiley, 1979.
37. Glöckner G. Polymer Characterization by Liquid Chromatography. Amsterdam: Elsevier, 1986.
38. Wu CS. Handbook of Size Exclusion Chromatography. New York; Marcel Dekker, 1995.
39. Garmon RG. End group determinations. Techn Methods Polym Eval 1975; 4(1):31.
40. Bassett DC. Principles of Polymer Morphology. Cambridge: Cambridge University Press, 1981.
41. Woodward AE. Understanding Polymer Morphology. Cincinnati: Hanser-Gardner, 1995.
42. Corradini P, Guerra G. Polymorphism in polymers. Adv Polym Sci 1992; 100:183.
43. Haward RN, ed. The Physics of Glassy Polymers. New York: Wiley, 1973.
44. Cheremisinoff NP, ed. Elastomer Technology Handbook. Boca Raton, FL: CRC Press, 1993.
45. Bartenev GM, Zenlenev YV, eds. Relaxation Phenomena in Polymers. New York: Halsted, 1974.
46. Strobl G. The Physics of Polymers, 2nd ed. Berlin: Springer-Verlag, 1997, Chapter 5.
47. Eisenberg A. The glassy state and the glass transition. In: Mark JE, Eisenberg A, Graessley WW, Mandelkern L, Samulski ET, Koenig JL, Wignall GD, eds. Physical Properties of Polymers, 2nd ed. Washington, DC: American Chemical Society, 1993:61–95.
48. Turi EA, ed. Thermal Characterisation of Polymeric Materials, 2nd ed. New York: Academic Press, 1982.
49. Mathot VBF, ed. Calorimetry and Thermal Analysis of Polymers. Cincinnati: Hanser, 1994.
50. Bershtein VA, Egorov VM. Differential Scanning Calorimetry of Polymers, Chichester: Ellis Horwood, 1973.
51. De Gennes P-G. Scaling Concepts in Polymer Physics. Cornell: Cornell University Press, 1979.
52. Guven O. Cross-Linking and Scission of Polymers. Dordrecht: Kluwer, 1990.
53. Burchard W, Ross-Murphy SB, eds. Physical Networks. London: Elsevier, 1990.
54. Guenet JM. Thermoreversible Gelation of Polymers and Biopolymers. London: Academic Press, 1992.
55. Tadokoro H. Structure of Crystalline Polymers. New York: Wiley, 1979.

56. Hall IH, ed. Structure of Crystalline Polymers. London: Elsevier, 1984.
57. Rhodes G. Crystallography Made Crystal Clear. A Guide for Users of Macromolecular Models. New York: Academic Press, 1993.
58. Mandelkern L. In: Mark JE, Eisenberg A, Graessley WW, Mandelkern L, Samulski ET, Koenig JL, Wignall GD, eds. The Crystalline State in Physical Properties of Polymers, 2nd ed. Washington, DC: American Chemical Society, 1993:145–200.
59. Fraser RDB, MacRae TP, Rogers GE. Keratins: Their Composition, Structure, and Biosynthesis. Springfield, IL: Charles C Thomas, 1972.
60. Bendit EG. In: Parry DA, Creamer LK, eds. Fibrous Proteins: Scientific, Industrial, and Medical Aspects. New York: Academic Press, 1980.
61. Ward IM, Hadley DW. An Introduction to the Mechanical Properties of Solid Polymers. Chichester: Wiley, 1993.
62. Nielsen LE, Landel RF. Mechanical Properties of Polymers and Composites, 2nd ed. New York: Marcel Dekker, 1993.
63. Bartener G. Mechanical Strength and Failure of Polymers. Engelwood Cliffs, NJ: Prentice-Hall, 1993.
64. Crompton TR. Practical Polymer Analysis. New York: Plenum Press, 1993.
65. Williams JG. Stress Analysis of Polymers. London: Longmans, 1973.
66. Aklonis JJ, MacKnight WJ. An Introduction to Polymer Viscoelasticity, 2nd ed. New York: Wiley, 1983.
67. Mark JE, Erman B. Rubberlike Elasticity: A Molecular Primer. New York: Wiley, 1988.
68. Matsuoka S. Relaxation Phenomena in Polymers. Cincinnati: Hanser-Gardner, 1992.
69. Flory JP. Principles of Polymer Chemistry. Ithaca: Cornell University Press, 1953.
70. Flory JP, Kriegbaum WR. J Chem Phys 1950; 18:1086.
71. Barton AFM. Solubility Parameters and Other Cohesion Parameters, Boca Raton, FL: CRC Press, 1983.
72. Small PA. J Appl Chem 1953; 3:71.
73. Hoy KL. J Paint Technol 1970; 42:76.
74. Grulke EA. In: Brandrup J. Immergut EH, eds. Polymer Handbook, 3rd ed. New York: Wiley, 1989:519–559.
75. Flory PJ. Disc Far Soc 1970; 49:7.
76. Morawetz H. Macromolecules in Solution, 2nd ed; New York: Wiley, 1975.
77. Kratochvil P. Classical Light Scattering from Polymer Solutions. Amsterdam: Elsevier, 1987.
78. Chu B. Laser Light Scattering. San Diego: Academic Press, 1990.
79. Glatter O, Kratky O. Small Angle X-Ray Scattering. New York: Academic Press, 1982.
80. Higgins JS, Benoit HC. Polymers and Neutron Scattering. Oxford: Clarendon Press, 1994.
81. Forsman WC, ed. Polymers in Solution, Theoretical Considerations and Newer Methods of Characterisation. New York: Plenum Press, 1983.
82. Mattice WL. Suter UW. Conformational Theory of Large Molecules. New York: Wiley, 1994.
83. Dubin P, ed. Microdomains in Polymer Solutions. New York: Plenum Press, 1982.
84. Stroeve P, Balazs AC, eds. Macromolecular Assemblies in Polymer Systems. Washington, DC: American Chemical Society, 1992.
85. Kurata M, Tsunashima Y. In: Bandrupt J. Immergut EH, eds. Polymer Handbook, 3rd ed. New York: Wiley, 1989:1–59.
86. Bohdanecky M, Kovar J. Viscosity of Polymer Solutions. Amsterdam: Elsevier, 1982.
87. Fuoss RM, Strauss UP. J Polym Sci 1948;3:246.
88. Barnes HA, Hutton JF, Walters K. An Introduction to Rheology. Amsterdam: Elsevier, 1989.
89. Glass JE, ed. Polymers as Rheology Modifiers. Washington, DC: American Chemical Society, 1991, Chapters 7 and 9.
90. Glass JE, ed. Polymers as Rheology Modifiers. Washington DC: American Chemical Society, 1991, Chapters 10, 13, and 14.

91. English RJ, Gulati HS, Jenkins RD, Khan, SA. Solution rheology of a hydrophobically modified alkali-soluble associative polymer. J Rheol 1997;41:427–444.
92. Bird RB, Stewart WE, Lightfoot EN. Transport Phenomena. New York: Wiley, 1960
93. Ferry JD. Viscoelastic Properties of Polymers, 3rd ed. New York: Wiley, 1980.
94. Graessley WW. Adv Polym Sci 1974; 16:1.
95. Tam KC, Tiu CJ. Non-Newt Fluid Mech 1993;46:275.

APPENDIX I: GLOSSARY

A	Arrhenius prefactor
a	Mark-Houwink coefficient
B	bulk modulus
c^*	overlap concentration
E	Young's modulus of elasticity
E'	storage modulus
E''	loss modulus
ΔG	change in Gibbs free energy
G	modulus
G	molar attraction constant (Small and Hoy)
G'	shear storage modulus
G''	shear loss modulus
ΔH	change in enthalpy
J	elongation compliance
K	Mark-Houwink coefficient
k	rate constant
M	modulus
M_n	number-average molecular weight
M_v	viscosity molecular weight
M_w	weight-average molecular weight
R	ideal gas constant
$\langle r^2\rangle^{1/2}$	average root mean square end to end distance
ΔS	change in entropy
$\langle s^2\rangle^{1/2}$	radius of gyration
T_g	glass transition temperature
T_m	melting point
x	molar fraction
α	expansion factor
β	compressibility
δ	solubility parameter (Hildebrandt)
γ	strain
η	viscosity
η_r	reduced viscosity
η_{rel}	relative viscosity
η_{sp}	specific viscosity
$[\eta]$	intrinsic viscosity
θ	Flory critical miscibility temperature
μ	dipole moment

ν	kinetic chain length
ρ	density
σ	tensile strength
τ	relaxation time
ϕ	volume fraction
ω	frequency
ξ	screening length
ζ	correlation length
χ_1	Flory-Huggins interaction parameter
CED	cohesive energy density
DP	degree of polymerization
DS	degree of substitution
DSC	differential scanning calorimetry
DTA	differential thermal analysis
GPC	gel permeation chromatography
IPN	interpenetrating network
LCST	lower critical solution temperature
MALDI-MS	matrix-assisted laser desorption ionization mass spectrometry
MWD	molecular weight distribution
NMR	nuclear magnetic resonance
TGA	thermal gravimetric analysis
UCST	upper critical solution temperature

APPENDIX II: Definitions of Terms Commonly Used in Polymer Science

Amorphous polymer: noncrystalline polymer or noncrystalline areas in bulk polymer.

Anionic polymerization: a polymerization initiated by an anion.

Bingham plastic: a polymer which does not flow until the applied stress exceeds a threshold stress value.

Blend: mixture of different polymers, in which the polymers are mixed intimately in either one or two phases.

Branched polymer: a polymer having extensions of the polymer chain attached to the polymer backbone (or main chain), such as in low-density polyethylene (LDPE).

Cationic polymerization: a polymerization initiated by a cation, such as sulfuric acid.

Chain-growth polymerization: a polymerization method that consists of a least three steps: initiation, propagation, and termination. The polymerization can be initiated by a free radical, a cation, or an anion.

Chain transfer: a process in which a growing chain becomes a dead polymer by abstracting a group from some other compound, thereby generating a new active site.

Cloud point: some systems, notably poly(ethylene oxide) in water, have an inverse solubility/temperature relation and exhibit a cloud point on heating. The cloud point is the temperature at which a polymer starts to precipitate from a solution when the temperature is raised.

Composite: mixture, on a macroscopic level of different polymers, one forming a continuous phase and another a discontinuous phase.

Conformations: various shapes of polymers resulting from the rotation of single bonds in the chain. Not to be confused with configurations, which are related chemical structures produced by the breaking and making of covalent bonds.

Contour length: the fully extended length of a polymer chain, equal to the product of the length of each repeat unit (l) times the number of units) (or mers, n), thus the product nl is the full contour length.

Copolymer: a polymer chain containing more than one monomeric species of different chemical structure.

Creep: cold flow of a polymer under stress.

Critical chain length: the minimum chain length required for entanglement of the polymer chains.

Crystalline polymer: a polymer with ordered structure, such as high-density polyethylene (HDPE) and cellulose. Semicrystalline polymers consist of regions of crystallinity or crystallites dispersed in amorphous regions.

Dipole-dipole interactions: moderate secondary forces between polar groups in different molecules or in different locations in the same molecule.

Elastomer: a polymer, such as polyisoprene, that readily undergoes deformation and exhibits large reversible elongations under applied stress.

End-to-end distance: the shortest distance between the ends of a polymer chain.

Excluded volume: the volume that must be disregarded because only one atom of a chain may occupy any specific space at any specific time.

Flory-Huggins parameter (or χ *parameter*): a quantity obtained by application of the lattice theory to polymer solutions. It describes the thermodynamic goodness of a solvent for a polymer.

Gel permeation chromatography: a type of liquid solution elution chromatography that separates solutions of polydisperse polymers into fractions by means of a sieving action through swollen cross-linked polymer beads of controlled pore sizes.

Glass transition temperature: a characteristic temperature at which glassy amorphous polymers become flexible or rubber-like because of segmental motion. It corresponds to the lowest temperature at which segmental motion of a polymer chain can take place.

HEUR polymers (*Hy*drophobe-modified *E*thoxylated *UR*ethane polymers): a class of rheology modifiers consisting of poly(ethylene oxide) fragments connected by isocyanate units. Aqueous solutions of HEUR polymers exhibit increased viscosity at low shear rate.

Homopolymer: a polymer made up of only one repeating unit, in contrast to a copolymer, which is made up of more than one repeat unit.

Hydrogen bonding: strong secondary force between a hydrogen atom in one molecule and an oxygen, nitrogen, or fluorine atom in another molecule. These forces may also exist between a hydrogen atom in one location and oxygen, nitrogen, or fluorine atoms in another location of the same molecule. Intermolecular hydrogen bonds are responsible for the high strength of fibers, such as keratin and nylon. Helices in some polymers are the result of intramolecular hydrogen bonds.

Impact modifier: a material that improves the resistance of polymers to stress.

Interfacial polymerization: a polymerization in which the reaction takes place at the interface of two immiscible liquids.

Interpenetrating networks: intimate combination of two polymers both in network form, where at least one of the polymers is synthesized or cross-linked in the presence of the other.

Ionomer: a water-insoluble polymer with relatively few electrically charged groups along the chain.

Latex: a stable dispersion in water of polymer particles produced by emulsion polymerization.

Lattice theory: a theory that describes solutions in terms of three-dimensional lattices, where each lattice site is occupied by a segment, either a monomeric unit or a solvent molecule.

Linear polymer: a polymer that consists of a linear chain without extending branches.

Living polymer: a charged polymer chain or macroion, which carries one ionic group, usually at one chain end.

Melt index: a measure of flow, related inversely to melt viscosity, the time for 10 g of a polymer to pass through a standard orifice at a specified time and temperature.

Modulus: the ratio of stress to strain, which is a measure of stiffness of a polymer. A high modulus polymer is stiff and has very low elongation. Some systems, especially solutions of high molecular weight or cross-linked polymers, show ''complex'' behavior under stress. They posses an elastic modulus, G', and a loss modulus, G'', representing the recoverable and irrecoverable strain, respectively.

Molecular weight distribution: a probability curve used to describe the distribution of molecular weights in a polydisperse sample. The number-average molecular weight is the simple arithmetic mean, determined experimentally from colligative properties of polymer solutions. The weight-average molecular weight is the second power average, determined experimentally by light scattering. For polydisperse samples the number-average molecular weight is smaller than the weight-average molecular weight.

Monodisperse: a polymer made up of molecules of one specific molecular weight, such as a protein.

Newtonian fluid: a fluid whose viscosity is proportional to the applied viscosity gradient.

Oligomer: very-low-molecular-weight polymer, usually with a degree of polymerization of 10 or less.

Overlap concentration: the concentration of a polymer solution where individual polymer coils begin to overlap without undergoing chain contraction. This concentration is frequently not very high; thus it is often called the semidilute regime.

Plasticizer: a nonvolatile liquid or solid, which is compatible with a hard plastic and which reduces the glass transition temperature of this polymer, and thus increases the flexibility of hard polymers.

Polydisperse: a polymer consisting of molecules of many different molecular weights, such as most commercial polymers.

Polyelectrolytes: water-soluble polymers with many electrically charged groups per molecule. They form polyions on dissociation, either polyanions, as in the case of dissociated polyacrylic acid, or polycations, as in the case of protonated poly(vinylamine). They may also be polysalts, as in the case of the sodium salt of polyacrylic acid.

Pseudoplastic: a system where the shear rate increases faster than the applied stress; also known as shear-thinning system.

Radius of gyration: the root-mean-square distance of a chain end to the center of gravity of a polymer coil.

Reactivity ratio: the relative reactivity of one monomer compared to another during a polymerization.

Reptation model: a theoretical model to account for the ability of long polymer chains to move through a polymer matrix. In this approach the chain is assumed to be contained in a hypothetical tube that is placed in a three-dimensional network formed by the entangled chains. The contours of the tube are defined by the position of the entanglement points in the network.

Rheopectic liquid: a liquid that exhibits an increase in viscosity as a function of time.

Shear: stress caused by planes sliding by each other, as in greasing or polishing a flat surface.

Solubility parameter: a numerical value, which can be used to predict solubility. It is equal to the square root of the cohesive energy density or heat of vaporization per unit volume.

Step-growth polymerization: a polymerization method, in which the polymer chain grows slowly in a step-like manner. Also known as polycondensation, the process used to prepare polyesters and polyamides, for example.

Stress: force per unit area.

Suspension polymerization: a process in which liquid monomers are polymerized as liquid droplets suspended in water.

Tacticity: a property that describes the steric order of a polymer chain. Polymers with a unique way of coupling the monomer units are called isotactic. If the coupling of monomer units varies, but in a regular way, the polymers are called syndiotactic. Atactic polymers are polymers with an irregular steric structure. Polystyrene, for example, can adopt all types of tacticities, depending on the process of synthesis.

Theta solvent: a solvent in which a polymer exists as a statistical coil. Under these conditions the χ parameter takes a value of 0.5.

Thixotropic liquid: a liquid that exhibits a decrease in viscosity as a function of time.

Viscoelastic: having the properties of a liquid and a solid.

2

Polymer Adsorption: Fundamentals

Timothy M. Obey
University of Bristol, Bristol, England

Peter C. Griffiths
Cardiff University, Cardiff, Wales

I. GENERAL FEATURES OF POLYMER ADSORPTION

The adsorption of a polymer from solution onto a surface is usually described in terms of an adsorption isotherm. This relates the amount of polymer at the particle surface (mg/m^2) with the amount of polymer in solution (ppm or mg/L). In contrast with the Langmuir-type low-affinity isotherms displayed by small molecules, polymers tend to show high-affinity isotherms of the type shown in Figure 1.

Initially all the polymer molecules are adsorbed from solution (point A). As the concentration of polymer is further increased, osmotic forces between neighboring molecules cause the polymer chains to start to repel each other. An equilibrium between the attraction of the surface for more polymer and the repulsive lateral osmotic forces between neighboring polymer segments results in the adsorption of an approximately constant amount of polymer at the surface and observation of the so-called *pseudo-plateau*.

Small molecules usually reach equilibrium adsorption levels relatively quickly, but for polymer molecules steady states may take much longer to achieve. Two factors contribute to this: first, polymer molecules have much lower diffusion coefficients compared to small molecules, and second, polymer molecules require a finite time to rearrange from their solution conformation to their adsorbed conformation. The first effect is rate determining at low concentration and the second is rate determining at high concentration. These effects are further complicated if the polymers are polydisperse since the more rapidly diffusing small molecules will gradually be replaced at the surface by the slower-diffusing large molecules (1).

The size of the polymer molecule makes it extremely unlikely that all the segments of the macromolecule will be in contact with the surface at any one time, and as a result the polymer adopts a conformation consisting of *tails*, *loops*, and *trains*, shown schematically in Figure 2.

Multipoint attachment of the molecule to the surface makes it difficult for all the

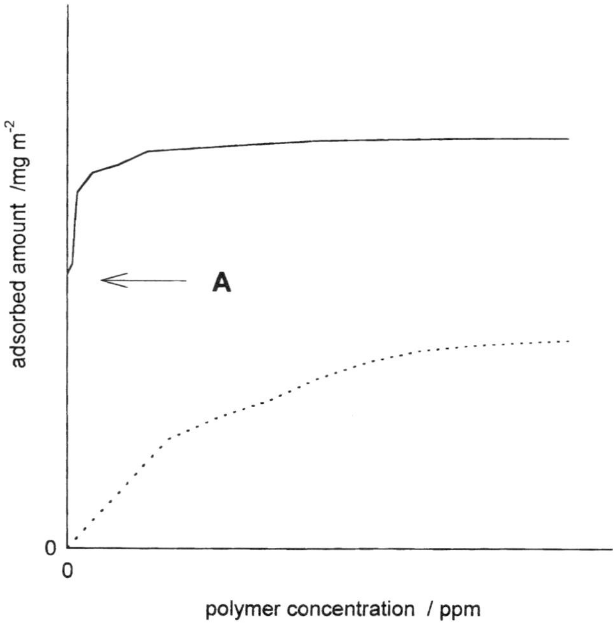

Figure 1 A high-affinity polymer adsorption isotherm, which relates the amount of polymer at the particle surface to the amount of polymer in solution (solid line) and a low-affinity Langmuir-type isotherm (broken line).

segments to desorb simultaneously. Polymer adsorption can, thus, be thought of as an essentially irreversible phenomenon even though each of the individual polymer segments may be reversibly adsorbed.

II. DRIVING FORCE FOR ADSORPTION

For any spontaneous process to occur chemical thermodynamics tells us that there must be a lowering of the free energy, ΔG, of the system. The driving force for polymer adsorption is thus the competition between the net energy change on adsorption (enthalpy of adsorption), the loss of conformational entropy of the adsorbed polymer, and the gain in entropy of solvent molecules released from the surface and polymer upon adsorption.

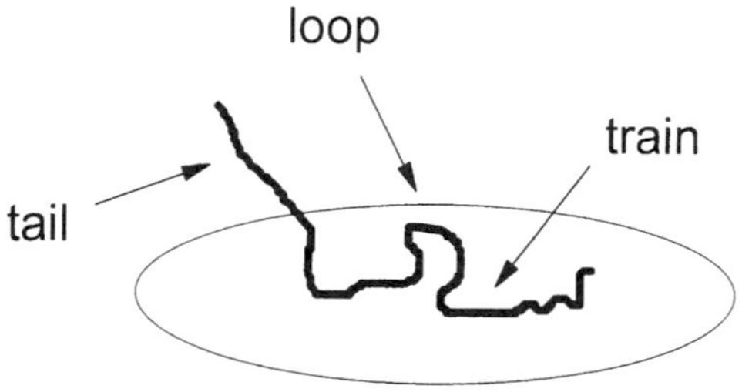

Figure 2 The *tails, loops, and trains* representation of the conformation of a polymer adsorbed at a surface.

These enthalpic and entropic segment-surface, solvent-surface, and segment-solvent interactions are generally described in terms of the exchange free energies, χ and χ_s (essentially the quality of the solvent and the affinity of the surface for the polymer, respectively). For adsorption to occur, the attractive energy must be larger than the loss in entropy. This leads to the idea of a critical adsorption energy, χ_{sc}, below which no adsorption will occur. The nature of the attractive energy is essentially a combination of electrostatic and van der Waals forces, though solvent effects also play an important role in the overall adsorption process.

III. COLLOIDAL FORCES

The forces of attraction and repulsion that control the adsorption process also determine the stability of colloidal dispersions. The stability of any colloidal dispersion consisting of particles, polymer molecules, or mixtures of particles and polymer molecules dispersed in a medium is determined by the balance between the attractive van der Waals forces and repulsive (or attractive) electrostatic forces.

A. van der Waals Forces

For the idealized case of spherical particles of radius a in a vacuum, separated by a distance h, the van der Waals force (V_A) at small interparticle separations (where h is of the order of 10 nm) is

$$V_A = -Aa/12h \quad (1)$$

A is the Hamaker constant (2). In real colloidal systems the particles are suspended in a medium or "solvent," in which case an "effective" Hamaker constant has to be used to describe the force operating between the particles. When two particles 1 and 2 separated by a solvent 3 are at large distances from one another, the interactions are particle-solvent interactions A_{13} and A_{23}. When the particles approach one another, particle-solvent *and* particle-particle interactions must now be considered. The effective Hamaker constant becomes

$$A_{132} = A_{12} + A_{33} - A_{13} - A_{23} \quad (2)$$

which can be simplified to

$$A_{132} = (\sqrt{A_{11}} - \sqrt{A_{33}})(\sqrt{A_{22}} - \sqrt{A_{33}}) \quad (3)$$

Equation 3 can be applied either to two particles composed of different materials, for instance, a polystyrene latex particle and a solvated polymer molecule, say poly(ethylene oxide), or to two particles composed of the same material, in which case Eq. 3 becomes

$$A_{131} = (\sqrt{A_{11}} - \sqrt{A_{33}})^2 \quad (4)$$

Hamaker constants tend to vary between 10^{-20} J and 10^{-19} J. So, for example, for polystyrene latex particles in water where the Hamaker constants are $A = 6.5 \times 10^{-20}$ J and $A = 3.7 \times 10^{-20}$ J, respectively, the effective Hamaker is 3.9×10^{-21} J.

When both A_{11} and A_{22} are either greater or less than A_{33}, the interparticle interaction A_{132} is predicted to be positive and, therefore, the van der Waals force attractive. If, however, A_{33} has an intermediate value between A_{11} and A_{22}, then A_{132} is negative and the van der Waals force is predicted to be repulsive. For particles of the same material A_{131} is always positive.

B. Electrostatic Forces

Electrostatic forces arise from the presence of charged groups on the particle surface or polymer molecule. For particles these may arise as a result of surface ionization (e.g., a silica sol), unequal dissolution of ions of which the crystalline particles are composed (e.g., a AgI sol), or may be the result of ionic species produced by the initiator used in the preparation of the particle dispersion (e.g., polystyrene latex). For polymers the electrostatic charge is due to ionization of (typically) carboxyl, sulfonate, or amino groups. Ionization of these groups may or may not be pH dependent.

Theories describing the distribution of ions near charged surfaces (Gouy-Chapman) or other ions (Debye-Hückel) assume a Boltzmann distribution of ions and, hence, a largely exponential decrease in electrical potential with increasing distance from the charge. The decay constant of this exponential decrease is the Debye-Hückel screening length (or thickness of the double layer), $1/\kappa$. For an aqueous solution of a 1:1 electrolyte the value of κ is given by

$$\kappa = 3.288\sqrt{I}\ \text{nm}^{-1} \tag{5}$$

where I is the ionic strength of the electrolyte.

For two differently sized spheres of radii a_1 and a_2 the repulsive interaction (V_R) due to a small overlap of the potentials generated by their surface charges is given by

$$V_R = \frac{64\pi\varepsilon a_1 a_2 k^2 T^2 \gamma_1 \gamma_2}{(a_1 + a_2)e^2 z^2} \exp(-\kappa h) \tag{6}$$

For equal spheres this reduces to

$$V_R = \frac{32\pi\varepsilon a k^2 T^2 \gamma^2}{e^2 z^2} \exp(-\kappa h) \tag{7}$$

where z is the counterion valency, e is the electronic charge, ε is the dielectric constant of the solvent, and

$$\gamma = \frac{\exp(ze\psi_d/2kT) - 1}{\exp(ze\psi_d/2kT) + 1} \tag{8}$$

ψ_d is the surface potential (strictly the Stern potential) (3). Using the Debye-Hückel approximation ($ze\psi/kT \ll 1$ or $z\psi \ll 25$ mV), Eq. 7 simplifies to

$$V_R = 2\pi\varepsilon a \psi_d^2 \exp(-\kappa h) \tag{9}$$

It can be seen then that not only does V_R decrease exponentially with distance, but it is also decreased by a rise in the solution electrolyte concentration (increase in κ). For a 10^{-3} mol/dm^3 solution of a 1 : 1 electrolyte the thickness of the double layer, $1/\kappa$, is approximately 10 nm, but if the electrolyte concentration increases to 10^{-1} mol/dm^3, then $1/\kappa$ falls to 1 nm.

IV. DLVO THEORY

The combination of the two energies of interaction, i.e., van der Waals and electrostatic, to produce an overall energy of interaction is commonly known as the DLVO theory (4,5). Figure 3 shows potential energy curves for such a combination. As V_R is lowered, by either lowering the surface potential or increasing the electrolyte concentration, the repulsive energy barrier is also lowered. If the energy barrier is large compared with the thermal energy (kT) of the colloidal dispersion, then the system will be stable; if not, flocculation will occur.

V. DISPERSION STABILITY

The presence of adsorbed polymer at the particle surface may modify these repulsive energy barriers, and hence affect the stability of the dispersion. For instance, the adsorbed layer may cause a significant lowering of the Hamaker constant and thus weaken the van der Waals attractive forces. If, however, the polymer is charged (i.e., is a polyelectrolyte), then the electrical double-layer forces may be enhanced if the charge is of the same sign or diminished if it is of opposite sign to the surface charge group.

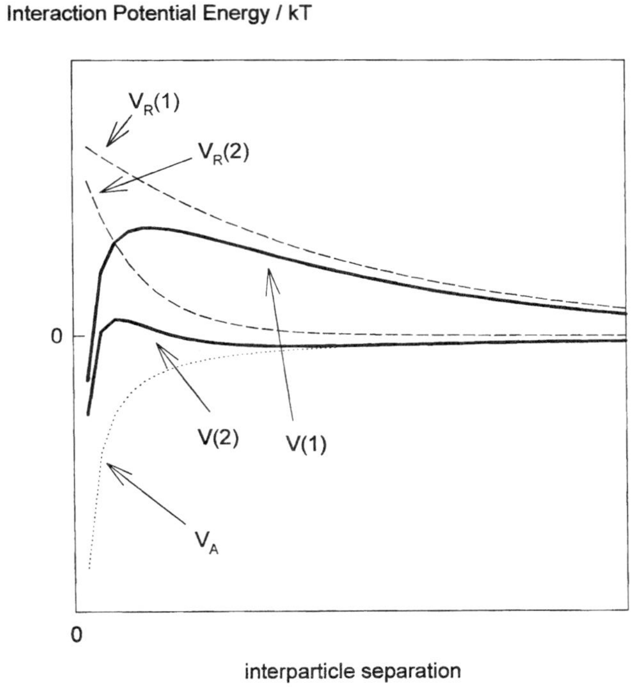

Figure 3 Theoretical DLVO potential energy curves. The dotted line, V_A, corresponds to a van der Waals attraction while the dashed lines, V_R, correspond to the electrostatic repulsion at a low electrolyte concentration, $V_R(1)$, and a high electrolyte concentration, $V_R(2)$. The solid lines are the total interaction curves.

A. Steric Stabilization

The basis for the so-called *steric* interaction is the observation that under good solvency conditions two polymer molecules of the same material repel each other. The steric interaction is, essentially, a combination of three effects.

1. The free energy change on adsorption of polymer onto a particle surface is negative. If collision between two polymer-coated particle results in desorption of polymer, then as ΔG for desorption is positive stability will be enhanced.
2. If the polymer layers become compressed on collision, then there will be a loss of configurational entropy and, hence, an increase in free energy.
3. When the adsorbed layers interpenetrate one another, there is a local increase in the polymer concentration. This leads to a repulsive osmotic force between the particles.

For sterically stabilized systems the total interaction energy now becomes

$$V = V_A + V_R + V_S \tag{10}$$

where V_S is the steric repulsion term. Figure 4 shows a schematic representation of the total interaction energy.

The basic equation for the steric interaction is given by Eq. 11 (6).

$$V_S = 2\pi k_B T a \Gamma^2 N_A [v_p^2/V_s^*] \times [0.5 - \chi][1 - h/2\delta_h]^2 + V_{\text{elastic}} \tag{11}$$

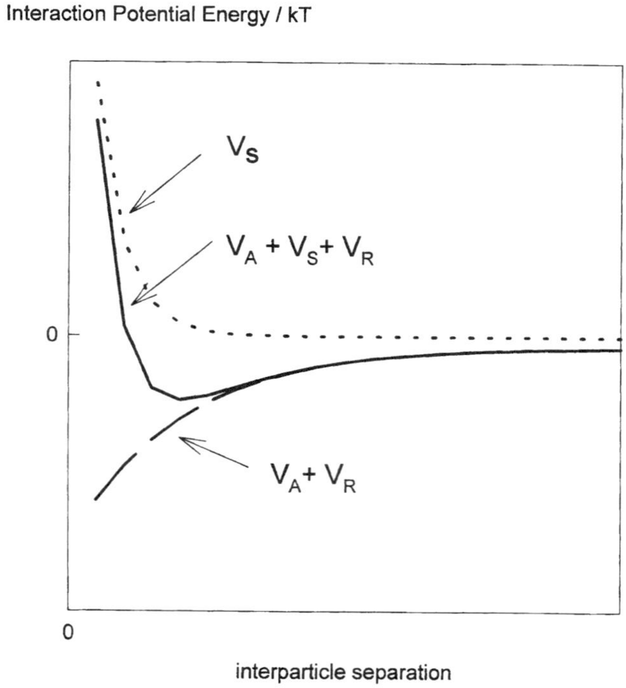

Figure 4 The total potential energy curve for a sterically stabilized system (solid line) comprising a steric interaction (dotted line) and a van der Waals/electrostatic term (dashed line).

where Γ is the amount of polymer adsorbed at the particle surface, v_p is the specific partial volume of the polymer, and V_s^* is the molar volume of the solvent. δ_h is the hydrodynamic thickness of the adsorbed polymer layer. V_{elastic} is the elastic contribution that comes about due to reconformation of the polymer chains on the two particle surfaces.

Two very distinct cases emerge from this equation depending on the value of the Flory-Huggins parameter χ. In a good solvent χ is less than 0.5 and the polymer chains repel each other, which enhances the stability of the system. When χ is greater than 0.5, the chains attract one another, enhancing flocculation. For water-soluble polymers added salt can also affect the value of χ (as well as, of course, the range of the electrostatic forces) and in many cases solvency of the polymer chains decreases with added salt. The value of χ is affected by temperature. If the temperature of the particle dispersion exceeds that of the θ-temperature (i.e., when $\chi = 0.5$) of the stabilizing polymer, the dispersion will become unstable (7). This critical flocculation temperature is also dependent on pressure (8).

From Eq. 11 several conditions for effective steric stabilization can be identified.

1. A high adsorbed amount of polymer
2. Good solvency conditions
3. A highly extended adsorbed polymer layer
4. Particle size $\gg$ radius of gyration of the polymer

The practical realization of these conditions can be met by using a variety of polymeric stabilizers. In practice steric stabilizers are usually block copolymers with lyophobic ''anchor'' groups, to provide firm attachment to the surface, and highly lyophilic ''bouy'' groups, to provide the requisite thick steric barrier (see Section VI.B).

B. Bridging Flocculation

The vast majority of polymeric flocculants are high-molecular-weight polyelectrolytes, which may be cationic or anionic. The charge densities of polyelectrolytes with weakly acidic or basic groups may be pH dependent. Some, with strongly ionized groups such as poly(styrene sulfonate), have charge densities independent of pH. Flocculation is brought about by the adsorption of a single polymer chain on more than one particle, i.e., by a bridging mechanism (9). Bridging flocculation occurs over a narrow range (of the order of several parts per million) of concentrations. The floc structures, which tend to be rather loose, sediment rapidly and are easily removed from solution by filtration. Particles and flocculants usually have opposite charges, though there is evidence of Ca^{2+} counterions facilitating the flocculation of negatively charged particles by anionic polymers. The Ca^{2+} counterions are thought to act as ''bridges'' to the polymer ''bridges.''

C. Charge Neutralization

When the polymeric flocculant and particle have opposite charges, flocculation may be brought about by neutralization of the particle surface charge. Bridging may still be operative in such a system. When overall neutralization of the charge has been achieved, there may still be patches of charge, both positive and negative, on the particle surface. These patches of charge may orient themselves in such a way as to promote aggregation of the particle. This process is known as ''charge patch flocculation'' (10).

D. Depletion Flocculation

In dispersions of particles and nonadsorbing polymer, flocculation may be induced at certain concentrations (11). At low concentrations the presence of free polymer has no effect on the dispersion stability, but as the concentration is raised flocculation occurs. As two particles approach each other, at separations corresponding to twice the radius of gyration of the polymer, polymer becomes excluded from the volume of solution between the particles. The particle separation is such that polymer is prevented from entering the interparticle space. The gap can now be considered as an osmotic membrane, permeable only to solvent molecules. The bulk solution thus exerts a compressive osmotic pressure and solvent drains from the space between the particles causing the particles to flocculate.

VI. POLYMER ADSORPTION

A. Homopolymer Adsorption

The most obvious place to start in choosing a stabilizer polymer is to use a homopolymer. Two restrictions apply here. First, the polymer must be strongly attached to the particle surface, and second, it must form a highly extended, dense layer. For a homopolymer these two requirements are working against one another. Figure 5 shows adsorption isotherms for poly(ethylene oxide) adsorbed on polystyrene latex. Typically, for physically adsorbed homopolymers the maximum level of adsorption, Γ_{max}, lies in the region between 0.3 and 3 mg/m^2.

From the adsorbed amount it is straightforward to calculate the adsorbed area per molecule. Multilayer adsorption is evident only if the polymer is close to phase separation

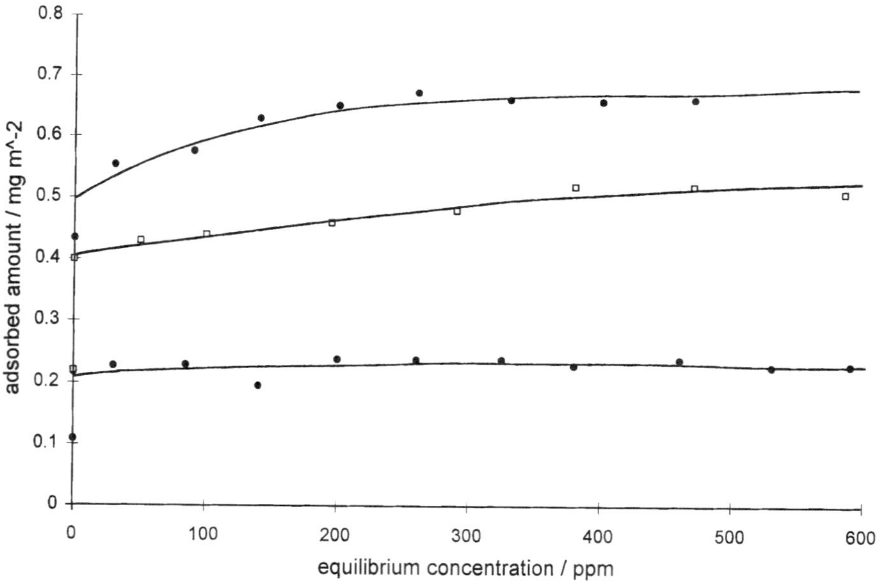

Figure 5 Adsorption isotherms for poly(ethylene oxide) adsorbed onto poly(styrene) latex. Molecular weights in order of decreasing maximum adsorbed amounts are: 930K, 114K, and 10.3K. (J. A. Shar, unpublished results.)

in the bulk solution, in which case the surface layer is acting as a nucleating center. Polydispersity can dramatically affect the shape of the isotherm, depending on the amount of surface area available. This is because high-molecular-weight chains adsorb preferentially, at least at low equilibrium concentrations.

If adsorption isotherms are obtained for a range of molecular weights, the basic relationship between Γ_{max} and molecular weight can be found. For poor solvents Γ_{max} varies as the logarithm of molecular weight, whereas in a good solvent the dependence is much weaker.

The layer thickness, the other important parameter when considering steric effects, can be obtained by photon correlation spectroscopy (see Section IX.D) and typical data for the same polymer system are shown in Figure 6. The hydrodynamic thickness of the adsorbed layer, δ_h, can be easily measured, but is difficult to calculate theoretically. Both the molecular weight and coverage dependence are important factors in designing effective steric stabilizers. At low coverages the thickness of the adsorbed layer is independent of chain length, but at a critical value extended tail segments are formed preferentially with increasing N, the number of segments. This strongly suggests δ_h is determined by the volume fraction of segments at the periphery of the adsorbed layer.

The molecular weight dependence of δ_h at full coverage has been determined from the data shown in Figure 6 and also theoretically. It has been found that $\delta_h \approx N^{0.8}$, though lower values have also been reported.

B. Copolymer Adsorption

Copolymer adsorption is more complex as the intimate structure of the chain determines the extent of adsorption. Random copolymers adsorb in an intermediate way to that of

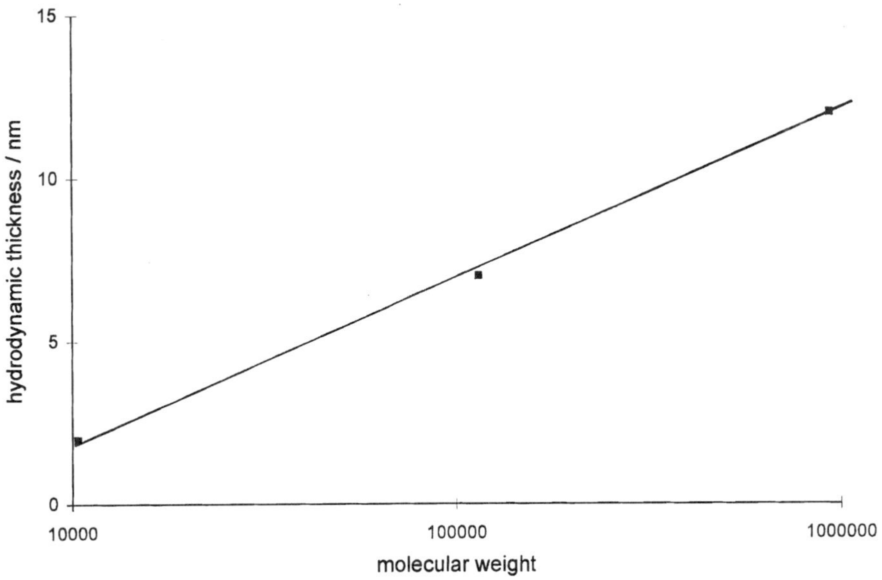

Figure 6 Hydrodynamic thicknesses for poly(ethylene oxide) adsorbed onto poly(styrene) latex measured at the plateaux of the adsorption isotherm, for the same systems in Figure 5. (J. A. Shar, unpublished results.)

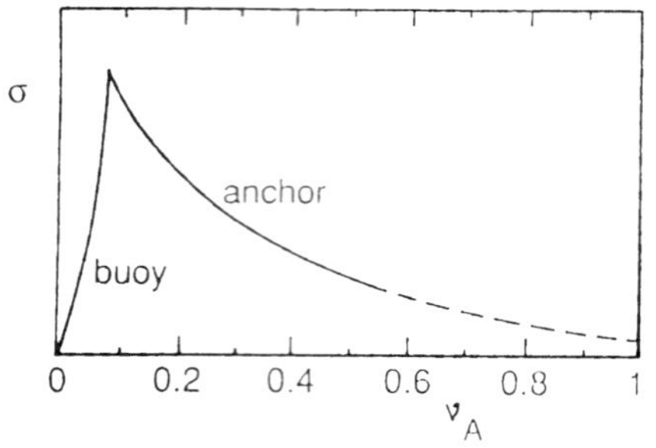

Figure 7 Predictions of Scheutjens and Fleer theory for the adsorption of diblock copolymers; surface density σ versus fraction of anchor segment ν_A. (Reproduced with permission from Ref. 16.)

their corresponding homopolymers, whereas block copolymers retain the adsorption preference of the individual blocks. The lyophilic block, the buoy, extends away from the particle surface into bulk solution, while the lyophobic anchor block provides firm attachment to the surface.

Figures 7 and 8 show the theoretical adsorption and hydrodynamic layer thickness behavior of an AB block copolymer, but as can be seen from these figures, they depend on the anchor/buoy composition. In general, the adsorbed amounts are higher than is the case for homopolymers and the adsorbed layer more extended and more dense. Maximum levels of adsorption are achieved when around 10% of the segments are anchors. In principle, then, these materials are better steric stabilizers than homopolymers.

Chain architecture also plays a role in determining the adsorption characteristics of copolymers. For instance, if we consider triblock ABA-type copolymers the relative positions of the anchor and buoy blocks become important. When there are two buoy blocks and a central anchor block, the copolymers show diblock AB-type behavior (see Fig. 9 and 10). If, however, there are two anchor blocks and a central buoy block, surface precipitation of the polymer molecule at the particle surface is generally observed. This precipitation (or multilayer formation) process is due to strong interaction between the anchor blocks themselves and manifests itself in the form of an ever-increasing adsorption isotherm (i.e., there is no plateau) of the type shown in Figure 11. When compared with

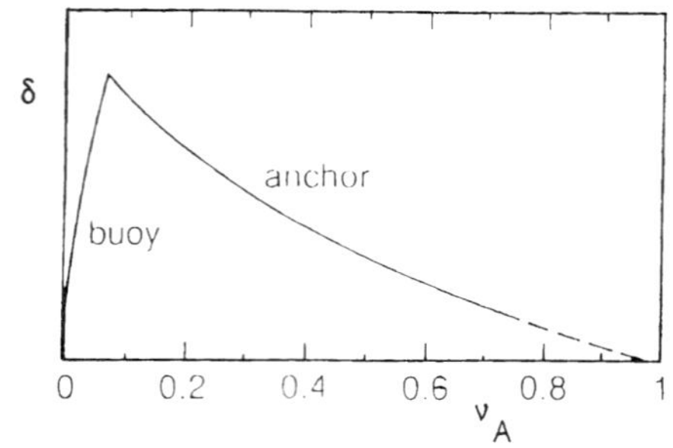

Figure 8 Predictions of Scheutjens and Fleer theory for the adsorption of diblock copolymers; layer thickness δ versus fraction of anchor segment ν_A. (Reproduced with permission from Ref. 16.)

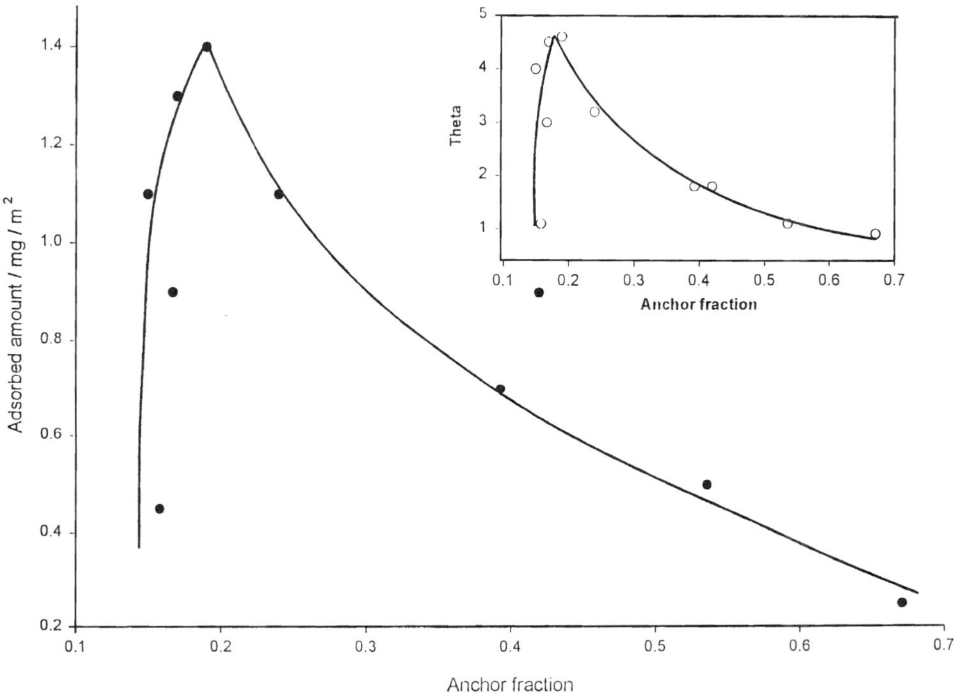

Figure 9 Adsorbed amount versus fraction of anchor segment ν_A for poly(ethylene oxide)-poly(propylene oxide)-poly(ethylene oxide) ABA triblock copolymers adsorbed onto poly(styrene latex). Inset shows the mean-field calculations of surface coverage versus fraction of anchor segment ν_A obtained using Scheutjens and Fleer theory. (J. A. Shar, T. Obey, and T. Cosgrove: Colloids and Surfaces. In press.)

ABA triblock copolymers that have two buoy blocks, these molecules have higher adsorbed amounts and layer thickness for a given molecular weight.

C. Polyelectrolyte Adsorption

The presence of charge groups along the polymer backbone can alter the adsorption process in a number of ways. If the charge groups are of the same sign as that of the particle surface, then the result is generally nonadsorption. If, however, the charge groups are of the opposite sign, then adsorption can occur through electrostatic attraction between the adsorbing particle and the polyelectrolyte. The strong attractive interaction has two consequences: the adsorbed configuration will tend to be rather flat and the adsorbed amount will be independent of molecular weight.

The adsorption process is affected by the presence of any background electrolyte in solution. An increase in ionic strength will shield both surface and polyelectrolyte charges with the consequence that the surface-polymer interaction will decrease. However, and more importantly, there will also be a decrease in the lateral interactions between segments in the adsorbed layer. This allows the adoption of a more compact adsorbed conformation with the result that the adsorbed amount will increase. In general, the adsorbed amount almost always increases with increasing ionic strength.

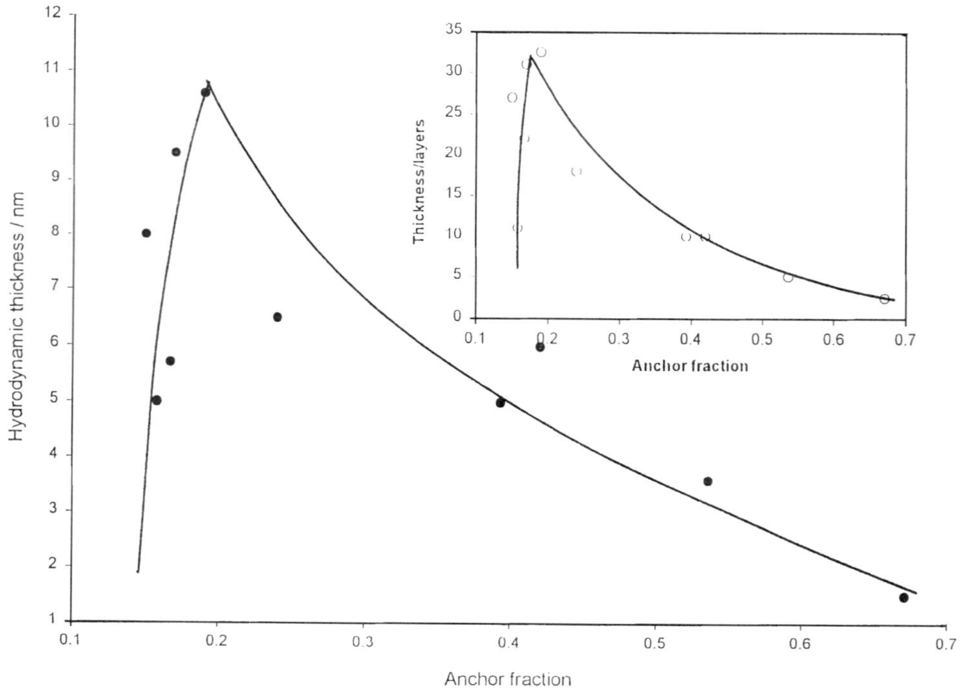

Figure 10 Hydrodynamic thickness versus fraction of anchor segment ν_A for poly(ethylene oxide)-poly(propylene oxide)-poly(ethylene oxide) ABA triblock copolymers adsorbed onto poly(styrene latex). Inset shows the mean-field calculations of thickness versus fraction of anchor segment ν_A obtained using Scheutjens and Fleer theory. (J. A. Shar, T. Obey, and T. Cosgrove: Colloids and Surfaces. In press.)

VII. KINETICS

The kinetics of polymer adsorption is a highly complex process. Several distinct processes occur simultaneously each with a characteristic time scale. Generally, it is difficult to separate these processes except under certain limiting conditions:

1. The first process is the mass transport of the polymer to the surface, which may be via either diffusion or convection.
2. Having reached the surface, the polymer must then attach itself to a surface site, which depends on any local activation energy barrier.
3. The polymer molecule is undergoing large-scale rearrangements as it changes from its solution conformation to a "tail-loop-train" conformation.

Once the polymer solution has been brought into contact with the surface, the adsorbed amount increases with time. This increase is rapid in the beginning but subsequently slows as the surface becomes saturated. The initial rate of adsorption is sensitive to the bulk solution polymer concentration and molecular weight as well as the solution viscosity. Nevertheless, all the polymer molecules arriving at the surface tend to adsorb

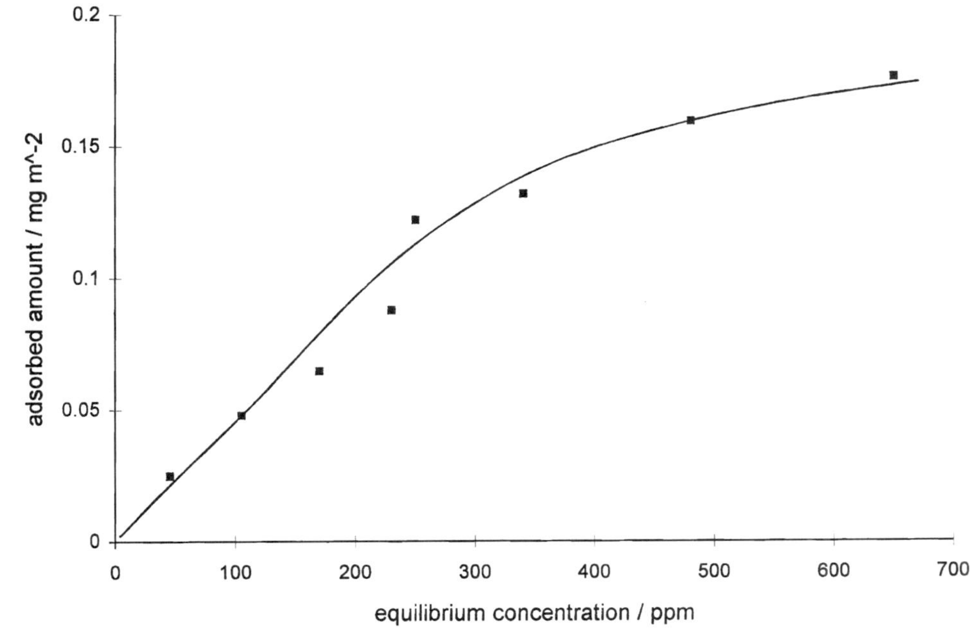

Figure 11 Adsorption isotherm for poly(propylene oxide)-poly(ethylene oxide)-poly(propylene oxide) ABA triblock copolymers adsorbed onto poly(styrene latex), molecular weight 3250 g/mol with 12 mol% ethylene oxide. (J. A. Shar, unpublished results.)

immediately. The concentration of unadsorbed polymer around the periphery of the forming layer—the *surface polymer solution*—is zero, and therefore, the concentration of polymer in the interfacial region is significantly greater than the bulk polymer solution concentration. Mass transport is found to dominate the kinetics of adsorption until 75% of full surface coverage.

At higher surface coverages, the rate of adsorption decreases since the polymer molecules arriving at the surface cannot immediately adsorb. Over time an equilibrium is set up between this interfacial concentration of polymer and the concentration of polymer in the bulk. Given that the adsorption isotherm is of the high-affinity type, no significant change in the adsorbed amount is expected, even over decades of polymer concentration. If the surface polymer solution concentration increases toward that of the bulk solution, the rate of adsorption decreases because the driving force for adsorption (the difference in concentration between the surface and bulk solutions) decreases.

Adsorption processes tend to be very rapid (an equilibrated polymer layer can form within several 1000 sec) but desorption is a much slower process. Even though there is rapid equilibration of polymer within the interfacial region, fully desorbing a polymer layer with pure solvent would take several hundreds of years!

Once the polymer has adsorbed onto the surface, it may subsequently chemically react with the surface. The rate of reaction can often be the limiting step in the overall adsorption kinetics.

VIII. LIQUID/LIQUID INTERFACES

The adsorption of polymers at the liquid/liquid interface is somewhat different from that at the solid/liquid interface as the polymer can penetrate both phases. χ determines the adsorption behavior of polymers at liquid/liquid interfaces. The presence of the polymer at the interface between the two immiscible liquids lowers the surface tension. Determination of the adsorption isotherm (see Section IX.B) is more straightforward compared to particulate dispersions as surface tension measurements, interpreted using the Gibbs equation, can be used to give accurate adsorbed amounts.

The driving force for adsorption for a homopolymer is the ability of the polymer to screen the unfavorable interactions between the immiscible solvents. The polymer layer thickness is generally equivalent to its solution radius of gyration and is equivalent to one or two monolayers. If the polymer has a very different solubility in the two phases, i.e., it is much more soluble in one phase compared with the other, the volume fraction profile attains a high plateau value in the phase in which the polymer is more soluble but falls off monotonically as the interface region is approached and traversed.

Random AB copolymer with different solvencies for the two segments will assemble in such a way as to minimize the unfavorable A segment/solvent interactions while maximizing favorable B segment/solvent interactions. The chain connectivity and short block sizes of the random copolymer mean that it cannot wander too far from the interface as this would entail an increase in the number of unfavorable segment/solvent interactions. Block copolymers are able to form a much thicker and more extended layer because of the increased size of the blocks and the associated greater penetration into the preferred solvent.

IX. EXPERIMENTAL APPROACHES TO THE STUDY OF POLYMER ADSORPTION

A. General Considerations

A multitude of experimental techniques are commonly used to study adsorbed polymer layers. Often, each technique is sensitive only to a particular facet of the adsorbed polymer layer, and thus, a detailed understanding of the structure of the polymer layer can often only be gained through a combination of techniques. Generally, the more information one particular technique provides, the more complex and involved that technique will be.

In any study of polymer adsorption three basic questions need to be answered:

1. What are the thermodynamic aspects of the adsorption process; i.e., what is the adsorbed amount per unit area and what is the enthalpy of adsorption?
2. What conformation does the polymer adopt at the surface; i.e., what is the thickness of the adsorbed layer and how does the distribution of segments normal to the surface vary?
3. What are the dynamic properties of the system; i.e., how long does it take for the polymer to diffuse to the surface and rearrange itself at the surface, and how much time to individual segments spend in contact with the surface?

When trying to answer these questions, it is desirable that a number of criteria be satisfied:

1. The polymers should be as well characterized and as monodisperse as possible.
2. Adsorbents should have a well-defined geometry and surface structure (planes or spheres are usually preferred). It is now possible to prepare a wide range of polymer lattices and inorganic particles for use as model surfaces. Any surface heterogeneity should be well characterized; e.g., the number density and type of any surface charge should be known.
3. Aggregation of disperse particle surfaces should be avoided at all times. At low surface coverages and where there is insufficient electrostatic or steric repulsion to overcome the van der Waals attraction this may be difficult.
4. To avoid variations in local polymer concentration when mixing the particle dispersion and the polymer solution, the particles should be added to the polymer.

B. The Adsorbed Amount, Γ

One of the simplest experiments is to establish how much polymer is adsorbed onto the surface. This is known as the *adsorbed amount* and is determined from the *adsorption isotherm* (see Fig. 1). The adsorption isotherm relates the amount of polymer adsorbed at an interface to its equilibrium solution concentration. Determination of the adsorbed amount almost always involves measurement of the polymer concentration in solution before and after equilibration with a dispersion of known surface area. This usually requires separation of the dispersion particles from the supernatant by centrifugation. Separation of the bound and free polymer by dialysis can also be used but it is difficult to determine the amount of polymer that may be adsorbed onto the dialysis membrane. As these techniques require a knowledge of the amount of polymer removed from solution, they are known as *depletion* methods.

The amount adsorbed per unit area, Γ, may be calculated from

$$\Gamma = \frac{(C_{\text{initial}} - C_{\text{equilibrium}})V}{A_s} \tag{12}$$

where V is the total volume of solution, A_s is the surface area of the dispersion, and C_{initial} and $C_{\text{equilibrium}}$ are the initial and equilibrium concentrations of polymer, respectively.

Over the years, various analytical methods have been developed for detecting small amounts of polymer in solution. These can be divided into two broad areas:

1. Complexation of the polymer in the supernatant with another chemical species (e.g., PEO and phosphomolybdic acid or PVA and boric acid/potassium iodide) and analysis of the amount of complex formed (usually by measuring the turbidity of the resultant solution).
2. Direct analysis of the polymer solution, e.g., by ultraviolet, infrared (IR), or fluorescence spectroscopy.

An alternative method of analysis is to monitor the increase in the weight of the dried particles and equate the increase to the amount of polymer adsorbed on the particle surface. Since typical adsorbed amounts are of the order of a few mg/m^2, the accuracy of these *gravimetric* methods can be questionable.

Certain spectroscopic techniques can be used *directly* on the dispersion, without the need to remove the particles, if the adsorbed and nonadsorbed polymer show different characteristic signals in the electromagnetic spectrum. *High-resolution* nuclear magnetic resonance (NMR) utilizes the fact that adsorbed polymer segments are in a different chemical environment than the free polymer molecules, and that the chemical shift of functional groups within the polymer chain are different in these two environments. This spectroscopic approach has commonly been used to determine isotherms of surfactants bound to polymer chains and can be used to determine conventional adsorption isotherms of polymer on particulate surfaces (12). However, the resolution is often somewhat low for polymer-particle systems.

C. The Enthalpy of Adsorption, ΔH_{ads}

The enthalpy of adsorption can be obtained from a study of the temperature dependence of the adsorption isotherm. A plot of the equilibrium concentration of polymer in solution against the reciprocal of absolute temperature at a constant adsorbed amount yields ΔH_{ads}.

D. The Thickness of the Adsorbed Layer, δ

The second most common parameter used to characterize the polymer layer is its *thickness*. The layer thickness is the principal factor in defining the effectiveness of the polymer as a steric stabilizer. The thickness of the adsorbed layer is usually defined as the distance of the plane of shear from the particle surface. This distance is generally referred to as the *hydrodynamic thickness*, δ_h, and is obtained from several different techniques such as measurement of the diffusion coefficient, sedimentation coefficient, or electrophoretic mobility of the particles with and without the presence of the adsorbed polymer layer.

The thickness of the layer may also be defined as a derived parameter from the volume fraction profile $\phi(z)$ of the adsorbed polymer layer the most common feature of which is the second moment or *root-mean-square thickness* of the layer:

$$\delta_2^2 = \frac{\int_0^\infty \varphi^a(z) z^2 dz}{\int_0^\infty \varphi^a(z) dz} \tag{13}$$

The most commonly used technique for determining δ_h is *photon correlation spectroscopy* (PCS) [also known as *quasi-elastic light scattering* (QELS)]. PCS has become one of the standard tools of the trade for the colloid chemist. In this technique concentration fluctuations arising from the diffusive motion of the dispersion particles give rise to fluctuations in the dielectric constant of the medium are monitored photometrically. These fluctuations decay exponentially with a time constant related to the *diffusion coefficient*, D_s, of the scatterer, which can in turn be related to its *hydrodynamic radius* through the Stokes-Einstein equation:

$$D_s = \frac{kT}{6\pi\eta a} \tag{14}$$

where η is the solvent viscosity and a is the particle radius. A value for the hydrodynamic thickness of a polymer layer can be obtained by measuring the apparent increase in size of the particle upon adsorption of the polymer. Typically, δ_h is twice the solution *radius of gyration* of the free polymer. Figure 12 shows a typical layout of a PCS machine.

The thickness of the adsorbed polymer layer may also be calculated from electrophoretic mobility measurements by calculating the zeta-potential at the plane of shear of the particle. This potential corresponds to the potential at the periphery of the adsorbed layer. By also measuring the zeta-potential of the bare particle and assuming a value of 4 Å for the Stern layer, use of Eq. 15 allows the calculation of δ_e, the electrokinetic thickness of the adsorbed layer (13).

$$\kappa(\delta_e - 0.4) = \ln\left[\frac{(\exp(ze\zeta/2kT) + 1)(\exp(ze\zeta_0/2kT) - 1)}{(\exp(ze\zeta/2kT) - 1)(\exp(ze\zeta_0/2kT) + 1)}\right] \tag{15}$$

where ζ and ζ_0 are the zeta potentials of the coated and bare particles, respectively. The electrophoretic determination of δ_e relies upon the assumptions that the presence of the polymer layer does not affect the surface charge density of the particle, the specific adsorption of ions in the Stern layer, or the charge distribution in the diffuse part of the double layer.

Surface force measurements are another method for measuring the thickness of polymer layers. The surface force apparatus consists of two flat surfaces onto which the polymer is adsorbed. One of these surfaces is directly connected to a piezoelectric crystal, the other to a motor via a double cantilever spring. Optically transparent mica surfaces are used as they can be cleaved easily to yield microscopically flat surfaces (~0.2 nm). Light is shone onto the bottom of one of the two surfaces that has been silvered on the back face. Constructive interference fringes are observed as the separation of the surfaces is varied. The absolute separation of the mica surfaces can be obtained once the fringe pattern has been calibrated. The force, on the other hand, is determined from deflections in the cantilever of known spring constant. A crossed cylinder geometry is used since this is

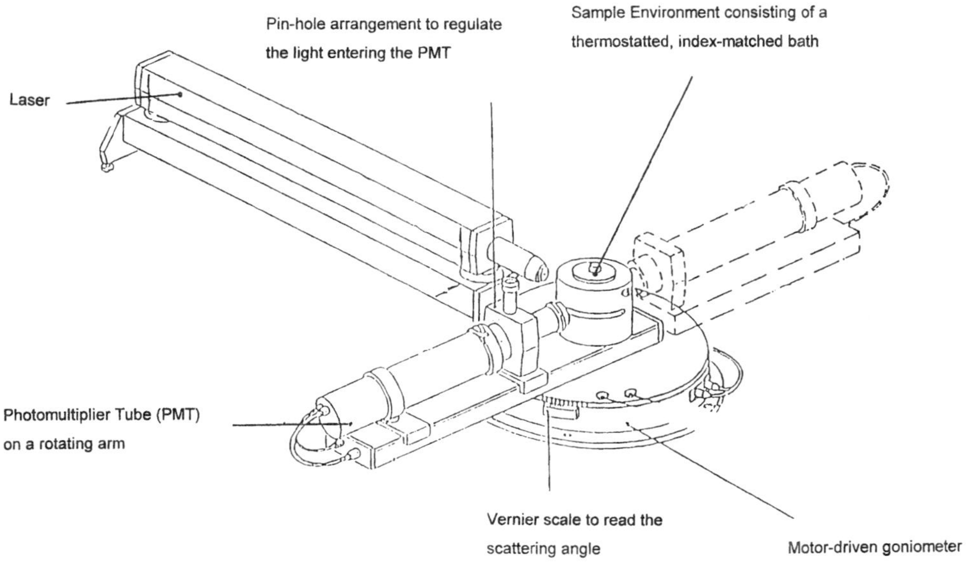

Figure 12 A typical photon correlation spectrometer.

experimentally facile. Furthermore, this geometry allows the use of the Deryagin approximation, which relates the measured force to the free energy of interaction. When the two polymer-bearing surfaces overlap, there is a change in the force (often a repulsion), which allows the layer thickness to be determined.

E. The Bound Fraction, $\langle p \rangle$

Several methods can be used to determine the fraction of segments, $\langle p \rangle$, of the polymer chain actually in contact with the surface. Small-angle neutron scattering (SANS) and neutron reflectivity (NR) ellipsometry, electron paramagnetic resonance (EPR), IR, and NMR spectroscopy have all been used. Most suffer from the drawback that the distinction between bound and free segments *close* to the interface is often difficult to define. This distinction is important as the bound fraction effectively determines how well anchored the polymer is to the surface.

The *bound fraction* is defined as the fraction of segments *physically* in contact with the surface;

$$\langle p \rangle = \frac{\Gamma_{\text{trains}}}{\Gamma_{\text{adsorbed}}} \tag{16}$$

where Γ_{trains} is the mass of polymer in direct contact with the surface.

The bound fraction is *easily* and *directly* accessible by only a few of the above techniques. IR spectroscopy utilizes the principle that the molecular bonds of the absorbed polymer segments are perturbed from their normal state when in contact with a surface. As a consequence the force constant defining the resonance frequency in the two domains bound (i.e., those with restricted mobility), and free (i.e., motionally unrestricted), are different. Absorption bands representing the bound polymer segments will, therefore, appear in a different part of the spectrum from those of free polymer. The spectrum of polymer in solution (i.e., no particles present) is subtracted from the overall adsorbed polymer spectrum to recover the signals from bound segments. The emergence of computer-based FT (Fourier Transform)-IR spectrometers has greatly facilitated this type of study since good quality data can now be acquired quickly and accurately. One drawback of this technique is, however, the limited range of solvents applicable: strongly adsorbing solvents such as water tend to mask the weaker polymer signals.

Polymer relaxation NMR studies are somewhat more involved and often require the use of a solid-state NMR machine. The bound components give rise to broad lines that cannot be detected on conventional (liquids) NMR spectrometers; only free segments are measured. Using a solid-state NMR machine, the complex line-shape can be deconvoluted into the bound and free components.

EPR is comparable to solid-state NMR but has the same principal limitation in that the distinction between the segments bound in trains and short loops close to the interface is not easily made. These limitations lead to an overestimation of the bound fraction. Nevertheless, EPR and NMR results generally show rather good agreement. Any perturbing effects due to the presence of the spin-active group are ignored.

Solvent relaxation NMR studies have, however, proved to be very informative and simple to perform on conventional NMR machines without the need for extra hardware. As with bound and free polymer, the solvent also has two distinct NMR environments. In the bulk phase, the solvent has a characteristic NMR relaxation time of several seconds. When the same molecule is constrained at an interface, this relaxation time is reduced by several orders of magnitude, typically to tens of microseconds. The average value of this relaxation time in a particle dispersion is a sum of the populations of solvent molecules in each environment. The population of the solvent molecules in the two environments changes dramatically upon adsorption of the polymer as solvent molecules are displaced from the surface. This change in the relaxation time can be related to the conformation of the adsorbed polymer, and hence, the bound fraction (14). Unlike other NMR experiments, deuterated solvents are not required.

F. The Volume Fraction Profile

The volume fraction profile can be obtained by scattering and reflection techniques. X-ray and neutron *scattering* are employed if the substrate is particulate, and X-ray, neutron, and light *reflection* is used when the substrate is a flat, homogeneous surface.

Reflectometry, where only the intensity of the reflected light is measured, requires a thin film adsorbed onto a reflecting substrate. The thin film has a different refractive index than both the bulk solution and the substrate; so interference occurs between the rays reflected from the substrate/film and film/bulk solution interfaces. By model fitting the refractive index-distance behavior, it is possible to extract the volume fraction profile of the adsorbed polymer layer (15).

If the polarization of the reflected light is also measured, the technique is known as *ellipsometry*. Measurements are usually carried out at the Brewster angle, where the parallel polarized, reflected light is at its minimum value. The measured quantity is the *ellipticity*—the ratio of the reflection coefficients of the parallel and perpendicularly polarized light:

$$\rho_{ell} = e^{i\Delta} \tan \psi \tag{17}$$

where Δ is the phase shift and $\tan \psi$ is the amplitude ratio of the reflected light perpendicular and parallel to the plane of incidence. These parameters are read from the ellipsometer. The ellipticity of the bare surface is first measured before the surface is exposed to the polymer solution. The adsorbed polymer layer modifies these reflection coefficients and, hence, alters the ellipticity. Measurements are taken at two angles, and from Eq. 17, the modified phase shift and amplitude ratio can be obtained. Ellipsometric data of this sort are usually interpreted in terms of an equivalent homogeneous film with an average refractive index and *ellipsometric* thickness. Alternatively, the modified values can be model-fitted by assuming a refractive index profile. The ellipsometric thickness is given by

$$\delta_{ell} = \frac{\left[\int_0^\infty \varphi^{a}(z)\,dz\right]^2}{\int_0^\infty (\varphi^{a}(z))^2\,dz} \tag{18}$$

Neutrons possess a unique combination of physical properties; their wavelength depends on their velocity and is typically 1 Å; their energy is typically of the order of kT, but they have no charge. The scattering event occurs due to a very short range repulsive interaction with the nucleus. Neutrons are thus ideal noninvasive probes. The efficiency of the scattering process depends on the *scattering length* of the nucleus. This parameter is akin to the optical refractive index in light-scattering studies. Fortunately for the colloid scientist, hydrogen and deuterium nuclei have very different *scattering length densities* (a combination of the scattering lengths of the constituent atoms) and a wide range of scattering length densities can be obtained. Most common materials lie within the extremes given by water and heavy water. An 80% deuterated polystyrene latex would therefore have the same scattering length density as a mixture of 90% D_2O and 10% H_2O; i.e., to the neutrons, the particles are no different from the solvent and are thus invisible. It is therefore possible to highlight certain constituents of the system e.g., the adsorbed layer. This index matching process is known as *contrast matching*.

The intensity of scattered radiation as a function of neutron wavelength depends on the size and shape of the scatterers and their concentration. The required information is contained within the *shape factor*, $P(Q)$

$$I(Q) = C_{\text{inst}} n_p(\rho_p - \rho_s)^2 P(Q) \tag{19}$$

where C_{inst} is the instrument constant, n_p is the concentration of particles, and ρ is the scattering length densities of the particles (p) and solvent (s). The general $P(Q)$ for an adsorbed polymer layer is

$$P(Q) = \frac{2\pi A_s}{Q^2} \left| \int_0^\infty \varphi(z) e^{iQz} dz \right|^2 \tag{20}$$

where $\varphi(z)$ is the volume fraction profile of the adsorbed layer and A_s is the surface area of each particle. The experimental approach often adopted is to measure $I(Q)$ and to model-fit the date by generating representative shapes for the volume fraction profile. The scattering from this ''model volume fraction profile'' is then compared to the measured data in an iterative manner. Both the optimum shape and parameters describing that shape can thus be obtained (16).

The *Guinier approximation* allows one to calculate the size, R, of the scatterers from the low Q region ($Qa \ll 1$):

$$I(Q) = I_0 \exp\left(\frac{-Q^2R^2}{3}\right) \tag{21}$$

while the high Q limit—the *Porod* region—allows the surface area of the particles to be calculated:

$$I(Q) = C_{\text{inst}} n_p(\rho_p - \rho_s)^2 2\pi A_s Q^{-4}. \tag{22}$$

Neutrons can also be totally externally reflected when incident at glancing angles. This forms the basis of the technique known as neutron reflectometry (or reflectivity). For a single interface between media i and j the ratio of the reflected and incident amplitudes defines the Fresnel coefficient:

$$r_{ij} = \frac{\mu_{ni} \sin \phi_i - \mu_{nj} \sin \phi_j}{\mu_{ni} \sin \phi_i + \mu_{nj} \sin \phi_j} \tag{23}$$

The reflectivity, $R = I_R/I_0$, of the measured quantity is a function of the Fresnel coefficients

$$R = \frac{r_{01} e^{i\delta} + r_{12} e^{-i\delta}}{e^{i\delta} + r_{01} r_{12} e^{-i\delta}} \tag{24}$$

where the media correspond to air (0), polymer layer (1), and solvent (2) and δ is the phase difference between the neutrons reflected from the 01 and 12 interfaces. The phase difference is given by

$$\delta = 2\pi\mu_{ni}(d_1/\lambda)\sin\phi \tag{25}$$

d_1 is the thickness of the first layer forming the multilayer model used to fit the measured data. Many such layers can be incorporated into the model in an analogous manner to the fitting of the SANS data (16).

REFERENCES

1. Cohen Stuart MA, Scheutjens JMHM, Fleer GJ. J Polym Sci Polym Phys 1980; 18:559.
2. Hamaker HC. Physica 1937; 4:1058.
3. Reerrink H, Overbeek JThG. Discuss Faraday Soc 1954; 18:74.
4. Deryagin BV, Landau L. Acta Phys Chim URSS 1941; 14:633.
5. Verwey EJW, Overbeek JThG. Theory of the Stability of Lyophobic Colloids. Amsterdam: Elsevier, 1948.
6. Napper DH. Polymeric Stabilisation of Colloidal Dispersions. New York: Academic Press, 1983.
7. Napper DH. J Colloid Interface Sci 1977; 58:390.
8. Croucher MD, Hair ML. J Phys Chem 1979; 83:1712.
9. Gregory J. In: Finch CA, ed. Chemistry and Technology of Water Soluble Polymers. New York: Plenum Press, 1983:307–320.
10. Gregory J. J Colloid Interface Sci 1973; 42: 448.
11. Asakura S, Oosawa F. J Chem Phys 1954; 22:1255.
12. Cosgrove T, Fergie-Woods J. Colloids and Surfaces, 1987; 25:91.
13. Kayes JB, Rawlins DA. Colloid Polym Sci 1979;257: 622.
14. van der Beek GP, Cohen Stuart MA, Cosgrove T. Langmuir 1991; 7:327.
15. Cosgrove T, Patel A, Semlyn JA, Webster JRP, Zarbakhsh A. Langmuir 1993; 9:2326.
16. Fleer GJ, Cohen Stuart MA, Scheutjens JMHM, Cosgrove T, Vincent B. Polymers at Interfaces. London: Chapman & Hall, 1993.

3

Polymeric Surfactants
Stabilization of Emulsions and Dispersions

Th. F. Tadros
Imperial College, London, England

I. INTRODUCTION

Personal care formulations are designed to have a number of benefits, both functional and aesthetic (1). For these reasons, many systems are designed to provide cleaning and protective barriers against damaging environments such as sunlight (sunscreens) and they should have a pleasant odor, make the skin feel smooth, and appeal to the customer on application. Because of these requirements many personal care formulations have complex recipes, which in many cases are arrived at by a trial-and-error procedure and using expert panels to assess their performance. However, in recent years there has been great demand to rationalize these compositions, clarifying their complex interactions and applying fundamental principles of colloid and interface science to these systems (2).

At present, many personal formulations are based on oil-in-water (o/w) or water-in-oil (w/o) emulsions ''structured'' (using gelling agents) to produce creams with the right consistency (rheology) that appeals to the customer. These systems are thermodynamically unstable, as their formation is accompanied by a large increase in interfacial energy (small droplets) and hence a large and positive interfacial energy (3). This can be understood if one considers the free energy of formation, ΔG^{form}, of an emulsion from a bulk oil, i.e.,

$$\Delta G^{form} = \Delta A \gamma_{12} - T\Delta S^{conf} \quad (1)$$

where ΔA is the increase in interfacial area, γ_{12} is the interfacial tension, T is the absolute temperature and ΔS^{conf} is the configurational entropy arising from the increase in the number of possible configurations due to the formation of a large number of droplets. With emulsions $|\Delta A_{12}| \gg |-T\Delta S^{conf}|$ and hence $\Delta G^{form} > 0$; i.e., the formation of an emulsion is nonspontaneous and with time the emulsion tends to break down by flocculation and coalescence to reduce ΔA and hence ΔG.

The above thermodynamic argument implies that to stabilize an emulsion against flocculation and coalescence, one needs to create an energy barrier between the droplets to prevent their close approach (whereby the van der Waals attraction is strong). Several methods may be applied to create such a high (repulsive) energy barrier. The most common procedure applied in many colloidal systems is to create an electrical double layer at the oil/water interface. When two droplets with such double layers (of the same charge sign) approach a separation distance that is twice the double-layer thickness, strong repulsion occurs and this counteracts the van der Waals attraction. The energy-distance curve for such systems shows an energy barrier (maximum) at intermediate distances of separation, which has to be overcome for flocculation and coalescence to occur. The height of this barrier depends on the surface (or zeta) potential and electrolyte type and concentration.

The above method of stabilization (referred to as electrostatic stabilization) can be produced by the use of ionic surfactants (of the anionic, cationic, or zwitterionic type). However, for a number of reasons this method of stabilization is not ideal for personal care formulations. First, the stabilization is influenced by the presence of electrolytes in the system, which reduces repulsion and may cause instability. In addition, many ionic surfactants cause skin irritation as a result of their penetration and interaction with the stratum corneum (4). The latter is the main barrier to water loss and it consists of lipids that are organized in a bilayer structure (liquid crystalline), which at high water content is transparent and soft (5). Surfactants that interact with the lipid bilayer and reduce its ''liquid-like'' nature (by disrupting the liquid crystalline structure) may cause crystallization of the lipids, and this has a drastic effect on the appearance and smoothness of the skin (''dry'' skin feeling).

For the above reasons, many personal care emulsions are formulated using nonionic surfactants of which the alcohol ethoxylates (the ICI ''Brij'' series), sorbitan esters (Spans), and their ethoxylates (Tween) are the most commonly used surfactants. These surfactants adsorb at the oil/water interface with the hydrophobic (alkyl) group pointing to (or dissolved in) the oil phase and the hydrophilic chain [mostly poly(ethylene) oxide (PEO)] remaining in the aqueous phase. These molecules produce a repulsive barrier as a result of the unfavorable mixing of the polar PEO chains (when these are in good solvent conditions) and the reduction in configurational entropy of the chains when these overlap. Such repulsion is usually referred to as steric stabilization (see below) (6). These nonionic surfactants, which are usually used in mixtures) have been successfully applied to prepare stable o/w and w/o emulsions. In addition, in some cases, they form liquid crystalline structures at the o/w interface and these prevent coalescence of the oil droplets (7).

As will be discussed later, one of the main features of effective steric stabilization is strong adsorption (anchoring) of the chains to the interface. This anchoring is produced by the use of polymeric surfactants, the main topic of this chapter. These materials have attracted considerable attention in recent years for stabilization of many o/w and w/o emulsions. Apart from their effectiveness in prevention of flocculation and coalescence of the droplets, they are also expected to cause no skin irritation. The high molecular weight of the surfactants prevents their penetration through the skin and hence they do not cause any disruption of the stratum corneum.

This chapter, will begin with a brief description of polymeric surfactants and their solution properties, followed by a description of the fundamental principles of using polymeric surfactants for stabilization of emulsions (as well as suspensions), starting with a section on the adsorption and conformation of these molecules at the interface. This is followed by a section on stabilization of dispersions by polymeric surfactants. Particular attention will be given to the criteria that need to be satisfied for effective steric stabilization. This is followed by a section on rheology of emulsions stabilized by polymeric surfactants. Both interfacial rheology of the surfactant film at the interface and the bulk rheological properties of the various systems will be described. Finally, a section will be devoted to the use of polymeric surfactants for preparation of stable multiple emulsions of the w/o/w type. These systems attracted considerable interest in recent years in cosmetic systems and a great deal of research has been carried out to prepare stable systems with the right consistency (rheology) for cosmetic applications.

II. GENERAL DESCRIPTION OF POLYMERIC SURFACTANTS

Polymeric surfactants of the block (AB or ABA) or graft (BA_n) type are essential materials for the preparation of many systems, e.g., dyestuffs, papercoatings, inks, agrochemicals, pharmaceuticals, personal care products, ceramics, detergents, etc.

A block copolymer is a linear arrangement of blocks of varying composition:

Diblock – poly A – block poly B ~~A~~~~~~ ~~~~~~B~~
Triblock – poly A – block poly B – poly A
~~A~~~~~~ ~~~~B~~~~ ~~~~~A~~

A graft copolymer is a nonlinear array of one B block on which several A polymers are grafted

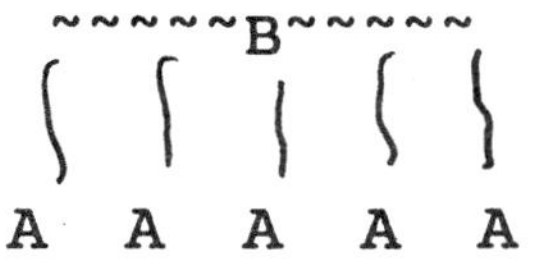

Block copolymers have gained considerable importance in the last three decades. Their special chemical structure (different A and B chains) yields unusual physical properties. Block copolymers frequently exhibit phase separation: one block type in a continuous matrix of the second block type. The fact that block copolymers are able to participate in different types of phases gives them special properties both colloidal and mechanical: surface activity, surface elasticity, impact modification.

Two types of investigations are essential to explain the behavior of block and graft copolymers: (1) properties in a solvent in which both the A and B blocks are soluble—this gives information on their conformation; (2) Properties in a solvent that is a nonsolvent for one of the blocks but a good solvent for the other block.

Block coplymers exhibit surface activity since one of the blocks is soluble in one of the phases and the other is miscible in the other phase, e.g., AB block, A hydrophilic, B hydrophobic

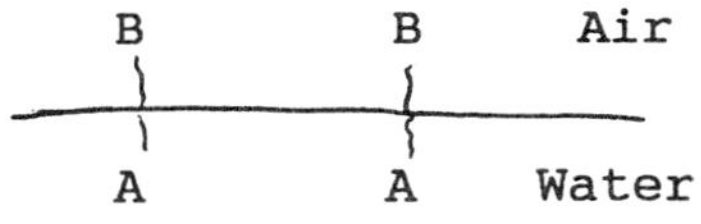

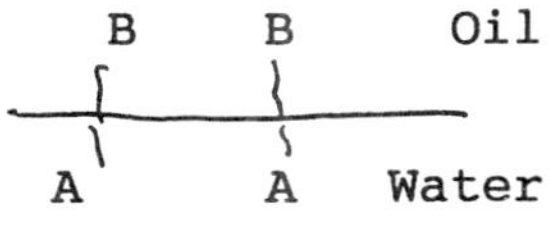

Since block copolymers are amphiphilic, they aggregate in solution to form micelles:

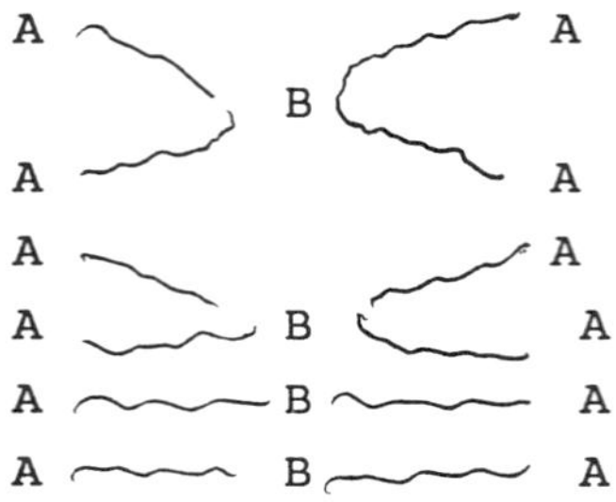

ABA block copolymer may form micelles with smaller aggregation number

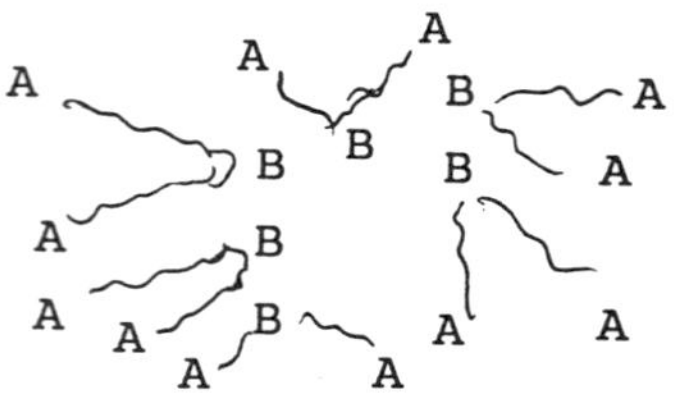

AB block can form simple micelles

Graft copolymers also aggregate in solution to form micelles, again with small aggregation numbers. A dimer may be the form of aggregation.

Most block and graft copolymers have low critical micelle concentrations (cmc) and in many cases it is not easy to measure the cmc for these block and graft copolymers. The aggregation process is also affected by temperature and solvency of the medium for the A chains. One of the most useful methods to follow the aggregation of block and graft copolymers is time average light scattering. By measuring the intensity as a function of concentration one can extrapolate the results to zero concentration and obtain the molecular weight of the micelle. This allows one to obtain the aggregation number from a knowledge of the molecular weight of the monomer.

III. GENERAL CLASSIFICATION OF POLYMERIC SURFACTANTS

The simplest type of polymeric surfactant is a homopolymer, which is formed from the same repeating units: for example, poly(ethylene oxide) (PEO), poly(vinylpyrrolidone) (PVP). Homopolymers have little surface activity at the oil/water (O/W) interface. However, homopolymers may adsorb significantly at the solid/liquid (S/L) interface. Even if the adsorption energy per monomer segment is small (fraction of kT, where k is the Boltzmann constant and T is the absolute temperature), the total adsorption energy per molecule may be sufficient (several segments are adsorbed at the surface) to overcome the unfavorable entropy loss of the molecule at the S/L interface. Homopolymers may also adsorb at the solid surface by some specific interaction, e.g., hydrogen bonding (for example, adsorption of PEO or PVP on silica). In general, homopolymers are not the most suitable emulsifiers or dispersants.

A small variant is use of polymers that contain specific groups that have high affinity to the surface, e.g., partially hydrolyzed poly(vinyl acetate) (PVAc), technically referred to as poly(vinyl alcohol) (PVA). Commercially available PVA molecules contain 4–12% acetate groups. The acetate groups give the molecule its amphipathic character: on a hydrophobic surface (such as polystyrene) the polymer adsorbs with preferential attachment of the acetate groups on the surface, leaving the more hydrophilic vinyl alcohol segments dangling in the aqueous medium. Partially hydrolyzed PVA molecules exhibit surface activity at the O/W interface.

The most convenient polymeric surfactants are those of the block-and-graft copolymer type: triblock polymeric surfactants—Pluronics (BASF) and Synperonic PE (ICI)—two poly-A blocks of PEO and one poly-B block of polypropylene oxide (PPO). Several chain lengths of PEO and PPO are available. Triblocks of PPO-PEO-PEO (inverse Pluronics) are also available. Polymeric triblock surfactants can be applied as emulsifiers and dispersants. The hydrophobic PPO chain resides at the hydrophobic surface, leaving the two PEO chains dangling in aqueous solution (providing steric stabilization).

The above triblocks are not the most efficient emulsifiers or dispersants—the PPO chain is not sufficiently hydrophobic to provide a strong ''anchor'' to a hydrophobic surface or to an oil droplet. The surface activity of the PEO-PPO-PEO triblock at the O/W interface is probably due to ''rejection'' anchoring: the PPO chain is not soluble in water or most oils. Several other di- and triblock copolymers have been synthesized: diblocks of polystyrene block–polyvinyl alcohol; triblocks of poly(methylmethacrylate)–block polyethylene oxide–poly(methyl methacrylate); diblocks of polystyrene-polyethylene oxide; triblocks of polyethelene oxide–polystyrene–polyethylene oxide.

An alternative (and perhaps more efficient) polymeric surfactant is the amphipathic graft copolymer consisting of a polymeric backbone B (polystyrene or polymethylmethacrylate) and several A chains (''teeth'') such as polyethylene oxide. The graft copolymer is referred to as a ''comb'' stabilizer—the polymer forms a ''brush'' at the solid/liquid interface. The copolymer is usually prepared by grafting a macromonomer such as methoxy polyethylene oxide methacrylate with polymethyl methacrylate. In most cases, some polymethacrylic acid is incorporated with the polymethylmethacrylate backbone: this leads to reduction of the glass transition of the backbone, which makes the chain more flexible for adsorption at the S/L interface. Typical commercially available graft copolymers are Atlox 4913 and Hypermer CG-6 (ICI).

The ''grafting into'' technique has also been used to synthesize polystyrene–polyethylene oxide graft copolymers. These molecules are not commercially available.

IV. SOLUTION PROPERTIES OF POLYMERIC SURFACTANTS

To understand the solution behavior of polymeric surfactants of the block-and-graft type, it is essential to consider the solution properties of the more simple homopolymers. The solution behavior of homopolymers was considered in the thermodynamic treatment of Flory and Huggins.

The Flory-Huggins theory considers the free energy of mixing of pure polymer with pure solvent, ΔG_{mix}, in terms of two contributions: the enthalpy of mixing, ΔH_{mix}, and the entropy of mixing ΔS_{mix}:

$$\Delta G_{mix} = \Delta H_{mix} + \Delta S_{mix} \tag{2}$$

Assuming that the polymer chain adopts a configuration on a lattice (provided by the solvent molecules) and considering that the mixing is ''random,'' ΔS_{mix} is given by

$$\Delta S_{mix} = - k[n_1 \, ln \, \phi_1 + n_2 \, ln \, \phi_2] \tag{3}$$

where k is the Boltzmann constant, n_1 is the number of solvent molecules with a volume fraction ϕ_1, and n_2 is the number of polymer molecules with a volume fraction ϕ_2.

The enthalpy of mixing, ΔH_{mix}, is given by the following expression:

$$\Delta H_{mix} = n_1 \phi_2 \chi kT \tag{4}$$

where χ is a dimensionless interaction parameter and χkT expresses the difference in energy of a solvent molecule in pure solvent compared to its immersion in pure polymer. χ is usually referred to as the Flory-Huggins interaction parameter.

Combining Eq. (2)–(4), one obtains,

$$\Delta G_{mix} = kT[n_1 \ln \phi_1 + n_2 \ln \phi_2 + \chi n_1 \phi_2] \tag{5}$$

The mixing of a pure solvent with a polymer solution creates an osmotic pressure, π, which can be expressed in terms of the polymer concentration c_2 and the volume fraction of the polymer:

$$\pi/c_2 = RT[(1/M_2) + (v_2^2/V_1)(1/2 - \chi)c_2 + \cdots] \tag{6}$$

where v_2 is the partial specific volume of the polymer ($v_2 = V_2/M_2$) and V_1 is the molar volume of the solvent.

The second term in Eq. 6 is the second virial coefficient:

$$\pi/c_2 = \mathrm{RT}\ [(1/M_2) + B_2 c_2 + \cdots] \tag{7}$$

$$B_2 = (v_2^2/V_1)(1/2 - \chi) \tag{8}$$

Note that $B_2 = 0$ when $\chi = 1/2$—the polymer behaves as ideal in mixing with the solvent. This condition was designated by Flory as the θ-point.

In a θ-condition, the polymer chains in solution have no attraction or repulsion and they adopt their unperturbed dimensions. When $\chi < 1/2$, B_2 is positive—mixing is nonideal, leading to positive deviation (repulsion). This occurs when the polymer chains are in ''good'' solvent conditions. When $\chi > 1/2$, B_2 is negative—mixing is nonideal, leading to negative deviation (attraction). This occurs when the polymer chains are in ''poor'' solvent conditions (precipitation of the polymer may occur under these conditions).

Since the polymer solvency depends on temperature, one can also define a θ-temperature at which $\chi = 1/2$.

The function $[(1/2) - \chi]$ can also be expressed in terms of two mixing parameters, an enthalpy parameter κ_1 and an entropy parameter ψ_1:

$$[(1/2) - \chi] = \kappa_1 - \psi_1 \tag{9}$$

The θ-temperature can also be expressed in terms of κ_1 and ψ_1:

$$\theta = (\kappa_1\ T)/\psi_1 \tag{10}$$

Alternatively one can write

$$[(1/2) - \chi] = \psi_1[1 - (\theta/T)] \tag{11}$$

Several experimental results cannot be accounted for by the Flory-Huggins theory: dependence of χ on polymer concentration, phase separation of many polymer solutions (e.g., PEO) on heating.

The solution properties of copolymers are much more complicated. The two copolymer components A and B behave differently in different solvents. When the two components A and B are both soluble in the same solvent, they exhibit similar solution properties, e.g., a nonpolar copolymer in a nonpolar solvent.

With branched polymers of high monomer density (e.g., star-branched polymers), the θ-temperature depends on the length of the arms and is in general lower than that of a linear polymer with the same molecular weight. Another complication arises from specific interaction with the solvent, e.g., hydrogen bonding between polymer and solvent molecules (e.g., with PEO and PVA in water). Aggregation in solution (lack of complete dissolution) may also present a problem in determining the solution properties of block-and-graft copolymers.

One of the most useful parameters for characterizing the conformation of a polymer in solution is the root-mean-square (rms) end-to-end length $\langle r^2 \rangle^{1/2}$, which represents a configuration character r as the distance from one end group to the other of a polymer chain molecule. Another useful parameter is the radius of gyration $\langle s^2 \rangle^{1/2}$, which is a measure of the effective size of a polymer molecule—it is the rms distance of the elements of the chain from its center of gravity.

For linear polymers,

$$\langle s^2 \rangle^{1/2} = [\langle r^2 \rangle^{1/2}]/6^{1/2} \tag{12}$$

The radius of gyration of a polymer molecule in solution can be determined from light-scattering measurements. Dilute solutions of copolymers in solvents that are good for both components exhibit similar behavior to homopolymer chains. In selective solvents, whereby the medium is a good solvent for one component, say A, and a poor solvent for the second component, B, one part of the amphipathic block or graft copolymer will separate as a distinct phase, while the other stays in solution. The insoluble portion of the amphipathic copolymer will aggregate reversibly to form micelles. It is believed that the micelles of block-and-graft copolymers are spherical. The critical micelle concentration of block-and-graft copolymers is usually very low.

Several methods may be applied to obtain the micellar size and shape of block-and-graft copolymers: light scattering, small-angle X-ray scattering, small-angle neutron scattering.

Dynamic light scattering (photon correlation spectroscopy, PCS) can also be applied to obtain the hydrodynamic radius of the micelle. By measuring the intensity fluctuation of scattered light by the micelles (when these undergo Brownian diffusion), one can obtain the diffusion coefficient of the micelles D, from which the hydrodynamic radius R can be obtained using the Stokes-Einstein equation:

$$D = \frac{kT}{6\,\pi\eta R} \tag{13}$$

where η is the viscosity of the medium.

V. ADSORPTION AND CONFORMATION OF POLYMERIC SURFACTANTS AT INTERFACES

Understanding the adsorption and conformation of polymeric surfactants at interfaces is key to knowing how these molecules act as stabilizers. Most basic ideas on adsorption and conformation of polymers have been developed for the solid/liquid interface (8). (See Chapter 2.) The same concepts may be applied to the liquid/liquid interface, with some modification whereby some parts of the molecule may reside within the oil phase, rather than simply staying at the interface. Such modification does not alter the basic concepts, particularly when one deals with stabilization by these molecules.

The process of polymer adsorption involves a number of interactions that must be separately considered. Three main interactions must be taken into account, namely the

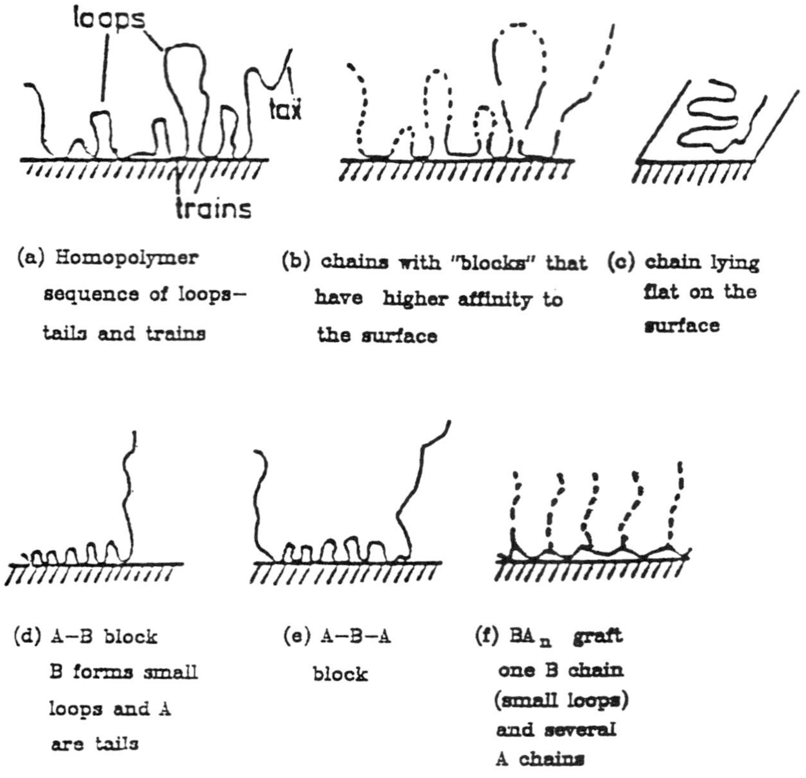

Figure 1 Various conformations of polymeric surfactants adsorbed on a plane surface. (a) Random conformation of loops-trains-tails (hompolymer); (b) preferential adsorption of ''short blocks''; (c) chain lying flat on the surface; (d) AB block copolymer with loop-train configuration of B and long tail of A; (e) ABA block as in d; (f) BA_a graft with backbone B forming small loops and several tails of A (''teeth'').

interaction of the solvent molecules with the surface (or oil in the case of oil/water (o/w) emulsions) that need to be displaced for the polymer segments to adsorb, the interaction between the chains and the solvent, and the interaction between the polymer and the surface. Apart from knowing these interactions, one of the most fundamental considerations is the conformation of the polymer molecule at the interface. These molecules adopt various conformations, depending on their structure. The simplest case to consider is that of a homopolymer that consists of identical segments [e.g., poly(ethylene oxide)], which shows a sequence of loops, trains, and tails, as illustrated in Figure 1a. For such a polymer to adsorb, the reduction in entropy of the chain as it approaches the interface must be compensated by an energy of adsorption between the segments and the surface. In other words, the chain segments must have a minimum adsorption energy, χ^s, otherwise no adsorption occurs. With polymers that are highly water soluble, such as poly(ethylene oxide) (PEO), the interaction energy with the surface may be too small for adsorption to occur, and if this takes place, the whole molecule may not be strongly adsorbed to the surface. For this reason, many commercially available polymers that are described as hompolymers, such as poly(vinyl alcohol) (PVA), contain some hydrophobic groups or short blocks (vinyl acetate in the case of PVA) that ensure their adsorption to hydrophobic surfaces. This is illustrated in Figure 1b. Clearly, if all the segments have a high affinity to the surface, the whole molecule may lie flat on the surface, as illustrated in Figure 1c. This situation is rarely the case, since the molecule will have very low solubility in the continuous medium.

The most favorable structures for polymeric surfactants are those represented in Figure 1d, 1e, and 1f, referred to as block-and-graft copolymers. The molecule shown in Figure 1d is an AB block, consisting of a B chain that has a high affinity to the surface (or soluble in the oil phase), referred to as the ''anchoring'' chain, and an A chain that has very low affinity to the surface and is strongly solvated by the medium. As will be discussed below, this is the most convenient structure, since the forces that ensure strong adsorption are opposite to those that ensure stability. A variance on the structure shown in Figure 1d is the ABA block copolymer, shown in Figure 1e. In this case, the anchor chain B contains two stabilizing chains (tails). Another variance is that shown in Figure 1f, which is described as a graft copolymer (''comb''-type structure) with one B chain and several A chains (tails or ''teeth'').

It is clear from the above description of polymer configurations that for full characterization of the process of adsorption, it is necessary to know the following parameters: the amount of polymer adsorbed per unit area of the surface, Γ(mole/m^2 or mg/m^2), the fraction of segments in close contact with the surface, p, and the distribution of polymer segments, $\rho(z)$, from the surface toward the bulk solution. It is essential to know how far the segments extend into solution, i.e., the adsorbed layer thickness δ. It is important to know how these parameters change with polymer coverage (concentration), the structure of the polymer, and its molecular weight. It is also essential to know how these parameters change with the environment, such as solvency of the medium for the chains and temperature.

Several theories describe the process of polymer adsorption, which have been developed using either the statistical mechanical approach or quasi-lattice models. In the statistical mechanical approach, the polymer is considered to consist of three types of structures with different energy states, trains, loops, and tails (9,10). The structures close to the surface (trains) are adsorbed with an internal partition function determined by short-range forces between the segment and surface (assigned an adsorption energy per segment χ^s). The segments in loops and tails are considered to have an internal partition function equivalent to that of segments in bulk solution and these are assigned a segment-solvent interaction parameter χ (Flory-Huggins interaction parameter). By equating the chemical potential of the macromolecule in the adsorbed state and in bulk solution, the adsorption isotherm can be determined. In the earlier theories, the case of an isolated chain on the surface (low coverage) was considered, but later the theories were modified to take into account the lateral interaction between the chains, i.e., at high coverage.

The quasi-lattice model was developed by Roe (11) and by Scheutjens and Fleer (12). The basis procedure was to describe all chain conformations as step-weighted random walks on a quasi-crystalline lattice that extends in parallel layers away from the surface. This is illustrated in Figure 2, which shows a possible conformation of a polymer molecule at a surface. The partition function was written in terms of number of chain configurations that were treated as connected sequences of segments. In each layer, random mixing (Bragg-Williams or mean field approximation) between segments and solvent molecules was assumed. Each step in the random walk was assigned a weighting factor p_i that was considered to consist of three factors: the adsorption energy χ^s, the configurational entropy of mixing, and the segment-solvent interaction parameter χ.

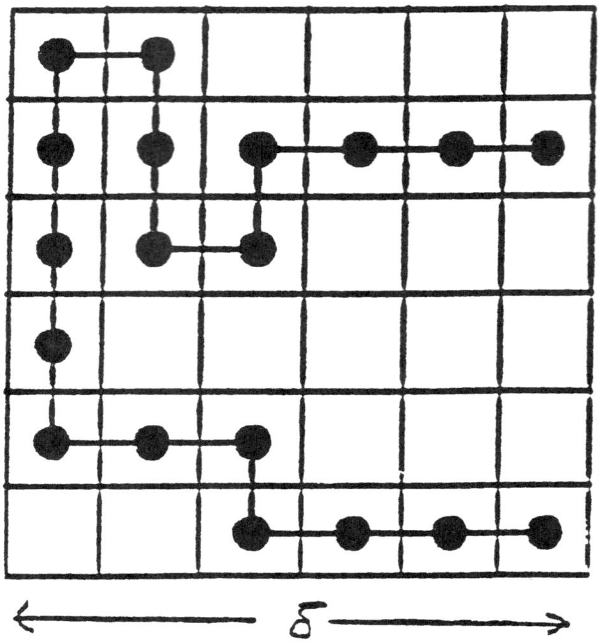

Figure 2 Possible conformation of a polymer molecule at an interface.

The above theories gave a number of predictions for polymeric surfactant adsorption, which are summarized as follows. As the number of segments in the chain increases from low (with few segments) to high (large number of segments) values, the adsorption isotherm changes from a Langmuirian type (characteristic for surfactant adsorption) to a high-affinity type. In the latter case, the first addition of polymer chains to the solution results in their virtual complete adsorption. Adsorption in this case is described as being "irreversible"; i.e., the equilibrium between adsorbed and free polymer is shifted toward the surface. This explains the strong anchoring of the polymer chains to the surface. As the solvency of the medium for the chains decreases, the amount of polymer adsorbed increases. This explains the relatively "weaker" adsorption of homopolymers that are highly solvated by the medium. It is now clear from these theories why block-and-graft copolymers are preferred for stabilization of dispersions. The poor solubility of the anchor chain B in the medium and its strong affinity to the surface ensures the strong adsorption of the molecule. In contrast, the high solubility of the stabilizing chain A ensures effective steric stabilization. Another prediction from the theories is that the higher the molecular weight of the polymer, the higher the amount of adsorption, when the latter is expressed in mg/m^2. The bound fraction, p, increases with increase of the adsorption energy, χ^s, but it decreases with increase in surface coverage and increase of the molecular weight of the polymer. The segment density distribution, $\rho(z)$, and the adsorbed layer thickness δ increase with increase of the molecular weight of the polymer. They also increase with increase of solvency of the medium for the chains.

Several experimental methods can be applied to study adsorption and conformation of polymers at interfaces. The amount of polymer adsorbed, Γ, can be directly determined by equilibrating a known amount of the disperse phase (particles or droplets) with a poly-

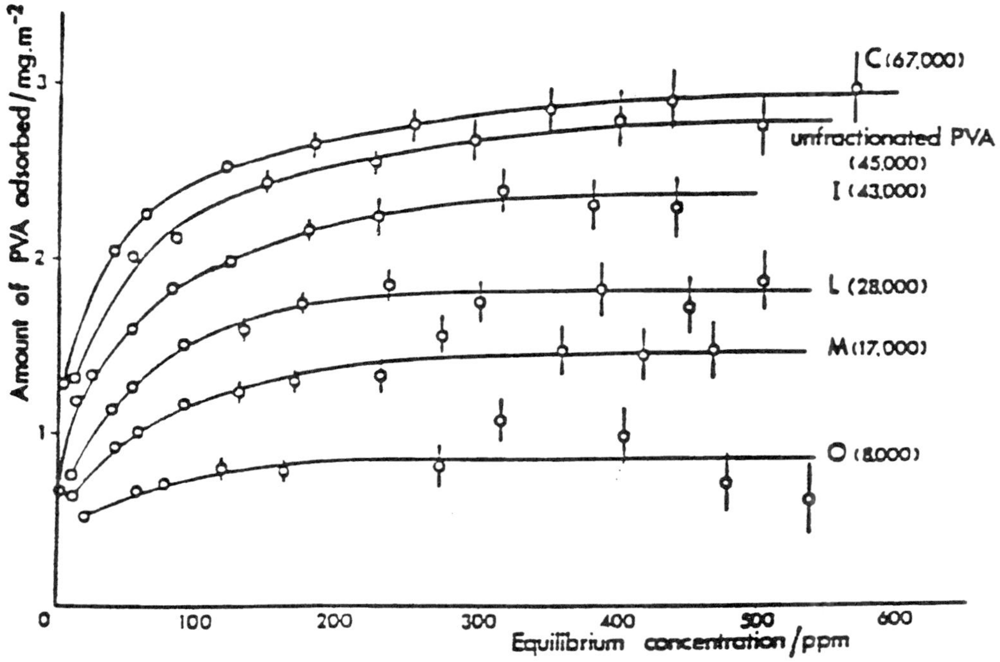

Figure 3 Adsorption isotherms of poly(vinyl alcohol) on polystyrene latex at 25°C.

mer solution of known concentration, C_1. When the system reaches equilibrium (that may take hours or even days with molecular-weight polymers), the disperse phase is separated (by filtration or centrifugation) and the equilibrium concentration of the polymer, C_2, is determined using a suitable analytical method. From C_1 and C_2 and the amount of disperse phase m and its surface area A (m^2/g, which may be obtained from a knowledge of the particle size distribution), Γ can be calculated; i.e.,

$$\Gamma = \frac{C_1 - C_2}{mA} \tag{14}$$

Figure 3 shows the adsorption isotherms at 25°C for poly (vinyl alcohol) (PVA) (containing 12% acetate groups) on polystyrene latex (13). Shown are the high-affinity isotherms for the polymers and the increase in adsorption of the polymer with increase of the molecular weight. Similar isotherms are expected for the adsorption of the polymer on oil droplets. However, in the latter case it is not possible to obtain the full isotherm since to produce the emulsion one requires a minimum amount of polymer. In addition, the surface area of the emulsion has to be determined at each point from the droplet size distribution.

As expected from theory, it was also shown that the adsorption of PVA increases with decrease of solvency of the medium for the chains, obtained either by increasing the temperature or by addition of electrolyte such as KCl or Na_2SO_4.

The polymer-bound fraction, p, can be directly determined using spectroscopic methods such as nuclear magnetic resonance (NMR). The method depends on the reduction in the mobility of the segments that are in close contact with the surface. By using a pulsed NMR technique one can estimate p. An indirect method for estimation of p is to use microcalorimetry. Basically one compares the enthalpy of adsorption per molecule with that per segment (8). The latter may be obtained by using small molecules of similar structure to a polymer segment.

Several methods may be used to determine the adsorbed layer thickness, δ (8). Most of the methods depend on measuring the hydrodynamic radius of the particles with and without the adsorbed polymer layer. For example, one may measure the relative viscosity, η_r, of a dispersion with an adsorbed polymer layer. Assuming that the particles behave as hard spheres (when δ is small compared with the particle radius R) of noninteracting units (low volume fraction of the disperse phase), η_r can be related to the effective volume fraction, ϕ_{eff}, by the Einstein equation:

$$\eta_r = 1 + 2.5\phi_{eff} \tag{15}$$

From ϕ_{eff} and ϕ(the core volume fraction), the adsorbed layer thickness, δ_h, can be calculated using the equation

$$\phi_{eff} = \phi\left[1 + \frac{\delta_h}{R}\right]^3 \tag{16}$$

To apply the above method one should use a dispersion with monodisperse particles with a radius that is not much larger than δ_h. This limits the method for direct use with emulsions, which are polydisperse and have relatively large radii. However, small model particles of polystyrene may be used and the assumption is made that the polymer conformation at the interface is similar to that at the o/w interface.

Another method for determining δ_h is to apply dynamic (quasi-elastic) light scattering, referred to as photon correlation spectroscopy (PCS). By measuring the intensity fluctuation of scattered light (using a laser) by the particles, as a result of their Brownian diffusion, one can determine the diffusion coefficient, D, of the particles (8). It is also necessary to use small particles in this case (which show Brownian motion) with a radius that is not much larger than δ_h. From D the hydrodynamic radius R_h of the particles can be obtained using the Stokes-Einstein equation:

$$D = \frac{kT}{6\ \pi\eta R_h} \tag{13,17}$$

By carrying out the measurements in the presence and absence of polymer layers one can obtain δ_h. In the presence of an adsorbed polymer layer the hydrodynamic radius is the sum of the core radius and the adsorbed layer thickness, whereas in the absence of the polymer layer, R_h is simply the core radius. Again, as with the viscosity technique, this method cannot be directly applied to emulsions, which are polydisperse and have a radius that is large for significant Brownian motion.

VI. INTERACTION BETWEEN PARTICLES (DROPLETS) CONTAINING ADSORBED POLYMER LAYERS (STERIC STABILIZATION)

When two particles or droplets containing adsorbed polymer layers (with an adsorbed layer thickness δ) approach a distance of separation h whereby these layers begin to overlap, i.e., when $h < 2\delta$, repulsion occurs as a result of two main effects (6). The first repulsive force arises from the unfavorable mixing of the polymer layers when these are present in a good solvent (i.e., the chains are strongly solvated by the medium). The unfavorable mixing of polymer solutions in good solvent conditions was considered by Flory and Krigbaum (14), whose theory was applied to the present case of interparticle interaction. A schematic representation of the mixing of polymer layers on close approach is shown in Figure 4, which shows the situation when two particles with polymer layers are forced to approach a distance h that is less than 2δ forming an overlap region with a volume element dV. Before overlap, the chains have a volume fraction ϕ_2 and the solvent has a chemical potential μ_1^α. In the overlap region, the volume fraction of the chains is ϕ_2', which is higher than the ϕ_2, and the solvent has a chemical potential μ_1^β, which is lower than μ_1^α. This is equivalent to an increase in the osmotic pressure in the overlap region. As a result, solvent diffuses from the bulk to the overlap region and the two particles or droplets are separated; this results in strong repulsion. The latter is referred to as mixing or osmotic repulsion.

Using the Flory-Krigbaum theory (14), one can calculate the free energy of mixing, G_{mix}, due to this unfavorable overlap, i.e.,

$$\frac{G_{mix}}{kT} = \frac{4\pi}{3V_1}\phi_2^2 N_{av}\left(\frac{1}{2} - \chi\right)\left(\delta - \frac{h}{2}\right)^2\left(3R + 2\delta + \frac{h}{2}\right) \tag{18}$$

where k is the Boltzmann constant, T is the absolute temperature, V_1 is the molar volume of the solvent, and N_{av} is the Avogadros constant.

It is clear from Eq. 18 that when the Flory-Huggins interaction parameter, χ, is less than 0.5, i.e., the chains are in good solvent conditions, G_{mix} is positive and the interaction is repulsive and it increases very rapidly with decreasing h, when the latter is lower than 2δ. This explains why polymeric surfactants such as Hypermer CG6 (a graft copolymer of polymethylmethacrylate backbone and PEO side chains, produced by ICI) are ideal for stabilizing dispersions in aqueous media. For stabilization of dispersions in nonaqueous media, such as water/oil (w/o) emulsions, the stabilizing chains have to be soluble in the oil phase (normally a hydrocarbon). In this case polyhydroxystearic acid (PHS) chains are ideal. A polymeric surfactant such as Aralacel P135 (an ABA block copolymer of PHS-PEO-PHS produced by ICI) is an ideal w/o emulsifier.

Equation 18 also shows that when $\chi > 0.5$, i.e., when the solvency of the medium for the chains becomes poor, G_{mix} is negative and the interaction becomes attractive. The condition $\chi = 0.5$ is referred to as θ-solvency and this denotes the onset of change of

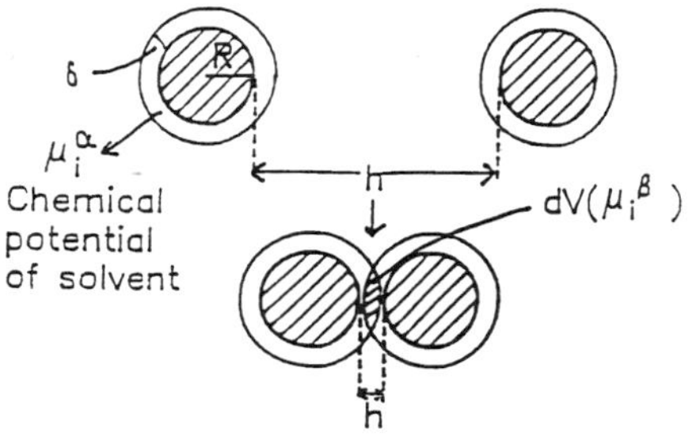

Figure 4 Schematic representation of overlap of two polymer layers.

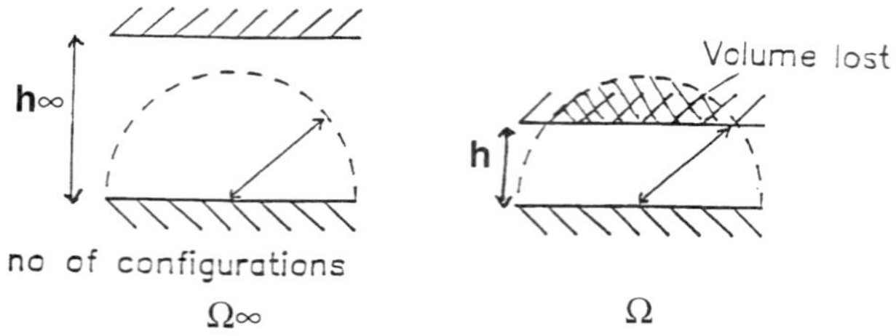

Figure 5 Schematic representation of the entropic, volume restriction, or elastic interaction.

repulsion to attraction. Thus to ensure steric stabilization by the above mechanism one has to ensure that the chains are kept in better than a θ-solvent.

The second repulsive force arises from the loss of configurational entropy when the chains overlap. This is schematically illustrated in Figure 5, whereby the polymer chain is represented by a simple rod with one attachment point to the surface. When the two surfaces are separated at infinite distance, each chain will have a number of configurations, Ω_∞, that are determined by the volume of the hemisphere swept by the rod. When the two surfaces approach a distance h that is smaller than the radius of the hemisphere swept by the rod, the volume available to the chains becomes smaller and this results in a reduction in the configurational entropy to a value Ω (which is less than Ω_∞). This results in strong repulsion and the effect is referred to as entropic, volume restriction, or elastic repulsion and is given by the following expression (6),

$$G_{el} = 2\nu \ln \frac{\Omega}{\Omega_\infty} \tag{19}$$

where ν is the number of polymer chains per unit area of the surface. G_{el} is always repulsive and it becomes very high on considerable overlap of the polymer chains.

Plots of G_{mix} and G_{el} versus h are illustrated in Figure 6, which shows that G_{mix} increases very rapidly with decrease of h as soon as h becomes smaller than 2δ (and $\chi < 0.5$). G_{el} also increases very rapidly with decrease of h on further overlap. Combination of G_{mix}, G_{el}, and G_A (the van der Waals attraction) results in the total $G_T - h$ curve shown in Figure 6. This curve shows a minimum (G_{min}) at $h \sim 2\delta$, but when $h < 2\delta$, G_T increases very rapidly with further decrease in h. The depth of the minimum, G_{min}, depends on the adsorbed layer thickness. With increase of δ, G_{min} decreases, and at sufficiently

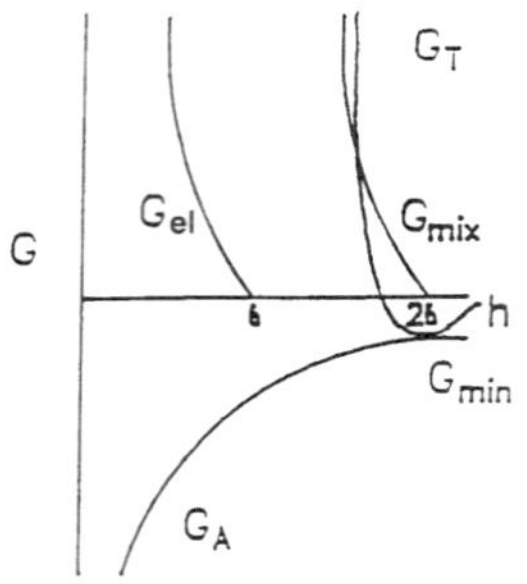

Figure 6 Schematic representation of the variation of G_{mix}, G_{el}, G_A, and G_T with h.

high values of δ (of the order of 5–10 nm), it reaches small values (fraction of kT units). This shows that with sterically stabilized dispersions, there is only weak attraction at relatively long distances of separation, which in most cases is overcome by the Brownian diffusion. Thus, one can say that the net interaction is repulsive and this ensures the long-term stability of the dispersion.

From the above discussion one can summarize the main criteria for effective steric stabilization. First, there should be enough polymer to ensure complete coverage of the surface by the chains. This will prevent any attraction between the bare patches or bridging by the polymer chains (which can adsorb simultaneously on more than one particle). Second, the chains must be strongly adsorbed (''anchored'') to the surface. This prevents any displacement on close approach. In this respect block-and-graft copolymers containing an anchoring chain [such as polystyrene or poly(methyl methacrylate) to hydrophobic surfaces] are the best stabilizers. In some cases strong adsorption may be achieved by a phenomenon referred to as rejection anchoring. If the B chain is insoluble in the medium (water or oil), it can adsorb by this rejection mechanism. This situation applies to poly(propylene oxide) (PPO), which is insoluble in water and in most oils. This explains the use of block copolymers of the PEO-PPO-PEO as emulsifiers.

The third criterion for effective steric stabilization is to ensure that the stabilizing chain A remains in good solvent conditions at all times and under all conditions. As discussed above, for systems where water is the continuous medium PEO is the most suitable A chain(s). The polymer chain is highly soluble in water and remains solvated up to high temperatures. It can also tolerate reasonable amounts of electrolyte. For dispersions, where the continuous medium is a hydrocarbon oil (e.g., w/o emulsions) polyhydroxystearic acid is the most suitable A chain(s).

The last criterion for effective steric stabilization is to have a sufficiently thick adsorbed layer to avoid any weak flocculation. This is particularly important for concentrated dispersions. As discussed above, a value of δ of the order of 5–10 nm is usually sufficient. Hence the side PEO chains need to have a molecular weight of the order of 1000–2000. With most graft copolymers, these side chains are extended and they provide a sufficiently thick layer.

VII. RHEOLOGY OF EMULSIONS STABILIZED WITH POLYMERIC SURFACTANTS

The flow characteristics (rheology) of emulsions is a subject of considerable importance from both a fundamental and applied point of view. At a fundamental level, the rheology of emulsions is a direct manifestation of the various interaction forces that occur in the system. The various processes that occur in emulsion systems, such as creaming and sedimentation, flocculation, coalescence, Ostawald ripening, and phase inversion, may be investigated using various rheological techniques. Various methods may be applied such as measurements of shear stress as a function of shear rate (steady state), strain as a function of time at a constant applied stress (creep), and oscillatory techniques. The principle of each of these methods will be briefly described. In addition, the properties of the interfacial film (polymeric surfactant) can be studied from investigations of the interfacial rheology of the film such as its viscosity and elasticity. Again, the principles of these measurements will be described. As we will see later, interfacial rheological investigations provide fundamental understanding of the various breakdown processes in emulsions such as thinning and disruption of liquid films and coalescence of droplets.

At an applied level, study of the rheology of emulsions is vital in many industrial applications of personal care products. It is useful to summarize the factors that affect emulsion rheology in a qualitative way. One of the most important factors is the volume fraction of the disperse phase, ϕ. In very dilute emulsions ($\phi < 0.01$), the relative viscosity, η_r, of the system may be related to ϕ using the simple Einstein equation (as for solid/liquid dispersions) (15); i.e.,

$$\eta_r = 1 + 2.5\phi \tag{15,20}$$

As the volume fraction of the emulsion is gradually increased, the relative viscosity becomes a more complex function of ϕ and it is convenient to use a polynomial representing the variation of η_r with ϕ; i.e.,

$$\eta_r = 1 + k_1\phi + k_2\phi^2 + k_3\phi^3 + \cdots \tag{21}$$

where k_1 is the Einstein coefficient (which is equal to 2.5 for hard spheres), k_2 is a coefficient that accounts for hydrodynamic interaction between the droplets, which arises from the overlap of the associated flow patterns and their eventual overlap at appreciable ϕ values (16); k_2 is equal to 6.2. The hydrodynamic interaction term is usually sufficient to describe the viscosity of dispersions up to $\phi = 0.2$. Above this volume fraction, higher-order interaction terms (k_3, ϕ^3) are necessary. As will be seen later, only semiempirical equations are available to describe the variation of η_r with ϕ over a wide range.

Another factor that may affect the rheology of emulsions is the viscosity of the disperse droplets. This is particularly the case when the viscosity of the droplets is comparable to or lower than that of the dispersions medium. This problem was considered by Taylor (17), who extended the Einstein hydrodynamic treatment for suspensions for the case of droplets in a liquid medium. Taylor (17) assumed that the emulsifier film around the droplets would not prevent the transmission of tangential and normal stresses form the continuous phase to the disperse phase and that there was no slippage at the o/w interface. These stresses produce fluid circulation within the droplets, which reduces the flow patterns around them. Taylor derived the following expression for η_r:

$$\eta_r = 1 + 2.5\left(\frac{\eta_i + 0.4\eta_o}{\eta_i + \eta_o}\right)\phi \tag{22}$$

where η_i is the viscosity of the internal phase and η_o is that of the external phase. Clearly, when $\eta_i \gg \eta_o$ (as with most o/w emulsions), the term between the brackets becomes equal to unity and Eq. 22 reduces to the Einstein equation. On the other hand, when $\eta_i \ll \eta_o$ (as with foams), the term between the brackets becomes equal to 0.4 and the Einstein coefficient becomes equal to 1. When η_i is comparable to η_o, Einstein's coefficient can assume values between 1 and 2.5 depending on the relative ratio of η_i/η_o. However, this analysis assumed a deformable droplet, which may not be the case when a surfactant or polymer film is present at the interface. In this case, interfacial tension gradients and/or surface viscosity will make these droplets appear as hard spheres and the emulsion behaves in a similar way to a solid/liquid dispersion.

The third factor that affects emulsion rheology is the droplet size distribution. This is particularly the case at high-volume fractions. When $\phi > 0.6$, η_r is inversely proportional to the reciprocal of the mean droplet diameter (18). The above equations do not show any dependence on droplet size and an account should be made for this effect by considering the average distance between the droplets in an emulsion. At high shear rate, the droplets are completely deflocculated (i.e., all structure is destroyed) and they are equidistant from each other. At a critical distance of separation between the droplets, which depends on droplet size, the viscosity shows a rapid increase. The average distance of separation between the droplets, h_m, is related to the droplet diameter, d_m, by the simple expression

$$h_m = d_m\left[\left(\frac{\phi_{max}}{\phi}\right)^{1/3} - 1\right] \tag{23}$$

where ϕ_{max} is the maximum packing fraction that is equal to 0.74 for hexagonally packed monodisperse spheres. With most emulsions, ϕ_{max} reaches a higher value than 0.74 as a result of polydispersity. Equation 23 indicates that with small droplets the critical value of h_m is reached at lower ϕ values than with larger droplets.

Several other factors that affect the rheology of emulsions may be considered that are related to the properties of the continuous phase and the interfacial film. Three main properties of the continuous phase may be considered. The first and most important is the viscosity of the medium, which is affected by the additives present such as excess emulsifier and thickeners (e.g., polysaccharides) that are added in many personal care emulsions to prevent sedimentation or creaming as well as to produce the right consistency for application. The second property of the medium that affects emulsion rheology is the chemical composition such as polarity and pH, which affects the charge on the droplets and hence their repulsion. The viscosity of the emulsion is directly related to the magnitude of the repulsive forces. The latter are also affected by the nature and concentration of electrolyte in the system, which represent the third important property of the medium. The influences of charge and repulsion between droplets in an emulsion are sometimes referred to as electroviscous effects. Two such effects may be distinguished. The first electroviscous effect arises from distortion of the double layers around the droplets as the latter are sheared. This effect is very small and it contributes a small increase in the relative viscosity. However, the secondary electroviscous effect arises from overlap of the double layers, which becomes significant in concentrated emulsions. The magnitude of the secondary electroviscous effect is proportional to ϕ^2. Thus, this effect can cause a large increase in the viscosity of the system. It is clear that by addition of electrolytes, the double layers are compressed, resulting in a large reduction of the electrosviscous effects. This could find application in many practical systems, where a high viscosity is undesirable.

The rheology of emulsions may also be influenced by the interfacial rheology of the emulsifier film surrounding the droplets. When shear is applied to an interfacial film, its constituent molecules as well as the molecules of the oil and water phases in its immediate vicinity are displaced from their equilibrium positions (19). The stress that develops depends on the associated molecular rearrangement. This will have an effect on the interfacial viscosity of the film, η_s, and affect the bulk rheology of the emulsion, if the latter is formed from large, deformable droplets. The viscosity of an emulsion in which the drops deform under shear increases more rapidly with ϕ than that with emulsions of identical size but surrounded by an elastic film that prevents deformation. Clearly, when the droplets are very small, deformation is less likely and the effect of interfacial rheology becomes less significant. In some cases the chemical nature of the emulsifier has an effect on the relative viscosity, particularly at high ϕ values. This has been demonstrated by Sherman (20) for food emulsions prepared using emulsifiers of different chemical nature. The nature and concentration of emulsifier can also have a dramatic effect or emulsion phase inversion (21,22). An excess emulsifier will have a pronounced effect on the viscosity of the continuous phase, resulting in an increase in the overall viscosity of the system. Under these conditions phase inversion may occur at relatively lower disperse volume fraction when compared with that at lower emulsifier concentration. The nature of the emulsifier, in particular its solubility and distribution in both phases also has a large effect on the rheology of the system. Unfortunately, there are no systematic studies of these effects on the rheology of emulsions.

Many personal care emulsions and creams are complex systems that are formulated to behave like "semisolids," being solid-like under ambient conditions and becoming transformed to a liquid-like consistency when stressed during application to the skin (23). The dominant colloidal structural elements of these semisolid preparations are three-dimensional colloidal solid networks in which a liquid is incorporated. Such a bicoherent (sponge-like) structure may be referred to as a gel. These gel structures may be in either a crystalline or liquid crystalline state whose properties are determined by the bulk rheology of the system. The bulk rheology is in turn determined by the structure of the liquid crystalline phases produced, which may be established using low-angle X-ray and freeze fracture techniques (23). The structure of the system and its rheological properties also determine the stability, interaction with the skin, and ingredient release.

VIII. INTERFACIAL RHEOLOGY

Interfacial rheology deals with the response of mobile interfaces to deformation (24). Emulsions contain a molecular or macromolecular surfactant film at the fluid interface, which, apart from being necessary for the stabilization of the dispersion, also initiates additional interfacial stresses beyond that stress already contributed by a homogeneous interfacial tension, γ. If a nonuniformity of surfactant concentration develops within the fluid interface, an interfacial tension gradient $d\gamma/dA$, where A is the interfacial area, is produced. This gradient is sometimes defined by the Gibbs elasticity, ε, which is simply equal to $d\gamma/d \ln A$, which induces both areal and volumetric liquid motion. The gradient-driven flow is the basis of the so-called "Marangoni effect." In addition to the possible existence of these interfacial tension gradients, other interfacial rheological stresses of a viscous nature may arise, such as those relating to interfacial shear and dilational viscosities (25). Many surfactant and polymer films also exhibit non-Newtonian interfacial rheological behavior that may be characterized by Bingham plastic models and interfacial viscoelasticity. Below a summary of the basic equations needed to describe the above-mentioned interfacial rheological parameters is given, followed by a brief description of some of the essential techniques required to measure interfacial rheology. Finally, some results will be given to correlate interfacial rheology with emulsion stability.

A. Basic Equations for Interfacial Rheology

The interfacial shear viscosity, η_s, is the ratio between the shear stress, σ, and shear rate, $\dot{\gamma}$, in the plane of the interface; i.e., it is a two-dimensional viscosity. The unit for surface viscosity is, therefore, $Nm^{-1}s$ (surface Pas). A liquid-liquid (or liquid-vapor) interface with no adsorbed surfactant or polymer shows only a negligible interfacial shear viscosity. However, in the presence of an adsorbed surfactant or polymer layer, an appreciable interfacial shear viscosity is obtained (which can be orders of magnitude higher than the bulk viscosity of the film). This appreciable shear viscosity can be accounted for in terms of the orientation of the surfactant or polymer molecules at the interface. For example, surfactant molecules at the o/w interface usually form a monolayer of vertically oriented molecules with the hydrophobic portion pointing to (or dissolved in) the oil, leaving the polar head groups pointing in the aqueous phase. A two-dimensional surface pressure, π, may be defined; i.e.,

$$\pi = \gamma_o - \gamma \tag{24}$$

where γ_o is the interfacial tension of the clean interface (i.e., before adsorption of surfactant or polymer) and γ is the corresponding value with the adsorbed film. Since γ_o is of the order of 30–50 mNm^{-1}, whereas γ can reach values as low as a fraction of a mNm^{-1} unit, it is clear that π can be high, reaching values of the order of 30–50 mNm^{-1}. Thus, any shear field applied across the interface containing these adsorbed surfactants or polymers (with high surface pressure) results in a large viscous interaction between adjacent molecules. With macromolecules that form loops and tails at the interface (11), the film resists compression as a result of the lateral repulsion between the loops and tails.

The interfacial dilational elasticity, ε, results from the presence of interfacial tension gradients due to inhomogeneous surfactant or polymer films. The regions that are depleted from the film have higher interfacial tension than those containing the adsorbed film. As a result, an interfacial tension gradient $d\gamma/dA$ is set and the Gibbs dilational elasticity may be defined as

$$\varepsilon = \frac{d\gamma}{d\ ln\ A} \tag{25}$$

The above situation may arise during emulsification or on approach of two emulsion droplets. As the interface is stretched, the film will no longer cover the whole interface and regions depleted from surfactant or polymer are created. This results in interfacial tension gradients and surfactant or polymer molecules tend to diffuse from the bulk to the interface to fill these depleted regions. During this process, liquid may be transported to the interface, a phenomenon usually referred to as the ''Marangoni'' effect (26). This Gibbs-Marangoni effect is sometimes believed to be the driving force for stabilization of thin liquid films between droplets, thus preventing their coalescence.

The interfacial dilational viscosity: η_s^d can be simply defined if one considers a uniform expansion of the interface at a constant-rate $d\ ln\ A/dt$; i.e.,

$$\eta_s^d = \frac{d\gamma}{dln\ Adt} \tag{26}$$

As mentioned above, interfacial films exhibit non-Newtonian flow, which can be treated in the same manner as for dispersions and polymer solutions. The steady-state flow can be described using Bingham plastic models. The viscoelastic behavior can be treated using stress relaxation or strain relaxation (creep) models as well as dynamic (oscillatory) models. The Bingham-fluid model of interfacial rheological behavior (27) assumes the presence of a surface yield stress, σ_s; i.e.,

$$\sigma = \sigma_s + \eta_s\dot{\gamma} \tag{27}$$

In stress relaxation experiments, a sudden strain is applied on the film, within a short period of time, and the stress σ followed as a function of time. If $\sigma(t)$ is the stress at time t and σ_o is the instantaneous value at the moment when the constant strain γ is applied, then,

$$ln \frac{\sigma(t)}{\sigma_o} = \frac{t}{t_r} \tag{28}$$

where t_r is the relaxation time that is given by the ratio η/G, where G is the relaxation modulus.

In strain relaxation (creep) experiments, a small constant stress is applied on the film and the strain or compliance J (where $J = \gamma/\sigma$) is followed as a function of time. The compliance at any time t, $J(t)$, is given by the expression

$$J(t) = \frac{\left[1 - \exp\left(-\frac{t}{t_r}\right)\right]}{G} \tag{29}$$

In dynamic (oscillatory) experiments, the stress or strain is varied periodically with a sinusoidal alteration at a frequency ω (rad/sec) and the resulting strain or stress is compared with the applied values. For a viscoelastic material, the stress and strain show a time shift Δt between the sine waves of the stress and strain. The product of this time shift and the frequency ω gives the phase angle shift δ (note that for a viscoelastic material $0 < \delta < 90°$). The amplitude ratio of stress and strain gives the complex modulus G^*, which is split into two components through the phase angle shift δ: the in-phase component G' (the real part of the complex modulus, referred to as the storage or elastic modulus) and the out-of-phase component G'' (the imaginary part of the complex modulus, referred to as the loss of viscous modulus); i.e.,

$$G' = |G^*| \cos \delta \tag{30}$$

$$G'' = |G^*| \sin \delta \tag{31}$$

and

$$|G^*| = G' + iG'' \tag{32}$$

The dilational modulus ε^*, for a sinusoidally oscillating surface dilation, can also be split into in-phase (referred to as the dilational elasticity) and out-of-phase components; i.e.,

$$|\varepsilon^*| = \varepsilon' + i\varepsilon'' \tag{33}$$

B. Basic Principles of Measurement of Interfacial Rheology

The simplest procedure to measure the interfacial shear viscosity is to use a torsion pendulum surface viscometer (28). In this technique, the damping of a torsion pendulum due to the viscous drag of a surface film is observed. The shearing element can be in the form of a ring, a disc, or a knife-edged disc, which is suspended by a torsion wire and positioned at the place of the interface, as shown in Figure 7. Measurements are made of the period of the pendulum and the damping as the pendulum oscillates. The apparent surface viscosity, η_s, is given by the expression

$$\eta_s = \eta_o\left(\frac{\Delta/\Delta_o}{t/t_o} - 1\right) \tag{34}$$

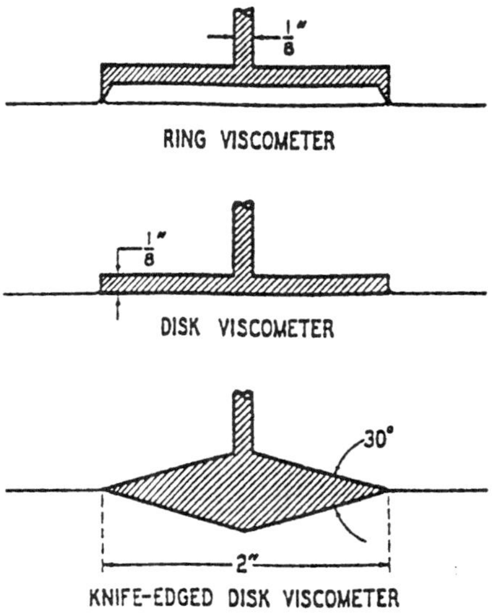

Figure 7 Surface viscometer designs.

where η_o is the sum of the bulk viscosities of the two phases forming the interface. Δ is the difference in logarithm of the amplitude of successive swings for the interface with adsorbed surfactant or polymer and Δ_o is the corresponding value without film. t is the period of the pendulum for the film-covered interface and t_o the corresponding value without film.

The surface viscosity may be related to the torsion modulus of the wire, C_w, the polar moment of inertia of the oscillating pendulum, I, and the dimensions of the viscometer by the expression (28)

$$\eta_s = \frac{C_w I}{2\pi} \frac{R_2^2 - R_1^2}{R_1^2 R_2^2} \left[\frac{\Delta}{7.4 + \Delta^2} - \frac{\Delta_0}{7.4 + \Delta_o} \right] \tag{35}$$

where R_1 is the radius of the surface viscometer and R_2 is the radius of the container.

One of the main drawbacks of the torsion pendulum viscometer is that it uses a range of shear rates and hence it is not suitable for measurement of non-Newtonian films. In the latter case, it is preferable to use the rotational torsional viscometer. The surface film is sheared between rotating concentric rings on a surface. The shear rate can be held constant by rotating one ring, while measuring the torque T on the other ring (28); i.e.,

$$\eta_s = \frac{T}{4\pi\Omega} \frac{R_2^2 - R_1^2}{R_1^2 R_2^2} + \frac{\sigma_s}{\Omega} \ln \frac{R_2}{R_1} \tag{36}$$

where Ω is the angular velocity.

Another convenient method for measuring the interfacial shear viscosity is to use the deep-channel surface viscometer (25), shown schematically in Figure 8. Basically it consists of two concentric brass cylinders (separated by a distance y_o) lowered into a pool of liquid contained within a brass dish, to a depth at which the brass cylinders nearly touch the bottom of the dish. The dish is rotated with a known angular velocity, ω_o, and the midchannel or "centerline" surface motion of the interface within the channel (formed

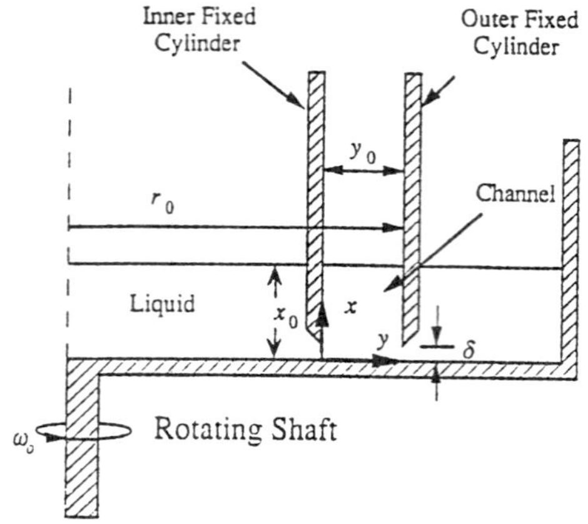

Figure 8 The deep-channel surface viscometer.

by the concentric cylinders) is measured using talc or teflon particles placed within the fluid interface; i.e.,

$$\frac{\eta_s \pi}{\eta y_o} = \frac{v_c^*}{v_c} - 1 \tag{37}$$

where η is the bulk shear viscosity, v_c^* is the center-line surface velocity in the presence of the film, and v_c is the corresponding value in the absence of the film.

Three techniques may be applied for measurement of the dilational surface elasticity and viscosity (25). The first method applies surface waves to the interface (with frequency ω). The dilational elasticity, ε', is given by the expression

$$\varepsilon' = \frac{\varepsilon_o[1 + (\tau/\omega)^{1/2}]}{[1 + 2(\tau/\omega)^{1/2} + 2(\tau/\omega)]} \tag{38}$$

where ε_o is the Gibbs elasticity and τ is a ''diffusion parameter'' that is related to the diffusion coefficient D of the surfactant molecule.

The relaxation elasticity, ε'', is given by the expression

$$\varepsilon'' = -\frac{\varepsilon_o(\tau/\omega)^{1/2}}{[1 + 2(\tau/\omega)^{1/2} + 2(\tau/\omega)]} \tag{39}$$

The tangential bulk-phase stress component evaluated at the interface combines an elastic (interfacial tension gradient) effect, ε', and an apparent viscous effect, $(\eta_s^d + \eta_s) + \varepsilon''/\omega$. One of the most convenient methods of measuring capillary waves is to use light scattering (29), which can yield information on both the tension and dilational modulus of the interface.

The second method for measuring dilational elasticity and viscosity is based on rotation, translation, or deformation of bubbles and droplets (25). Agarwal and Wasan (30) have suggested that the translational velocity of bubbles or droplets in a quiescent liquid might be used to determine the apparent dilational viscosity. Unfortunately, this simple method is not suitable since the settling velocity is not sensitive enough to assess the magnitude of the apparent surface viscosity. Wei et al. (31) suggested that measurements of the circulation velocity of a tracer particle in the equatorial plane of a spherical droplet rotating within a shear field might provide a means for deducing a combination of shear and dilational viscosities. The study of droplet shape deformation in a shear field provides another method for measuring the apparent interfacial dilational viscosity (32). Such a method was applied by Phillips et al, using the spinning drop technique.

The third method for measuring dilational elasticity and viscosity is the maximum bubble pressure method (33). Although this method overcomes some of the problems encountered in the surface wave and droplet deformational methods, it can only be applied for measurement at the air/liquid interface.

Several methods were suggested for measurement of the non-Newtonian rheological behavior of surfactant and polymer films. For example, Biswas and Haydon (34) constructed a special apparatus for measurement of the two-dimensional creep and stress relaxation of adsorbed protein films at the o/w interface. In creep experiments, a constant torque (in mNm^{-1}) was applied and the resulting deformation (in radians) was recorded as a function of time. In the stress relaxation experiments, a certain deformation γ was produced in the film by applying an initial stress, and the deformation was kept constant by gradually decreasing the stress.

The deep-channel viscometer could also be adapted for measurement of the nonlinear interfacial rheological behavior of the film (25). In this case several small tracer particles are placed on the fluid interface at different radial positions and the angular velocities are determined from measurements of the period of revolution. When used for the purpose of measuring viscoelastic properties, the deep-channel viscometer is operated in an oscillatory mode, in which mode of operation the floor of the viscometer is oscillated sinusoidally. Simultaneous measurements of the phase angle between the surface motion and the oscillating motion of the bottom dish, and the ''surface-to-floor'' amplitude ratio, may permit determination of the viscoelastic properties of the fluid interface, presuming knowledge of an appropriate rheological model (25).

C. Correlation of Interfacial Rheology with Emulsion Stability

Several examples may be quoted to illustrate the correlation between interfacial rheology and emulsion stability. One of the first observations was made by Cockbain and Roberts (35), who found that addition of an alcohol such as lauryl alcohol to an emulsion stabilized by an anionic surfactant increased the emulsion stability. This was attributed to an increase in the interfacial shear viscosity. Later, Prince et al. (36) found that the dilational elasticity of the film increased markedly in the presence of the alcohol and they, therefore, attributed the enhanced stability to such high surface elasticity. Other authors attributed the enhanced stability to a high interfacial viscosity (37), although Prince et al. (36) argued against this since they found that the film stability was not very sensitive to either temperature changes or the concentration of alcohol, which had a pronounced effect on η_s. Wasan et al. (37,38) claimed correlation between interfacial shear viscosity and emulsion stability. Among the most convincing examples of the correlation of interfacial rheology with emulsion stability are the results of Biswas and Haydon (34). These authors have systematically investigated the rheological characteristics of various proteins, namely albumin, poly (ϕ-L-lysine), and arabinic acid, at the o/w interface and correlated these measurements with stability of the oil droplets at a planar o/w interface. As mentioned above, the viscoelastic properties of the adsorbed films were studied using creep and stress relaxation measurements. Figure 9 shows a typical creep curve for bovine serum albumin at the petroleum ether/water interface. The curve shows an initial, instantaneous deformation characteristic of an elastic

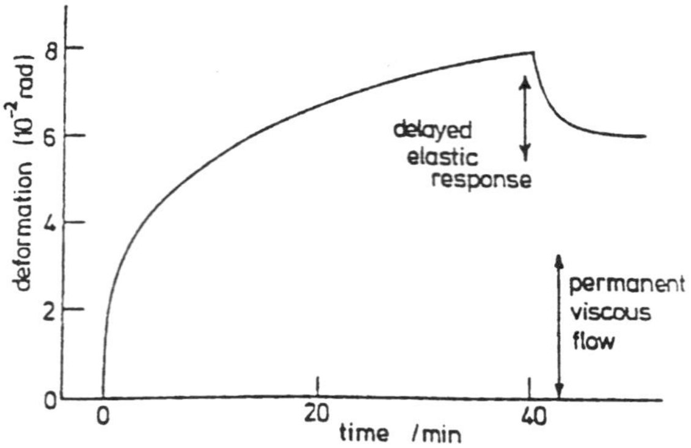

Figure 9 Creep curve of an adsorbed bovine serum albumin film (pH = 5.2) at a petroleum ether/water interface, at a constant stress of 0.0116 Nm^{-1}.

body, followed by a nonlinear flow that gradually declines and approaches the steady state of a viscous body. After 30 min, when the external force was withdrawn, the film tended to revert toward its initial state, with an initial instantaneous recovery followed by a slow one. The original state was not obtained even after 20 hr, and the film seemed to have undergone some irreversible flow. This behavior illustrates the viscoelastic properties of the bovine serum albumin.

Biswas and Haydon (34) also found a striking effect of pH on the rigidity of the protein film. This is illustrated in Figure 10, where the shear modulus G and surface viscosity η_s are plotted as a function of pH. The elasticity of the film is seen to be at a maximum at the isoelectric point of the protein. Biswas and Haydon (34) then measured the rate of coalescence of petroleum ether drops at a planar o/w interface by measuring the lifetime of a droplet resting beneath the interface. The half-life of the droplets was plotted as a function of pH, as shown in Figure 10, which clearly illustrates the correlation with G and η_s. Biswas and Haydon (34) derived an equation relating the time of coales-

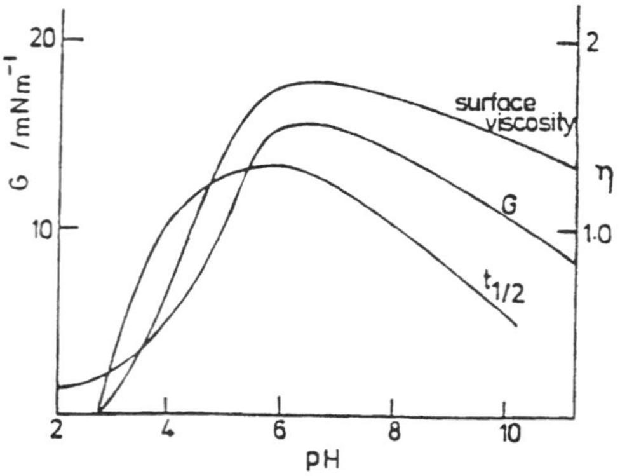

Figure 10 Shear modulus, surface viscosity, and half-life of petroleum ether drops beneath a plane petroleum ether/0.1 mol/dm^3 aqueous KCl interface, as a function of pH.

cence τ with the viscoelasticity of the film, the thickness of the adsorbed film h, and the critical distortion of the plane interface under the weight of the drop; i.e.,

$$\tau = \eta_s \left[3C' \frac{h^2}{A} - \frac{1}{G} - \phi(t) \right] \tag{40}$$

where G is the (instantaneous) elasticity, η_s is the long-time viscosity (i.e., for an infinite time of retardation), $\phi(t)$ is the elastic deformation per unit stress, and $3C'$ is a critical deformation factor. Equation 40 predicts that: (1) the lifetime of the drop, τ, increases with increase of the viscosity of the protective film; (2) the rate process of coalescence is not influenced by the instantaneous elasticity, but this parameter is likely to set a limit on the process through the critical deformation factor $3C'$; (3) the lifetime should depend on the film thickness and vary linearly with h^2 if the retarded elasticity $\phi(t)$ is neglected; (4) τ should be a fixed but not a fluctuated quantity.

The results of Biswas and Haydon (34) indicate clearly that no significant stabilization occurred in the case of nonviscoelastic films. However, the presence of viscoelasticity is not sufficient to confer stability when drainage is rapid. For example, it was found that the highly viscoelastic films of bovine serum albumin or pepsin could not stabilize w/o emulsions; the same was found with pectin and gum arabic. It was clear that in these cases the drainage was rapid even from rigid films, e.g., w/o droplets in the case of bovine serum albumin. In fact, as expected, it was only after solvent drainage had taken place, and the disperse phases were still separated by a film of high viscosity, that enhanced stabilization occurred. It was concluded from these investigations that, in agreement with the prediction of theory, the requirement for stability against coalescence was the presence of a film with appreciable thickness. It was also necessary that the main part of the film be located on the continuous side of the interface.

Several other examples may be found in the literature, in which a correlation between the interfacial viscosity of macromolecular stabilized films with droplet stability was found. However, there are also a number of cases where stable emulsions could be prepared without any significant interfacial viscosity or elasticity. It can be concluded, therefore, that one should be careful in using interfacial rheology as a predictive test for emulsion stability. Other factors, such as film drainage and thickness, may be more important. In spite of these limitations, interfacial rheology offers a powerful tool for understanding the properties of surfactant and macromolecular films at the liquid/liquid interface. In cases where a correlation between the interfacial viscosity and/or elasticity and emulsion stability is found, one could use these measurements to screen various other components that have a marked effect on these parameters.

IX. INVESTIGATIONS OF BULK RHEOLOGY OF EMULSION SYSTEMS

As discussed in the introduction, the bulk rheology of emulsion systems can be investigated using steady-state (shear stress as a function of shear rate), constant stress, and oscillatory techniques. These methods are the same as those described for interfacial rheology. In this section, some results on various emulsion systems will be described to illustrate the use of rheological measurements in investigating the interaction between emulsion droplets. First, the viscosity-volume fraction relationship for o/w and w/o emulsions will be discussed to show the analogy with suspensions. This is then followed by a section on the viscoelastic properties of concentrated emulsions. The third section will deal with the case of flocculated emulsions, which may be produced, for example, by the addition of a "free" (nonadsorbing) polymer or by van der Waals attraction.

A. Viscosity-Volume Fraction Relationship for o/w and w/o Emulsions

The relative viscosity (η_r)–volume fraction (ϕ) curves for paraffin oil/water emulsions are shown in Figure 11. Four emulsion systems were prepared using nonionic surfactants, namely Synperonic NPE 1800 and its analogs (39). These surfactants have the following structural formula: $C_9H_{19}—C_6H_5—(CH_2—CH(CH_3)—O)_m—(CH_2—CH_2—O)_n—OH$. They all contain the same hydrophobic chain (nonyl phenyl and 13 moles propylene oxide), but have different moles of ethylene oxide: 27 for Synperonic NPE 1800, 48 for NPE A, 80 for NPE B, and 174 for NPE C. The average droplet diameter for each emulsion was determined using the Coulter Counter, and the volume mean diameter (VMD) is given in the legend of Figure 11. The molecular weight (M_w and hydrodynamic thickness (δ_h) of these surfactant molecules was determined before and the results were as follows:

	Synperonic NPE 1800	NPE A	NPE B	NPE C
M_w	2180	3080	4460	8650
δ_h(nm)	5.8	6.4	8.5	11.6

The above emulsion system is fairly simple, since it is likely that the nonyl phenyl and propylene oxide chain is on the oil side of the interface, whereas the poly(ethylene oxide) chain is on the aqueous side of the interface. The hydrodynamic thickness of the surfactants, given above, is much smaller than the droplet radius and hence these sterically stabilized emulsions may approximate hard-sphere dispersions very closely (with an effective radius $R_{eff} = R + \delta_h$). This can be tested by fitting the data to the hard-sphere model suggested by Dougherty and Krieger (40,41).

By application of the theory of corresponding states, these authors derived the following equation for the relative viscosity:

$$\eta_r = \left[1 - \left(\frac{\phi}{\phi_p}\right)\right]^{-[\eta]\phi_p} \tag{41}$$

where [η] is the intrinsic viscosity, which has a theoretical value of 2.5 for rigid spheres, and ϕ_p is the maximum packing fraction, which is equal to 0.64 for random packing and 0.74 for hexagonal close packing of monodisperse spheres. However, Krieger (41) showed that, with hard-sphere dispersions, ϕ_p is close to 0.6. Since the emulsions are polydisperse, a higher value for ϕ_p is to be expected. The value of ϕ_p for each emulsion was estimated from plots of $\eta^{-1/2}$ versus ϕ, which gave a straight line. Extrapolation to $\eta^{-1/2} = 0$ (i.e., $\eta = \infty$) gave ϕ_p. The values obtained were 0.73, 0.73, 0.79, and 0.69 for Synperonic NPE 1800, NPE A, NPE B, and NPE C, respectively. Using the calculated ϕ_p values, plots of η_r were constructed. These are shown in Figure 11. It can be seen from these results that

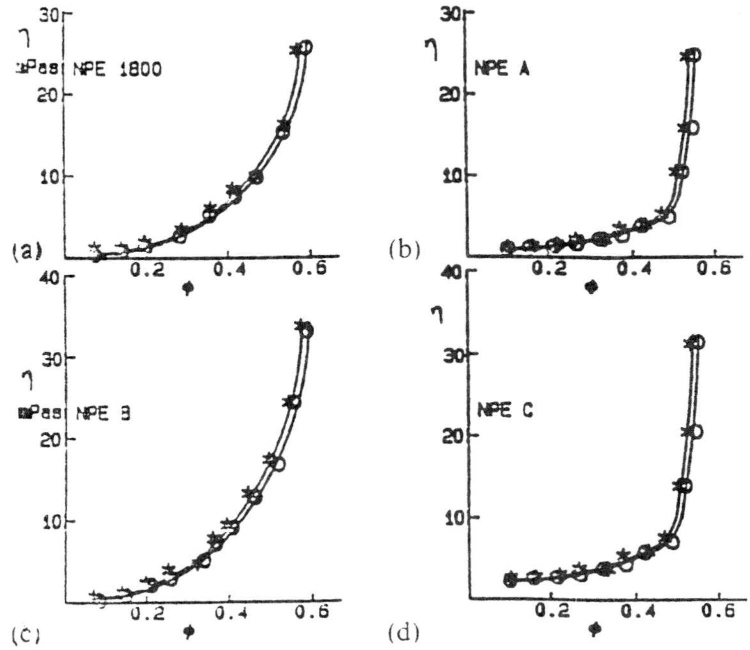

Figure 11 $\eta_r - \phi$ curves for paraffin oil/water emulsions. (a) Synperonic NPE 1800, VMD = 3.5 μm; (b) NPE A, VMD = 4 μm; (c) NPE B, VMD = 4.5 μm; (d) NPE C, VMD = 5 μm. (x) Experimental results; (o) theoretical values according to the Dougherty-Krieger equation.

the emulsions stabilized with the Synperonic NPE surfactants closely approximate hard-sphere dispersions.

The relative viscosity-volume fraction curve for water-in-oil emulsions (42) is shown in Figure 12. Isoparaffinic oil (Isopar M) was used in this case and the emulsions were prepared using an A-B-A block copolymer of PHS-PEO-PHS (Arlacel P135, supplied by ICI; PHS refers to poly-12-hydroxystearic acid and PEO refers to polyethylene oxide).

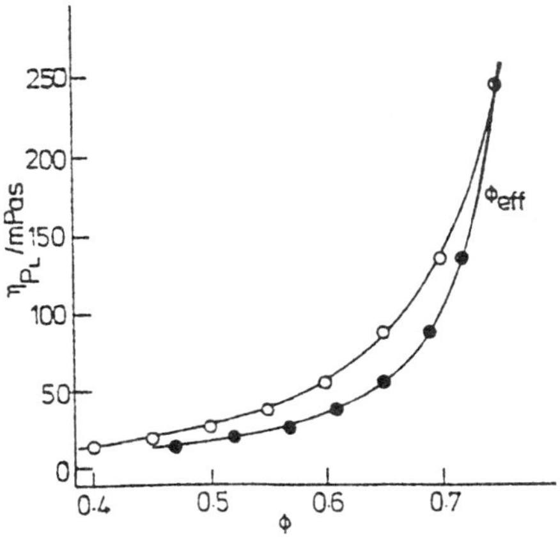

Figure 12 Viscosity-volume fraction curve for w/o emulsions.

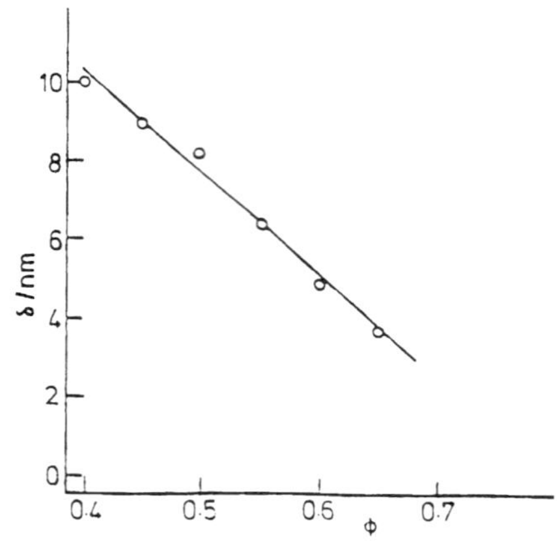

Figure 13 Variation of δ with ϕ.

The weight-average molecular weight of the polymer is 6809; its number-average value is 3499. The emulsion had a narrow size distribution with a z-average radius R of 183 nm, as determined by photon correlation spectroscopy. As shown before (43), the viscosity-volume faction curve may be used to obtain the adsorbed layer thickness as a function of ϕ. Assuming that the w/o emulsions behave like near-hard-sphere dispersions, it is possible to apply the Dougherty-Krieger equation (40,41) to obtain the effective volume fraction. Using Eq. 41, ϕ_{eff} can be calculated from η_r provided a reasonable estimate can be made of $[\eta]$ and ϕ_p. $[\eta]$ was taken to be equal to 2.5, whereas ϕ_p was estimated from a plot of $\eta^{-1/2}$ versus ϕ, as described above. ϕ_p was found to be 0.84, which is a reasonable value considering the polydispersity of the emulsions. Figure 12 shows the ϕ_{eff} values. From ϕ_{eff} and ϕ, the adsorbed layer thickness, δ, was calculate using the following expression:

$$\phi_{eff} = \phi\left[1 + \left(\frac{\delta}{R}\right)\right]^3 \tag{42}$$

A plot of δ versus ϕ is shown in Figure 13. It can be seen that δ decreases linearly with increase in ϕ. The value at $\phi = 0.4$ in 10 nm, which is a measure of the fully extended PHS chain. At such relatively low ϕ, there will be no interpenetration of the PHS chains since the distance between the droplets is relatively large. This value of δ obtained from rheology is in close agreement with the results obtained from thin-liquid film measurements between two water droplets (44). It is also in close agreement with the results obtained by Ottewill and co-workers (45,46) using compression cells and small-angle neutron scattering. The decrease in δ with increase in ϕ is similar to the results obtained using latex dispersions stabilized with grafted PEO chains (43). This reduction in δ with increase in ϕ may be attributed to the interpenetration and/or compression of the chains on increasing ϕ. If complete interpenetration is possible, the δ value can be reduced by half its value in dilute dispersions. Indeed, the results of Figure 13 show that δ is reduced to 4 nm at $\phi = 0.65$. This reduction in δ can also be attributed to compression of the chains on close approach, without the need to invoke any interpenetration. It is also probable that a combination of both mechanisms may occur on approach of the droplets in a concentrated dispersion.

B. Viscoelastic Properties of Concentrated o/w and w/o Emulsions

The viscoelastic properties of concentrated o/w and w/o emulsions were investigated using dynamic (oscillatory) measurements. For that purpose a Bohlin VOR (Bohlin Reologie, Lund, Sweden) instrument was used. Concentric cylinder platens were used and the measurements were carried out at 25 $\pm$ 0.1°C. In oscillatory measurements, the response in stress of a viscoelastic material subjected to a sinusoidally varying strain is monitored as a function of strain amplitude and frequency. The stress amplitude is also a sinusoidally varying function in time, but for a viscoelastic material it is shifted out of phase with the strain. The phase angle shift between stress and strain, δ, is given by

$$\delta = \Delta t \omega \tag{43}$$

where ω is the frequency in radians/sec ($\omega = 2\pi\nu$, where ν is the frequency in Hertz). From measurement of the angular deflection (using a transducer) and the resulting torque on the detector shaft (the inner cylinder is connected to interchangeable torque bars) used for monitoring the stress, the phase angle shift and stress and strain amplitudes (τ_o and γ_o, respectively) are determined and one can determine the following rheological parameters: G^* (the complex modulus), G' (the storage modulus), G'' (the loss modulus), and η' (the dynamic viscosity). G' is a measure of the energy stored elastically in the system (the elastic component of the complex modulus), whereas G'' is a measure of the energy dissipated as viscous flow.

In viscoelastic measurements, one measures the viscoelastic parameters as a function of strain amplitude (at a fixed frequency) to obtain the linear viscoelastic regions. The strain amplitude is gradually increased from the smallest possible value at which a measurement can be made and the rheological parameters are monitored as a function of γ_o. Initially the rheological parameters remain virtually constant and independent of the strain amplitude. However, above a critical value of strain amplitude (referred to as γ_{cr}), the rheological parameters show a change with further increase in γ_o. G^* and G' show a decrease with increase in γ_o above γ_{cr}, whereas G'' usually shows an increase. This behavior is attributed to the effect of strain amplitude on the structure of the concentrated dispersion. At $\gamma_o < \gamma_{cr}$, the structure of the concentrated dispersion is not perturbed, whereas at $\gamma_o > \gamma_{cr}$, some breakdown of the structure may occur. For example, in a flocculated system, some flocs are broken down above γ_{cr}. Similarly, for a stable dispersion, the regular arrangement of the particles in the system is disturbed above γ_{cr}. It is therefore necessary to carry out the viscoelastic measurements in the linear region (i.e., at $\gamma_o < \gamma_{cr}$) to obtain information on the structure of the system without any appreciable perturbation of that structure. Once the linear region is established, measurements are made as a function of frequency. By fixing the frequency range, while changing the parameters of the system, such as its volume fraction, solvency of the medium for the stabilizing chains, etc., one can obtain information of the interparticle interaction in the concentrated dispersion (47). This is illustrated in Figure 14.

Figure 14 shows typical plots of G^*, G', G'', and η' as a function of frequency (Hz) for an isoparaffinic o/w emulsion (48) with $\phi = 0.6$, which is stabilized using an ABA block copolymer of PEO-PPO-PEO (Synperonic PE), with an average of 47.3 polypropylene oxide (PPO) units and 41.6 polyethyleneoxide (PEO) units. The volume mean diameter of the droplets was 0.98 μm (as determined by the Coulter Counter). It can be seen from Figure 14 that below a certain frequency $G'' > G'$, whereas above that frequency

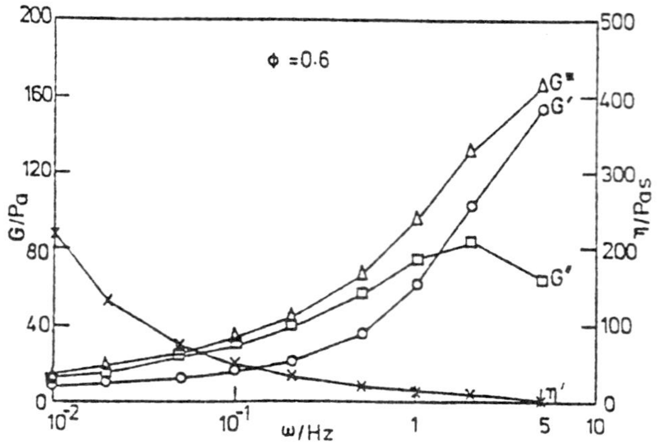

Figure 14 Variation of G^*, G', G'', and η' with frequency (Hz) for an o/w emulsion; $\phi = 0.6$.

$G' > G''$. This behavior is typical of a viscoelastic system. In the low-frequency regime, the system shows more viscous than elastic response, since in this region (relatively long time scale) the energy dissipation is relatively greater than the elastic energy stored in the system. In the high-frequency regime (relatively short time scale), this energy dissipation is not significant and the system stores most of the energy showing a predominantly elastic response. The characteristic frequency, ω^* (rad/sec) at which $G' = G''$ (the crossover point), is related to the relaxation time of the system; i.e., $t_r = l/\omega$. Thus by carrying out oscillatory measurements as a function of frequency at various volume fractions, one can obtain the variation of relaxation time with ϕ. As expected, ω^* shifts to lower frequency values as ϕ increases; i.e., t_r increases with increase in ϕ. This is illustrated in Figure 15, which clearly shows the rapid increase in t_r with ϕ, when the latter exceeds 0.54. This increase in relaxation time is the result of the strong elastic interaction between the droplets, which increases in magnitude with increase in ϕ. In addition, on increasing ϕ, the diffusion coefficient of the droplets decreases. Both effects result in an increase in t_r.

The above trend is also observed if G^*, G', and G'' are plotted versus ϕ. This is illustrated in Figure 16 for the above emulsions at a frequency of 2 Hz. At $\phi < 0.56$, $G'' > G'$, whereas at $\phi > 0.56$, $G' > G''$. This reflects the increase in steric interaction with increase in ϕ. At $\phi < 0.56$, the droplet-droplet separation is probably larger than twice the adsorbed layer thickness and hence the adsorbed layer are not forced to overlap or compress. In this case, the repulsive interaction between the adsorbed layers is relatively weak and the emulsion shows a predominantly viscous response. However, when $\phi >$ 0.56, the droplet-droplet separation may become smaller than twice the adsorbed layer thickness and the chains are forced to interpenetrate and/or compress. This leads to strong steric repulsion and the emulsion shows predominantly elastic response. The higher the ϕ value, the smaller the distance between the droplets and the stronger the steric interaction. This explains the rapid increase in G' as ϕ increases above 0.56 and the progressively larger value of G' relative to G''.

Similar results were obtained for w/o emulsions stabilized by the ABA block of PHS-PEO-PHS (42). Figure 17 shows the variation of relaxation time t^* with ϕ, whereas Figure 18 shows the variation of G' and G'' (at $\omega = 1$ Hz) with ϕ. Figure 17 shows that t^* increases rapidly with increase in ϕ, when the latter is greater than 0.67. As mentioned

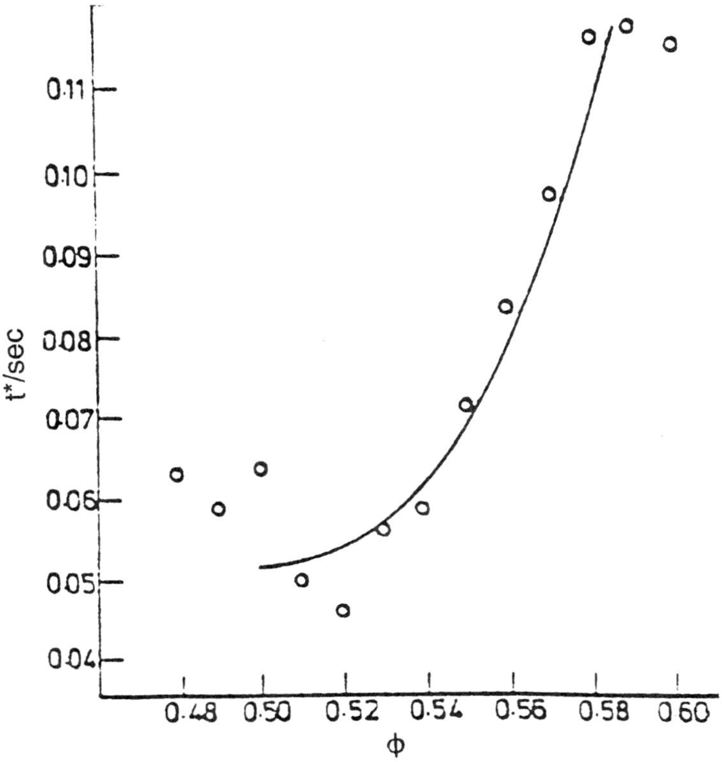

Figure 15 Variation of t_r with ϕ for an o/w emulsion.

above, this is the result of reduction in diffusion coefficient of the droplets and increase in steric repulsion as the surface-to-surface separation between the droplets becomes smaller than twice the adsorbed layer thickness. The results of Figure 17 also show a transition from predominantly viscous to predominantly elastic response as ϕ exceeds 0.67. This is a direct manifestation of the strong elastic interaction that occurs at and above this critical ϕ. Comparison of the results obtained using o/w versus w/o emulsions shows that the critical volume fraction, ϕ_{cr}, at which the emulsion shows a change from predominantly viscous to predominantly elastic response is higher for w/o emulsions than for o/w water emulsions. Both systems are polydisperse and the difference in droplet size distribution is unlikely to be the cause of this difference. The most likely reason is the difference in interaction between the two systems. With the w/o system, such interaction is short range and is governed by the adsorbed layer thickness, which, as mentioned above, is of the order of 5–10 nm depending on the volume fraction. The PHS chains in this case are in a medium of low permittivity (~2 for isoparaffinic oil) and there will be no contribution from double layers. The o/w emulsions, on the other hand, are stabilized by PEO and these chains are in an aqueous medium with a high permittivity (~78 for water). The PEO chains are relatively short (41.6 units for two A chains, i.e., ~21 EO units per chain) and, therefore, the adsorbed layer thickness is not large (probably at most of the order of 5 nm). However, in this case there will be some contribution from double-layer repulsion (since no electrolyte was added to the system) and the interaction is longer range when compared to that of the w/o system.

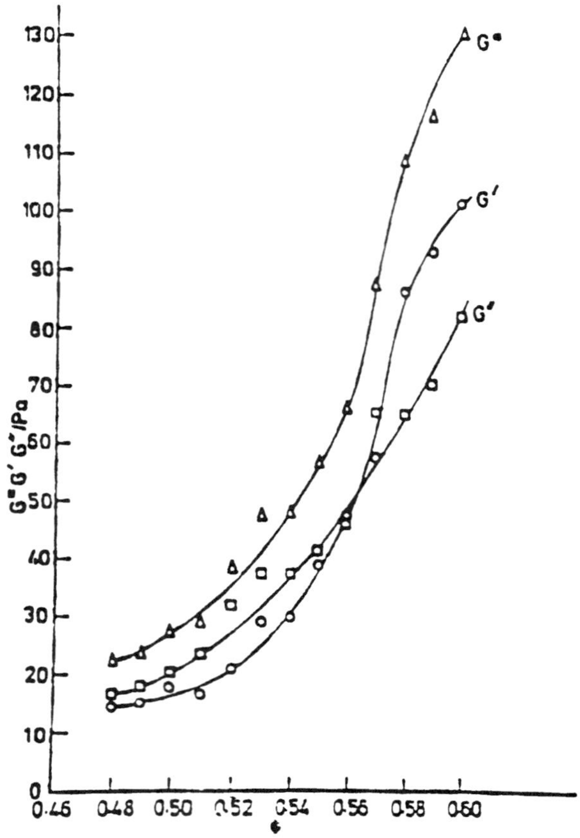

Figure 16 Variation of G^*, G', and G'' with ϕ (at w = 2 Hz) for an o/w emulsion.

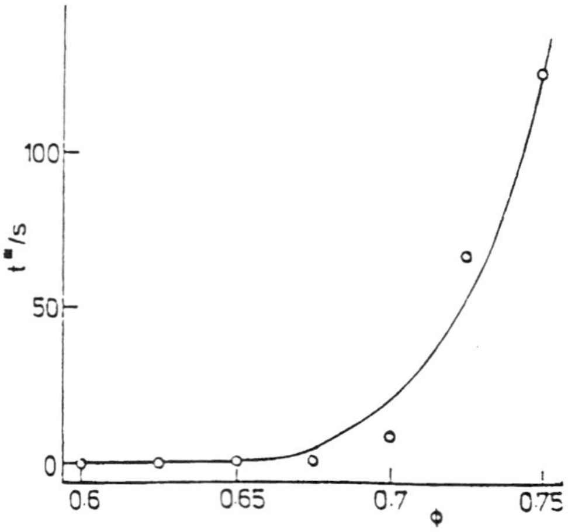

Figure 17 Variation of t* with ϕ for w/o emulsions.

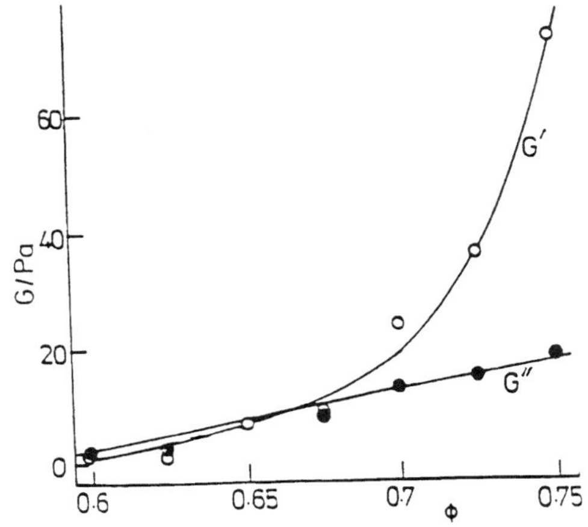

Figure 18 Variation of G' and G'' with ϕ for w/o emulsions.

The effect of droplet size and its distribution on the adsorbed layer thickness may be inferred from a comparison of the results obtained with the o/w emulsions with those recently obtained using polystyrene latex dispersions containing grafted PEO chains of (molecular weight 2000) (49). As discussed earlier, the viscoelastic behavior of the system (which reflects the steric interaction) is determined by the ratio of the adsorbed layer thickness to the particle radius (δ/R). The larger this ratio, the lower the volume fraction at which the system changes from predominantly viscous to predominantly elastic response. With relatively polydisperse systems, ϕ_{cr} shifts to higher values when compared to monodisperse systems with the same mean size.

C. Viscoelastic Properties of Weakly Flocculated Emulsions

A weakly flocculated emulsion may be produced by the addition of a "free" (nonadsorbing) polymer to a sterically stabilized emulsion. This has been illustrated by addition of PEO to an emulsion stabilized by Synperonic NPE 1800 (50). The stabilizing chain in this case is also PEO and the added "free" polymer does not adsorb on the droplets. This system is, therefore, similar to polystyrene latex with grafted PEO to which "free" PEO is added (51,52). Above a critical volume fraction of the free polymer, ϕ_p^+ (which depends on the molecular weight), flocculation of the dispersion occurs. The origin of flocculation is illustrated schematically in Figure 19. As the free polymer concentration is gradually increased, a critical concentration is reached, whereby the polymer coils can no longer fit in between the particles or droplets. In other words, the polymer coils are "squeezed out" from between the particles or droplets. This results in a polymer-free zone between the particles, and the osmotic pressure of the polymer solution outside the particles becomes higher than that in the regions between the particles (which are depleted from free polymer). This causes attraction of the particles or droplets in the dispersion, a phenomenon that is referred to as depletion flocculation. The free energy of attraction due to depletion is given by the following expression (53,54):

$$G_{dep} = 2\pi R\left(\frac{\mu_i - \mu_1^{\circ}}{v_1}\right)\Delta^2\left(1 + \frac{2\Delta}{3R}\right) \qquad (44)$$

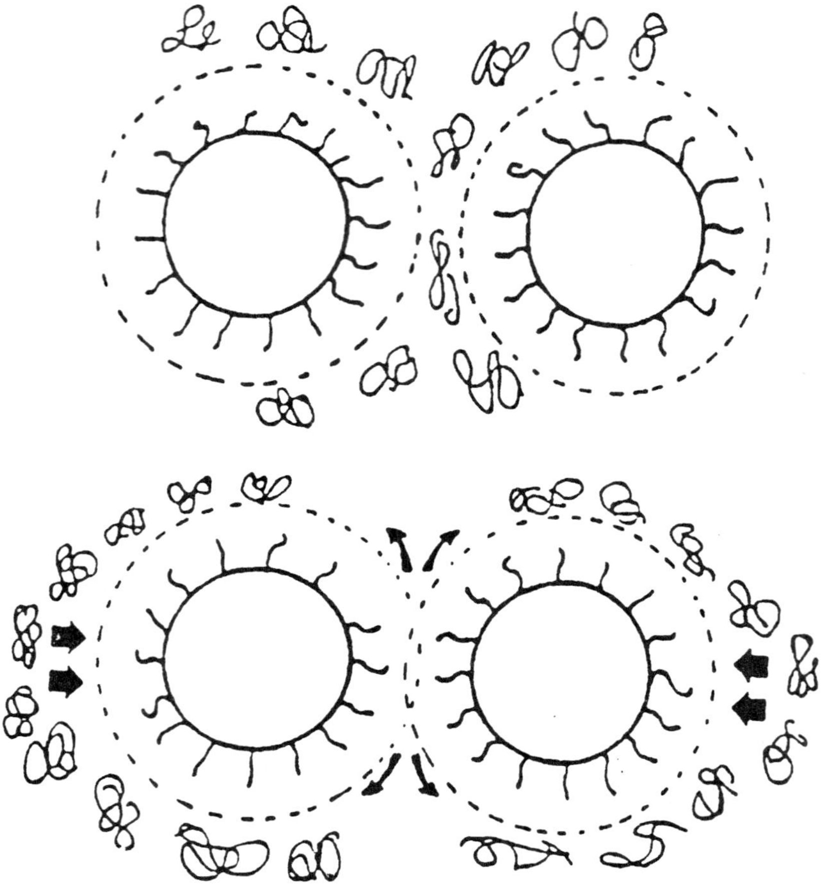

Figure 19 Schematic representation of depletion flocculation.

where v_1 is the molecular volume of the solvent, μ_1 is the chemical potential of the solvent in the presence of the free polymer, and μ_1^o that before the addition of the free polymer. The term $(\mu_1 - \mu_1^o)/v_1$ is a measure of the osmotic pressure of the polymer solution. Since $\mu_1 < \mu_1^o$, then G_{dep} will be negative (i.e., equivalent to an attractive force). Δ is the thickness of the depletion layer, which is determined by the radius of gyration of the free-polymer coil. Thus, G_{dep} has a magnitude that is determined by the osmotic pressure of the polymer solution and a range that is determined by the radius of gyration of the free-polymer coil. Since G_{dep} is proportional to the osmotic pressure, it is clear that, for a given molecular weight, as the free-polymer concentration is increased above ϕ_p^+, G_{dep} also increases. Since G_{dep} is proportional to Δ^2, the higher the molecular weight, the lower the value of ϕ_p^+. As discussed before (52), ϕ_p^+ also decreases with increase of the volume fraction of the dispersion.

Weak flocculation of an emulsion, produced by the addition of a free polymer, is expected to affect the viscoelastic properties of the emulsion. This is illustrated in Figure 20, which shows the variation of G^*, G', G'', and η' with frequency for an emulsion with $\phi = 0.6$ and at a volume fraction of free polymer (PEO with molecular weight M = 20,000) that is above ϕ_p^+ (0.159). It can be clearly seen that the emulsion shows the

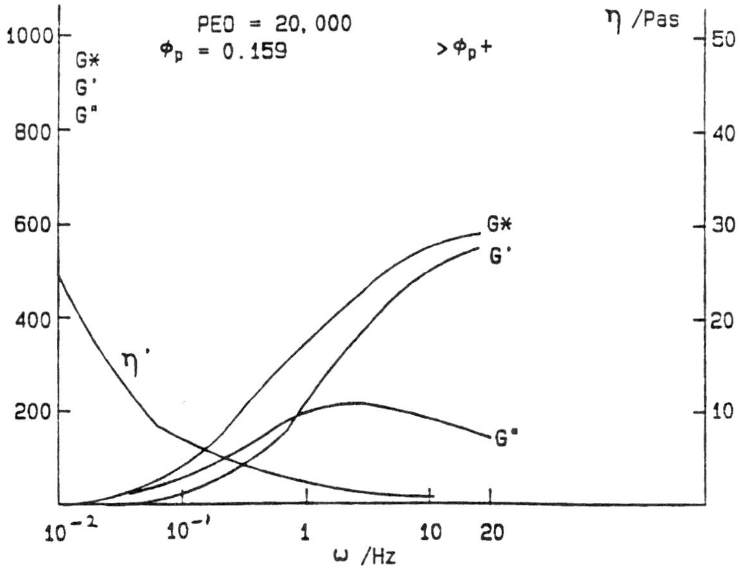

Figure 20 Variation of G^*, G', G'', and η' with frequency (Hz) for an o/w emulsion ($\phi = 0.6$) with added PEO (M = 20,000) at $\phi_p = 0.159$.

typical behavior of a viscoelastic system. At a frequency < 1 Hz, $G'' > G'$, whereas above 1 Hz, $G' > G''$ and G' approaches G^* at high frequency. G'', on the other hand, becomes equal to G' at 1 Hz, reaches a maximum at 1–2 Hz, and then falls gradually with increase in frequency. The characteristic frequency (at which $G' = G''$) is ~6 rad/sec giving a relaxation time of the order of 0.15 sec. This reflects the flocculation of the emulsion, since before addition of the free polymer, the emulsion was predominantly viscous over the whole frequency range. Similar results were obtained with the other flocculated systems. Plots of G^* and G' versus ϕ_p are shown in Figure 21. It can be seen that both G^* and G' show a rapid increase at $\phi_p > \sim 0.03$. Similar trends were obtained with emulsions flocculated by PEO with M = 35,000 and 90,000, but the free-polymer concentration above which the moduli showed a rapid increase was lower. The values of ϕ_p^+ obtained were 0.03, 0.022, and 0.012 for PEO with M = 20,000, 35,000, and 90,000 respectively. These values are comparable to those obtained using polystyrene latex dispersions (51,52). Thus, viscoelastic measurements can be applied to study the flocculation of emulsions in the same manner as for suspensions.

X. POLYMERIC SURFACTANTS IN MULTIPLE EMULSIONS

As discussed before (2), multiple emulsions (w/o/w or o/w/o) are ideal systems for application in personal care products for the following reasons. First, one can dissolve ingredients in three different compartments. For example with w/o/w multiple emulsions, one can incorporate two different water-soluble additives (proteins, enzymes, and vitamins) and an insoluble ingredient (e.g., perfume). Second, they can be applied for sustained release by control of the breakdown process that occurs on application. Third, they allow one to produce the same cream consistency required for many cosmetics, e.g., by incorporation of a thickener or gelling agent in the outer continuous phase.

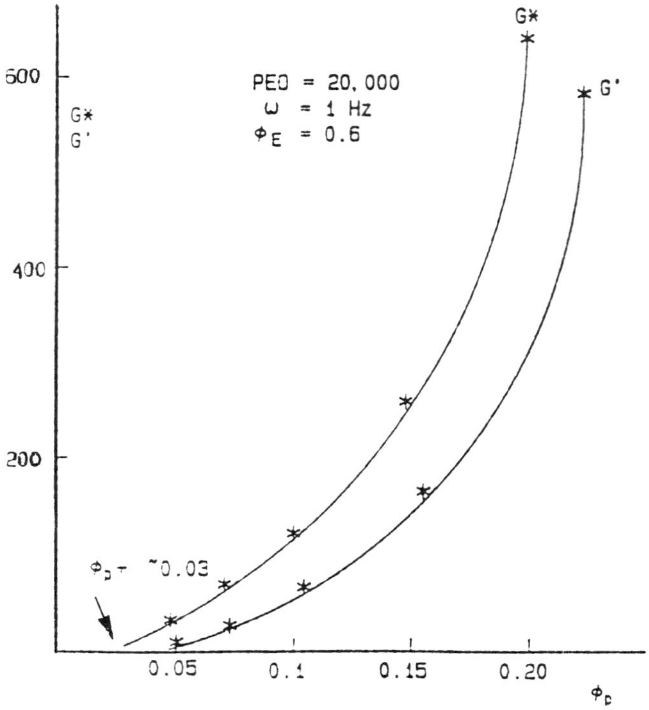

Figure 21 Variation of G^* and G' with ϕ_p (PEO, M = 20,000) for an o/w emulsion (ϕ = 0.6).

The main criteria for the preparation of stable multiple emulsions are as follows (2). First, one needs two optimum emulsifiers, one with a low and one with a high HLB number. Emulsifier 1 (with a low HLB number), which is used to prepare the primary w/o emulsion (for the case of w/o/w multiple emulsion), should prevent any flocculation or coalescence of the emulsion droplets. This emulsifier should ideally produce a viscoelastic film at the w/o interface that ensures the stability of the emulsions and prevents any transport of components from the internal droplets to the outer continuous medium during storage. Recent work in our laboratory (55) showed that Aralacel P135 satisfies this criterion. It produces a viscoelastic film, and the w/o emulsions prepared using this polymeric surfactant are stable over a long period of time and at various temperatures. The secondary emulsifier, with a high HLB number, should also produce an effective barrier to prevent flocculation and coalescence of the resulting multiple emulsion drops. Again a polymeric surfactant, such as Synperonic PF 127 (an ABA block of PEO-PPO-PEO produced by ICI), is ideal in this case.

The second criterion for stabilization of the multiple emulsion on storage is that there must be an optimum osmotic balance between the internal (water droplets) and the external continuous medium. This can be achieved by the use of electrolytes or nonelectrolytes. Usually, one keeps the osmotic pressure in the external continuous medium slightly lower than that of the internal water droplets.

The multiple emulsion is prepared by a two-stage process, as schematically illustrated in Figure 22. The primary emulsion is prepared by adding the aqueous phase to an oil solution of the polymeric emulsifier 1 with a low HLB number, e.g., Aralcel P135, using

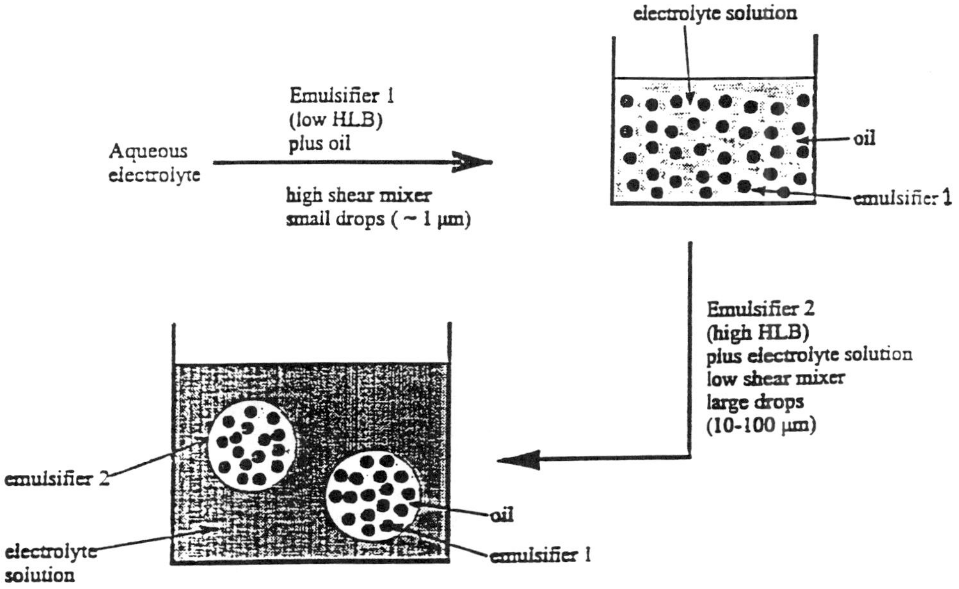

Figure 22 Schematic representation of the preparation of a w/o/w multiple emulsion.

a high-speed stirrer. Using this polymeric emulsifier, primary water droplets that are smaller than 1 μm in diameter can be produced. The size of the droplets in the primary emulsion can be determined using photon correlation spectroscopy (56).

This primary emulsion is then emulsified into aqueous solution of the high HLB polymeric surfactant (Synperonic PEF 127) using a low-speed stirrer (paddle stirrer) to produce multiple emulsion drops of the order of 10–100 μm in diameter.

A schematic representation of the multiple emulsion drop is shown in Figure 23, which illustrates the various components. In some cases a polymer coating (produced using, for example, polymethacrylic acid) may be used to ensure the long-term physical stability of the multiple emulsion. Using polymeric surfactants, multiple emulsions that are stable for more than one year could be produced (17). By incorporating a gelling agent such as Carbopol in the aqueous continuous phase, creaming of the multiple emulsion could be prevented. This gelling agent also produced the right consistency (rheology) for application as a cream.

XI. SUMMARY

This chapter described the basis principles involved in stabilization of dispersions by polymeric surfactants. The first part described polymeric surfactants and their solution properties. The second part described the adsorption of polymeric surfactants and their conformation at the interface. The methods that can be applied to determine the adsorption and conformation of polymeric surfactants were briefly described. The third part dealt with the stabilization mechanism produced using polymeric surfactants. Two main repulsive forces were considered. The first arises from the unfavorable mixing of the chains on close approach of the particles or droplets, when these chains are in good solvent conditions. This is referred to as mixing or osmotic repulsion. The second force of repulsions

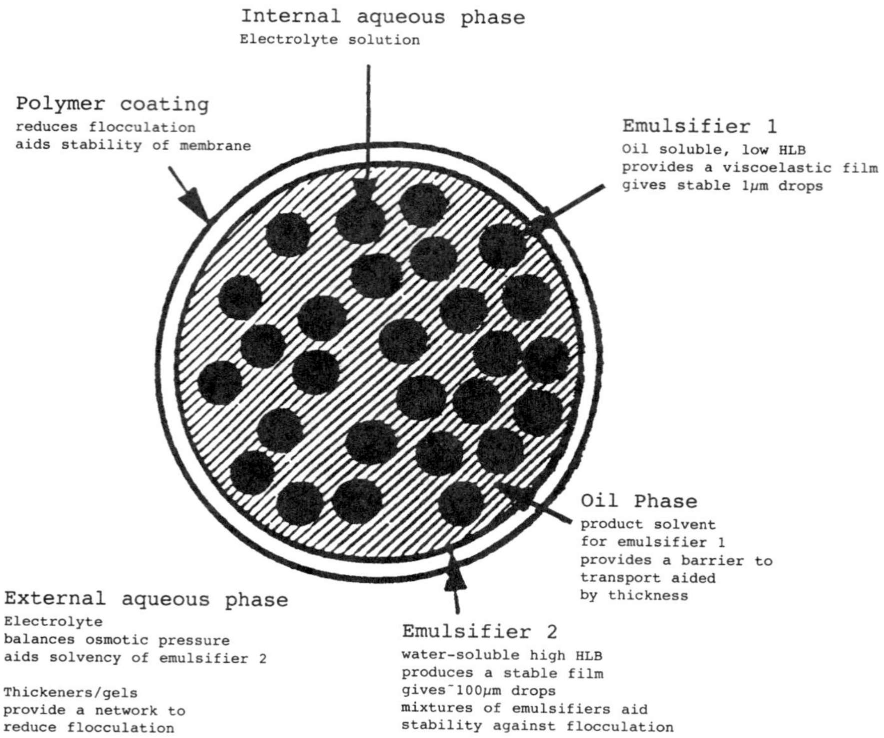

Figure 23 Schematic representation of the multiple emulsion drop showing the role of the various components.

arises from the reduction in configurational entropy of the chains on considerable overlap, referred to as elastic, volume restriction or entropic repulsion. Combination of the mixing and elastic repulsions with the van der Waals attraction results in an energy-distance curve that shows weak attraction at a separation distance, h, comparable to twice the adsorbed layer thickness, 2δ. However, when $h < 2\delta$, very strong repulsion arises when h is further reduced. The main criteria for effective steric stabilization were summarized. These are: complete coverage of the particle surface by the polymeric surfactant, strong adsorption (anchoring) of the chains to the surface, good solvency of the chains by the continuous medium, and reasonably thick adsorbed layers. These criteria are best satisfied by using block and graft copolymers consisting of two components, a B chain (the anchoring chain) that is insoluble in the medium and has a strong affinity to the surface and one or more A chains that are strongly solvated by the medium and have low affinity to the surface. AB, ABA block copolymers and BA_n graft copolymers can be used and examples are given.

The chapter next dealt with the rheology of emulsions stabilized by polymeric surfactants. The factors affecting the rheology of emulsions were briefly discussed. This was followed by a section on interfacial rheology and its correlation with emulsion stability. The bulk rheology of oil-in-water and water-in-oil emulsions stabilized by polymeric surfactants was described. Both steady-state and viscoelastic investigations were described. These emulsions show a transition from predominantly viscous to predominantly elastic response as the frequency of oscillation exceeds a critical value. This allows one to obtain the relaxation time of the emulsion system, which was shown to increase with increase in the volume fraction ϕ of the disperse phase. Plots of the complex modulus G^*, the storage modulus G', and loss modulus G'' as a function of ϕ showed a transition from predominantly viscous to predominantly elastic response at a critical ϕ value. This reflected the steric interaction with increase in ϕ. When the surface-to-surface separation between the droplets become smaller than twice the adsorbed layer thickness, the steric repulsion became strong, increasing in magnitude with increases in ϕ. The rheology section also described the viscoelastic properties of weakly flocculated emulsions. These were obtained by addition of a ''free'' (nonadsorbing) polymer to a sterically stabilized emulsion (depletion flocculation). Again the viscoelastic behavior reflected the weak attraction between the droplets in the emulsion. Above a critical volume fraction of free polymer (which decreased with increase of the molecular weight of the polymer) there was a rapid increase in the storage modulus and this determined the onset of depletion flocculation.

The last part of the chapter dealt with the preparation of stable water-in-oil-in-water (w/o/w) multiple emulsions that are suitable for application in cosmetics. The main criterion for producing stable w/o/w systems is to use two polymeric surfactants: one with a low HLB number for preparation of the primary w/o emulsion and one with a high HLB number for preparation of the final w/o/w multiple emulsion. The primary emulsifier should produce a viscoelastic film that prevents leakage from the internal water droplets to the outside continuous phase. It will also ensure high stability (minimum coalescence) of the internal water droplets. The secondary emulsifier should also provide an effective barrier to prevent flocculation and coalescence of the multiple emulsion droplets on storage. It is also essential to balance the osmotic pressure of the internal aqueous droplets and the outside continuous medium.

REFERENCES

1. Bruer MM. Cosmetic emulsions. In: Becher P, ed. Encyclopedia of Emulsion Technology, Vol 2. New York: Marcel Dekker, 1985:385–424.
2. Tadros ThF. Int J Cosmet Sci 1992; 14:93.
3. Tadros ThF, Vincent B. In: Becher P, ed. Encyclopedia of Emulsion Technology, Vol 1. New York: Marcel Dekker, 1983, Chapter 3.
4. Friberg SE. J Soc Cosmet Chem 1990; 41:155.
5. Kligman AM. In: Montagna W, ed. Biology of the Stratum Corneum in Epidermis. New York: Academic Press, 1964:421–446.
6. Napper DH. Polymeric Stabilization of Dispersions. London: Academic Press, 1983.
7. Friberg SE, Jansson PO, Cederberg E. J Colloid Interface Sci. 1976; 55:614.
8. Tadros ThF. Polymer colloids. In: Buscall R, Corner T, Stageman J, eds. Applied Sciences. London: Elsevier, 1985:105.
9. Silberberg A. J Chem Phys 1968; 48:2835.
10. Hoeve CA. J Polym Sci 1970; 30:361; 1971; 34:1.
11. Roe RJ. J Chem Phys 1974; 60:4192.
12. Scheutjens JMHM, Fleer GJ. Adv Colloid Interface Sci 1982; 16:341.
13. Garvey MJ, Tadros ThF, Vincent B. J Colloid Interface Sci 1974; 49:57.
14. Flory PJ. Principles of Polymer Chemistry. New York: Cornell University Press, 1953.
15. Einstein A. Investigations on the Theory of the Brownian Movement. New York: Dover, 1906.
16. Batchelor GK. J Fluid Mech 1977; 83:97.
17. Taylor GI. Proc Roy Soc 1932; A138:41.
18. Richardson EG. Kolloid Z 1933; 65: 32; J Colloid Sci 1950; 5:404; 1953; 8: 367.

19. Sherman P. Rheology of emulsions. In: Sherman P, ed. Emulsion Science. London: Academic Press, 1968, Chapter 4.
20. Sherman P. J Colloid Sci 1955; 10:63.
21. Sherman P. J Soc Chem Ind (Lond.) 1950; 69.
22. Becher P. J Soc Cosmet Chem 1958; 9:141.
23. Krog N. In: Sjoblom J, ed. Emulsions—A Fundamental and Practical Approach. NATO ASI Series, Series C, Vol 363. Kluger Academic Publishers, 1992:61.
24. Junginger HE. In: Sjoblom J, ed. Emulsions—A Fundamental and Practical Approach. NATO ASI Series, Series C, Vol 363. Kluger Academic Publishers, 1992:189.
25. Edwards DA, Brenner H, Wasan DT. Interfacial Transport Processes and Rheology. Boston: Butterworth-Heinemann, 1991.
26. Marangoni CGM. Ann Phys 1871; 3:337.
27. Mannheimer RJ, Schechter RS. J Colloid Interface Sci 1970; 32:225.
28. Criddle DW. The viscosity and elasticity of interfaces. In: Eirich FR, ed. Rheology, Theory and Applications, Vol 3. 1960:429, Chapter 11.
29. Langevin D. J Colloid Interface Sci 1981; 80:412.
30. Agarwal SK, Wasan DT. Chem Eng J 1979; 18:215.
31. Wei L, Schmidt W, Slattery JC. J Colloid Interface Sci 1974; 48:1.
32. Phillips WJ, Graves RW, Flumerfelt RW. J Colloid Interface Sci 1980; 76:350.
33. Bendure RL. J Colloid Interface Sci 1971; 35:238.
34. Biswas B, Haydon DA. Proc Roy Soc 1963; A271:296, 317.
35. Cockbain EG, McRoberts TS. J Colloid Sci 1953; 8:440.
36. Prince A, Arcuri C, van den Tempel M. J Colloid Interface Sci 1967; 24:811.
37. Wasan DT, McNamara JJ, Shah SM, Sampath K, Aderangi N. J Rheol 1979; 23:181.
38. Campanelli JR, Cooper DG. J Chem Eng 1989; 67:851.
39. Tadros ThF, Winn PD. To be published.
40. Krieger IM, Dougherty M. Trans Soc Rheol 1959; 3:137.
41. Krieger IM. Adv Colloid Interface Sci 1972; 3:111.
42. Tadros ThF, Thomas PK. To be published.
43. Prestidge C, Tadros ThF. J Colloid Interface Sci 1988; 124:660.
44. Aston MS, Herrington TM, Tadros ThF. Colloids Surfaces 1989; 40:49.
45. Cairns RJ, Ottewill RH. J Colloid Interface Sci 1976; 54:45.
46. Ottewill RH. Personal communication.
47. Tadros ThF. Langmuir 1990; 6:28.
48. Cutler JL, Tadros ThF. To be published.
49. Liang W, Tadros ThF, Luckham PF. J Colloid Interface Sci 1992; 153:131.
50. Tadros ThF, Winn PD. To be published.
51. Prestidge C, Tadros ThF. Colloids Surfaces 1988; 31:325.
52. Liang W, Tadros ThF, Luckham PF. J Colloid Interface Sci 1993; 155:156.
53. Asakura S, Oosawa F. J Polym Sci 1958; 33:245.
54. Fleer GJ, Scheutjens JHMH, Vincent B. ACS Symp Ser 1984; 240:245.
55. Lucel A, Tadros ThF. To be published.
56. Tadros ThF, PyC, Rouviere J, Taelman MC, Loll P. Colloids Surfaces 1994; 91.

4

Polymer/Surfactant Interaction
Manifestations, Methods, and Mechanisms

E. Desmond Goddard
*Union Carbide Corporation, Tarrytown, New York**

I. INTRODUCTION

The use of polymers and surfactants in the cosmetics industry is widespread. In fact, in many formulations, e.g., shampoos, lotions, and so forth, these ingredients occur together. Practitioners in this field are increasingly aware that, through interaction, these ingredients can affect each other's properties and, hence, the overall properties of the formulation, sometimes beneficially and sometimes adversely. Hence it is important to have basic information on the factors that govern the interaction of polymers and surfactants and on the alteration in properties that can be expected as a result of the products formed by interaction. Indeed, there has been a recent upsurge of interest in this field and it is significant that activity on this subject in the academic sector has been vigorous and continues to grow.

This field of study is actually quite old. Interaction and complex formation between natural polymers (proteins) and "surfactants" (lipids) were recognized early in this century, and much study on mixtures of proteins and synthetic surfactants was carried out in the 1940s and 1950s (1,2). Work on mixtures of synthetic uncharged polymers and ionic surfactants was initiated by Saito in the 1950s and on various (mostly natural) anionic polymers and cationic surfactants by Scott and co-workers at about the same time. For summaries of this early work several reviews are available (3–5).

The purpose of this chapter is to examine the four main types of interaction system by first describing results obtained using a variety of experimental techniques and to introduce several aspects of the interaction phenomenon and prepare the way for later discussion of models and applications. First, we will briefly review the pertinent properties of the single components.

A. Surfactants

Surfactants are the ultimate example of an amphipathic structure. They combine a long-chain alkyl group, which is hydrophobic, with an ionic group (sometimes polar group),

* Former Corporate Research Fellow.

which is highly hydrophilic. Such groups are normally incompatible—for example, a salt has virtually no solubility in a hydrocarbon liquid. In ionic surfactants, however, the two moieties are constrained by covalent bonds to coexist in the same molecule. If such a molecule is exposed to water, the powerful forces of hydration will attempt to drive the molecule into solution, but at the expense of exposing the attached hydrocarbon chains to an unfavored aqueous environment. There are many well-known consequences of this situation. In trying to minimize contact of their alkyl chains with water, surfactant molecules will adsorb at:

1. Solid/water interfaces (as in wetting and detergency)
2. Air/water interfaces, lowering the surface tension (as in foaming and wetting)
3. Oil/water interfaces, lowering interfacial tension (as in emulsification)

In these processes of adsorption, the hydrocarbon groups lose energy by (1) reducing contact with water and (2) associating with one another. Frequently the extent of available surface is limited and the number of surfactant molecules involved in adsorption is a small percentage of the total. The process is, of course, more favorable if the interface is highly extended, as in foams and emulsions. The ultimate process, however, for reduction of hydrocarbon/water contact is micellization. Above a certain critical concentration, the "c.m.c.," surfactant molecules spontaneously aggregate into roughly spherical assemblies, of diameter approximately two molecular lengths of the surfactant molecule. (See Fig. 1.) In more concentrated solutions of ionic surfactants other micellar shapes, e.g., cylinders and discs, form but we shall not be concerned with these here.

There are a number of important aspects of micellization.

1. The processes of aggregation and deaggregation, at least for pure surfactants like sodium dodecyl sulfate (SDS), are extremely fast—in the microsecond to millisecond range (6).

2. The enthalpy change, measured calorimetrically, of micellization is generally small (7,8). A realistic, if simplistic, explanation is that the energy lost in reducing the

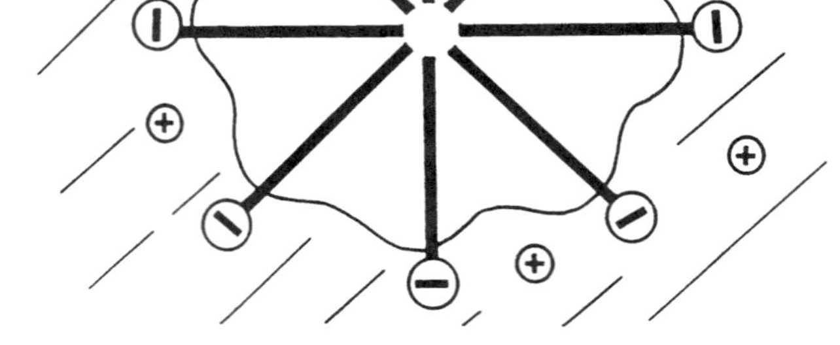

Figure 1 Schematic drawing of anionic surfactant micelle.

contact between hydrocarbon chains and water is offset by the energy gained in the electrical repulsion of ionic head groups brought into proximity in the micelle periphery.

3. The net result is that micellization represents a very delicate balance of forces. For example, adding salt, which reduces the micellar head group repulsive forces, or lengthening the "R" group of the surfactant, which increases the energy loss on eliminating the hydrocarbon chain/water interface, can sharply reduce the c.m.c. In any event, there will always be a high level of counterion binding by ionic surfactant micelles because of electrostatic attraction.

4. Nonionic surfactants are a special case. Because of the absence of electrical repulsive forces at the micellar periphery, aggregation takes place at a much lower concentration. For the same R group the c.m.c. of a nonionic surfactant can be two orders of magnitude lower than that of an ionic surfactant. Also, micellar shapes other than spherical, e.g., ellipsoids, are frequently encountered. All of the above factors, as will be seen, have a bearing on the subject of polymer/surfactant interaction.

B. Polymers

Polymers are materials composed of repeating units whose molecular weight is generally in the range of tens to hundreds of daltons. As the degree of polymerization (i.e., number of monomer units) can range from tens to thousands to even hundreds of thousands, the molecular weight of polymers can span a range of hundreds to millions of daltons. The vast majority of water-soluble polymers, whether of natural or synthetic origin, are carbon based. They generally owe their solubility to the presence of polar oxygen groups, such as —O—, —OH—, or, —COOH, which offset the hydrophobicity of $\equiv$CH, $=CH_2$, or CH_3 groups. Sometimes the polar groups are nitrogen based, such as =NH, $—NH_2$, or $—CONH_2$. As will be pointed out later, both the polar sites and the hydrophobic centers on the polymer represent sites for possible interaction with added surfactant. Polymers can be homopolymers, based on one repeating monomer unit, or copolymers, based on two or more repeating monomer units. Some water-soluble polymers, viz., "polyions," contain ionic groups leading to categories known as "polycations" and "polyanions," or, if of mixed composition, "polyampholytes." All of the above-mentioned categories of polymer are used in the cosmetics industry.

Of relevance to the present subject is the mobility of the polymer or the polymer segments in aqueous solution. Because of their high molecular weight the diffusion coefficient of polymers can be lower than that of simple solutes by a hundred- or thousandfold or more. However, the mobility of individual monomer groups within the polymer can be substantial, especially in polymer molecules that adopt a random configuration in solution. This point, as will be shown later, is one of much significance to the mechanism(s) of polymer/surfactant interaction. "Open" configurations and higher monomer mobility are encouraged in "good" solvents; more closed configurations and lower mobility are encountered in "poor" solvents. (See discussion of Flory-Huggins theory in Chapters 1–3.) The presence of charged groups along the polymer backbone, as in polyanions and polycations, tends to lead to "open" configurations and higher solution viscosity; the addition of salt to these solutions tends, by electrostatic screening, to favor more "closed" configurations and reduced viscosity.

C. Interaction: Preliminary Remarks

As stated in the Introduction, the field of polymer/surfactant interaction continues to be very active among colloid scientists, who have employed over two dozen experimental

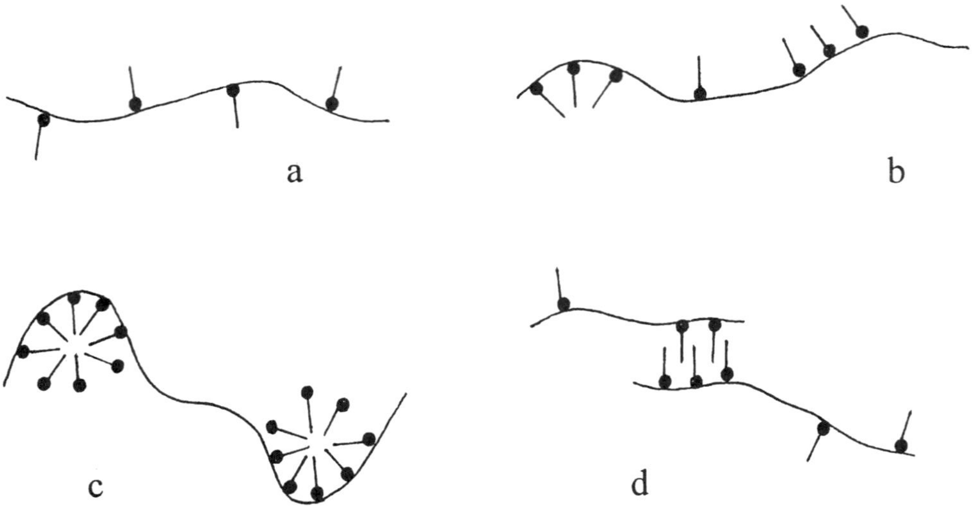

Figure 2 Schematic drawing of various modes of ''binding'' surfactant molecules by a polymer: c is the ''necklace'' model. See text.

techniques for its study. (See reviews, Refs. 1–5,9,10.) These methods and the results obtained have provided convincing evidence of the widespread existence of such interaction. The early interpretations of mechanism, starting with the protein/surfactant system, invoked a ''binding'' process of surfactant to sites along the polymer chain (a). Interpretation of more recent data has increasingly been made in terms of interaction involving ''cooperativity'' in binding of surfactant molecules (b) or, indeed, involving a perturbation of aggregation or micellization of the surfactant (c) brought about by the presence of the polymer. As will be discussed, elements of all three mechanisms are likely to be correct. (See Fig. 2.) Another possible variation (d) of the above schemes is where hydrophobic forces act between surfactant molecules adsorbed on different polymer chains.

II. SOME EXPERIMENTAL METHODS AND BASIC OBSERVATIONS

The early observations that led to concepts of binding were based on such techniques as dialysis equilibrium, electromethods, surface tension, viscosity, and so on. Methods such as fluorescence, nuclear magnetic resonance (NMR), and dye solubilization yielded data supporting perturbed micellization mechanisms. All of these techniques are still used to study polymer/surfactant interaction. To illustrate the current state of knowledge in this field, results from a half dozen or so methods, drawn mostly from the above, will be outlined and interpreted. For convenience, the material will be presented for four different categories of water-soluble polymer: (a) uncharged polymer, (b) charged polymer, (c) hydrophobically modified polymer, and (d) protein.

Categories a and b, because of their prevalence and wide use, are covered more fully than category c, because of its relative newness, and category d, because of its more limited current use and investigation. It is not our purpose to provide an extensive literature review—several are already available. Our purpose is to provide a description of fundamentals with emphasis on ''accessible'' methods that have been used to develop data, mechanisms, and interaction models.

A. Uncharged Polymers

Uncharged polymers are often used (and regarded) as ''nonspecific thickeners'' in cosmetic formulations. As will be shown, it cannot be assumed that they are ''passive'' agents in this respect as they can be affected by other formulation ingredients, notably surfactants. Evidence from a number of experimental techniques shows this.

1. Dialysis Equilibrium

This method has been widely and traditionally used for the study of the interaction of proteins in solution with smaller molecules and ions including surfactants. The principle rests on the fact that a membrane can be chosen such that, while the macromolecule is contained in the dialysis bag made from the membrane, the smaller molecule (and water) can move freely between the bag and the solution in the outer container. When equilibrium is established, analysis reveals the degree of ''binding'' of the smaller molecule by the macromolecule. [One complication is the Donnan membrane effect (11,12) but this can be overcome if the measurements are done in the presence of salt, e.g., 0.1 M NaCl.]

The method was first employed for an uncharged polymer/charged surfactant pair by Fishman and Eirich to study the polyvinylpyrrolidone (PVP)/sodium dodecyl sulfate (SDS) system (13). No identifiable interaction was observed below a certain concentration of surfactant (''T_1'' according to the Jones convention—see below) after which, with increase in concentration, there was a sharp rise in apparent binding of SDS, which eventually leveled when the SDS bulk concentration reached or exceeded concentration ''T_2'' (see below). Such effects are illustrated in Figure 3, which depicts data of Shirahama (14) for the polyethyleneoxide (PEO)/SDS system. There are several other references in the 1970s to use of the dialysis technique on systems related to the above, with results in general terms following the pattern of Figure 3. Polymers investigated, in addition to PEO (14,15) and PVP (12,13), include methylcellulose (MeC) and polyvinylalcohol (PVA) (16). These data reinforced the notion, first fostered for proteins, that soluble macromolecules are able to ''bind'' surfactants in solution, presumably by providing favorable sites for their attachment.

2. Specific Ion Electrodes

The advent of electrodes that are specific to ionic surfactants, e.g., $Na^+(DS^-)$ or $(DTA^+)Br^-$ (SDS and DTAB), has made the determination of ''binding'' curves of surfactants by polymers much easier. These yield results in much the same way as the glass electrode allows electrometric determination of hydrogen ions. The electrodes are often ''home-made'' (17–19) but some are now available commercially (Orion Research, Model 93-42). A test of the reliability of the electrode is to check its conformity to the dictates of the Nernst equation, viz., that a 10-fold change in concentration of the metered surfactant ion should yield an emf change of 59 mV at 25°C (17–19). In any case, it is advisable to calibrate the electrode by metering the surfactant in the appropriate concentration range. The great advantage of this method is that it allows binding of an ion by the polymer to be determined without added salt required by the dialysis membrane method.

Results illustrating the use of a ''decyl sulfate'' electrode to study interaction with PVP are given in Figure 4 (20). Note that the surfactant by itself (lowest plot) leads to an emf/log concentration plot, up to the c.m.c., with the required Nernstian slope. Before the breakpoints (T_1) that occur in the presence of the polymer one can see that the slope is virtually unaffected by polymer; beyond T_1, i.e., in the ''binding'' zone, the slope is lower, implying binding of surfactant. After saturation, i.e., at concentrations above T_2

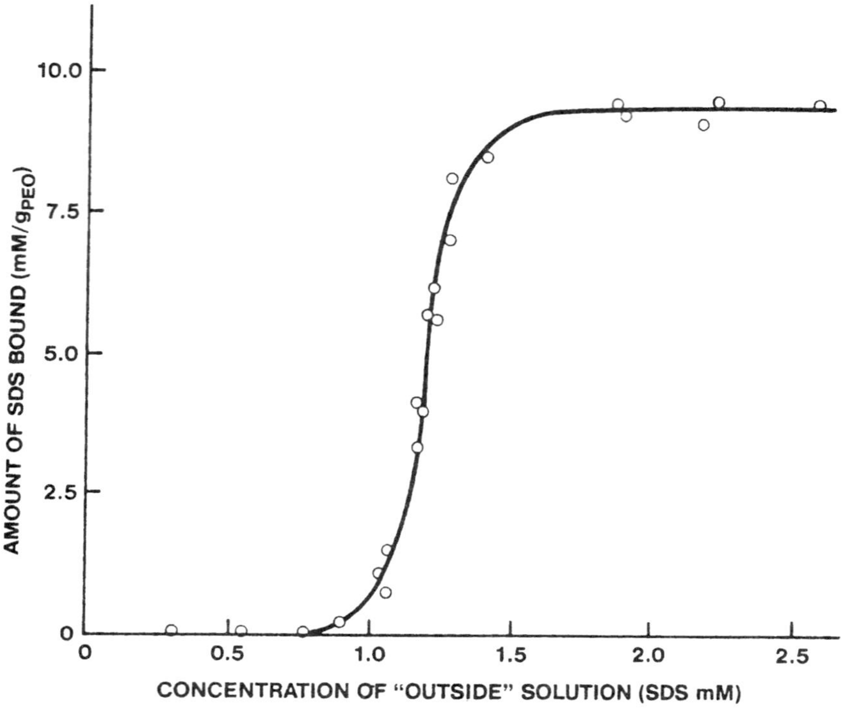

Figure 3 Binding isotherm of PEO/SDS system in 0.1 M NaCl: solid line from Hill equation (170). (From Ref. 14.)

($cmc_{apparent}$) the slopes reverse in sign in all cases implying formation of micelles. It is of interest that T_1, the concentration for onset of interaction, is virtually independent of polymer concentration while, as expected, T_2, the concentration for saturation of added polymer, increases linearly with it.

Historically, the first use of a specific surfactant ion electrode for polymer/surfactant studies seems to have been that of Birch et al. (17), who used a DS electrode to investigate the PVP/SDS and PEO/SDS systems, followed by Gilanyi and Wolfram (21), who studied the PVA/SDS and PEO/SDS systems.

Another way to study the aggregation process is to use an electrode specific to the surfactant's counterion. As depicted in Figure 1, there is considerable binding of counterions by an ionic micelle and this would be affected by association with a polymer. (See Fig. 11 and later discussion.) This method has been applied to studies of the PEO/SDS and PVA/SDS systems (17,21–23) and confirms results obtained by other methods.

Finally, a third ''electromethod,'' namely electrical conductivity (κ), has been employed. It is well known that micellization of an ionic surfactant like SDS leads to a slope change in its κ versus concentration plot. Work by Jones (24) on the PEO/SDS system showed that introduction of PEO into the surfactant solution led to pre- and postmicellar breakpoints consistent with the T_1 and T_2 concepts mentioned above. Furthermore, interpretation of the conductivity data for PEO/SDS and PVP/SDS systems by Zana et al. provided confirmation that the degree of counterion (Na) binding for the ''complexes'' was considerably lower than that observed with simple SDS micelles (25).

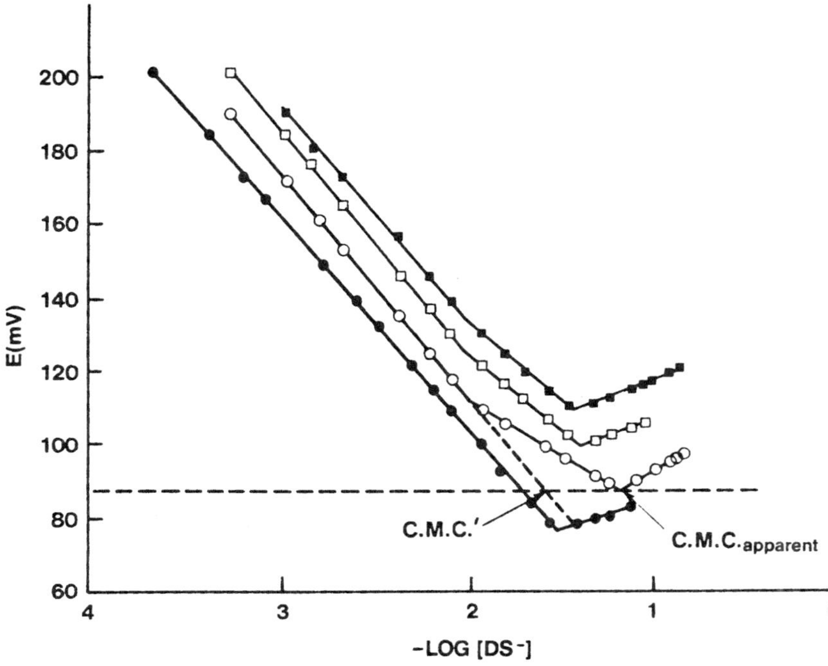

Figure 4 Emf/concentration plots of SDS in the presence of PVP: (○) 1.2% PVP; (□) 0.5% PVP; (■) 0.25% PVP; (●) 0% PVP. Each upper curve is raised progressively by 10 mV. (From Ref. 20.)

3. *Surface Tension*

A very simple and informative technique for the study of polymer/surfactant pairs involves ordinary measurements of surface tension. In these mixtures, it is often the case that the polymer is feebly surface active; hence, the measured surface tension will be a sensor essentially of the free or uncomplexed surfactant in solution. Departure of the mixed systems from the surface tension behavior of polymer-free surfactant solutions would then be an indication of binding of the surfactant by the polymer, or of complex formation.

An ideal system is illustrated in Figure 5. Here, as the surfactant concentration is increased, the with- and without-polymer curves will coincide until a critical concentration (T_1) for binding is reached. If the binding energy is high enough (and constant), the surfactant concentration, and hence the surface tension, will remain constant until the polymer binding sites are saturated. The resultant plateau will end at the saturation concentration T_2'. Beyond this point the concentration of free surfactant will rise and the surface tension will drop along the line $T_2'T_2$ until regular micelles form, i.e., rejoin the curve of the polymer-free system. Despite the fact that polymers generally have some surface activity, the surface tension method has proved to be very useful for studying polymer/surfactant interaction. (The implicit assumption that the "complex" has low surface activity is, however, *not* true in the case of many polyion/surfactant mixtures. See below.)

The concept of transitions, T_1 and T_2, was introduced by Jones (24) on the basis of his surface tension data on PEO/SDS mixed systems. His findings were confirmed and extended by Schwuger (26). Another system widely studied by the surface tension method

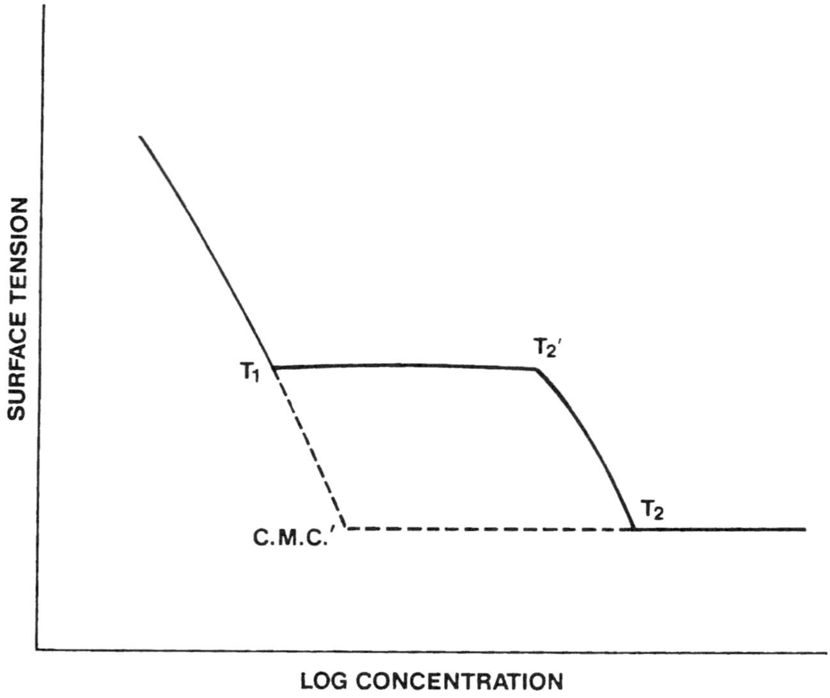

Figure 5 Schematic surface tension/concentration plot (T_1-T_2'-T_2) of a surfactant in the presence of a complexing polymer. See text.

comprises PVP/SDS pairs (12,27–29). Features essentially similar to those noted with PEO were obtained (Fig. 6) and are summarized as follows:

1. Transition concentrations T_1 and T_2 straddled the c.m.c. of SDS.
2. T_2 increased directly with the amount of polymer, whereas T_1 varied very little.
3. Constancy of surface tension, implying constant SDS activity, in the "interaction" zone was more evident at higher polymer concentration.
4. In the low surfactant concentration regime increasing departures from the "surfactant alone" curve are evident as the polymer concentration is increased, but the essential features showing "T_1" and "T_2" transitions are maintained.

The picture that emerges is that an association reaction of surfactant takes place in the presence of polymers. Since the association reaction starts at a lower concentration than the c.m.c., it can be deduced that it is energetically more favorable than simple micelle formation. Only when the polymer is saturated will regular micelles form (on further addition of surfactant).

4. *Viscosity*

The configuration of a dissolved polymer affects the rheology of its solution: symmetric configurations, such as spheres, would lead to relatively low viscosity; anisometric configurations, for example rods, would favor high viscosity. Most neutral polymers in solu-

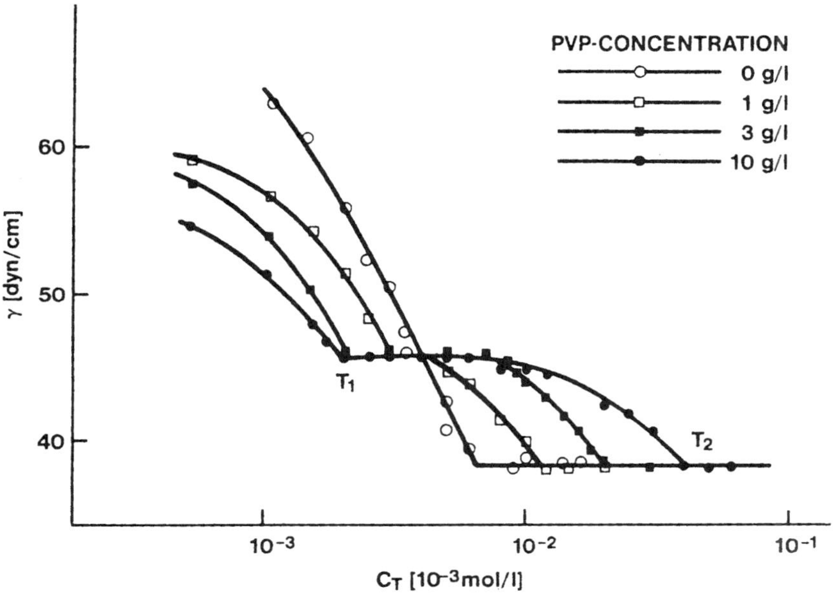

Figure 6 Surface tension (γ)/concentration plot of SDS in the presence of PVP at various concentrations; *T* assignments follow those of Figure 5. (From Ref. 27.)

tion would have configurations between these extremes; on the other hand, polyelectrolytes tend, because of backbone charge repulsion, to adopt a linear configuration, unless the ionic strength of the solution is high. This configuration favors an increase in viscosity of the solution.

When an unionized polymer binds an ionic surfactant, the polymer will acquire a charge and hence, on the basis of the "polyelectrolyte effect," an increase in viscosity would be anticipated. This area has been investigated by a number of authors, e.g., Jones (24) and Francois et al. (30), who examined the effect of adding SDS to a series of PEO polymers. A sudden increase in viscosity occurs at a certain concentration (T_1) of added surfactant, independent of polymer molecular weight, and this increase can be as high as fivefold, which is consistent with a polymer-charging effect. (See Fig. 7.)

Actually, the viscosity method can be considered a "traditional" method to study polymer/surfactant interaction and its first use was by Saito, who reported increases in viscosity of PVP and MeC solutions on adding SDS (31). Its subsequent popularity is, undoubtedly, connected with the simple nature of the equipment that can be used for its measurement.

5. *Solubilization: Oil-Soluble Dyes*

A traditional property of micellar surfactant solutions is their ability to dissolve water-insoluble, oil-soluble materials such as hydrocarbons, esters, and certain dyes and perfumes. This property, in fact, gave early support to the concept that micelles do indeed exist in aqueous solutions of surfactants, the core of the micelles in effect providing microdroplets of liquid hydrocarbon in solution with solvent properties.

A discovery of fundamental importance was made by Saito in 1957 (31). He reported that a number of water-soluble polymers can enhance the capacity of various surfactants

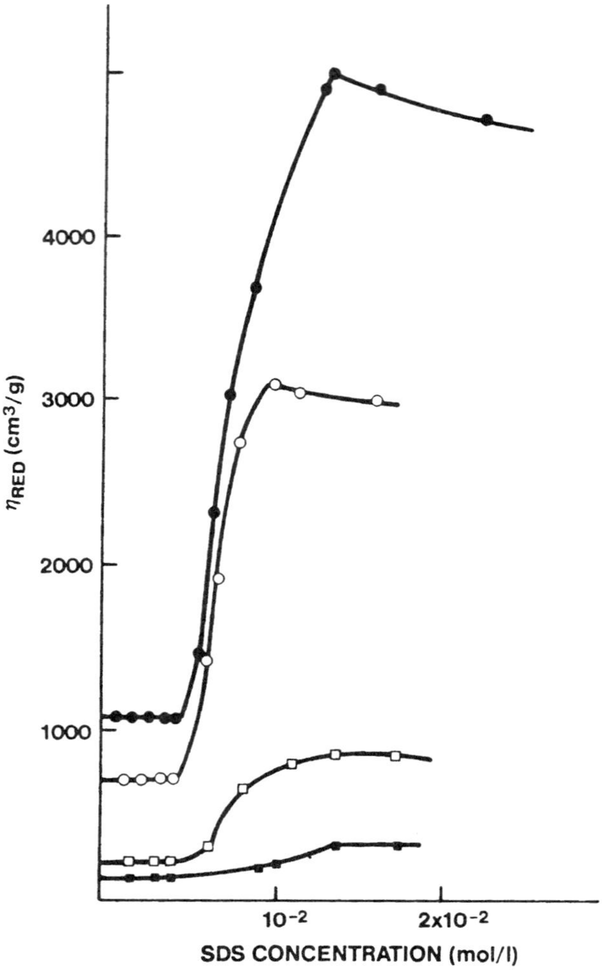

Figure 7 Reduced viscosity of PEO as a function of SDS concentration: (●) mol wt = 2×10^6, concentration, Cp = 6×10^{-1} g/L; (○) mol wt = 10^6; Cp = 6×10^{-2} g/L; (□) mol wt = 2×10^5, Cp = 5×10^{-1} g/L; (■) mol wt = 7×10^4, Cp = 5×10^{-1} g/L. (From Ref. 30.)

to solubilize the oil-soluble dye Yellow OB. This enhancement was manifested as an initiation of solubilization activity below the formal c.m.c. of the surfactant. If solubilization indeed requires the presence of ''microdroplets of hydrocarbon'' in solution, it has to be concluded that the combination of polymer and ''bound'' surfactant is tantamount to the presence of aggregates of surfactant molecules akin to micelles or premicelles. In other words, the data support model b or, more likely, model c given in the Introduction (Fig. 2).

This discovery has led to much subsequent activity in this field (27,28,32). For example, in studying solubilization of the dye Orange OT by PEO/SDS mixtures, Jones (32) found good agreement between the point of initial solubilization and the T_1 value obtained from electrical conductance measurements; deduced T_2 values by the two methods were also in good agreement.

The above type of behavior can also be seen in Lange's data for the solubilization of Orange OT by mixtures of PVP and a series of alkyl sulfates (27). (See Fig. 8.) These data provide a useful illustration of two effects that show that, while the T_1 values are lower than the corresponding c.m.c.'s (C_{10} and C_{12}), they systematically follow the same dependence pattern that c.m.c.'s do on surfactant chain length. The data thus point to a similarity between micellization and polymer-assisted surfactant aggregation.

6. Fluorescent Dyes

The above picture is reinforced by results obtained from a related technique. During the last 20 years the use of fluorescent probes to study micellization and aggregation phenomena has become widespread, because of the sensitivity and simplicity of the basic method. In essence, this method is based on the fact that selected fluorescence "probes," e.g., pyrene, pyrene aldehyde, and so forth, exhibit different fluorescence characteristics in aqueous ("polar") and nonaqueous ("nonpolar") environments (33). Probes are generally (but not always) chosen that are sparingly soluble in water so that if aggregates of surfactant form they will tend to distribute toward the latter and the overall fluorescence characteristics of the solution will change (34,35). Typically, measured fluorescence characteristics will be of the form shown in Figure 9.

For example, in the case of pyrene (the most widely used fluorescent dye) the measured parameter is I_1/I_3, the ratio of intensity of the first (372 nm) and third (385 nm) fluorescence peaks; for pyrene aldehyde it is λ_{max}, the wavelength of maximum absorption (36,37). In the presence of interacting polymer the plot is displaced to lower surfactant concentration: this implies that a surfactant aggregation process, formally akin to micelli-

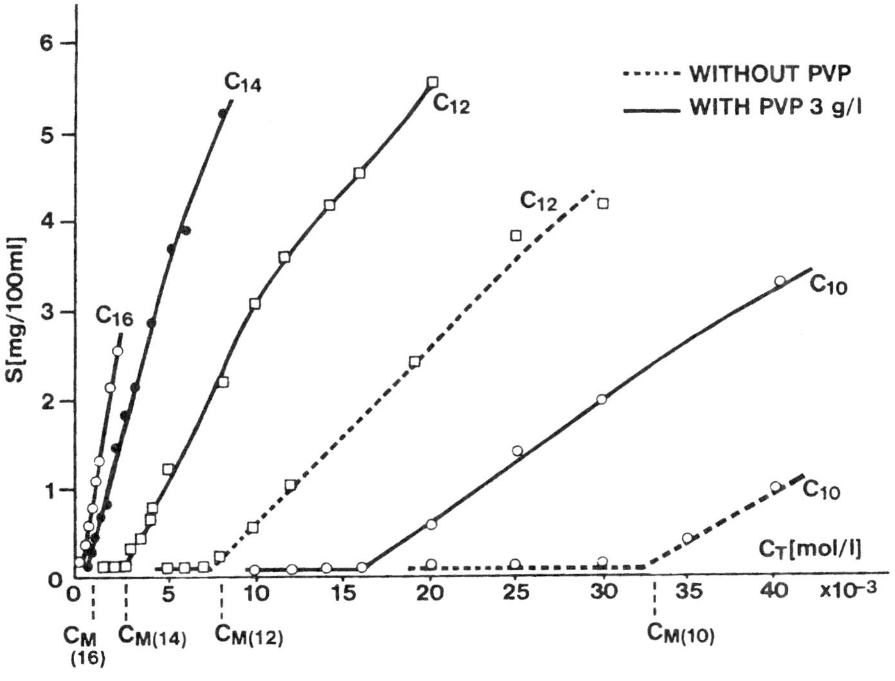

Figure 8 Effect of PVP on the solubilization/concentration plots of sodium alkyl sulfates of different chain lengths and indicated c.m.c. (C_M). Dye is Orange OT. (From Ref. 27.)

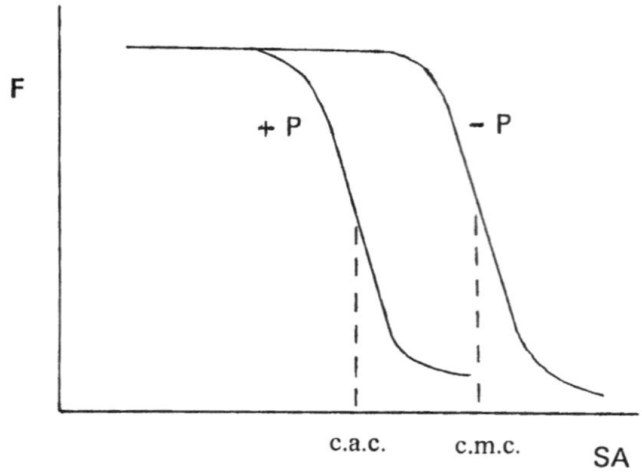

Figure 9 Schematic plot of change, with added surfactant concentration, of fluorescence (F) of added probe, in the presence (+P) and absence (−P) of interacting polymer.

zation, occurs, but below the c.m.c. Conventionally, by the fluorescence technique, the c.m.c. is taken to be at the midpoint (highest slope point) of the plot: a "critical association concentration" (c.a.c.) can be derived from the "with polymer" plot. The literature on the fluorescence method applied to the study of polymer/surfactant systems is extensive and only a few additional points are made here:

1. Behavior similar to that in Figure 9 has been authenticated for well-studied systems like PEO/SDS and PVP/SDS (34,35,38,39).
2. The designations "c.m.c." and "c.a.c." seem to signify a similar phenomenon, i.e., the onset of aggregation and hence solubilizing power.
3. While lower than that of water, the polarity of polymer/surfactant aggregates is sometimes higher than that of micelles, showing that there are residual differences in the aggregated state.
4. Using methods designed to give information on cluster size [e.g., by the use of fluorescence quenchers (34,40,41) and the study of steady-state fluorescence or its decay (42)] it has been shown that the surfactant aggregates that first form (at the c.a.c.) tend to be smaller than regular micelles (ca. 20 vs. 60–80 monomers) but they will have approximately doubled in size when the "T_2" concentration is reached (40,41,43).

The interested reader is referred to a number of excellent and comprehensive recent reviews on the subject of fluorescence (34,43–45).

7. Nuclear Magnetic Resonance

In 1977 a paper by Cabane appeared that has had a major impact on thinking in this field (46). In an extensive NMR study of the PEO/SDS system Cabane investigated the ^{13}C NMR shifts of the different carbons in the SDS molecule on adding increasing amounts of PEO to micellar solutions of SDS. Substantial chemical shifts were noted for the three carbon atoms, (C_1, C_2, C_3) closest to the sulfate headgroup, but were virtually absent for carbons C_4–C_{12}. Furthermore, the shifts for C_1, C_2, and C_3 atoms were linear up to a concentration of added PEO corresponding to the T_2 condition, i.e., where the polymer is just saturated with surfactant. (See Fig. 10a,b.) When the experiment was done in reverse, i.e., SDS was added in increasing amounts to a fixed concentration (1%) solution of PEO, a linear shift in the ^{13}C line of PEO was observed up to a concentration corresponding to the T_2 value of the system.

One can draw a number of conclusions from Cabane's work. First, the environment experienced by surfactant carbons C_4–C_{12} in the polymer/surfactant aggregate is indistinguishable from that in regular surfactant micelles suggesting that the aggregates themselves are modified micelles. On the other hand, the NMR data show that carbons C_1–

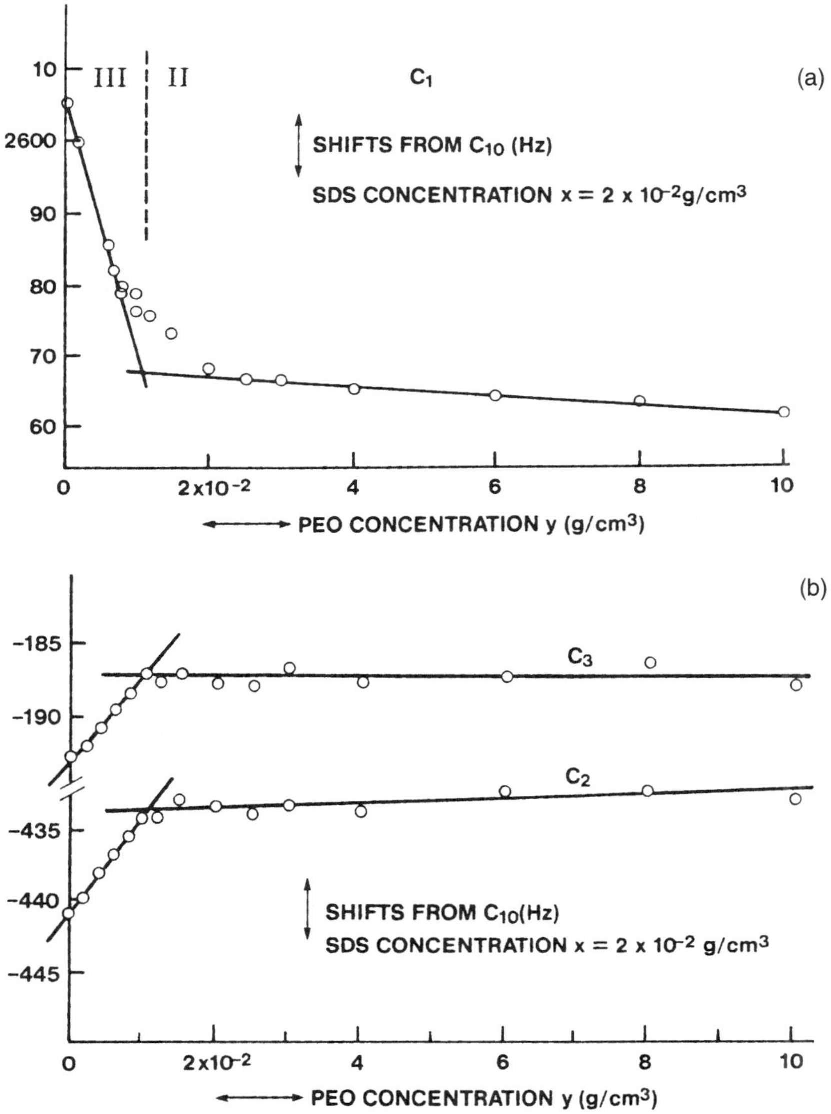

Figure 10 (a) Effect of PEO on the difference in chemical shift between carbons C_1 and C_{10} of the SDS chain. (b) Difference of chemical shifts between C_2 and C_{10} of the SDS chain and between C_3 and C_{10}. (From Ref. 46.)

C_3 of SDS in the polymer/surfactant aggregate are in a different environment and Cabane suggests that EO groups of the polymer replace water molecules in the outer region of the micelles. These ideas, which will be discussed later, are illustrated in Figure 11: they reinforce the "necklace" model proposed by Shirahama.

The first use of NMR methods to study polymer/surfactant interaction was by Muller and Johnson (47), who studied the NMR shift (δ) of the fluorine atom in PEO/F_3 SDS mixtures and obtained results in harmony with the foregoing (F_3 SDS is a modification of SDS in which the terminal CH_3 group is replaced by CF_3). Thus, in the presence of PEO (constant amount) at a certain concentration (T_1) of added F_3 SDS, lower than its c.m.c., a slope change in the δ versus reciprocal concentration plot was observed. At a second concentration (T_2), above the c.m.c., the slope changed again to a value close to that observed in polymer-free micellar F_3 SDS solutions. T_1 was found to be independent of polymer concentration while T_2, again, increased with it.

A recent review of the use of NMR as applied to polymer/surfactant systems can be found in the chapter by Stilbs in Ref. 48.

8. Other Investigation Methods

A large number of other methods have been used to study the interaction of uncharged water-soluble polymers and charged surfactants. The reader is referred to review articles for further information (4,5,9,48). Methods include ultracentrifugation (30), gel filtration (49), electro-optics (50), calorimetry (51), small-angle neutron scattering (52), electron spin resonance (53), diffusion (pulsed gradient spin echo NMR) (54), and finally, fast kinetics studies (55,56), which showed that the kinetics of formation and disintegration of polymer-surfactant aggregates are as fast as those of ordinary micellization, i.e., in the micro- to millisecond range (6).

B. Polyelectrolyte/Surfactant Mixtures

Conditioning polymers applied from aqueous solution are generally positively charged. The reason for this, as discussed in Chapter 10, is that keratin substrates (especially hair)

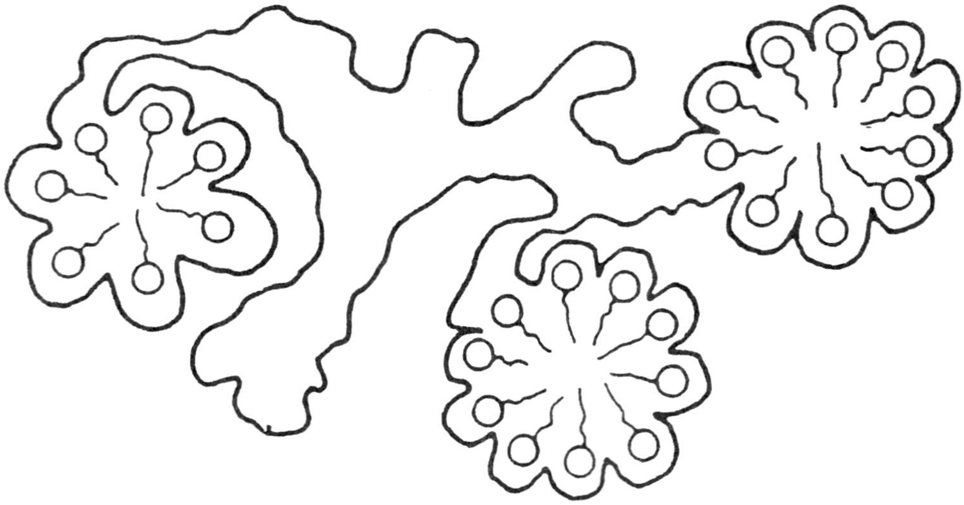

Figure 11 Schematic diagram of a polymer-surfactant complex. (From Ref. 162.)

usually carry a net negative charge. The successful development of "2-in-1" shampoos i.e., compositions that clean and condition, created interest in another phenomenon involving the strong forces of electrostatic interaction, namely the interaction between cationic polymers and anionic surfactants. (Attraction between polyanions and anionic surfactants can be assumed to be negligible—except in special situations, for example when the polymer is hydrophobically modified. See next section.)

1. Solubility Characteristics

One of the primary properties of mixtures of polyion and oppositely charged surfactant systems is their tendency to form insoluble precipitates. Indeed, if stoichiometric amounts (based on charge/charge equivalence) of a polycation and an anionic surfactant are mixed, precipitation of the polymer/surfactant can be expected. Thus, a knowledge of the solubility characteristics of such combinations chosen for a formulation becomes desirable, if not essential. A detailed study (57–59) of the Polymer JR 400/TEALS, and other, surfactant systems led to "solubility diagrams" of the type shown in Figure 12. (Polymer JR is a polycation based on HEC, supplied by Amerchol Corp.) In this log-log diagram, the fact that the line of maximum precipitation has a 45° slope signifies that the complexes formed under these conditions have a constant composition, actually of 1:1 stoichiometry based on charge. [Earlier results by Scott and co-workers on mixtures of various polyanions and cationic surfactants should be acknowledged (60). This group had also demonstrated the formation of 1:1 complexes.] Actually, Figure 12 suggests that a series of

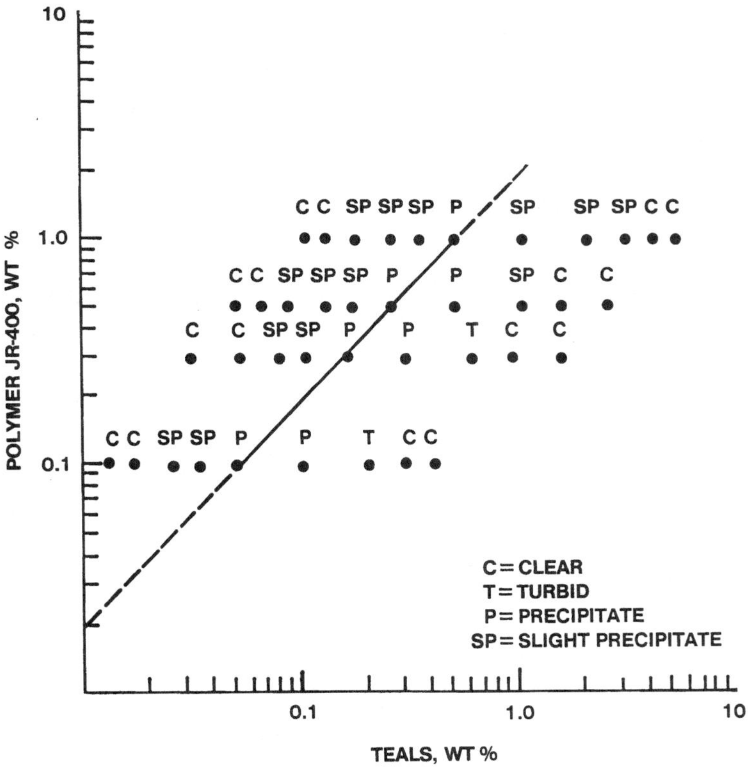

Figure 12 Solubility diagram of Polymer JR 400/TEALS system. (From Ref. 57.)

insoluble complexes of varying stoichiometry can be formed. Evidence for this was obtained from electrophoresis studies that showed that the precipitate particles on the left-hand (polymer rich) side of the stoichiometric line were positively charged whereas those on the right-hand (surfactant rich) side were negatively charged (58). The variety of structures that form, including bilayers, vesicles, threads, and globules, have recently been examined by Goldraich et al. (61) using light and cryotransmission electron microscopy. It is apparent that, for a given level of polycation, clear systems can be formulated at both relatively low and relatively high levels of surfactant—a fact of great importance to formulators. Actually, in real systems, the behavior observed can be less ideal than that of Figure 12. For instance, if the charge density of the polycation is very high, or if "irregularities" are introduced into the surfactant structure, such as chain branching, wing-shaped alkyl groups, or EO moieties in the head group, the "resolubilization area" illustrated in Figure 12 can be more restricted (59). Furthermore, a feature of interest in the solubility diagram of Polymer JR/alkyl sulfate systems was that, at lower concentrations than shown, the 45° maximum insolubility line tends to bend toward the surfactant axis (59). This feature, as will be discussed in Chapter 5, is of potential significance to mechanisms of conditioning in 2-in-1 shampoos.

In recent years much work aimed at determining complete phase diagrams of various combinations of polyion/oppositely charged surfactant pairs has been carried out by the groups of Lindman (9,62) and of Kwak (63). Their diagrams considerably refine the simple concepts referred to above. Furthermore, these workers have successfully modeled the phase behavior using Flory-Huggins concepts (64) and spinodal/binodal phase demarcations (63). The interested reader is referred to the original publications for details.

Successful attempts have been made to modify/minimize precipitation in polyelectrolyte/oppositely charged surfactant systems. Laurent and Scott (65) reported such an effect with the addition of simple salts and defined a "critical electrolyte concentration" (c.e.c.) at which precipitation is totally inhibited. (See Chapter 5 and also Section III.E below.) Likewise, Dubin et al. (66,67) have found inhibitory effects on adding nonionic surfactants to these mixed polymer/surfactant systems, presumably a result of mixed micelle formation.

Results essentially similar to those given in Figure 12 have been reported recently by Manuszak-Guerrini et al. (68) for the Polymer JR/SDS and aminocarbamoylcellulosic/SDS systems. From what follows it will be seen that there is abundant evidence that in the preprecipitation (and in the postprecipitation) zone the surfactant associates with the polymer to form soluble complexes in which the bound surfactant exists in aggregated form.

2. Specific Ion Electrodes to Study Surfactant Binding

Kwak (and co-workers) (10) were the first to employ the electrode method to study interactions involving ionic polymer systems—in their case a series of polyanions of both synthetic and natural origin, and the cationic surfactants, alkyltrimethylammonium and alkylpyridinium halides (69,70).*

---

* The fact that there are more investigations of binding isotherms of cationic surfactants by anionic polymers than vice-versa undoubtedly reflects the fact (71) that it has been found easier to "home-make" electrodes for these surfactants than for anionic surfactants. (See, however, Chapter 10 and Section II.A.2 above.) A typical electrode, employing a cell with a PVC membrane impregnated with a 1:1 complex of DTAB and SDS, showed Nernstian response to DTAB over three decades of concentration (18,19).

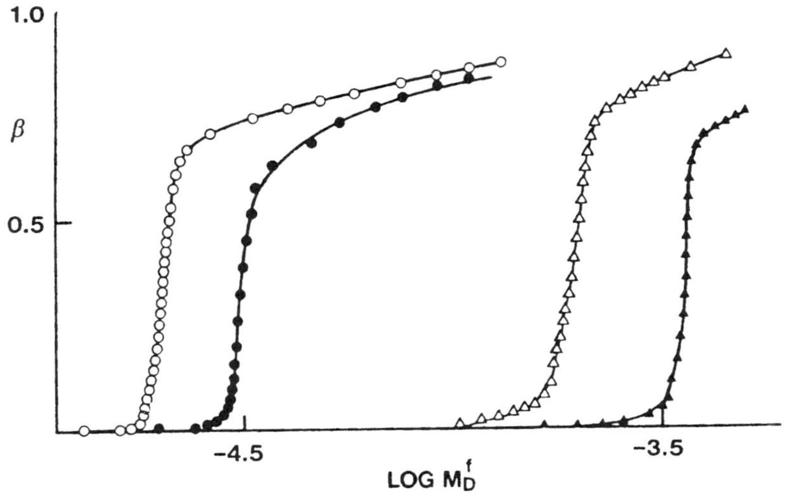

Figure 13 Binding isotherms of polacrylate (5×10^{-4} M): comparison of alkylpyridinium and alkyltrimethylammonium ions. (△) DPy Cl; (○) T Py Br; (▲) DTABr; (●) TTABr. β is the degree of binding. (From Ref. 70.)

Representative results of Hayakawa et al. (70) are given in Figure 13. Several important conclusions can be drawn from these data: (1) The initial concentration for binding is extremely low, appreciably lower than the c.m.c. of the surfactant. (2) The binding curves are sigmoidal, again indicating that a cooperative process, i.e., clustering of the bound surfactant, is involved. This means that the presence of the polyion renders binding and cluster formation of the surfactant much more favorable than in self-clustering of the surfactant alone (simple micelle formation). Evidently, the strong electrostatic attraction of the ionic sites on the polymer leads to the adsorption of individual surfactant ions, which then initiate and promote the aggregation process. (3) As for simple micellization, there is a major reduction in critical aggregation concentration (c.a.c.) as the chain length of the surfactant is increased (from C_{12} to C_{14}). (4) Other data of Hayakawa and Kwak (72,73) demonstrate that added simple electrolyte has a strong influence, in the sense of increasing the c.a.c., i.e., weakening the interaction. (See Section III.E.) The above data were all obtained on clear systems, i.e., below the stoichiometric equivalent concentration of the surfactant. An important corollary is that, in these oppositely charged systems, extensive interaction and formation of intermolecular complexes can occur even with no formation of insoluble species, as stated in the introduction to this section.

3. *Surface Tension*

Surface tension provides a particularly useful and informative approach to studying interaction in polymer/surfactant pairs in the case where the polymer alone is inactive or only feebly active at the air/water interface. Such is the case with many polyelectrolytes including the well-known conditioning agent Polymer JR 400. Goddard and co-workers, in their studies of this polymer in combination with SDS, showed that a strong synergistic reduction of surface tension occurred (57,58). This behavior is quite different from that observed in systems with nonionic polymers. The effect is evident at low concentrations of SDS (Fig. 14) and implies that the polymer of normally feeble surface activity is transformed,

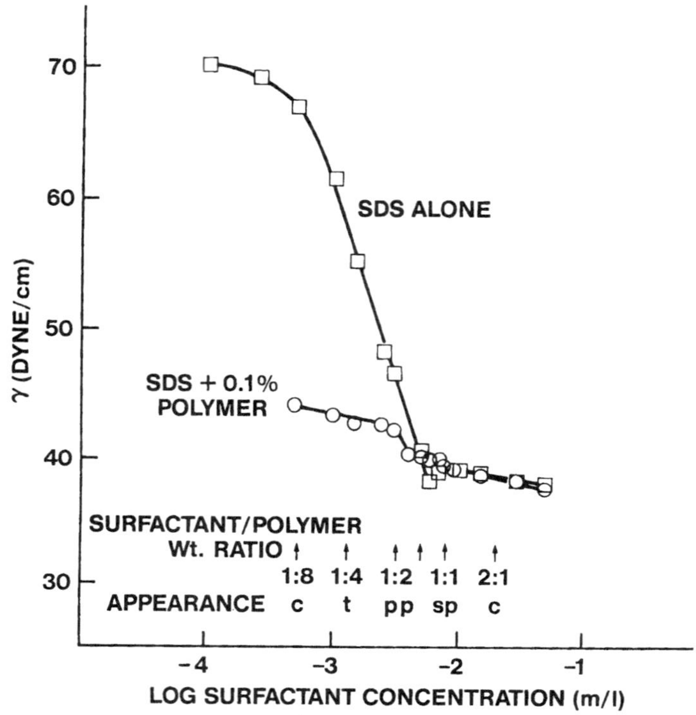

Figure 14 Surface tension/concentration curves of SDS with and without Polymer JR 400. (c) Clear; (t) turbid; (p) precipitate; (sp) slight precipitate. (From Ref. 57.)

on addition of small amounts of SDS, into a much more hydrophobic entity (''complex'') by virtue of the hydrocarbon chains of the bound surfactant. The importance of electrostatic attraction between surfactant and polycation is further attested by the fact that no interaction, as judged by surface tension criteria, was observed between SDS and the parent polymer, hydroxyethylcellulose (HEC). Neither did a nonionic surfactant, Tergitol 15-S-9 (Union Carbide), nor a charge-neutral tetradecylbetaine surfactant (57) show any interaction with Polymer JR.

Figure 15 depicts the changing conditions in the solution and surface of the system as the concentration of added SDS is increased. Even under conditions of maximum precipitation, when most of the polymer and added surfactant are out of solution, the surface tension is still low. This result illustrates the high intrinsic surface activity of the complex. Eventually, when the solutions are sufficiently concentrated in surfactant and become clear, their surface tension becomes the same as that of the corresponding polymer-free systems. The interpretation is that the polymer under these conditions is totally associated with bulk phase micelles, i.e., in effect is stripped from the surface. While this interpretation was advanced many years ago (57,58), it is only recently that direct experimental support for the hypothesis was developed (74). On the basis of *surface* viscosity measurements it was shown that the latter conditions, like those obtained with simple micellar solutions, correspond to surfaces with high fluidity. On the other hand, at lower surfactant concentrations, including those where precipitation takes place, high surface viscosity and even surface viscoelasticity were observed showing the presence of polymer in the ad-

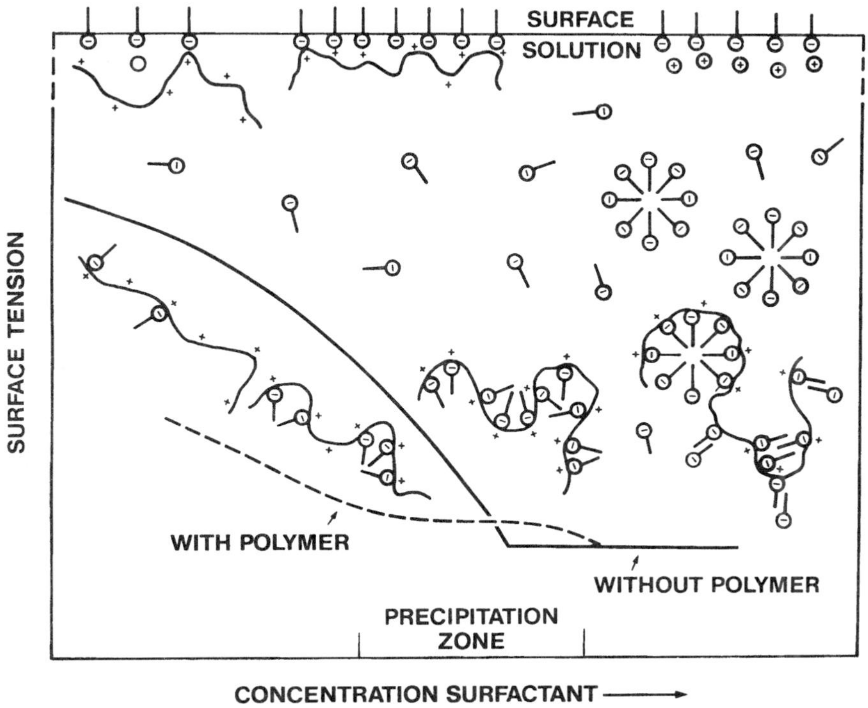

Figure 15 Conditions in bulk and surface containing a polycation (fixed concentration) and anionic surfactant. Full line is hypothetical surface tension/concentration curve of the surfactant alone: dotted line is that of mixture with polycation. Simple countercations are depicted only in surface zone.

sorbed phase. (See Fig. 16.) These results have direct relevance to the subject of foaming and will be discussed further in Chapter 5.

Surface tension studies, yielding results similar to the above, have been obtained on other combinations of polyelectrolyte/oppositely charged surfactant systems. These include poly-L-lysine/SDS (75), carboxymethylcellulose/alkyl TAB surfactants (76), and sulfonated polyacrylamide/DTAB (77,78) combinations.

4. *Viscosity*

It has been pointed out that, through electric repulsion of charges along their backbone, polyelectrolytes tend to adopt a rod-like configuration in solution and, hence, to promote high solution viscosity. Accordingly, the anticipated interaction between polyelectrolyte and oppositely charged surfactants should, in principle, be readily assessed by viscosity measurements, which will register the effects of backbone flexibility, ionic bonding, and also bound alkyl chain association. The virtue of such measurements is that viscometers are standard bench-top equipment, available in most laboratories. As will be seen, very different types of behavior have been observed with different polymer/surfactant systems.

Mixtures of the cationic cellulosic Polymer JR 400 and SDS showed the following characteristics. At a level of 0.1% polymer, no increase in solution viscosity (indeed, a small decrease prior to the precipitation zone) was registered on addition of SDS (79). By contrast, at the higher level of 1.0% polymer a very substantial increase was registered

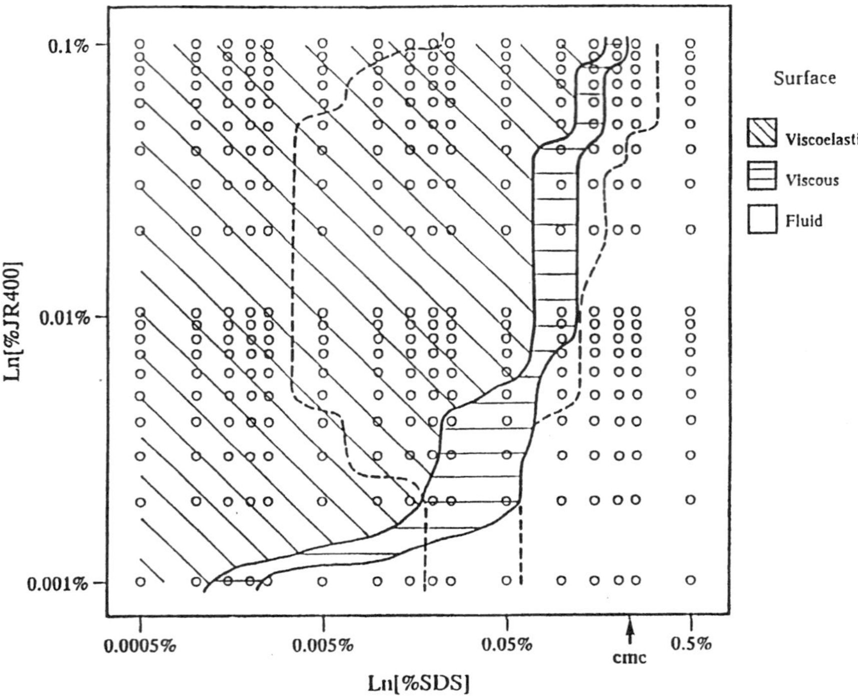

Figure 16 Surface "phase map" of the Polymer JR 400/SDS system. (From Ref. 74.) Dashed line encloses area of bulk precipitation or turbidity.

especially in the immediate preprecipitation zone of the phase diagram (see Fig. 17) together with a modest increase in the postprecipitation zone. This behavior suggests different structures in these two zones, as already discussed (Fig. 15). In particular, in the preprecipitation zone a network is invoked in which surfactant molecules bound to one macromolecule associate with similarly linked surfactant molecules on other polymer chains. These structures would be expected to be shear thinning. Indeed, rheological data on the 1% Polymer JR/0.1% SDS system confirmed this picture (80). Thus, at low shear rates, up to about 25 sec^{-1}, the system had a high viscosity and was Newtonian. Thereafter, it was markedly shear thinning, until at about 400 sec^{-1} it was again Newtonian with a comparatively low differential viscosity. The inference is that the energy input at shear rates >400 sec^{-1} is sufficient to break the intermolecular association bonds. Another expectation is that the effects would be magnified as the molecular weight of the polymer is increased. This effect was confirmed with the system Polymer JR 30M, and will be described in the section on gel formation in Chapter 5.

By contrast with the above, corresponding data obtained for another polycation, acrylamide/β-methacryloxyethyltrimethylammonium chloride (Reten, Hercules), at 1% concentration, showed no change in viscosity with added SDS in the preprecipitation zone (80). There is thus little doubt that the clustering of bound SDS that takes place is *intra*-polymolecular in this case. A similar situation was reported by Abuin and Scaiano (81) for mixtures of polystyrene sulfonate and DTAB in which an observed 10-fold *reduction* of viscosity was ascribed to coiling of the polymer around small clusters of surfactant molecules that formed. On the other hand, McCormick and Johnson (82) reported that

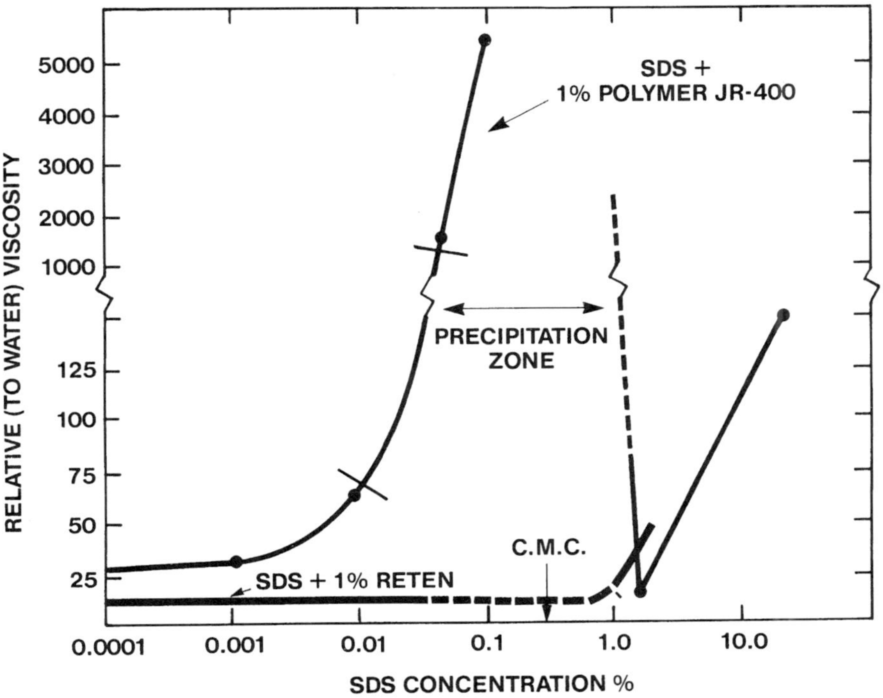

Figure 17 Relative viscosity of 1% Polymer JR 400 and 1% Reten 220 as a function of SDS concentration. (From Ref. 80.)

addition of SDS to the copolymer diallylalkoxybenzylmethylammonium chloride/diallyldimethylammonium chloride resulted in a large *increase* in solution viscosity and ascribed this result to the formation of intramolecular polymeric micelles.

In general, one can argue that two opposing effects will accompany the addition of a charged surfactant to an oppositely charged polyelectrolyte. First, binding of surfactant will reduce the overall charge of the polyion and lead to contraction of the coil and, probably, further contraction by condensation around micellar clusters that will form. Second, bonding between surfactant molecules linked to *different* polymer chains will constitute cross-links leading to increased viscosity. These effects will be concentration and molecular weight dependent, and, a priori, in a particular system difficult to predict. Nonetheless, it is clear that simple measurements of solution viscosity will often be a sensitive indicator of interaction in a particular polyelectrolyte surfactant system, especially if carried out over a range of concentration and reactant ratios. At high surfactant concentration the solution viscosity often falls. To a large extent the properties are now dominated by surfactant micelles, which no longer have to be ''shared'' by the polymer molecules and, hence, cross-linking effects, which are responsible for viscosity elevation, would disappear. (See Fig. 18.)

5. *Solubilization: Oil-Soluble Dyes*

Kwak's work using specific ion electrodes, referred to earlier, had given evidence of the cooperative binding of cationic surfactants by several polyanions (69). This phenomenon implies cluster formation of the bound surfactant molecules, which, as outlined above,

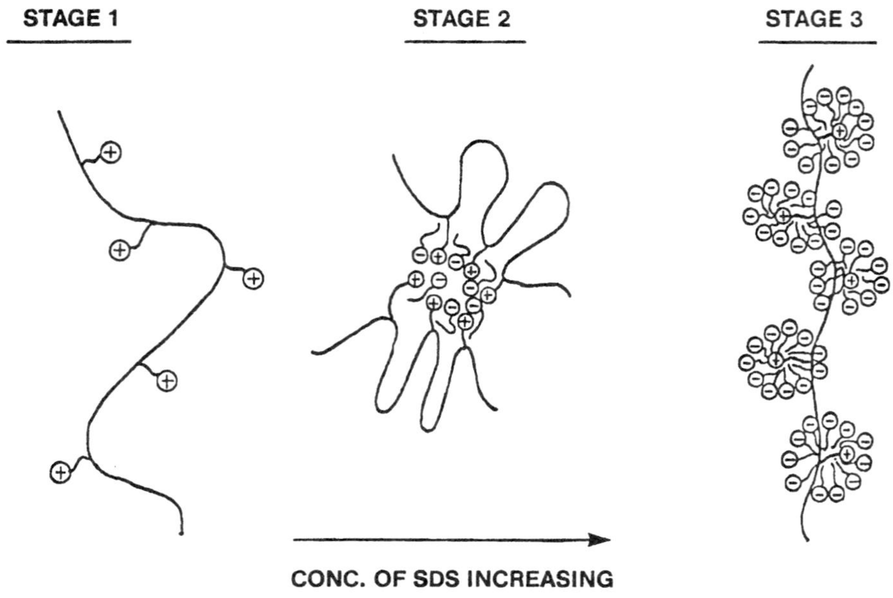

Figure 18 Different stages of binding of SDS by a polycation—ultimately resembling a "necklace." (From Ref. 85.)

carries the connotation of potential solvent activity of the "microdroplets" (hydrocarbon clusters) so formed. Earlier work (79) on Polymer JR/SDS combinations had confirmed this: at concentrations about two orders of magnitude lower than the c.m.c. of the surfactant its mixtures with the polymer were shown to solubilize the oil-soluble dye Orange OT (region 1). This confirms a low value of the c.a.c. (See Fig. 19.) It is interesting that, as

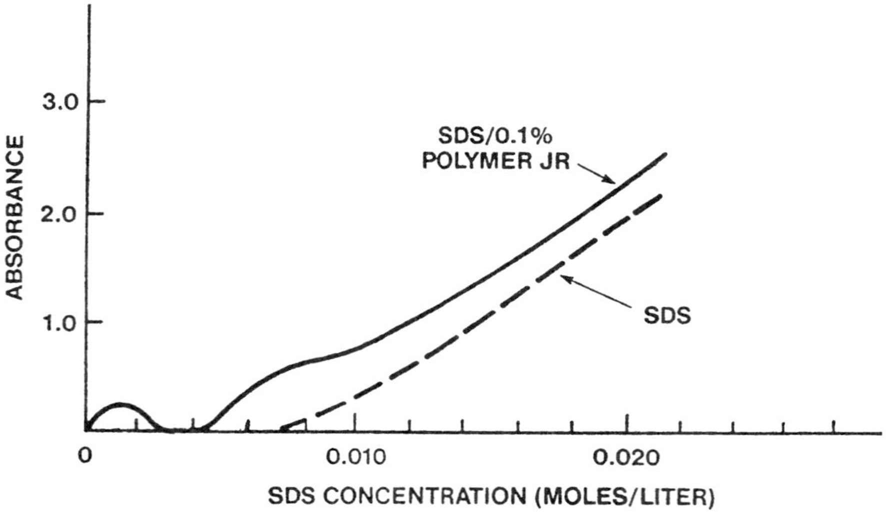

Figure 19 Solubilization of Orange OT by SDS alone and in the presence of 0.1% Polymer JR 400. Region 2 (zero solubilization) lies between region 1 (low SDS) and region 3 (high (SDS). (From Ref. 80.)

a function of SDS concentration, for a fixed level of Polymer JR, the solubilization value falls to near zero: this corresponds to the region 2 where insoluble precipitates form. (See Fig. 12.) It is significant that in the resolubilization zone at higher SDS concentrations, the amount of dye solubilized actually surpassed that of the corresponding polymer-free micellar systems emphasizing residual differences between simple and polymer-covered micelles (region 3). (See Fig. 19.) Tests carried out (83) with the micelle-disclosing dye Pinacyanol allowed the conclusion that micelle-type structures were present in regions 1 and 3 but not in region 2. Hayakawa et al. (84) developed some insight into the role of the polymer in the solubilization process of polymer/surfactant systems by comparing data for complexes formed by dextran sulfate and polystyrene sulfonate in combination with DTAB and TTAB cationic surfactants. The oil-soluble dyes used were *o*-(2-amino-1-naphthylazo) toluene and pyrenecarbaldehyde. Dextran sulfate exhibits highly cooperative binding of these cationic surfactants; binding to polystyrene sulfonate occurs at lower surfactant concentration but is less cooperative. These results probably reflect greater flexibility of the dextran sulfate polymer but also a hydrophobic contribution to the process of surfactant clustering in the case of polystyrene sulfonate. The fact that the dextran sulfate complexes were found to have a higher solubilization capacity (expressed per bound mole of surfactant) than the polystyrene sulfonate complexes for both the above dyes seems to be in harmony with this explanation. The effects of polyion structure on the binding of oppositely charged surfactants are presented in a broader sense later.

Many other reports of the solubilization of oil soluble dyes by polyelectrolyte/oppositely charged surfactant pairs can be found in the literature. For example, solubilization of Yellow OB has been reported for cationic cellulosic/SDS systems (85) and for polyvinylsulfonate/RTAB systems (86). Likewise, solubilization of Sudan III by PEI/SDS systems has been studied (87).

6. *Fluorescent Dyes*

Early work on conditioning polyelectrolyte/surfactant systems using fluorescent dyes was carried out on the Polymer JR 400/SDS system with pyrene and pyrene aldehyde (83). It was shown, for example, that pyrene is more efficiently solubilized by the ''low concentration'' SDS aggregates than the ''high concentration'' SDS aggregates referred to in the last section. From these results the authors concluded that there are distinct structural differences between the two, the former corresponding to hemimicelle-type assemblies of low surfactant aggregation number, and the latter to more conventional micelles—the ''beads'' in the entangled necklace structure. (See Fig. 18.)

In measurements with pyrene aldehyde, the position of λ_{max}—the wavelength of maximum fluorescence—yields *D*, the dielectric constant of the absorbing medium (micelles) according to $\lambda_{max} = 0.582D + 431.5$. For SDS micelles, a *D* value of 50 was deduced, indicating the probe experiences an environment comparable in polarity to ethanol. In the immediate pre- and postprecipitation zones of Polymer JR/SDS mixture with 0.01 and 0.1% polymer, pyrene aldehyde was shown to experience a much lower polarity medium, of dielectric constant down to as low as 30, indicating a less open and less hydrated palisade layer of the aggregated surfactant phase as compared to regular micelles (83). With Reten 220, on the other hand, the corresponding solubilizing environments have a *D* value almost identical to that of regular micelles, suggesting a more open and hydrated structure in this case. Specific contributions of the polymer structure to the nature of the association complex are thus clearly established. Well into the postprecipitation zone the properties in both cases approximated those of SDS micellar solutions.

Historically, the use of fluorescent dyes to study the interaction of polyelectrolyte/surfactant systems seemed to lag behind their use for studying their uncharged polymer/surfactant counterparts. In the last decade, however, their use in the former systems has become widespread. These developments are summarized in the comprehensive review articles of Winnik (43,44). A partial listing of systems studied includes polystyrene sulfonate/DTAB (88), polymethacrylate/C_{10}TAB (89), polyacrylate/DTAC (90), polyacrylate/DTAC, DTAB, CTAC (91), and PVMMA/DTAC (92). In general, but with one or two exceptions (81), the number n of surfactant molecules per aggregate in the presence of polyelectrolyte has been found to be roughly the same (viz., ~50 monomers) as in their absence. However, the microviscosity experienced by the fluorescent probe in the former case can be substantially higher (92); i.e., the polymer can influence the fluidity within the surfactant aggregate. Another finding of interest is that n can depend strongly on the degree of ionization in systems where the polyion has weak electrolyte character. For example, in the PVMMA/DTAC system just cited (92) n was found to vary from 50 in ionized systems (COO^-) to 10 in unionized systems (COOH). Of course, the actual fluorescence characteristics of a weak polyelectrolyte by itself can change with pH (33).

C. Hydrophobically Modified Water-Soluble Polymers

About 50 years ago Strauss and co-workers (93,94) developed the notion of "zero c.m.c" polymeric materials that would spontaneously form/possess micelle-like assemblies when dissolved in water, regardless of the solution concentration. Strauss referred to the materials as "polysoaps." They were, in essence, water-soluble ionic polymers with a suitable degree of hydrophobic substitution. Thus, consistent with the overall requirement of being water soluble, the polymer could possess a small number of long hydrocarbon chains, or a larger number of shorter hydrocarbon chains, or a mixture of both. For water solubility, the polymer had to contain a number of ionic or ionizable groups, nominally along or offset from the polymer backbone. Because of hydrophobic interactions there would be a natural tendency of hydrocarbon groups in the aqueous environment to associate, hence spontaneously creating the "micelles" of Strauss. It was to be expected that this process would endow the solutions with properties typical of micellar soap solutions, such as the ability to solubilize hydrocarbons, as has been clearly demonstrated by Strauss (93).

Interest in these "alkyl modified" polymeric structures was relatively low for some time, but about 20 years ago was heightened when it was realized that interalkyl chain association, as well as intrachain association, could take place, effectively increasing the molecular weight of the polymer and, therefore, the viscosity of the solution. Hence the term "associative thickener" evolved and now includes polyamphiphilic structures, i.e., not necessarily only polyionic structures. The presence of hydrophobic groups endows these polymers with surface and interfacial activity and hence with potential as foam, emulsion, and suspension stabilizers as well as surface conditioners.

From the viewpoint of the subject of this chapter it is clear that the hydrophobic groups on these polymers also represent sites for attraction of surfactants in solution and, hence, interaction. As with the other categories of polymer, summaries of various techniques to study such interaction will be presented, starting with viscosity because of the rheological importance of these systems.

1. *Viscosity, Phase Separation, Gelation*

Extensive work on the self-association and thickening properties of hydrophobically modified (HM) polymers was reported in the 1980s. For example, see the compilation of papers in Ref. 95. One such polymer of relevance to cosmetics is HM-HEC, or, more correctly, a series of HM-HECs, in which the hydrophobic (HM) group has ranged from C_8 to C_{16} (96,97) and has also included alkyl phenyl groups (98). Illustrative rheological data for this type of polymer are shown in Figure 20. While the solution viscosity characteristics of such a polymer in combination with surfactant will clearly depend on a number of factors, e.g., the degree of substitution, type and chain length of the substitution, absolute concentration of polymer (96,97), and so forth, under practical conditions the viscosity response to added surfactant can typically be of the form shown in Figure 21. It is interesting that such data can actually be obtained with a *nonionic surfactant* additive (96,97). Similar results have been obtained by other workers (99). They show that HM-polymers, unlike the categories of polymer described earlier, are sensitive to interaction with uncharged (as well as charged) surfactant molecules through what are termed *hydrophobic forces*. Mechanistically, one can explain the maximum in viscosity depicted in Figure 21 as being due to surfactant micelles acting as "cross-linkers." (See Fig. 22.) At higher surfactant concentration, when micelles are in abundance, they are no longer shared by the hydrophobic groups of the polymer and the viscosity falls. (See below.) Increments in viscosity in the more conventional combination of HM-HEC and anionic surfactant (such as SDS) have been reported by several authors (99–101). Mechanisms involved are essentially similar to those just described but can involve, in addition, the adsorption of single surfactant ions (or small clusters) onto the hydrophobic centers of the polymer, which would in this way acquire the characteristics of a polyion. A cautionary note was introduced regarding the above effects when it was reported (98,100) that *phase separation*

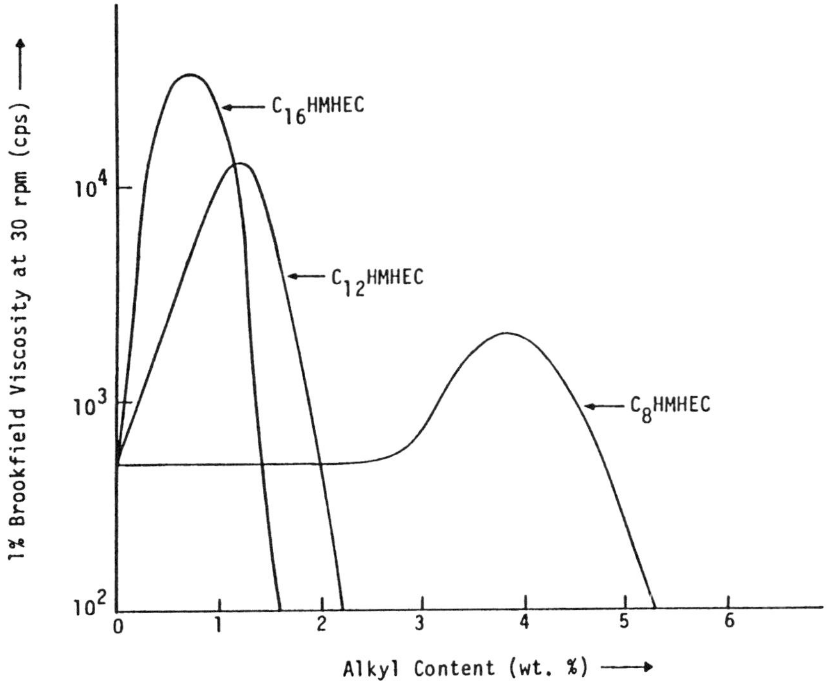

Figure 20 Brookfield viscosity (at 30 rpm) of 1% HM-HEC solutions versus alkyl group content of hydrophobe. (From Ref. 97.)

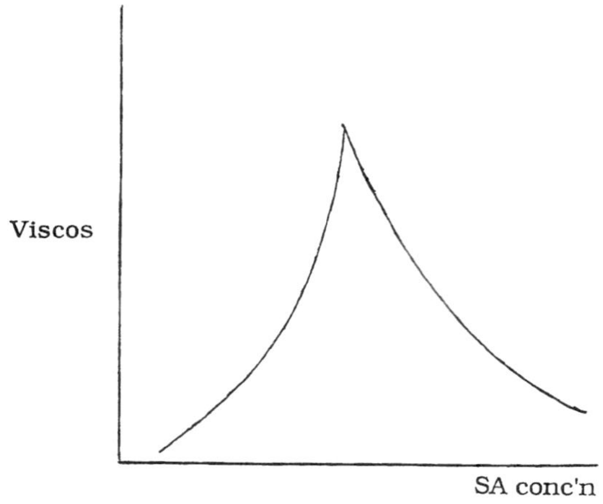

Figure 21 Schematic plot of viscosity response of a HM-polymer solution to added surfactant.

can be encountered in mixed HM-HEC/surfactant systems, whether the surfactant be anionic, cationic, or nonionic. Such phase separations, which can seriously complicate manifestations of an apparent viscosity change, are probably best explained on the basis of the Flory-Huggins theory. (See below and Chapters 1–3.)

As an example of a hydrophobically modified polycation we cite the cationic cellulosic polymer Quatrisoft Polymer LM-200, which has pendant dodecyl groups. Its rheological properties in combination with SDS (and other anionic surfactants) have been examined in some detail (102). In common with its ''parent'' cationic cellulosic Polymer JR, when combined with anionic surfactants, it can lead to zones of phase incompatibility (precipitation). (See Fig. 23.) However, in this case, enhanced viscosity (and gelling) effects are found not only in the region prior to the precipitation zone (the lower gelling range), but also in the region just beyond it (the upper gelling range). This general topic is discussed further in Chapter 5. Although no special viscosity effects were noted after addition of nonionic or cationic surfactants to this polymer, interaction with them was detected by other methods (see below). Related work on HM- and cationic-cellulosic polymer/surfactant mixtures has been reported by Hoffmann and co-workers (103).

Turning to hydrophobically modified (HM)-anionic polyelectrolytes, one finds a great deal of work reported on the rheological properties of their mixtures with surfactants. As illustration, we may refer to the extensive work of Audebert, Iliopoulos, and Zana and their co-workers (90,104,105), whose research has included several studies on ionized copolymers of acrylic acid and alkyl (C_{12} or C_{18}) acrylamide (HM-PA). For example, increases in solution viscosity of C_{12}HM-PA with added surfactants, DTAB or DTAC, were found (90) at low levels of addition ($\sim 10^{-4}$ M), culminating in substantial increases (up to three or four orders of magnitude!) prior to micelle formation and phase separation at higher surfactant concentration (ca. 10^{-2} M). This behavior is reminiscent of that of combinations of polycation and anionic surfactant referred to previously. A representative depiction (90) of this sequence of events is given in Figure 24. These rheological effects eclipse those seen with the unmodified, ''parent'' polyacrylate homopolymer, illustrating how important the ''hydrophobic effect'' can be in polymer/surfactant interaction.

Further, and more compelling, illustrations of the hydrophobic effect came from other sets of measurements on HM(C_{18})-PA by Iliopoulos, Audebert, and co-workers (104). In

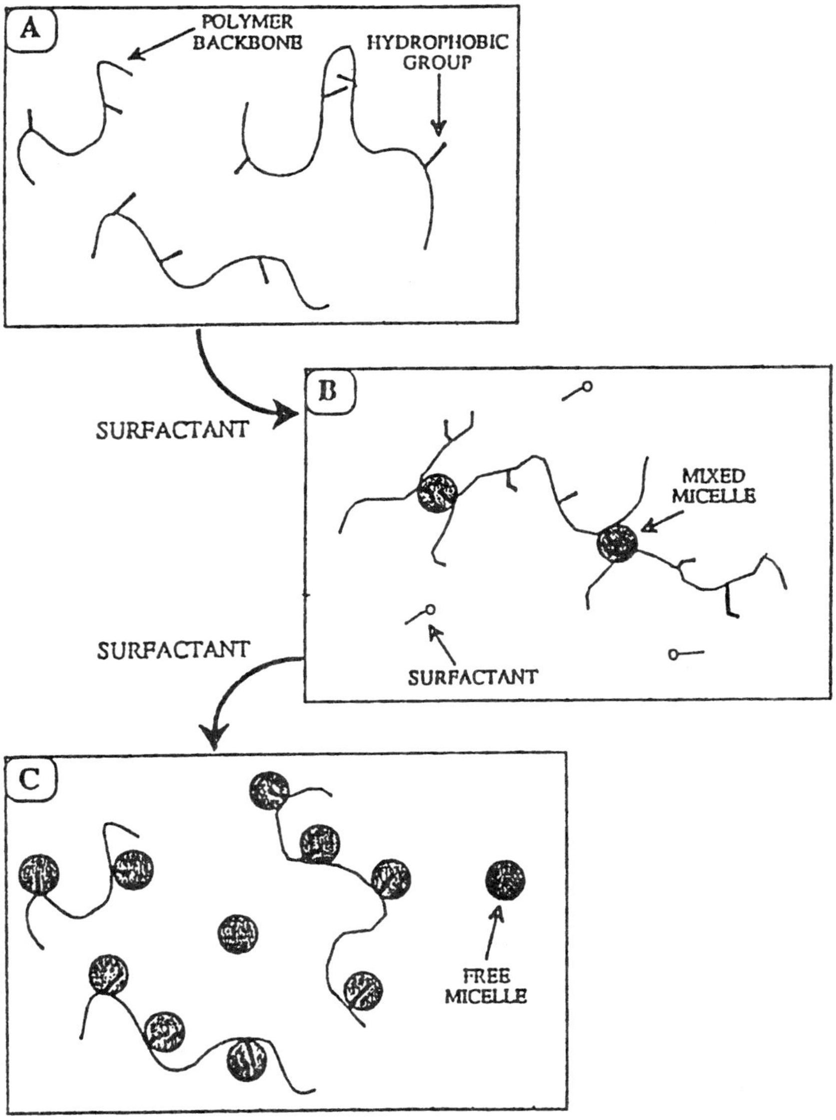

Figure 22 Schematic molecular representation of the interaction of a HM-polymer with an added surfactant. (From Ref. 104.)

the first set, the presence of (normally unreactive) nonionic surfactants, $C_{12}E_4$, $C_{12}E_5$, and $C_{12}E_6$, led to substantial increases in the viscosity of the polymer solution of as much as three decades! The effect was maximal at concentrations ($\sim 10^{-2}$ M) that considerably exceed the c.m.c. of the surfactants, suggesting that preformed micelles may have been involved in the aggregation process; also, the effect was largest with $C_{12}E_4$, which formed the largest micelles at the chosen temperature (25°C). (See Chapter 5, Fig. 18.) Even stronger evidence came from mixtures of HM(C_{18})-PA with the "standard" anionic surfactant, SDS: Despite unfavorable electrical repulsion, the forces of hydrophobic attraction again led to increases in viscosity—as much as a thousandfold—with the maximum in

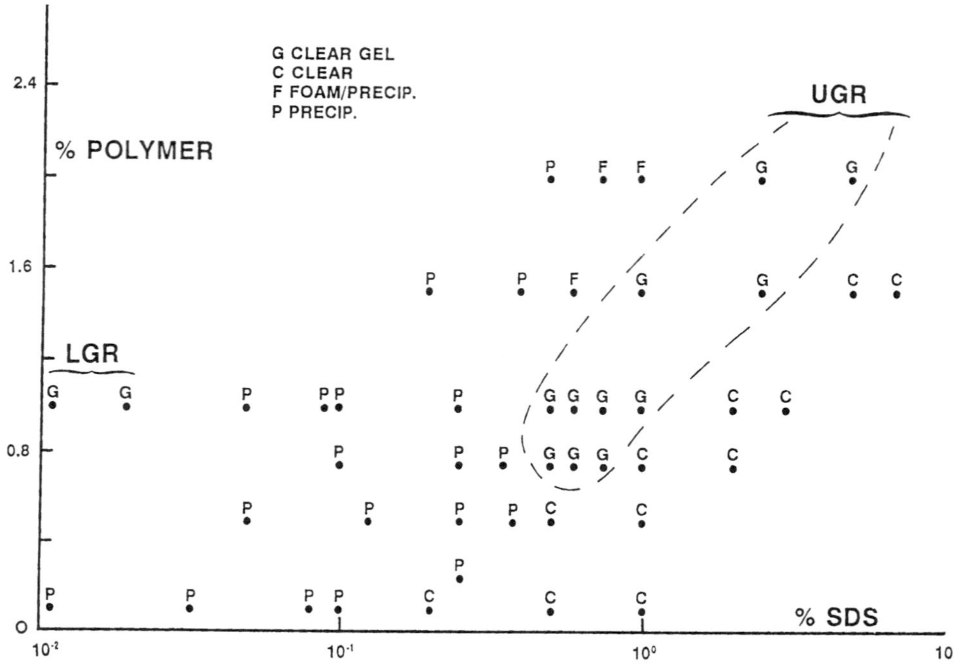

Figure 23 Solubility diagram of Quatrisoft LM 200/SDS system. Results show an upper gelling range (UGR) as well as a lower gelling range (LGR). Compare with Figures 12 and 17. (From Ref. 102.)

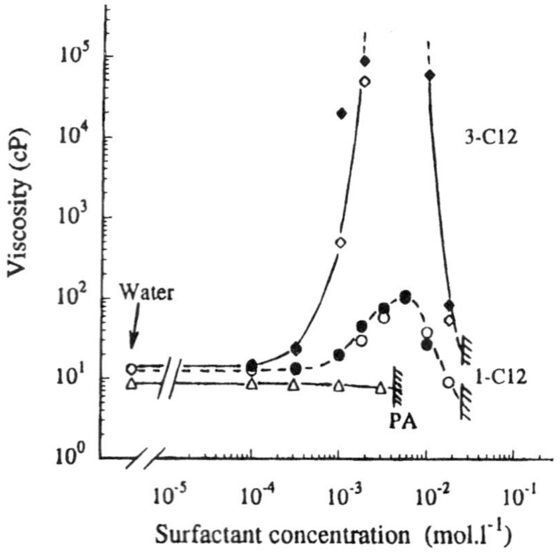

Figure 24 Viscosity of 1% solutions of sodium polyacrylate and polyacrylate hydrophobically modified within 1% ($1 - C_{12}$) and 3% ($3 - C_{12}$) alkyl side groups, in combination with added DTAB (open symbols) and DTAC (filled symbols) surfactants. (From Ref. 90.)

this case occurring near the c.m.c. of SDS (105). The former situation is illustrated in Figure 22, which also applies to the latter one.

Results similar to the above have been reported by Senan et al. for a related HM-PA polymer (106) in combination with various anionic surfactants. Likewise Petit et al. (107) have shown recently that interaction with anionic surfactants is maintained when the side chains in HM-PA polymers are changed to perfluoroalkyl groups.

2. *Surface Tension*

Early in this chapter it was pointed out that the surface tension method is most useful and discriminating for the study of polymer/surfactant interaction when the polymer has a low level of surface activity (at the air/water interface). This would evidently not be the case with HM-substituted polymers. Conversely, if it were possible to demonstrate interaction by this technique in a case rendered even more unfavorable by electrical repulsion between the two components, the evidence for *overall* mutual attraction would be especially convincing. Such was the case in two systems examined by McGlade et al. (108), who found clear evidence of interaction between SDS and poly(1-decene-co-maleic acid) or poly(1-octadecene-co-maleic acid), which are both anionic polyelectrolytes. The evidence was based on the observed crossover of the ''with-'' and ''without-polymer'' surface tension curves of SDS, implying a loss of surfactant from the surface by complex formation in the bulk phase, analogous to Figure 6. (See Fig. 25.) McGlade et al. were in fact the first to demonstrate interaction between a charged surfactant and a like-charged HM-polymer, and, therefore, the great potential importance of hydrophobic forces in such interactions.

Surface tension work on solutions of the HM-cationic cellulosic Quatrisoft Polymer LM-200 in combination with a series of surfactant types has been reported (102). With an oppositely charged surfactant (SDS) the surface tension results showed there was strong interaction but these results were complicated by phase separation effects. Evidence was obtained of some interaction with members of the cationic surfactant RTAB family but the effects were, in general, small at best. On the other hand, with the nonionic surfactant Tergitol NP 10, a crossover of the two surface tension curves for the surfactant, i.e., with and without polymer, was clearly evident. (See Fig. 26.) Although the shape of the curve with polymer present differs from the classic interaction case (see Figs. 5,6), inasmuch as no surface tension plateau is present, it is clearly consistent with binding of the surfactant and concomitant depletion of surfactant from the air/water interface. These results provide another example of how normally inert nonionic surfactants can be rendered ''interactive'' if the polymer present possesses hydrophobic groups.

3. *Fluorescent Dyes*

The fluorescence method has been used extensively for studying the interaction between hydrophobically modified (HM) polymers and surfactants, as is the case with the other categories of polymer already discussed. This is because of its sensitivity and versatility and the relative inexpensiveness of, at least, the basic measuring equipment. Again, because of extensive literature available (43,44), only highpoints and few illustrations are presented here.

Our starting point is again with ''unfavorable'' systems in which hydrophobic forces of attraction must overcome the forces of electrostatic repulsion between a polymer and a surfactant with a like sign of charge, as in the combination cationic cellulosic polymer/cationic surfactant. Measuring (109) the I_1/I_3 ratio of dissolved pyrene as a function of surfactant (DTAB) concentration, at a constant level of polymer, showed no apparent

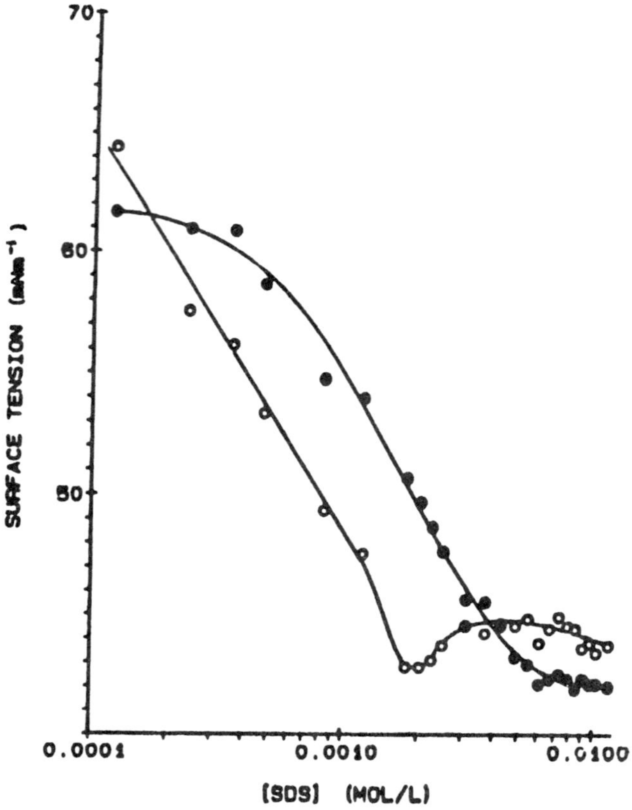

Figure 25 Surface tension as a function of SDS concentration for pH 8.0 buffer (○) and 0.5% poly (1-octadecene-comaleic acid)/pH 8.0 buffer (●) systems. (From Ref. 108.)

influence of Polymer JR (other than perhaps an effect similar to that of a simple electrolyte, like NaCl). On the other hand, a substantial influence was exercised by the hydrophobically modified Quatrisoft Polymer LM-200, suggesting a considerable drop in the apparent c.m.c. of the surfactant. (See Fig. 27.) Equally interesting is the evidence, from the pyrene fluorescence characteristics, of association of several other cationic surfactants (DTAC, TTAB, and CTAC), all at *much* lower concentrations (ca. one-hundredth) than their c.m.c. in the presence of this polymer, and also of preassociation of the HM-polymer molecules themselves (110). Data such as the foregoing have led to the currently accepted interpretation that in HM-polymer/surfactant systems these preassociation sites provide the nuclei for interaction with added surfactant molecules (104–107,110,111). Results similar to the above have been obtained by McGlade et al. (108) for a system charged in the opposite sense. (See above.)

When hydrophobic group interaction between a HM-polymer and a surfactant is reinforced by electrostatic interaction, as in HM-P^{n+}/SA^- or HM-P^{n-}/SA^+ systems, fluorescence methods show that association takes place at minute concentrations of added surfactant (112). This can be seen for the Quatrisoft/SDS system in Figure 28, which also illustrates the (somewhat less) potent interaction of the unsubstituted cationic cellulosic

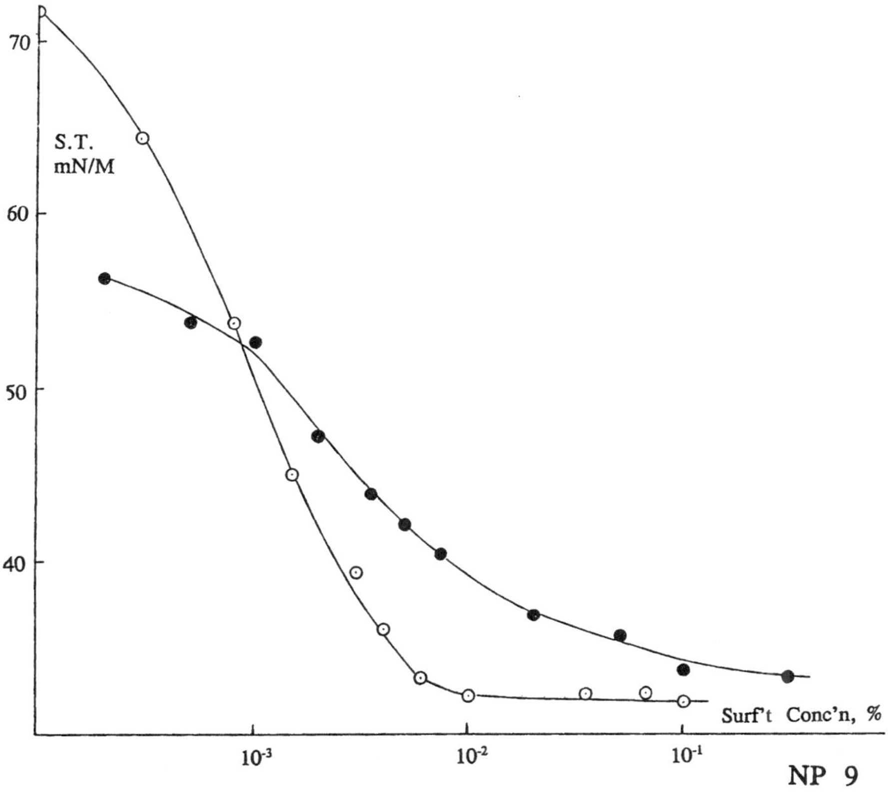

Figure 26 Surface tension curves of Tergitol NP10 in the presence (filled symbols) and absence (open symbols) of 1% Quatrisoft LM 200 polymer. (From Ref. 102.)

Polymer JR 400 with SDS. The former data have been confirmed by Guillemet and Piculell (113).

For systems charged in the opposite sense ($HM\text{-}P^{n-}/SA^{+}$) an excellent example and summary of fluorescence results is provided in a compilation by Magny et al. (90,114) for a series of hydrophobically modified polyacrylate copolymers, viz., $AA/C_{12}AAm$ and $AA/C_{18}AAm$. (In the first case the molar amounts of the modifying dodecylacrylamide monomer were 1 and 3%; in the second it was 1% octadecylacrylamide.) The interacting surfactant chosen was dodecyltrimethylammonium chloride (DTAC). (See Fig. 29.) The results show that the already strong interaction between the surfactant and the parent polyacrylate polymer is further reinforced by the presence on the polymer of dodecyl groups, that it is increased when the content of the latter is enlarged, and that the increase is even higher when the alkyl substitution is changed to octadecyl. Clearly, in the latter cases, the alkyl groups now appear to direct the micellization process. A point of much interest is that, using steady-state and time-resolved fluorescence methods, the authors were able to demonstrate that the total number of surfactant molecules and alkyl groups in the mixed micelles is close to the aggregation number of the free surfactant micelles. Similar work for a poly(maleic acid-coalkyl vinyl ether) group of polyanions in mixture with DTAC has been presented by Anthony and Zana (115). Finally, we refer to work by McCormick

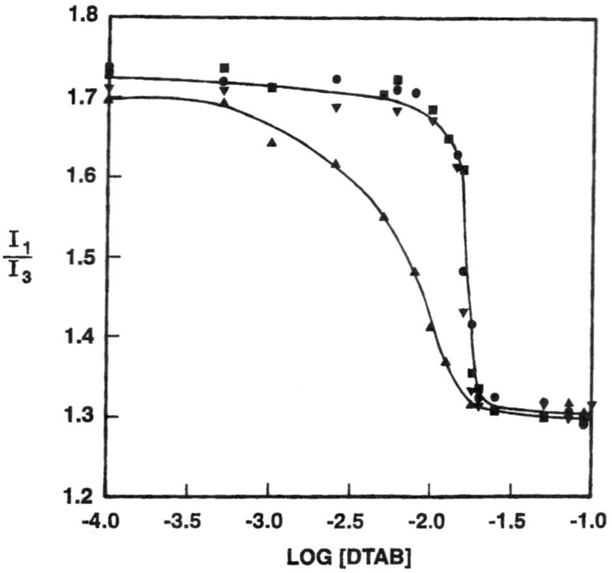

Figure 27 Plots of I_1/I_3 for the emission of pyrene in aqueous solutions of Quatrisoft LM 200 (1 g/L) (▲), Polymer JR 400 (1 g/L) (▼), water (●), and aqueous NaCl (6.0×10^{-4} mol/L) (■), as a function of DTAB concentration. (From Ref. 109.)

et al. (82,116), who used a fluorescence method to demonstrate the formation of mixed micelles when SDS was added to certain cationic copolymer solutions, studied for their solution-thickening behavior.

While hydrophobically modified nonionic polymers are encountered far less frequently than their ionic counterparts, one can find several fluorescence studies of their interaction with surfactants. These include investigations of the HM-HEC/SDS system by Dualeh and Steiner (100) and by Sivadasan and Somasundaran (117) of the same polymer with added SDS and also the nonionic surfactant $C_{12}EO_8$. A comprehensive study,

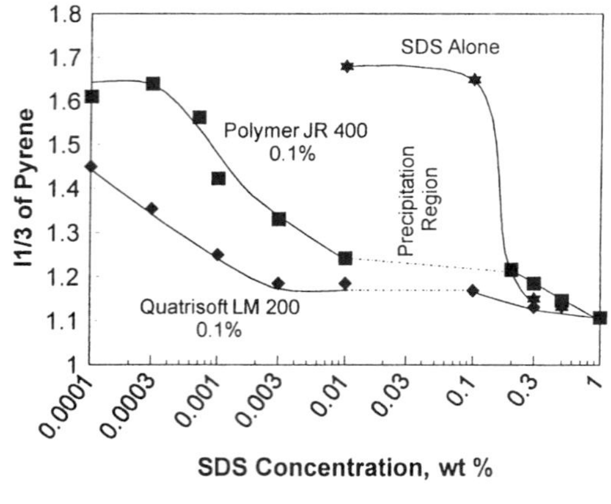

Figure 28 Plots of I_1/I_3 for pyrene as a function of SDS concentration in the absence and presence of Quatrisoft LM 200 and Polymer JR 400. (From Ref. 112.)

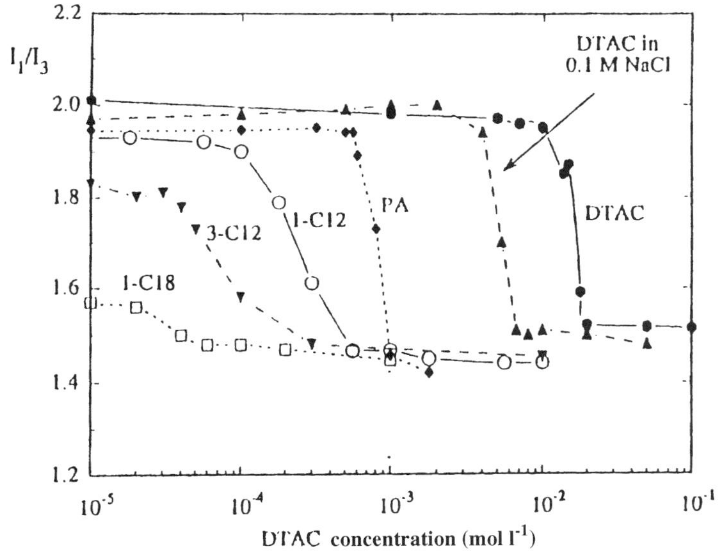

Figure 29 Plots of I_1/I_3 for pyrene as a function of DTAC concentration in the absence of polymer in water and 0.1 M NaCl, and in the presence of polyacrylate, unmodified (PA) or modified with 1% or 3% C_{12} groups, or 1% C_{18} groups. (From Ref. 90.)

by fluorescence with added pyrene, of the interaction of a family of hydrophobically modified poly-isopropyl acrylamides (HM-PNIPAM) with SDS, TTAC, and CTAC surfactants was reported by Winnik et al. (118). The modifying *N*-*n*-alkylacrylamide monomers included C_{10}, C_{14}, and C_{18} alkyl groups. Interaction was found to be strong in all cases and resulted in the formation of mixed clusters of alkyl group and surfactant molecules (~30 per n-alkyl group for the C_{12} and C_{14} surfactants, and ~15 for the C_{16} surfactant). Interaction between (C_{18}) HM-PNIPAM copolymer and the nonionic surfactant OTG (*n*-octyl β-D-thioglucopyranoside) has also been reported by these authors.

4. "Pseudo" Hydrophobically Modified Polymers

An elegant innovation to aid the study of polymer/surfactant interaction was the introduction of a fluorescent label directly onto the polymer molecule by covalent bonding. [See reviews by Winnik (43,44).] This approach has been particularly useful in systems, such as combinations of nonionic polymers and nonionic surfactants, where interaction is weak. For example, pyrene-labeled hydroxypropylcellulose (HPC) gave evidence of association with weakly reactive OTG (*n*-octyl-β-D-thioglucopyranoside) but only at concentrations near its c.m.c. (119). Experiments with pyrene-labeled PNIPAM have been reported by Winnik et al. (120), who obtained evidence of "noncooperative" association of this polymer with anionic and cationic surfactants. A polymer that has been terminally labeled with pyrene groups is PEO (121); in mixtures with SDS at lower concentrations fluorescence data indicated the polymer chain cyclized. At higher concentration the pyrene groups were located in separate micelles.

In a general sense it must be realized that pyrene itself is a large and relatively hydrophobic moiety. Accordingly, the introduction of pyrene groups into a water-soluble polymer structure can be regarded as rendering the latter more hydrophobic and thereby changing it to a "pseudo" hydrophobically modified polymer with properties different from those of the starting polymer. This term can be applied to other situations in which, for example, the polymer has been rendered more hydrophobic, not by the introduction of a small number of large alkyl (or other hydrocarbon) groups, but by a large number of small alkyl groups, e.g., methyl, ethyl, propyl, or even hydroxpropyl. For example, while polyacrylamide is inert its *N*-isopropyl derivative, PNIPAM, has been shown, by fluorescence (122) and other methods, to react readily with anionic surfactants. Likewise, while HEC is known to be relatively unreactive toward surfactants, methylcellulose (MeC) and hydroxypropylcellulose (HPC) are reactive (123,124). The most widely studied derivative in this respect has been ethylhydroxyethylcellulose (EHEC), which has been shown by fluorescence methods to react with both anionic (125) and cationic surfactants (126). By use of fluorescence quenching techniques it was shown that SDS micelles bound by EHEC are much smaller than regular SDS micelles (N_{agg} = 20 vs. 70), in common with similar effects found for bound cationic surfactant micelles (125). Further discussion of the effect of polymer structure on interaction with surfactants will be given later.

D. Proteins

All proteins are polymers, namely polypeptides, which are based on α-amino fatty acid building blocks. If a single amino acid were involved in formation of the polypeptide chain the structure could be represented as

$$H_2N\!-\!\!\left[\overset{\displaystyle R}{\underset{}{\overset{|}{C}H}}\!-\!C(O)NH\right]_n\!\overset{\displaystyle R}{\overset{|}{C}H}\!-\!COOH$$

Actually 20 common amino acids are found in nature with R groups ranging in character from acidic to basic, and polar to nonpolar. (See Table 1.)

The overall composition of α-amino fatty acids, together with their sequence, gives proteins their individual characteristics, including isoelectric point, solubility, secondary structure (random coil, helix, sheet, etc.), and tertiary structure (degree of folding, globular state, etc.). The forces involved in these structural manifestations include hydrogen bonding, "hydrophobic" bonding, ion-ion attraction, ion-dipole attraction, and so on. It is easy to understand, a priori, that a multitude of structures exist within the protein family, and why proteins are generally reactive toward surfactants, and why such interaction can lead to substantial changes in configuration and properties of proteins in solution. Indeed, in the realm of polymer/surfactant interaction, proteins were the first category of polymer investigated—about 100 years ago! A spurt of activity occurred in the 1940s with the advent of purified proteins and surfactants, and their interaction was studied by a variety of techniques including ultrafiltration, dialysis equilibrium, electrophoresis, spectral methods, solubility/precipitation behavior, and so on. Because of this, the literature on this subject is substantial and the interested reader is referred to comprehensive reviews of this early work (1,2). Here, as with the other categories of polymer, we will discuss results obtained using a few selected techniques to illustrate the current state of knowledge. By far the most popular systems studied are based on the proteins bovine serum albumin (BSA), gelatin, and lysozyme.

1. Solubility Characteristics

The precipitation phenomena encountered on mixing polyion/oppositely charged surfactant mixtures, at certain ratios, have already been referred to. These have direct relevance

Table 1 Properties of Amino Acid Residues in Proteins

Amino acid	Symbol	Side chain	pK	Hydrophobicity
Alanine	Ala	$—CH_3$		3.1
Arginine	Arg	$—(CH_3)_2NHC(NH_2)_2^+$	12	3.1
Asparagine	Asn	$—CH_2CONH_2$		~0
Aspartic acid	Asp	$—CH_2CO_2^-$	4.4–4.6	
Cysteine	Cys	$—CH_2SH$	8.5–8.8	4.0
Glutamic acid	Glu	$—(CH_2)_2CO_2^-$	4.4–4.6	
Glutamine	Gln	$—(CH_2)_2CONH_2$		~0
Glycine	Gly	$—H$		0
Histidine	His	$—CH_2(C_3N_2H_3)^+$	6.5–7.0	2.0
Isoleucine	Ile	$—CH(CH_3)CH_2CH_3$		12.3
Leucine	Leu	$—CH_2CH(CH_3)_2$		10.0
Lysine	Lys	$—(CH_2)_4NH_3^+$	10.0–10.2	6.3
Methionine	Met	$—(CH_2)_2SCH_3$		5.4
Phenylalanine	Phe	$—CH_2(C_6H_5)$		11.0
Proline	Pro	$—(CH_2)_3^-$		10.9
Serine	Ser	$—CH_2OH$		
Threonine	Thr	$—CH(CH_3)OH$		1.9
Tryptophan	Trp	$—CH_2(C_8NH_6)$		12.5
Tyrosine	Tyr	$—CH_2(C_6H_4)OH$	9.6–10.0	11.9
Valine	Val	$—CH(CH_3)_2$		7.1

Source: Ref. 186.

to corresponding mixtures involving proteins in view of their characteristic polyampholytic nature. In simplistic terms, below and above their isoelectric point proteins behave in effect like polycations and polyanions, respectively, and hence would be expected to display precipitation behavior with added anionic and cationic surfactants. This behavior was demonstrated many years ago by Pankhurst (127) for the combination, gelatin/SDS at low pH values. At constant gelatin concentration, and SDS concentration increasing from left to right, the appearance of the mixed solution could be represented as follows:

Clear/Turbid/Precipitate/Turbid/Clear

This behavior, which is similar to that displayed by polyion/oppositely charged surfactant mixtures (see Fig. 12), has been observed with other protein/surfactant systems, for example, in BSA mixtures with SDS (128). An important point is that, in the resolubilization (surfactant rich) zone, considerable restructuring of the dissolved protein molecules must be involved. There is evidence, at least for some proteins, that this restructuring can be irreversible (129,130).

Another important point, and one of fundamental significance, is that above the isoelectric point, although no precipitation is observed with added SDS, definite indications of interaction can still be obtained: see, for example, the surface tension data for gelatin/SDS presented below, calorimetric data for BSA/SDS (128), and other information to be given later. This means that proteins, like many HM-polyions, are able to interact with ionic surfactants against an unfavorable (overall) electrical gradient. For this reason many studies involving anionic surfactants have been executed above the i.e.p. of the protein, as illustrated below.

2. *Surfactant Binding Studies*

As stated in the introduction to this section, binding studies of surfactants to proteins have provided one of the traditional ways of examining their interaction. It is again emphasized that, in view of the ampholytic nature of proteins, it is important to specify the pH chosen for studying them. In principle, any means for determining the level of ''free'' surfactant in mixed solution with a protein can be used, such as specific ion electrodes referred to earlier, spectroscopic measurements, and so on. It is, however, important to emphasize that the ''traditional'' method used for these studies, i.e., dialysis equilibrium, requires that the ionic strength of the solutions be high enough to eliminate Donnan membrane effects. Furthermore, one must remember that the presence of salt will modulate ion/ion interaction—a major driving force in polyelectrolyte/charged surfactant interaction. (See below.)

A typical illustration comes from the binding isotherms of SDS to hen egg lysozyme (131) obtained *below* the isoelectric point, viz., at pH 3.2. (See Fig. 30.) It is seen that, well below the c.m.c. of SDS, binding occurs and is manifested in an initial steep rise of uptake with concentration. This is indicative of a highly cooperative association and has been ascribed by Jones to ionic bonding of the surfactant anion to the cationic lysine, histidine, and arginine residues of lysozyme. (This behavior is analogous to that of the BSA/SDS system discussed earlier; correspondingly, when these high-energy binding sites are saturated, precipitation of the protein occurs.) Further addition of surfactant causes redissolution of the precipitate and this corresponds to the second sharp rise in binding of the surfactant near to, but still below, its c.m.c. The steepness of binding again suggests a cooperative process and, in fact, progressive unfolding of the protein occurs in this region involving hydrophobic interaction with the surfactant.

The influence of ionic strength on the binding isotherm merits mention. In the initial (''electrostatic'') binding segment, increasing ionic strength weakens the interaction and shifts binding to higher surfactant concentrations. In the subsequent (''hydrophobic'') segment, a crossover occurs and secondary or ''nonspecific'' binding occurs at lower

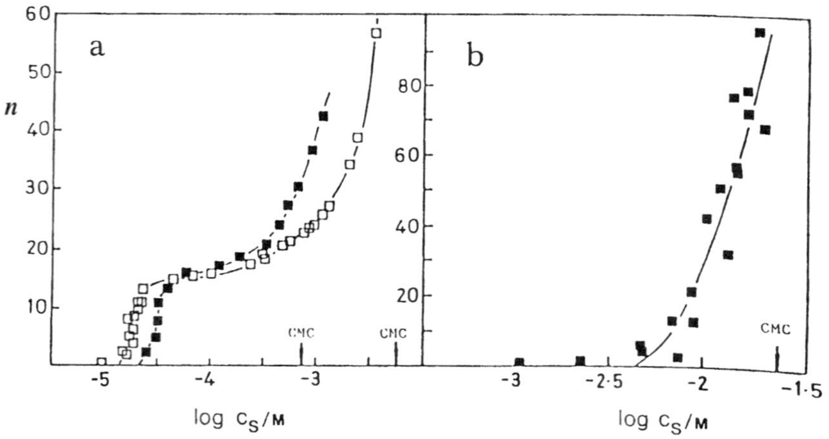

Figure 30 Binding isotherms of surfactants to lysozyme at 25°C. The average number *n* of ligands bound per protein molecule is plotted against the logarithm of the surfactant. (a) SDS: (□) pH 3.2, ionic strength 0.012 M; (■) pH 3.2, ionic strength 0.212 M. (b) *n*-Octyl β-glycoside: pH 6.4, ionic strength 0.132 M. (From Ref. 131.)

surfactant concentrations in this case. In harmony with the above interpretation, only a "nonspecific" binding region near the c.m.c. was observed by Jones and Brass for the interaction of lysozyme with the nonionic surfactant octyl-β-glycoside (131), implying a weaker interaction in this case (186).

In general, it should be emphasized that the uptake of an ionic surfactant by a protein can exceed the weight of the protein.

3. *Surface Tension*

The surface tension method has been employed by several workers to study protein/surfactant interaction. Figure 31 presents data of Knox and Parshall (132) that illustrate the behavior of mixtures of SDS and gelatin (above its isoelectric point). Interaction is evident from the existence of a surface tension plateau signaling the initiation (T_1) and completion (T_2) concentrations of SDS, according to the model for interaction described earlier. These arrests, together with the characteristic crossover of the with- and without-polymer curves, clearly support such a picture. Two explanations of the observed interaction are (1) SDS

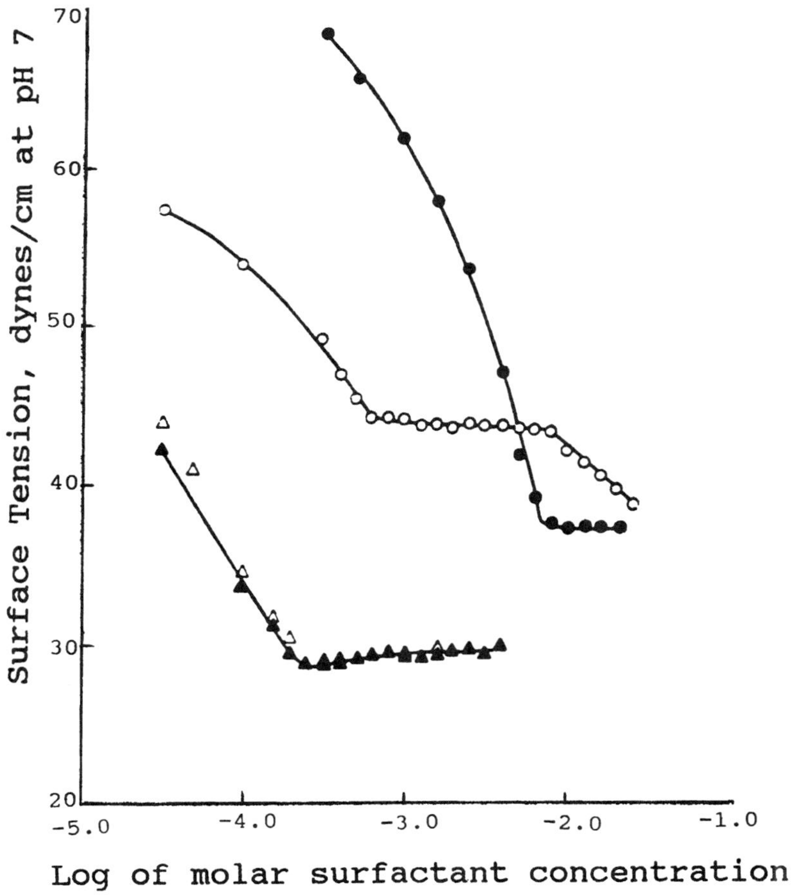

Figure 31 The effect of gelatin on the surface tension of SDS and Triton X100. (●) SDS in distilled water; (○) SDS in 1% gelatin; (▲) Triton X-100; (△) Triton X-100 in 1% gelatin. (From Ref. 132.)

molecules are able to sense and react with residual positive sites on the protein, even though the overall charge is negative; (2) "hydrophobic forces" of interaction with nonpolar side chains in the protein molecule are involved. The fact that no interaction was observed between gelatin and the nonionic surfactant Triton X-100 (a polyoxyethylated octylphenol) suggests that the second alternative does not provide a complete explanation. On the other hand, the fact that globular proteins such as BSA and lysozyme have been reported to interact with nonionic surfactants does lend support to mechanism 2. Such an example may be seen in the surface tension data of Nishikido et al. (133) for the combination BSA,C_{12} E_6. The form of the plots is different from the plateau and crossover pattern of Figure 31 and suggests that the protein may be part of a surface "complex."

(Historical note: The first use of a boundary tension method to study protein/surfactant interaction was in 1953 by Cockbain (133a), who, because of an interest in emulsions, employed *interfacial* tension measurements, but with both interacting components (BSA and SDS) in the aqueous phase. Despite the fact that the oil/water method is less favorable than its air/water counterpart (the measurements are less facile, the protein itself is interfacially quite active, and interfacial tension values with and without surfactant do not differ much), it was possible to identify T_1 and T_2 values, the beginning and the end of the interaction zone, as defined subsequently by Jones (24).)

4. *Viscosity*

Reference was made above to interaction between an anionic surfactant and a protein above its isoelectric point. A further illustration comes from viscosity characteristics of gelatin solutions above its isoelectric point (4.8) in the presence of added SDS. Greener et al. (134) have presented data covering a wide range of concentrations of this protein. Initial additions of SDS have little effect on its viscosity. (See Fig. 32.) However, at a certain concentration of SDS, and independent of the gelatin concentration, an increase in viscosity is observed. This behavior is consistent with the T_1 concept previously described. In all cases there follow a viscosity maximum and viscosity minimum, at SDS concentrations that increase with gelatin concentration. The increase in viscosity above T_1, in harmony with interpretations provided earlier, can be ascribed to a cross-linking of the polypeptide chains and, specifically by Greener et al. (134), to bonding via "micelle-like" aggregates. Results similar to the above have been obtained by Schwuger and Bartnik (135) for egg albumin/SDS systems. These authors explain the initial viscosity increase by a different mechanism, namely electrical charging of the protein by the bound SDS—and the subsequent minimum as the effect of surfactant counterions on the polymer coil. It is the secondary increase in viscosity in this interpretation that is attributed to a cross-linking mechanism involving micellar aggregates. Support for their interpretation of the first viscosity maximum actually comes from the observation of Greener et al. that an increase of ionic strength reduces the viscosity observed at the first maximum.

Other instances of the use of viscometry to study protein/surfactant interaction have been reported, for example by Jones and co-workers (136).

5. *Spectral Methods*

Both dye solubilization and fluorescence probe methods have been used to study protein/surfactant interaction. For example, data of Steinhardt et al. (137), who studied the solubilization of dimethylaminoazobenzene in ovalbumin-SDS mixtures, are shown in Figure 33. Solubilization occurs at concentrations of SDS well below the c.m.c., indicating that in the presence of ovalbumin the formation of nonpolar clusters is highly favorable. Unlike

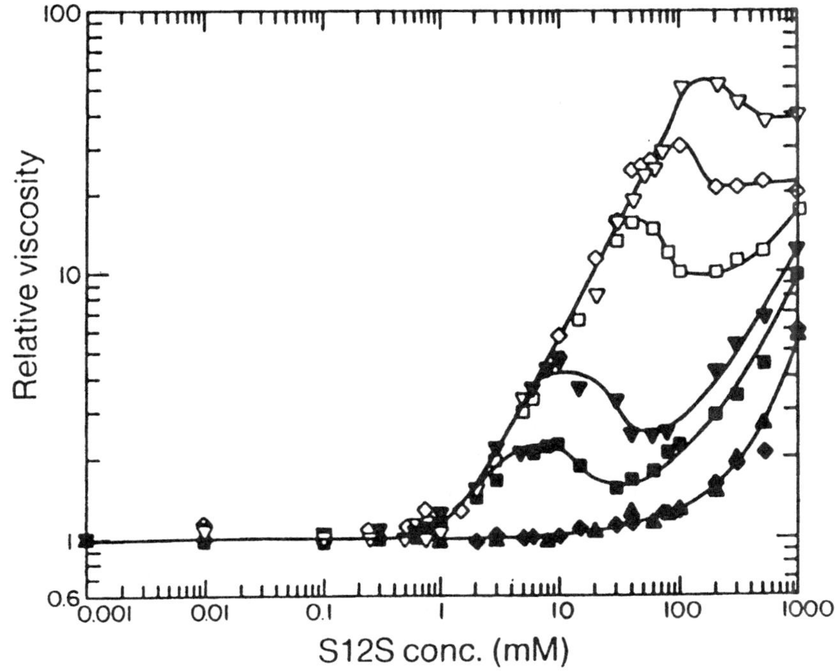

Figure 32 Relative viscosity of gelatin solutions versus SDS concentration. (▲) 0% gelatin; (◆) 0.1%; (■) 2.0%; (▼) 3.0%; (□) 5.0%; (◇) 7.0%; (▽) 10%. (From Ref. 134.)

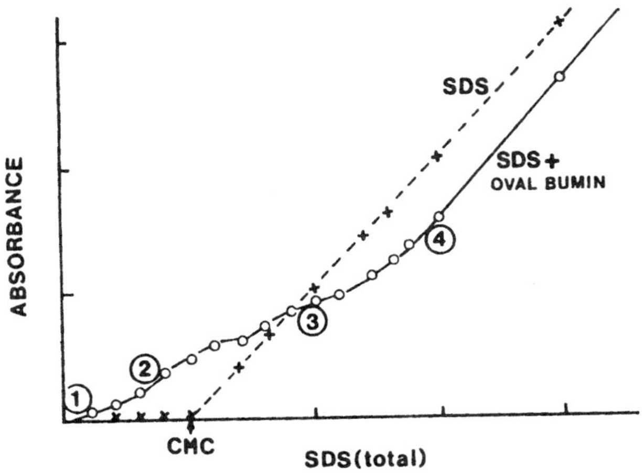

Figure 33 Solubilization (increase in absorbance) of dimethyl-aminoazobenzene by ovalbumin-SDS complexes in pH 7.4 (0.033 ionic strength) phosphate buffers at 25°C. (From Ref. 137.)

the case of Polymer JR-SDS systems previously described, above the c.m.c the solubilization curve of the protein-SDS mixtures crossed that of SDS alone, showing that the mixed clusters in this case have a lower solubilization capacity than that of regular SDS micelles.

Investigation of the gelatin-SDS system by Greener et al. (see above) included fluorescence measurements in which pyrene aldehyde was the probe. The characteristic sigmoidal response referred to earlier (Fig. 9) was obtained, but the fluorescence data also showed that:

1. The polarity of the protein-surfactant aggregates is lower than that of regular SDS micelles, as revealed by the shorter wavelength for maximum absorption by the probe. In this respect the behavior is similar to that of Polymer JR/SDS systems.
2. Unlike the viscosity data, the fluorescence results showed that the c.a.c. apparently decreases with increasing protein concentration, possibly indicating that the fluorescence method is the more sensitive of the two.

A variety of fluorescence techniques were employed by Whitesides and Miller (138) to examine the interaction of gelatin and SDS, to determine the size of the aggregates within the protein/surfactant complexes. The interested reader is referred to their original paper.

Miller et al. (139) have used NMR techniques to study the same system. ^{13}C NMR results suggest that only the ''outer'' carbons (near the headgroup) of SDS are affected by association with the gelatin polypeptide [as was found in the PEO/SDS system examined by Cabane (46) and referred to earlier]; diffusion coefficients measured by the pulsed gradient spin echo (PGSE) NMR method indicated that interaction with gelatin lowers the diffusion rate of SDS by an order of magnitude.

Small-angle neutron scattering (SANS) measurements on the gelatin/SDS system by Cosgrove et al. (140) showed that binding of SDS at low concentration results in a decrease in mesh size of the gel that this protein forms; above the c.m.c., however, the gelation mesh is destroyed and the ''bound'' SDS micelles assume a more elliptical shape than that of regular SDS micelles. Finally, a comprehensive spectroscopic probe analysis of the BSA/SDS system was made by Turro et al. (141). Fluorescence, electron spin resonance, and NMR investigations yielded results consistent with the ''necklace and beads'' model for the complexes of Shirahama. (See below.)

6. *Other Methods*

For a summary of methods used to study protein/surfactant interactions the reader is referred to recent reviews (129,130).

III. FACTORS AFFECTING THE ASSOCIATION REACTION

The process of ''complex formation'' between polymers and surfactants has increasingly come to be viewed as one that involves ''assisted'' or ''perturbed'' aggregation of the surfactant molecules. (See Section IV.) Hence it is not surprising that several factors influence association of surfactants with polymers the same way as they do micellization of surfactants, confirming the similarity of the two processes. As will be seen, however, there are a few important differences.

A. Surfactant Chain Length

For uncharged polymers one finds that the initial binding concentration T_1 (or c.a.c.) in a homologous series of ionic surfactants decreases with increasing chain length of the surfactant. (See, for example, Fig. 8.) In fact, there is a linear relationship between log T_1 and n, the number of alkyl chain carbons of the surfactant, just as there is between log c.m.c. and n. For PVP/SDS mixtures in 0.1 M NaCl solution, Arai et al. (12), using the relationship $ln\ T_1 = nw/kT +$ constant, found a value of w of $-1.1\ kT$. This corresponds to the free energy change per CH_2 group on transferring the surfactant from the unassociated state in solution to the complex, and is comparable to the value for the analogous transfer of the surfactant molecule to a micelle, confirming the analogy between the two processes. The logarithmic dependence of c.a.c. (and c.m.c.) can also be regarded as another manifestation of Traube's rule for the lowering of the surface tension of water by a homologous series of surfactants.

One can find similar chain length dependence in the interaction of charged surfactants with oppositely charged polyelectrotytes, as, for example, in the results of Kwak and co-workers (19,69,70,72). They studied the binding of families of homologous cationic surfactants to a variety of polyanions. The free energy of binding was obtained from the values of $(C_d^f)^{1/2}$ (the surfactant concentration at half saturation of the binding sites). The average value obtained, 1.2 kT/CH_2 group, while slightly higher than those of Arai, is still comparable to the free energy of micellization of the surfactants, again suggesting similarity of these aggregation processes. An illustration of the influence of alkyl chain length in surfactant binding can be seen in Figure 13.

Similar conclusions to the above, and an estimated value of w equal to 1.1 kT, were obtained from solubility studies on the Polymer JR/alkyl sulfate systems (59). Further details appear in Section IV.

There is much information in the literature on chain length effects in the binding of surfactants to proteins. For example, effects similar to those described above can be seen in the data of Kaneshina et al. (142) in the binding of C_{10}, C_{12}, and C_{14} TAB to BSA; and, likewise, in data of Jones (143–145) for the binding of C_8, C_{10}, and C_{12} sulfates to lysozyme. A good illustration of the influence of chain length and structure for a variety of anionic surfactants interacting with BSA is provided in data of Rendall (146). (See Fig. 34.) The measure of interaction affinity chosen here is the parameter, $\log_{10}C_{50}$, the concentration of surfactant required for 50 molecules to bind to a single BSA molecule. This parameter was found to vary directly (but not quite linearly) with surfactant c.m.c., again providing evidence of the similarity of binding and micellization.

B. Surfactant Structure

The influence of structural factors, including the nature of the headgroup (and its charge), in the surfactant can be expected to be most noticeable in interactions with "simple" uncharged water soluble polymers, i.e., those that lack hydrophobic groups to intensify interaction with surfactants, as discussed earlier. Examples are the extensively studied polymers PEO and PVP, which are known to react readily with a variety of surfactants such as alkyl sulfates, alkane sulfonates [including ABS (147)], and soaps (148), but not readily with alkyl phosphates (149). (In the latter case the lack of reactivity may be connected with the formation of a hydrogen-bonded structure involving partially ionized phosphate groups at the periphery of the micelle.)

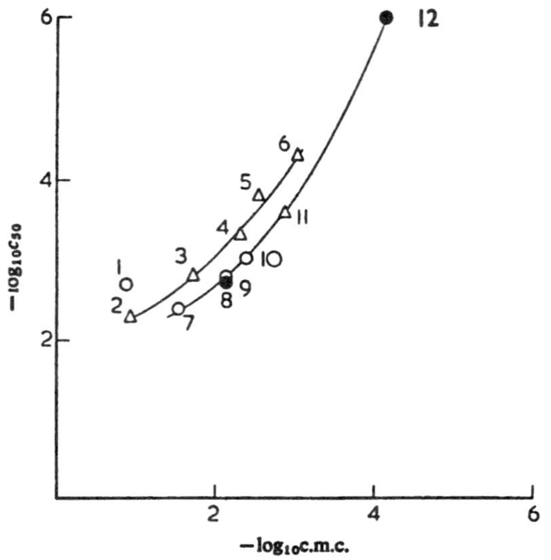

Figure 34 Plot of log C_{50} (concentration required to bind 50 surfactant molecules to a BSA molecule) versus surfactant c.m.c. (△) Sulfate: 2, C_8; 3, C_{10}; 4, C_{12}; 5, C_{12}; 6, C_{14}; 11, C_{12}. (○) Sulfonate: 1, C_8; 7, C_{10}; 9, C_{12}; 10, C_{12}. (●) Benzene sulfonate: 8, OBS (octyl benzene sulfonate); 12, DBS (dodecyl benzene sulfonate). (From Ref. 146.)

A structural variation of much interest to cosmetic scientists is represented by the well-known ethoxysulfate family of surfactants. Whereas interaction of this structural type of surfactant with a typical polycation remains strong (59), resolubilization by excess surfactant of insoluble complexes that form can be somewhat restricted. This is also the case with branched alkyl group anionic surfactants (59). In the former case (i.e., ethoxysulfates), however, interaction with uncharged polymers is weakened vis-à-vis simple alkyl sulfates, as illustrated by Saito's data on PVP and $C_{12}(EO)_4SO_4$ or $C_{12}(EO)_{12}SO_4$(150).

An early discovery, which has had abundant subsequent confirmation, was that anionic surfactants are much more reactive than cationic surfactants toward "simple" uncharged water soluble polymers (3). Several explanations of this interesting difference in reactivity have been attempted, but none is completely satisfactory, as is evident in various review articles (3,5,9). In a similar vein it is also now accepted that nonionic surfactants are generally unreactive toward "simple" uncharged (and also charged) polymers. These effects are summarized in Table 2, which also includes other combinations of polymer and surfactant. For example, Table 2 shows that an anionic surfactant will react strongly with a polycation but will not react, or will react only weakly, with a polyanion, illustrating the potent effect of electrostatic forces. It must be stressed that Table 2 applies to polymers that are not hydrophobically modified: as pointed out already, such modification can com-

Table 2 Surfactant Reactivity[a]

P^o:	SA^-	$>$	SA^+	$\gg$	SA^o
P^{n+}:	SA^-	$\gg$	SA^o	$\gg$	SA^+
P^{n-}:	SA^+	$\gg$	SA^o	$\gg$	SA^-

[a] Does not include HM-polymers.

pletely offset the effect of electrostatic forces. In any case, only limited investigation of the effect of surfactant structure on interactions with HM-polymers has been carried out. This is actually also the case with polyion/oppositely charged surfactant systems. [For example, the illustration of an apparent structure effect in Fig. 13, viz., higher apparent activity of R-pyridinium versus RTAB ions, may merely reflect an apparent increase in chain length of the former due to residual hydrophobicity of the pyridine ring (70).]

The effect of surfactants' structure on their reaction with proteins, on the other hand, has been more widely studied (2,146,151). In general, the reactivity sequence of the main surfactant types toward proteins is anionic > cationic > nonionic surfactants. Within the anionic surfactant family, alkyl sulfates appear to bind more strongly than alkyl benzene sulfonates ($-\varnothing SO_3$) and alkane sulfonates. (See data of Rendall in Fig. 35.) Overall one can set up the following binding efficiency sequence for proteins (129).

$$SO_4^- > SO_3^- > \varnothing SO_3^- > COO^-$$

The binding of ionic surfactants by a protein generally involves both electrostatic and hydrophobic attraction and can be accompanied by unfolding and sometimes denaturation of the protein. Uptakes can exceed 100% by weight, as mentioned previously.

C. The Polymer

1. Molecular Weight of the Polymer

There are many allusions (5) in the literature to the requirement of a minimum molecular weight of a polymer (nonionic) to support "complete" interaction with a surfactant (ionic). Several authors have placed this figure at ca. 4000 daltons for PEO and PVP, the most widely investigated nonionic polymers. Below a molecular weight of 1500 daltons interaction with these polymers is restricted (152).

By intuition one would expect that an increase in the affinity of interaction, achieved by hydrophobic substitution or the introduction of ionic groups in the polymer, would lower this molecular weight requirement. Although this aspect has not received much study, one can quote results for PPO (a "pseudo" HM-modified polymer): at a molecular weight of 1000 (the maximum value allowing water solubility) this polymer displays ready

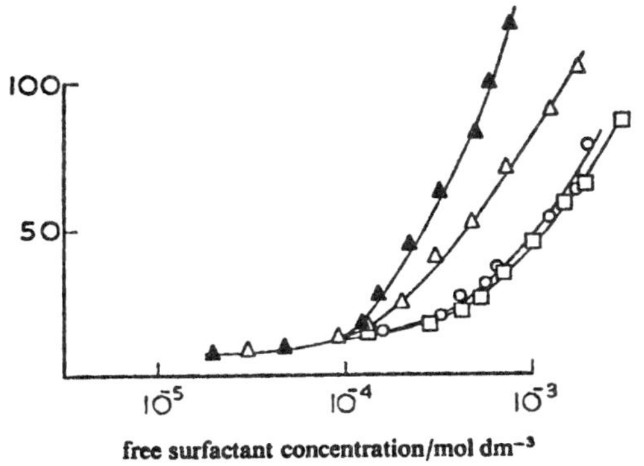

Figure 35 Surfactant binding to BSA in 10^{-2} M NaCl (open symbols) and in 10^{-1} M NaCl (filled symbols). (△) SDS; (○) sodium dodecane sulfonate; (□) octyl benzene sulfonate. (From Ref. 146.)

interaction not only with anionic and cationic surfactants but even with certain nonionic surfactants (153).

2. Amount of Polymer

The general concept of critical association (aggregation) concentration, T_1 or c.a.c., and of a saturation concentration, T_2, of surfactant in its reaction with a polymer has persisted. Generally T_1 lies below the c.m.c. of the surfactant and T_2 above the c.m.c. (See Figures 5, 6, and 36 for a summary of these concepts.) Experimentally, T_1—the ''initiation concentration''—is largely independent of polymer concentration whereas T_2—the ''saturation concentration''—increases linearly with polymer concentration, [P]. Thus $T_2 - T_1 = k[P]$ or, more precisely, $T_2^1 - T_1 = k[P]$, following the terminology of Figure 5. [While these simple concepts have ready applicability to the case of uncharged water-soluble polymers, there are complications in systems where precipitation and/or gross configurational changes can occur, as in reactions with polyelectrolytes and proteins. Often the solubility (59) or phase (62,154) diagram in these systems is not symmetric (see Fig. 40) and the c.a.c. changes in an irregular way with polymer concentration. A simple rule of thumb to formulators is that the higher the level of polycation, the higher the (anionic) surfactant level to achieve solubilization in the surfactant-rich region of the phase diagram. See Figure 12.]

To describe and ''summarize'' conditions prevailing in homogeneous mixtures of an interacting (nonionic) polymer/ionic surfactant pair, where the concentration of both components changes, we utilize a phase diagram constructed by Cabane and Duplessix (155) for the PEO/SDS system. (See Fig. 36.) In field I no complex formation occurs

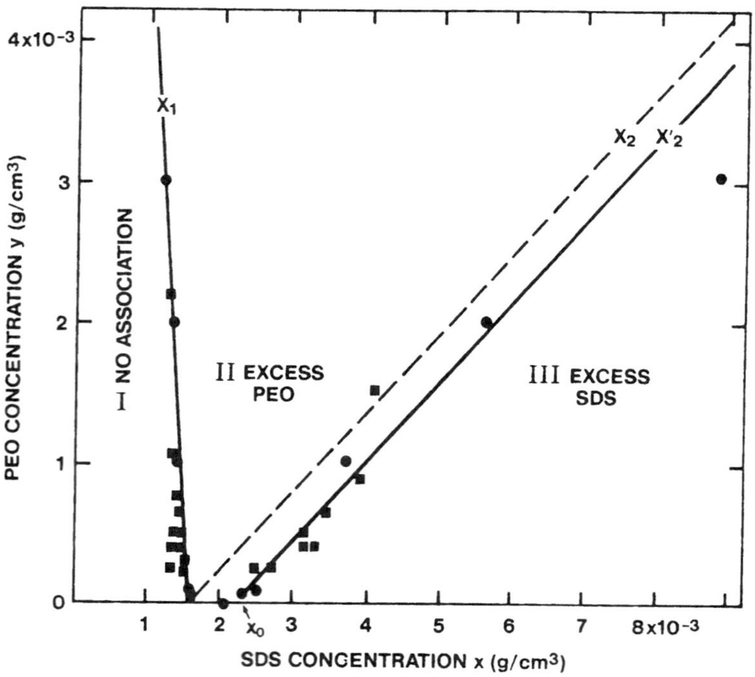

Figure 36 ''Phase diagram'' of PEO/SDS. X_0 refers to the c.m.c. of SDS; see text for explanation of other terms. (From Ref. 155.)

because c_{SDS} does not reach the c.a.c. In field III, monomeric SDS, micellar SDS, and saturated complexes exist. Field II is the domain of monomeric SDS and unsaturated complexes. The amount of complexes formed is proportional to the level of PEO present (and the concentration of available SDS). Near the X_2 boundary the complexes approach saturation; near the X_1 boundary the situation is reversed. This diagram illustrates the equivalence of the two ways of estimating the amount of complex at a given polymer level, viz., $(X_2' - X_0)$ and $(X_2 - X_1)$, or (T_2 − c.m.c.′) and $(T_2' - T_1)$, respectively. (See Figs. 5,36.) Discrepancies would occur at higher polymer levels because of the slight reductions of X_1 with polymer concentration, i.e., the slight negative tilt of the X_1 line. On the basis of data from a number of techniques, such as SANS (52), sedimentation (30), and gel filtration (49), it has been demonstrated (52) that in the "unsaturation" zone II SDS is shared equally among the polymer molecules, rather than being distributed according to the "all or none" model that has been proposed (156).

D. Polymer Structure

During and after the pioneering work of Saito (3–5) on the interaction between ionic surfactants and uncharged polymers it has been appreciated that there are definite differences in reaction affinity among polymers toward a given surfactant. For example, in cellulosic water soluble polymers it was known that MeC is more reactive than HEC; that PPO is more reactive than PEO; and that PVAc completely hydrolyzed (i.e., PVA) is less reactive than PVAc with lower degrees of hydrolysis (157). Attempting to rationalize the information available at the time (1972), Breuer and Robb (3) assigned a "reactivity" sequence to a group of six polymers as follows. For interaction with anionic surfactants the order of increasing reactivity was PVA $<$ PEO $<$ MeC $<$ PVAc $\leq$ PPO $\sim$ PVP; and for cationic surfactants the order was PVP $<$ PEO $<$ PVA $<$ MeC $<$ PVAc $<$ PPO. In this way the notion of correlation between the "hydrophobicity" of the polymer and its reactivity had its inception.

The position of PVP in the two series is noteworthy. This polymer is known to be weakly cationic: its slight residual positive charge promotes interaction with anionic surfactants and does the opposite with cationic surfactants.

Early support for the role of polymer hydrophobicity came from a study (158) of the interaction of a series of nonionizable polypeptides (poly-DL-alanine and three derivatives of poly-L-glutamine) with SDS. Strongest interaction, as judged from the lowest T_1 value (from dye solubilization and electrical conductivity measurements) and highest ionic dissociation (α, from sodium ion activity measurements) of the complex, was obtained with the most hydrophobic member, viz., poly-DL-alanine, and vice versa.

The notion of an interplay between polymer reactivity and hydrophobicity led Goddard, Leung and Ananthapadmanabhan (159,160) to propose an empirical method to assess such reactivity: it is based on measuring the extent of surface tension lowering brought about by the polymer alone in water (e.g., at 0.1 or 1% concentration). Polymers with negligible surface activity (HEC, PAAm, dextrose) are generally unreactive; those with intermediate surface activity (PNIPAM, PVA, PEO) are more reactive; and those with pronounced surface activity (PPO, PVAc) are most reactive. Other examples are EHEC, MeC, and HPC, which are all reactive (and surface active), versus HEC, which is not. Of course, as indicated earlier, the introduction of hydrophobic groups, however small, which the above conversions entail, would be expected to increase the polymer's "reactivity." We will see later how these concepts tie in with interaction modeling.

Another parameter possibly affecting polymer reactivity is the flexibility of the macromolecule. This is illustrated by the relatively strong interaction of SDS with amylose (which can undergo a helix-coil transition) and the relatively weak interaction with amylopectin (which cannot) (3,161). However, attempting to assign the lack of reactivity of HEC to its low level of flexibility is only partly convincing as the much more flexible polysaccharide dextran also shows little reactivity with surfactants like SDS (17) and SDDBS (162).

The advent of water-soluble polymers with well-defined hydrophobic centers, such as dodecyl or nonylphenyl side chains (or even pyrene groups), has continued to formalize the concept of a relationship between the hydrophobicity of a polymer and its reactivity. As mentioned earlier, reactivity in a series of alkyl-substituted polyacrylate polymers was shown, in the fluorescence measurements of Magny et al. (90,114), to correlate with the number and chain length of the substituent groups, as was the case for alkyl-substituted maleic anhydride copolymers (115). It is easy to understand that hydrophobicity introduced in this way can lead to interaction through the formation of mixed micelles with the surfactant. (See Fig. 22.) Indeed, as we have pointed out, the interaction affinity in some cases can be so large as to overcome unfavorable electrostatic forces.

Turning to the case of polyelectrolyte/oppositely charged surfactant pairs, one can also find reported cases of a definite influence of polyion structure on reactivity. The studies of Kwak et al. (69,73) on polyanion/cationic surfactant systems are the most complete. For example, from measurements of the binding affinity of a series of polyanions for the DTA^+ surfactant ion, the following binding sequence can be assigned: PSS > DexS > PAA > DNA > alginate ≥ pectate > NaCMC. There are also substantial differences in the "cooperativity" of binding within this series, and it is clear that the specifics of the polymer structure are involved. For example, PSS, the most strongly interacting polyanion of the series, is also the most hydrophobic but, curiously, binding is less cooperative with it than with the more hydrophilic DexS. Flexibility of the backbone is evidently a possible factor, which may also explain the somewhat stronger binding observed with alginate over the less flexible pectate. The flexibility factor undoubtedly operates in limiting interaction with the stiff-backboned NaCMC. Hayakawa et al. (70) have pointed out that the "linear charge density" parameter, ξ, and "detailed local structure" (unspecified) are also involved in determining the ultimate binding characteristics of a surfactant to a polyion. In summary: though much progress has been made in relating structure factors in polymers, both charged and uncharged, to their reactivity with surfactants, a need still exists for further detailed inquiry, especially when new structures are being considered. The case of proteins is much more complex in view of the multitude of structures involved (primary, secondary, and tertiary), the interplay of electrostatic and hydrophobic forces, chain unfolding, and so on. [A simplified analogy is provided in results reported for the PMA/TTAB system (163): under pH conditions of low charge density the polymer is coiled through hydrophobic (methyl group) and hydrogen bonding forces, and initial bonding involves only the exposed sites; continued binding, however, opens up the structure for further binding, as is observed with proteins.] Review articles (129,130) are recommended for further information on specific systems.

E. Added Salt

Salt effects on the micellization of ionic surfactants are well known: they can be substantial. It would therefore be no surprise to find related effects in the interaction of ionic surfactants with polymers where surfactant aggregation is also involved. For uncharged polymers, these effects are well illustrated in data of Murata and Arai (28) shown in Figure 37. In the same way as the c.m.c. of an ionic surfactant like SDS is substantially lowered by the addition of simple salt, so too is its c.a.c. in the presence of an interacting polymer like PVP. In both cases the unfavorable electrical potential at the periphery of the aggregate is mitigated by the sodium counterions. (The data shown in Fig. 37 show there is no dependence of the "saturation" concentration, T_2, on added salt.) These results represent extensions of earlier work by Saito (164,165). Results from recent studies of the effect of counterions on the interaction of an anionic surfactant (like SDS) with a nonionic polymer (like PEO or PVP) emphasize that it is the degree of binding of the *counterion* to the polymer that determines the influence of added salt, the extent of interaction, the size of the aggregate that forms, and its degree of ionic association (38,166–168).

A very different picture emerges as regards the effect of added salt on the association reactions in polyelectrolyte/oppositely charged surfactant systems. In this case the added ions will reduce the electrical attractive force by shielding, and the c.a.c. should *increase*. This effect is shown in data of Kwak (72,73), presented in Figure 38, which reveal not only an increase in c.a.c. but also an increase in cooperativity (steepness of binding) as the concentration of salt increases. In further investigations of the effect of added salt on polyanion/cationic surfactant systems Kwak's group showed that divalent cation salts, e.g., $MgCl_2$, $ZnCl_2$, $CaCl_2$, had a larger effect than NaCl, and trivalent $LaCl_3$ a still larger effect. Specific ion effects were sometimes found: as an example, for DexS, added $CaCl_2$ caused a larger increase in c.a.c. than $MgCl_2$ whereas no differences in this series were found for PSS. These data show the sensitivity of the association phenomena to the specific properties of the ions involved (169), as is well known in micellization. These results demonstrate unequivocally that electrostatic forces are a primary driving element in the

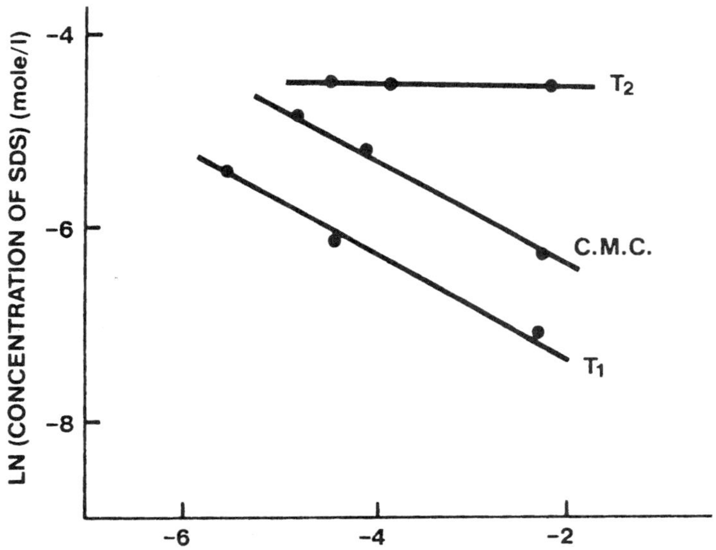

Figure 37 Effect of salt on the transition concentrations of 0.1% PVP/SDS systems; corresponding salt effect on c.m.c. of SDS is included. (From Ref. 28.)

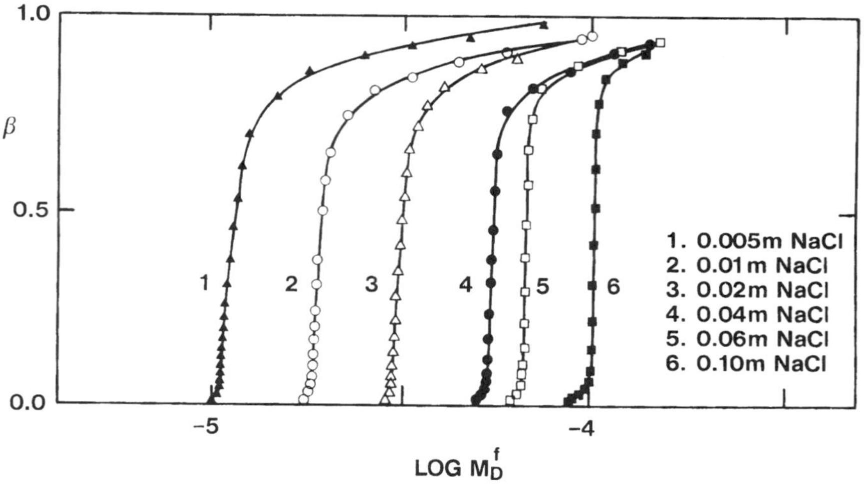

Figure 38 Binding isotherms for sodium dextran sulfate (5×10^{-4} M)–dodecylpyridinium chloride (DPyCl)–NaCl systems. M_D^f is the equilibrium concentration of DPyCl. (From Refs. 72, 73.)

adsorption/nucleation process of the surfactant ions onto the polymer and that shielding, by added electrolyte, diminishes the electrical potential for adsorption.

Reference has already been made to the interesting finding by Laurent and Scott (65) that precipitation of various polyanion/cationic surfactant systems can be totally inhibited by the addition of a sufficient amount of simple salt. This work allowed the definition of a critical electrolyte concentration (c.e.c.), which was found to vary from system to system. Clearly, electrostatic screening effects are again involved. This phenomenon has been confirmed and examined in some detail by Lindman and co-workers (see next section). Less work has been carried out in this respect on polycation/anionic surfactant systems and, at least in some systems involving cationic cellulosic polymer/SDS combinations, resolubilization by salt addition was found not to be facile (59,103).

Salt effects in protein/surfactant systems have been widely studied. As may be imagined, the effects can be quite complex and they vary considerably from system to system, with pH, with absolute ionic strength, and so on. For a system showing fairly simple behavior one may cite the combination of lysozyme and SDS described earlier: see Figure 30 (131). For a brief review of the field, with references, the reader is referred to Ref. 129.

IV. INTERACTION MODELS

A. Early Work

The early work done by protein chemists established the generality of the phenomenon of binding of ionic surfactants by proteins and ascribed it to a "site binding" mechanism. In a general sense, the sites on the protein for binding were considered to be the positive ionic centers of the polypeptide backbone (e.g., from lysine, arginine, etc., side chains) for anionic surfactants, and the negative sites (from glutamic acid, etc.) for cationic surfactants. It has been pointed out that it was realized that the electrostatic attraction at these sites is strong enough that binding can occur even against a *net* electric field that is unfavorable; i.e., an anionic surfactant can bind onto a protein above its isoelectric point, and a cationic surfactant below the isoelectric point.

When it was first established that the formation of polymer/surfactant complexes is a more general phenomenon, inasmuch as interaction can occur between ionic surfactants and several uncharged water-soluble polymers, the notion of site binding persisted although it was less easy to specify the adsorption sites in this case. Nonetheless, as for proteins, there were again indications of ''cooperativity'' in the binding process in the sense that the first bound surfactant ion aids the binding of the second, both aid the binding of the third, and so on. Evidence of this mechanism is the steepness of the binding curve (14) and the ability of the ''complexes'' to solubilize oil-soluble materials, such as dyes and fluorescent dyes, suggesting that the clusters of surfactant form microdroplets of hydrocarbon.

B. Uncharged Polymers

1. Simple Mass Action Equilibrium

It has been mentioned that Muller and Johnson (47), by NMR studies of terminally fluorinated SDS (i.e., F_3 SDS)/PEO mixtures, showed that the CF_3 groups in the aggregates experienced a similar environment to that in regular F_3 SDS micelles. Since their interaction data did not seem to obey a Langmuirian adsorption process, Smith and Muller (152) developed a different, simple model. They assumed that each polymer molecule consists of a number of ''effective segments'' of mass M_s, and total concentration [P], that act independently, M_s being the minimum molecular weight required for interaction. Each segment binds a cluster of n surfactant ions, D^- in a single step, the binding equilibrium being represented as

$$\mathrm{P} + n\mathrm{D}^- \rightleftharpoons \mathrm{PD}_n^{n-}$$

and the equilibrium constant being given by

$$\mathrm{K} = [\mathrm{PD}_n^{n-}]/[\mathrm{P}][\mathrm{D}^-]^n$$

K is obtained from the half-saturation condition, viz.,

$$\mathrm{K} = [\mathrm{D}]_{1/2}^{-n}$$

With trial values of n, and calculated ''theoretical'' isotherms, the best fit with the experimental data yielded values of the parameters M_s, n, and k.

The data of Smith and Muller indicated the cluster size, n, to be about 15, and M_s to be 1830, thus providing an explanation of the finding of these authors that PEO 1500, unlike higher molecular weights, is relatively ineffective for surfactant binding. The free energy of binding,

$$\Delta G^{\circ} = -RT \ln K^{1/n}$$

yielded a value of −5.07 Kcal/mol, which is close to that of micelle formation of F_3 SDS, again suggesting that ''binding'' and micellization are related processes.

2. Modified Langmuir (Hill) Equation

It is of interest that Shirahama, in an earlier paper (14) concerned with the binding of SDS by PEO, found that his data fitted a Langmuir-type adsorption equation if provision were made for cluster formation (n ≈ 20) of the bound surfactant molecules. The equation took the form

$$\theta = KC^n/(1 + C^n)$$

where θ is the degree of binding, n is an empirical constant, C is the (equilibrium) concentration of SDS, and K is the equilibrium constant. [This form of the adsorption equation had been proposed in 1910 by Hill (170).]

Another important contribution of Shirahama was his ''string of beads'' model for the structure of the complexes. (See Figs. 11, 18.) This, as it once seemed, somewhat unlikely model is now generally accepted. It is able to explain the NMR results of Muller and Johnson (47) and of Cabane (46), the experimentally observed pronounced cooperativity in binding, and the fast kinetics of formation and breakdown of the complexes, comparable to those of ordinary micelles, as observed by Wyn-Jones (55,56).

3. *Complex Mass Action Equation*

Nagarajan (162,171) developed a very general form of a mass balance equation governing the equilibrium in a solution in which surfactant can exist as single ions, regular micelles, or aggregates associated with a dissolved polymer. The total surfactant concentration X_t is partitioned into singly dispersed surfactant, X_1, surfactant in free micelles X_f, and surfactant bound as aggregates, X_b, in the mass balance equation

$$X_t = X_1 + g_f(K_fX_1)^{g_f} + g_bnX_p\left[\frac{(K_bX_1)^{g_b}}{1 + (K_bX_1)^{g_b}}\right] \tag{1}$$

In Eq. 1, the second and third terms represent X_f and X_b, respectively; g_f is the average aggregation number of the free micelles; and K_f is the intrinsic equilibrium constant for their formation. Furthermore, each polymer molecule is assumed to have n binding sites for surfactant aggregates of average size g_b. K_b is the intrinsic equilibrium constant for the binding of the surfactant on the polymer. It can also be visualized as the intrinsic equilibrium constant for the formation of polymer-bound micelles. X_p is the total concentration of polymer molecules in solution. The polymer influences Eq. 1 through the term nX_p, its effective mass concentration, which is independent of polymer molecular weight.

The relative magnitudes of K_b, K_f, g_b, and g_f determine whether or not complexation with the polymer occurs. If $K_f > K_b$, and $g_b \approx g_f$, the formation of free micelles occurs in preference to complexation. If $K_f < K_b$, and $g_b \approx g_f$, complexation/aggregation on the polymer takes place first and upon saturation of the polymer, free micelles form. If $K_f < K_b$, and g_b is much smaller than g_f, then formation of free micelles can occur even prior to saturation of the polymer.

Data obtained by Gilanyi and Wolfram (21) for the PEO/SDS system using a specific ion electrode verified the essential features of the Nagarajan equation. In Figure 39 the data are plotted according to the format of Eq. 1: the influence of polymer concentration can be clearly seen. The region AO corresponds to the conditions leading to the formation of ordinary micelles (no polymer present). The regions AB correspond to the preformation of polymer/surfactant aggregates, saturation at point B, and then a buildup of monomer concentration to the point C where ordinary micelles start to form. One can see that, if the concentration of polymer is high enough (e.g., at 1 g/L and especially, 4 g/L), the amount of surfactant is inadequate to saturate the polymer and no regular micelles form.

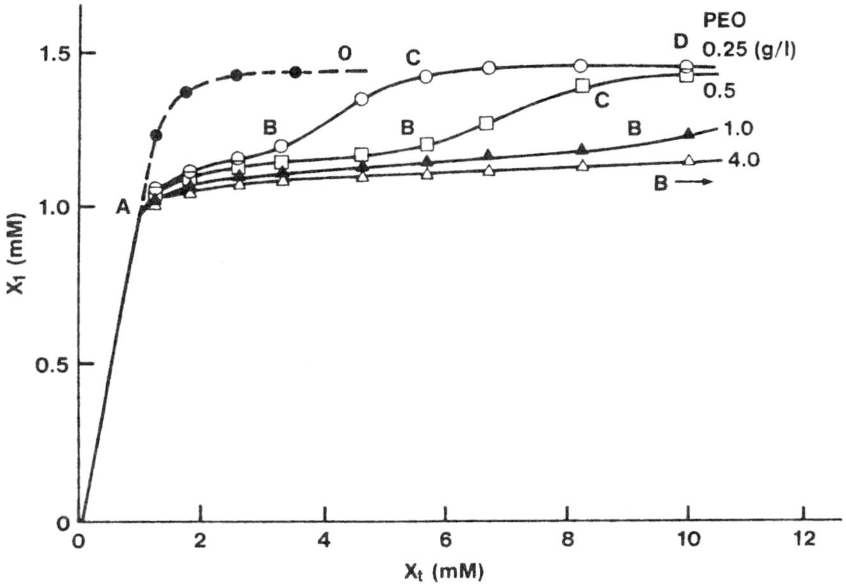

Figure 39 Experimental data of Gilanyi and Wolfram (21) for PEO/SDS solutions containing 0.1 M $NaNO_3$, and theoretical curves of Nagarajan. (From Refs. 162, 171, 172.)

4. *Other Models*

Several other theoretical treatments and models of binding of ionic surfactants by uncharged polymers have been developed recently. They include one by Hall (156) based on a Donnan equilibrium approach; related treatments by Nagarajan (172) and Ruckenstein et al. (173) that include a (differing) interfacial energy term in the free energy equation of special significance with "hydrophobic" HM-polymers; and the so-called "dressed micelle" model of Evans et al. (174). These are specialized treatments and interested readers are referred to the original papers or a brief review by Lindman and Thalberg (9) for further information. It seems that the case of HM-polymers could be accommodated in the above models by inclusion of suitable interfacial energy terms in view of the dominant nature of the latter in such systems.

C. Polyelectrolytes

1. *Shirahama-Schwarz Binding Model*

We turn next to charged polymer systems. As stated earlier, in systems of polymer and surfactant involving opposite charges, the concept of site binding (the "nucleation" event") of surfactant ions and aggregation of subsequently bound surfactant ions (the "cooperative process") was accepted at an early stage. This approach, which had been developed for the binding of dyes (175), was applied to the binding of surfactant ions by polyelectrolytes by Shirahama and co-workers (176,177). Only main results are presented here illustrated by Shirahama's derived expressions for binding.

$$K = [u(C_d^f)_{1/2}]^{-1}$$

Table 3 Cooperative Binding Constant *Ku* and Cooperative Parameter *u* at 30°C

		TTABr		DTABr	
Polymer	[NaCl] (mol/kg)	10^{-3} *Ku* (mol^{-1} kg)	*u* (±20%)	10^{-3} *Ku* (mol^{-1} kg)	*u* (±20%)
PAA		245	20	26.9	15
	0.01	30.5	600	2.69	500
Alginate		29.9	150	2.45	70
	0.01	7.5	2000		
Pectate		28.8	60	2.24	70
	0.01	7.2	2000		
NaCMC		25.1	7	1.78	4
	0.01	6.9	30		
DNA		107	20	9.3	6
	0.01	16.6	200	1.38	70
DexS	0.01			24.0	650
PSS[a]	0.01			(200)	(200)

[a] Interpolated from previous data from Ref. 73.
Source: Data from Ref. 69.

and

$$(d\beta/d \ln C_d^f)_{1/2} = \sqrt{u/4}.$$

In these expressions, *K* is the constant for binding to an isolated site on the polymer; *u* is a cooperativity parameter; $(C_d^f)_{1/2}$ is the equilibrium surfactant concentration at the half-saturation point, i.e., $\beta = 0.5$. *Ku* would represent the "cooperative binding constant." Similar relationships were derived by Satake and Yang (178).

A compilation of values of parameters *Ku* and *u* from extensive data of Hayakawa and Kwak (69,73) for a number of polyanions is given in Table 3. While the considerable variation in binding behavior has already been commented on (in Section III.D), it is pointed out that there is a range in both *Ku* and *u* of over two orders of magnitude; and furthermore that the addition of salt always reduces the value of *Ku* and increases the value of *u*. The review by Hayakawa and Kwak (10) can be consulted for further information in this field.*

2. *Stoichiometric Complex Separation Model*

The second (and third) models for polyelectrolyte/surfactant interaction are based on the solubility and phase characteristics of the mixed systems. The general form of the solubility diagram of a polyelectrolyte/oppositely charged surfactant system, as illustrated by the Polymer JR/TEALS combination, has been referred to (57). It showed an intermediate zone of precipitation, but clarity for high (and low) concentrations of the surfactant. The line representing systems of maximum insolubility in the log polymer/log surfactant concentration plot had a 45° slope indicating constant composition of the insoluble complexes,

* A recent series of papers by T. Wallin and P. Linse describe approaches to polyelectrolyte/surfactant interactions based on Monte Carlo simulations and mean field calculations (Langmuir 1996; 12:305; J Phys Chem 1996; 100:17873; J Phys Chem 1997; B101:5506; Langmuir 1998; 14:2490).

corresponding to 1:1 charge stoichiometry (Fig. 12). An interesting feature of the plot, however, was that the slope of the maximum insolubility line increased as the polycation concentration was decreased below a certain value, and eventually it became vertical, i.e., independent of polymer concentration. Furthermore, when the experiment was repeated with alkylsulfates of different chain lengths, it was found that although this pattern was common to all of them, the surfactant concentration corresponding to the vertical precipitation line changed substantially (but systematically) with chain length. [See Fig. 40 (59).]

This situation can be analyzed to yield an estimate of the energy of association as follows: for conditions of maximum precipitation, the equilibrium can be described by

$$C_t - C_e = \text{constant} \times [P]$$

where C_t and [P] are total concentrations of surfactant and polymer, respectively, and C_e, obtained from the position of the vertical lines of Figure 40, represents the equilibrium concentration of surfactant required to maintain the existence of the stoichiometric, precipitated complex. Under conditions corresponding to high polymer concentration, i.e., in the 45° slope region, C_e represents a small fraction of C_t and hence the relation C_t = constant × [P] holds. At lower concentrations of added polymer, especially when the surfactant is more weakly bound (as with octyl sulfate), the fraction C_e/C_t becomes pro-

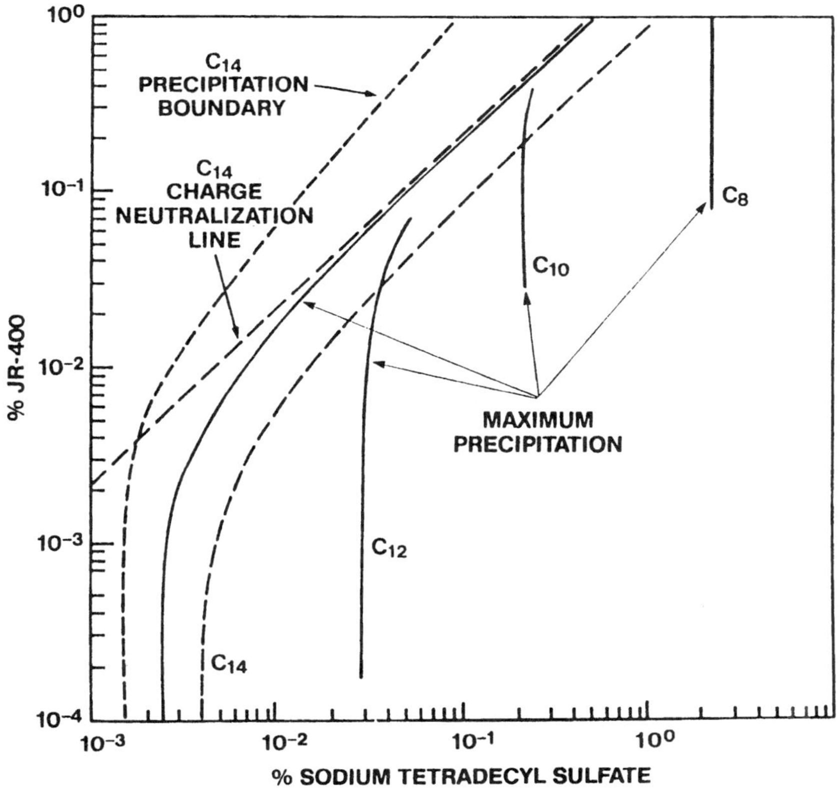

Figure 40 Solubility diagrams of the Polymer JR 400/sodium tetradecyl sulfate system. Maximum precipitation lines for the corresponding C_{12}, C_{10}, and C_8 sulfates are included. (From Ref. 59.)

gressively larger and finally approaches unity, when most of the added surfactant is required to maintain equilibrium with the precipitated stoichiometric complex. That is,

$$C_e \rightarrow C_t \text{ when } [P] \rightarrow 0$$

It is obvious from Figure 40 that the affinity of the association reaction increases strongly with increased chain length of the surfactant. In fact, the variation of C_e with alkyl chain lengths, which may be represented as a linear semilog plot, allows a quantitative estimate of the interaction energy of the surfactants with the polymer to be made.

The equilibrium governing the adsorption of an anionic surfactant onto a positively charged polymer can be expressed as

$$C_{ads} = C_b \exp\{(e\psi_o + n\phi)/kT\}$$

where C_b is the equilibrium concentration of surfactant in solution, C_{ads} is the concentration of adsorbed surfactant in undefined units, ψ_o is the electrical potential around the polymer, n is the number of CH_2 groups, in the surfactant chain, ϕ is the adsorption energy per CH_2 group, and k and T are the Boltzmann constant and absolute temperature, respectively. For conditions of maximum precipitation (i.e., charge neutralization), the equation simplifies to

$$C_{ads} = C_e \exp\{n\phi/kT\} = \text{a constant}$$

Hence, the slope of the $\log_{10} C_e$ versus n plot is $\phi/2.3\ kT$, and from the data a value of ϕ of 1.1 kT was obtained, somewhat higher than the value for the free energy of micelle formation of this type of surfactant, but close to the value for hemimicelle formation on oppositely charged mineral solids (179).

Support for these views was obtained from electrophoresis measurements referred to earlier (58) on fine particles of precipitate withdrawn from a series of aqueous compositions containing a constant concentration (0.1%) of Polymer JR and varying amounts of SDS. In brief, below the stoichiometric SDS concentration the particles bear a positive charge, and above it a negative charge. Near the stoichiometric ratio, the particles in suspension have zero or little charge. Ohbu et al. (85) have reported similar findings.

3. *Binary Polymer Model*

A completely different approach to modeling the behavior of systems of the above type was developed by Lindman and co-workers (64). It draws on the Flory-Huggins treatment of polymer solutions (see Chapters 1–3) and utilizes careful determinations of the phase diagrams of these systems—approaches that have recently been refined, analyzed, and extended by Ranganathan and Kwak (63).

In outline, the treatment, based on an energy minimization procedure, is as follows: The interaction energy expression uses one interaction parameter w_{ij} for each interaction species, i and j, in the system. For a combination of water (1), polymer A (2), and polymer B (3), there are three interaction parameters, w_{12}, w_{13}, and w_{23}, and two polymerization numbers, L_2 and L_3. The free energy expression is obtained by combining the entropy (mixing) and energy (contact dissimilarity) terms, the free energy being given by

$$\begin{aligned} A = {} & RTM_o\{\phi_1 \ln \phi_1 + (\phi_2/L_2)\ln \phi_2 + (\phi_3/L_3)\ln \phi_3\} \\ & + M_o\{w_{12}\phi_1\phi_2 + w_{13}\phi_1\phi_3 + w_{23}\phi_2\phi_3\} \end{aligned}$$

where M_0 is the total number of "cells" and ϕ is the volume fraction of component i in the phase. The interaction parameters are related to the normal Flory-Huggins interaction parameters (χ) through

$$w_{12} = \chi_{12}RT$$

Phase diagram calculations are carried out for a given set of the five parameters by the conventional procedure of minimizing the total free energy with respect to the content of the three components in the different phases. Despite the need for severe assumptions (for example, component 2, the surfactant, *has* to be treated as a second polymer) and the large number of adjustable parameters, it was found possible to obtain reasonable approximations to the actual behavior of mixed systems.

Several important findings were made by the Lindman group in their extensive phase studies of polyelectrolyte/oppositely charged surfactant systems. Thus, while precipitation zones were obtained in all mixed systems, it was not found that maximum precipitation occurred always at the 1:1 stoichiometric ratio (64). Furthermore, by carrying out the phase determinations in the presence of increasing amounts of salt it was confirmed that precipitation could be inhibited (by "electrical screening"). While this finding was itself not new (see Scott's definition of *c*ritical *e*lectrolyte *c*oncentration above), an interesting discovery was that further addition of salt beyond the c.e.c. could again lead to phase separation (62). These effects are illustrated in Figure 41.

The different behavior above and below the c.e.c. led Piculell and Lindman (180) to define two types of segregation (phase separation). One is *associative* separation when both solutes (i.e., polymer and surfactant) separate in one phase and the other phase contains mostly water (as seen in the tie lines that run *from* the water corner). This behavior is tantamount to "complex coacervation" observed by Bungenberg de Jong on mixing oppositely charged macromolecules, including proteins (181). The other is *segregative* separation in which the solutes collect in separate phases, and the tie lines run *across* the water corner. (See Fig. 42.) [This behavior is similar to that observed on mixing two nonionic polymers, e.g., dextran and polyethyleneglycol (182).]

Reference has already been made to the unusual behavior, e.g., lowering of surface tension (57,58,75), development of surface viscosity (74), and so forth, observed in mixed solutions of polycations and anionic surfactants. Buckingham et al. (75) arrived at the following form of the Gibbs adsorption equation for their system (poly-L-lysine/SDS):

$$d\gamma \approx -RT\,\Gamma d\,\ln[\mathrm{SDS}]$$

an implication being that the surface excess, Γ, of the DS anion, though highly influenced by the presence of polycation, is rather insensitive to its actual concentration. This equation (or, more strictly, its equivalent form) has recently been rederived by Asnacios et al. (78) for a system charged in the opposite sense, viz., the combination acrylamide-acrylamidesulfonate (AM-AMPS copolymer)/DTAB. The high value of the derived area per molecule of the DTA^+ ion (~80 A^2/mol) compared with that observed for DTAB alone (~45 A^2/mol) just prior to, or at, the c.a.c. and c.m.c., respectively (77,78), again suggests surface complex formation, analogous to that depicted in Figure 15, in which the polymer affects/imposes the packing arrangement of surfactant molecules in the surface (74). Implications regarding foaming are discussed in Chapter 5.

D. Proteins

1. *Multiple Equilibrium Model*

Traditionally, the interaction of a protein and a surfactant has been considered to involve a binding process. In addition to early reviews of this subject (1,2), one may cite more recent ones by Ananthapadmanabhan (129) and by Jones (130). Here it is pointed out that

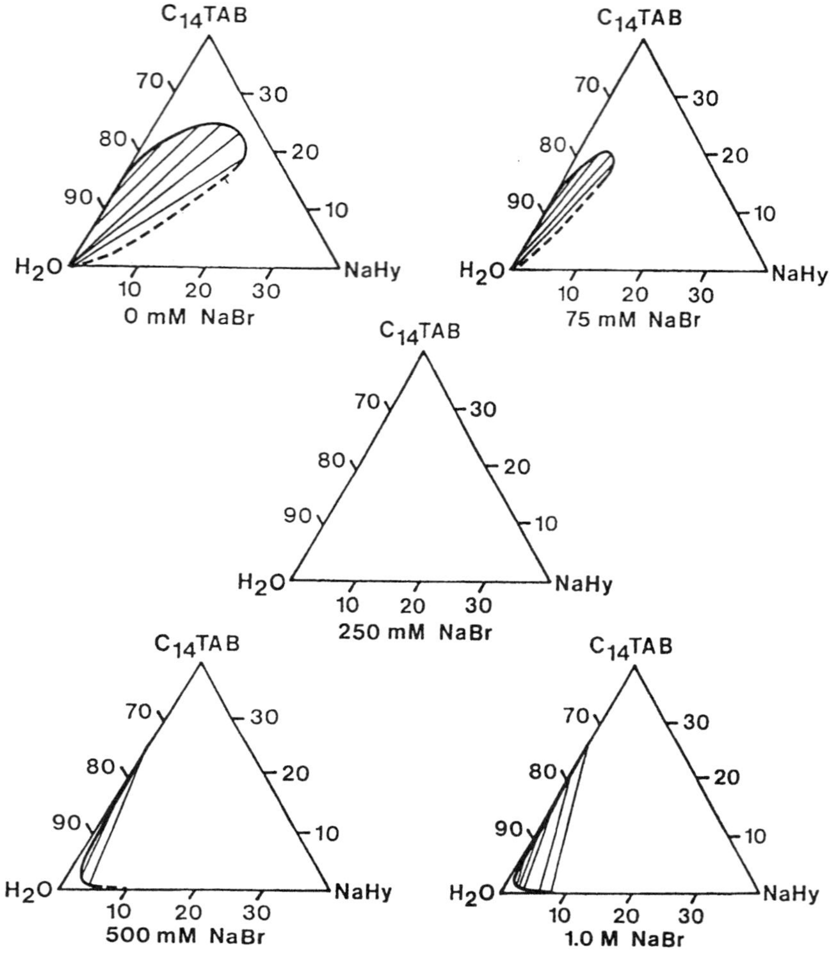

Figure 41 Pseudo three-component phase diagrams for the system sodium hyaluronate/C_{14}TAB/H_2O at different concentrations of added electrolyte. (From Ref. 62.)

the binding of a surfactant (D) by a protein (P) can be treated as a multiple equilibrium phenomenon which can be represented by

$$P + D \rightleftharpoons PD_1$$

$$PD_1 + D \rightleftharpoons PD_2$$

|

|

|

$$PD_{n-1} + D \rightleftharpoons PD_n$$

where n represents the maximum number of binding steps. If the equilibrium constant K for each binding step is the same, it follows that

$$K^n = \frac{[PD_n]}{[P][D]^n}$$

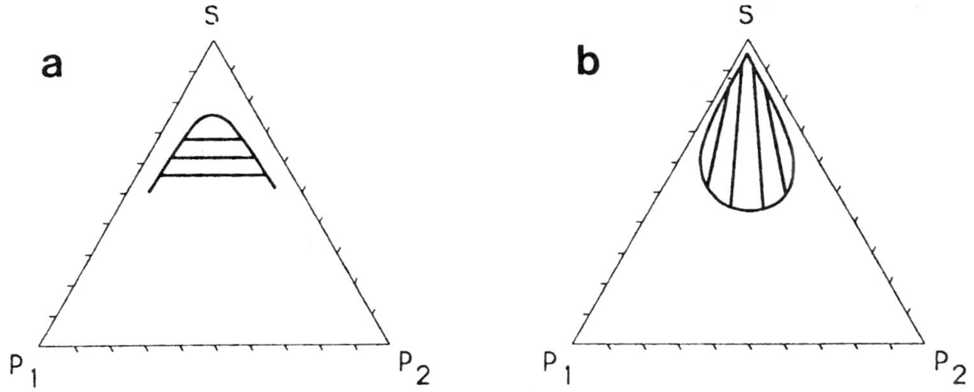

Figure 42 Segregative (a) and associative (b) phase separation in mixed polymer (P_1 and P_2) solutions according to Piculell and Lindman. S represents the solvent. (From Ref. 180.)

which is an equation of the same form as that derived by Smith and Muller (152). The average number, ν, of surfactant molecules bound per protein molecule would then be given by

$$\nu = \frac{n[PD_n]}{P + [PD_n]} = \frac{n(K[D])^n}{1 + (K[D])^n}$$

The above assumption is somewhat improbable, especially for proteins. It is, in fact, more likely that binding of one surfactant ion will lead to an increase or a decrease in binding affinity of the next one, corresponding to positive or negative "cooperativity," respectively. Such an effect is allowed for in the equation suggested by Hill (170):

$$\nu = \frac{n(K[D])^{n'}}{1 + (K[D])^{n'}}$$

A value of unity of n' implies no cooperativity in binding. A value greater than unity indicates positive cooperativity, and vice versa. Calculated isotherms illustrate the trends: for example, Jones (131,183), using the hypothetical case of a macromolecule with 50 binding sites and an assigned binding constant K of 10^4, constructed a family of isotherms corresponding to different values of the cooperativity coefficient n'. (See Fig. 43.) The correlation between cooperativity and steepness of the isotherms is readily seen.

A point of interest is that the Scatchard equation (2,184), which has been widely applied to the adsorption of surfactants to proteins (185), is readily derivable from the Hill equation. Thus, placing n' equal to unity, we have

$$\nu/[D] = K(n - \nu)$$

or

$$1/\nu = 1/n + 1/nK[D]$$

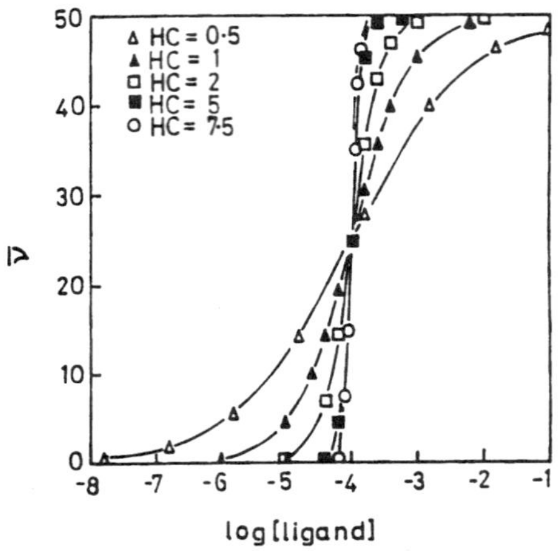

Figure 43 Binding isotherms, ν versus logarithm of ligand (surfactant) concentration, calculated from the Hill equation with 50 binding sites (intrinsic binding constant, 10^4) for a range of Hill coefficients, n', from 0.5 to 7.5. (From Refs. 131, 183.)

which has a similar form to the Langmuir equation. Plotting 1/ν against 1/[D] yields the values of n and K, and the latter in turn yields the free energy of binding through the expression

$$\Delta G^\circ = -RT \ln K$$

Applying this equation to the lysozyme/SDS data of Figure 30 (up to an n value of 18) yielded a ΔG° value of 6 kcal/mole (186), which is again comparable to the free energy of micelle formation of this surfactant and consonant with an aggregation process. Other methods to determine binding energy along the adsorption isotherm have been proposed, for example by Tanford (187,188), Bull (189), and Sen et al. (190).

The actual binding isotherm in many cases is much more complicated than that suggested in the simple reaction scheme above. It will also vary considerably from system to system. However, a schematic representation of binding prepared by Jones (191) is a reasonable representation of the behavior of a number of actual systems. (See Fig. 44.) The different types of observed behavior have also led to a number of pictorial attempts to depict the molecular pattern in reacted protein/surfactant systems. These will also vary with the particular polymer/surfactant combination chosen and with the degree of binding (192). A representative idea of thinking in this area is seen in the schematic drawings of Guo and Chen (193) (Fig. 45).

V. FINAL REMARKS

A general rationale of the foregoing would attempt to answer the question "why and how do polymer/surfactant complexes form?" In this respect it is appropriate to again consider salient properties of the two interacting species.

For a charged surfactant, the self-aggregation properties are of paramount importance. Thus, in the formation of regular ionic surfactant (spherical) micelles, a major resisting force is the crowding together of ionized head groups at the periphery of the micelle and

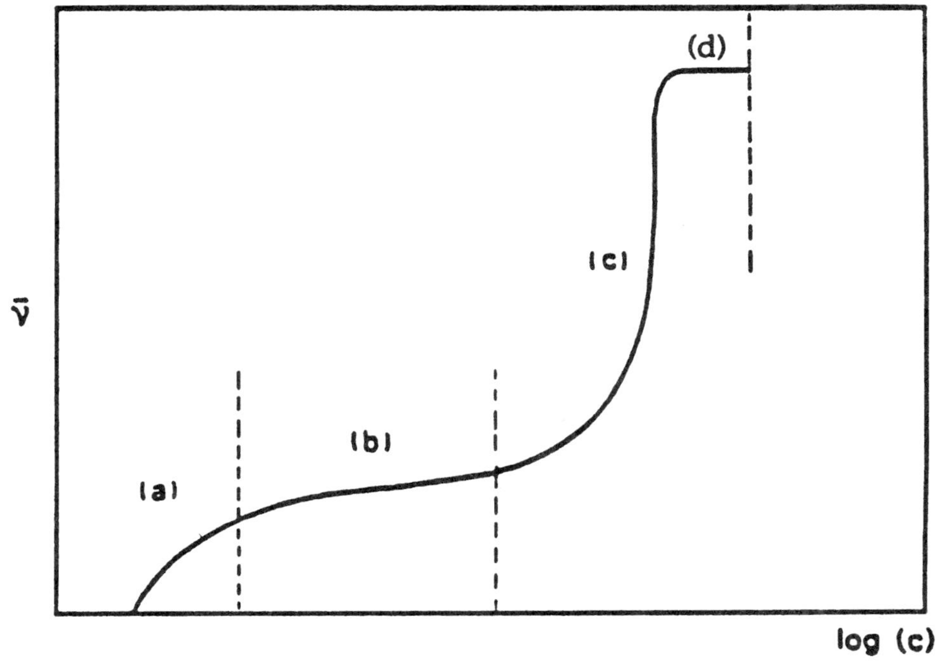

Figure 44 Schematic plot of the number of ligands per protein molecule (ν) versus the logarithm of the free ligand (surfactant) concentration, [c]. Region a, specific binding; region b, noncooperative binding; region c, cooperative binding; region d, saturation. (From Ref. 191.)

the development of a high electrostatic potential that can be offset only partially by counterion binding. Furthermore, in the well-accepted spherical, or Hartley, micelle (Fig. 1) there is a considerable distance, on a molecular scale, between the headgroups at the periphery, if only for geometrical reasons of packing. Some of this space will accommodate counterions, but most will comprise areas of the hydrocarbon chains exposed to water, an obviously unfavorable situation. Early NMR data indicated that the first few carbons (measured from the headgroup) of micellized molecules of SDS remain in contact with water. In contrast, let us consider a typical nonionic surfactant, say $C_{12}E_6$ or $C_{12}E_8$. Here there are no formal electrostatic forces resisting aggregation and the flexible PEO headgroups can readily position themselves so as to reduce contact of the radial array of micellar hydrocarbon chains with water. With these two unfavorable elements diminished, micelle formation is facilitated to the point that the c.m.c. is lowered about a hundredfold vis-à-vis that of ionic surfactant counterparts. A nonionic surfactant, in a sense, can be considered to be the analog of a preformed polymer/surfactant complex! The well-known lack of reactivity of nonionic surfactants toward most polymers is a further indication of this (Fig. 46a).

Another ''analog'' is found in the alkylpolyoxyethyleneoxide sulfate ($R(EO)_n$-$SO_4^-Na^+$) family of surfactants. Here the ''polymer'' is again part of the surfactant molecule but interposed before the headgroup. (See Fig. 46b.) Although these surfactants do remain interactive with polymers, such as PVP (150), the interaction tendency is considerably weaker than that of the parent alkyl sulfate surfactant. However, their self-association tendency (194) is again increased as illustrated by a progressive *reduction* in c.m.c (up to

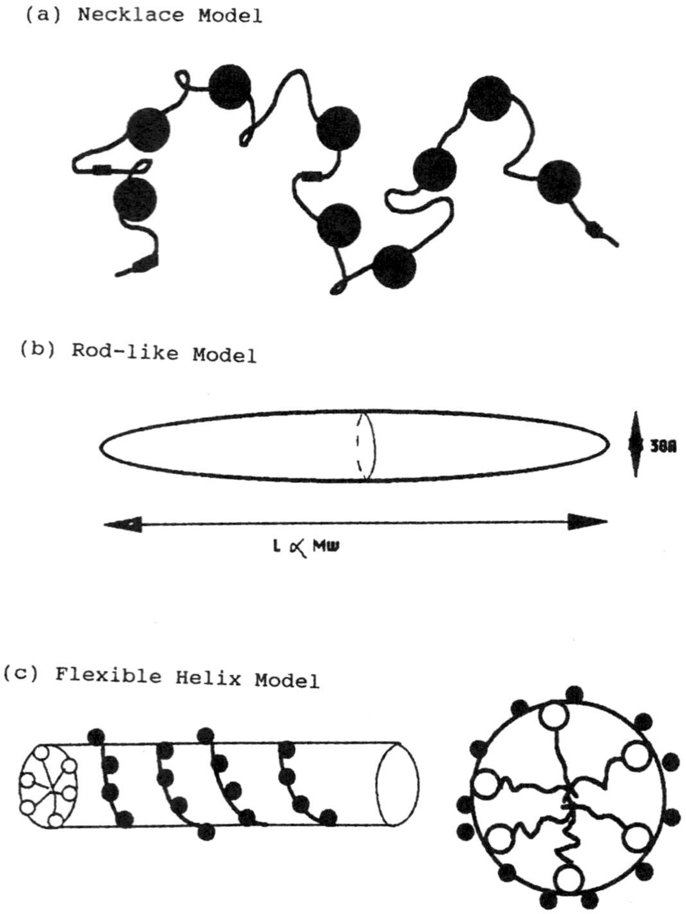

Figure 45 Schematic representation of the three types of structure proposed for the polymer-surfactant aggregates. (From Ref. 193.)

fourfold) accompanying the introduction $(EO)_n$ groups ($n = 1$–4) in the $C_{12}(EO)_nSO_4^-Na^+$ family (even though this increases the intrinsic hydrophilicity of the molecules) and by an increase in ionic dissociation of their micelles (by a factor of 2).

Let us now turn to a simple association surfactant, such as SDS, and consider first the effect of adding a ''simple'' interacting polymer to it. One can easily imagine a ''loopy'' configuration of the water-soluble polymer, associating with a micellar array of the surfactant, which allows ion-dipole association of the hydrophilic groups of the polymer and the ionic headgroup of the surfactant and, in addition, contact between the hydrophobic segments of the polymer and the exposed hydrocarbon areas of the micelle, in effect resulting in screening of the electrical charges and diminution of the extent of these exposed areas. Consequences of the above would include several features already observed, such as

1. A more favorable free energy of association, as manifested in a lowered ''c.m.c.'' (i.e., $T_1 <$ c.m.c.).

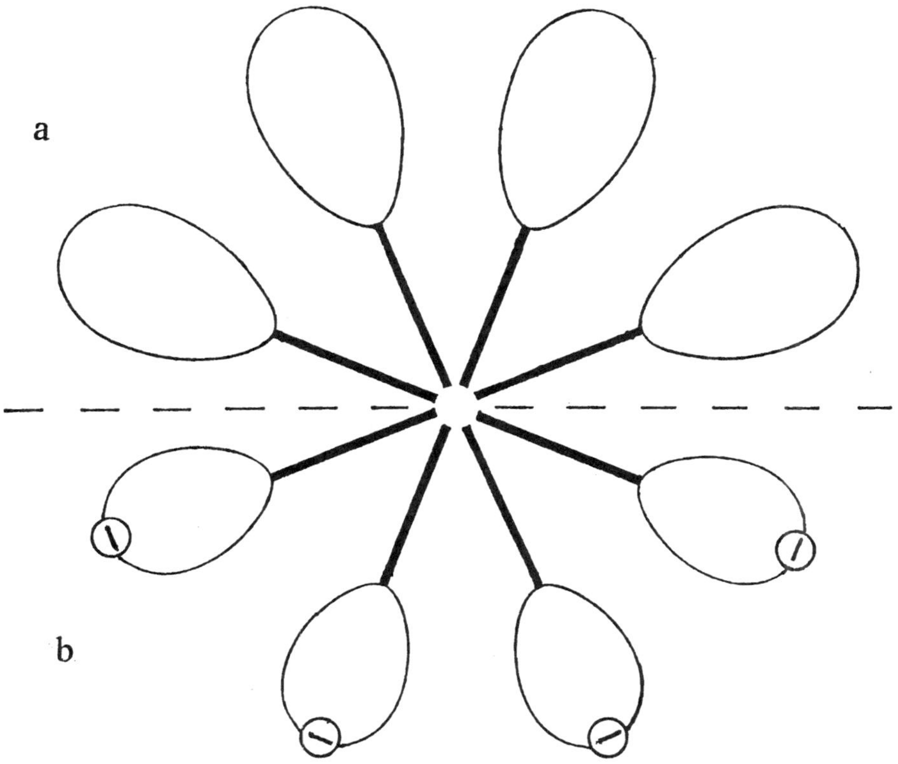

Figure 46 Schematic diagram of micelle in (a) nonionic surfactant, (b) alkylethoxysulfate surfactant. Compare with Figure 1.

2. Increased ionic dissociation of the aggregates.
3. An altered environment in the CH_2 groups of the surfactant near the headgroup, as seen in ^{13}C-NMR results. (See Figs. 10,11.)
4. Increased association tendency as the polymer becomes more hydrophobic (Breuer-Robb) (3).

Based on the current state of knowledge, a brief summary of the properties of ''conventional'' nonionic polymers that are reactive toward ionic surfactants is as follows. They should have:

1. Alternating hydrophilic and hydrophobic zones—hydrophilic for water solubility and ion binding, hydrophobic for filling peripherical micellar ''voids''
2. Flexibility, to be able to coat micelles and respond to the rapid disintegration and reformation of surfactant micelles
3. A minimum molecular weight, which will vary from polymer to polymer

Although it is currently not known whether the polymer *initiates* the interaction by instantaneous site binding of surfactant molecules or merely *responds* to ephemeral cluster formation of surfactant molecules, the above category of interaction can be considered as *micelle-directed* association.

The categories of polyelectrolyte and hydrophobically modified (HM) polymers are very different from the above. In these the association with the surfactant is considered to be *polymer directed* in view of the strong adsorption sites they provide for the said surfactant. This is borne out by extremely low c.a.c. values frequently observed in these systems, which confirm the high affinity of the adsorption processes. Conceptually (at least) interaction mechanisms in these systems are more straightforward.

First, in polyelectrolyte/oppositely charged surfactant systems one must decide between the likelihood of adsorption of surfactant on single sites and nucleation of aggregates at those sites versus adsorption at all sites. The latter is probably the normal mechanism in view of the high adsorption energy of these sites and, frequently, the positive/negative charge stoichiometry of the complexes that ultimately form. Nonetheless, there is also much evidence on the cooperativity of the overall interaction process, suggesting that surfactant ions adsorbed on different sites can associate to form aggregates. Fine points governing the detailed adsorption include the chemical structure of the polyelectrolyte (10) and its actual charge density (129,163,195).

In the case of HM-polymers abundant evidence exists that the alkyl groups in the dissolved polymer can be *preassociated*. This means that centers will be provided for the adsorption/association of surfactant ions (and molecules). Their composition and size will change with surfactant concentration, as will their nature—intermolecular and/or intramolecular. Fine points in this case include the number, type, chain length, and distribution of hydrophobic groups and, again, the detailed structure of the base polymer. In fact, the number of possible variations on this structural theme is vast!

Conceptually, proteins represent a combination of the two types of polymer just described. If one adds secondary and tertiary (and perhaps quaternary) structure effects in the protein, and also the possibility of unfolding, the number of possible variations in the interaction patterns with surfactants again becomes very large. Fortunately, the literature on this subject is substantial (2,129,130,185) and, as indicated in this chapter, many of the interaction patterns have been analyzed and are now well understood.

REFERENCES

1. Putnam FW. Adv Protein Chem 1948; 4:79.
2. Steinhardt J, Reynolds J. Multiple Equilibria in Proteins. New York: Academic Press, 1969.
3. Breuer MM, Robb ID. Chem Ind 1972; 530.
4. Robb ID. In: Lucassen Reynders EH, ed. Anionic Surfactants in Physical Chemistry of Surfactant Action. New York: Marcel Dekker, 1981.
5. Goddard ED, Ananthapadmanabhan KP. Interactions of Surfactants with Polymers and Proteins. Boca Raton, FL: CRC Press, 1992.
6. Aniansson EAG, Wall SN. J Phys Chem 1976; 80:905.
7. Goddard ED, Hoeve CAJ, Benson GC. J Phys Chem 1957; 61:593.
8. Goddard ED, Benson GC. Can J Chem 1957; 35:986.
9. Lindman B, Thalberg K. In: Goddard ED, Anathapadmanabhan KP, eds. Interactions of Surfactants with Polymers and Proteins. Boca Raton, FL: CRC Press, 1992.
10. Hayakawa K, Kwak JCT. In: Rubingh DN, Holland, PM. eds. Cationic Surfactants. New York: Marcel Dekker, 1991.
11. Shaw DJ. Introduction to Colloid and Surface Chemistry. London: Butterworths, 1966, Chapter 2.

12. Arai H, Murata M, Shinoda K. J Colloid Interface Sci 1971; 37:223.
13. Fishman ML, Eirich FR. J Phys Chem 1971; 75:3135.
14. Shirahama K. Colloid Polym Sci 1974; 252:978.
15. Shirahama K, Ide N. J Colloid Interface Sci 1976; 54:540.
16. Lewis K, Robinson CP. J Colloid Interface Sci 1970; 32:539.
17. Birch BJ, Clarke DE, Lee RS, Oakes J. Anal Chim Acta 1974; 70:417.
18. Hayakawa K, Ayub AL, Kwak JCT. Colloids Surfaces 1982; 4:389.
19. Malovikova A, Hayakawa K, Kwak JCT. In: Rosen MJ, ed. Structure/Performance Relationships in Surfactants. Symposium Ser. Washington, DC: American Chemical Society, 1984: 253, Chapter 15.
20. Kresheck GC, Constantinidis I. Anal Chem 1984; 56:152.
21. Gilanyi T, Wolfram E. Colloids Surfaces 1981; 3:181.
22. Botré C, Crescenzi VL, Mele A. J Phys Chem 1959; 63:650.
23. Botré C, DeMartis F, Solinas M. J Phys Chem 1964; 68:3624.
24. Jones MN. J Colloid Interface Sci 1967; 23:36.
25. Zana R, Lang J, Lianos P. Polym Prep Am Chem Soc Div Polym Chem 1982; 23:39.
26. Schwuger MJ. J Colloid Interface Sci 1973; 43:491.
27. Lange H. Kolloid Z Z Polym 1971; 243:101.
28. Murata M, Arai H. J Colloid Interface Sci 1973; 44:475.
29. Chari K, Hossain T. J Phys Chem 1991; 95:3302.
30. Francois J, Dayantis J, Sabbadin J. Eur Polym J 1985; 21:165.
31. Saito S. Kolloid Z 1957; 154:19.
32. Jones MN. J Colloid Interface Sci 1968; 26:532.
33. Kalyanasundaran K, Thomas JK. J Am Chem Soc 1977; 99:2039.
34. Zana R. In: Zana R, ed. Surfactants in Solution: New Methods of Investigation. New York: Marcel Dekker, 1987, Chapter 5.
35. Turro NJ, Baretz BH, Kuo P-L. Macromolecules 1984; 17:1321.
36. Kalyanasundaran K, Thomas JK. J Phys Chem 1977; 81:2176.
37. Turro NJ, Okubo T. J Phys Chem 1982; 86:159.
38. Zana R, Lianos P, Lang J. J Phys Chem 1985; 89:41.
39. Lissi EA, Abuin E. J Colloid Interface Sci 1985; 105:1.
40. Witte FM, Engberts JBFN. Colloids Surfaces 1989; 36:417.
41. Winnik FM, Winnik MA. Polymer J 1990; 22:482.
42. Zana R, Yiv S, Strazielle C, Lianos P. J Colloid Polym Sci 1987; 265:42.
43. Winnik FM. In: Goddard ED, Ananthapadmanabhan KP, eds. Interactions of Surfactants with Polymers and Proteins. Boca Raton, FL: CRC Press, 1992.
44. Winnik FM, Regismond STA. Colloids Surfaces 1996; 118:1.
45. Thomas JK. J Phys Chem 1987; 91:267.
46. Cabane B. J Phys Chem 1977; 81:1639.
47. Muller N, Johnson TW. J Phys Chem 1969; 73:2042.
48. Stilbs P. In: Kwak JCT, ed. Polymer Surfactant Systems. New York: Marcel Dekker, 1998.
49. Sasaki T, Kushima K, Matsuda K, Suzuki H. Bull Chem Soc Jpn 1980; 53:1864.
50. Rudd PJ, Jennings BR. J Colloid Interface Sci 1974; 48:302.
51. Olofsson G, Wang G. Pure Appl Chem 1994; 66:527.
52. Cabane B, Duplessix R. Colloids Surfaces. 1985; 13:19.
53. Shirahama K, Tohdo M, Murahashi M. J Colloid Interface Sci 1982; 86:283.
54. Carlsson A, Karlstrom G, Lindman B. J Phys Chem 1989; 93:3673.
55. Bloor DM, Wyn-Jones E. J Chem Soc (Faraday Trans 2) 1982; 78:657.
56. Gettings J, Gould C, Hall DG, Jobling PL, Rassing J, Wyn-Jones E. Chem Soc (Faraday Trans 2) 1980; 76:1535.
57. Goddard, ED, Phillips TS, Hannan RB. J Soc Cosmet Chem 1975; 26:461.
58. Goddard ED, Hannan RB. J Colloid Interface Sci 1976; 55:73.

59. Goddard ED, Hannan RB. J Am Oil Chem Soc 1977; 54:561.
60. Scott JE. Chem Ind 1955; 168.
61. Goldraich M, Schwartz JR, Burns JL, Talmon Y. Colloids Surfaces 1997; 125:231.
62. Thalberg K, Lindman B. In: Mittal KL, Shah DO, eds. Surfactants in Solution. New York: Plenum Press, 1991; 11:243.
63. Ranganathan S, Kwak JCT. Langmuir 1996; 12:1381.
64. Thalberg K, Lindman B, Karlström G. J Phys Chem 1991; 95:3370.
65. Laurent TC, Scott JE. Nature 1964; 202:661.
66. Dubin PL, Oteri R. J Colloid Interface Sci 1983; 95:453.
67. Dubin PL, Davis D. Colloids Surfaces 1985; 13:113.
68. Manuszak-Guerrini M, Smith-Wright L, Lochhead RY, Daly WH. J Soc Cosmet Chem 1997; 48:23.
69. Hayakawa K, Santerre JP, Kwak JCT. Biophys Chem 1983; 17:175.
70. Hayakawa K, Santerre JP, Kwak JCT. Macromolecules 1983; 16:1642.
71. Kwak JCT. Personal communication.
72. Malovikova A, Hayakawa K, Kwak JCT. J Phys Chem 1984; 88:1930.
73. Hayakawa K, Kwak JCT. J Phys Chem 1982; 86:3866.
74. Regismond STA, Winnik FM, Goddard ED. Colloids Surfaces A 1996; 119:221.
75. Buckingham JH, Lucassen J, Hollway F. J Colloid Interface Sci 1978; 67:423.
76. Barck M, Stenius P. Colloids Surfaces 1994; 89:59.
77. Bergeron V, Langevin D, Asnacios A. Langmuir 1996; 12:1550.
78. Asnacios A, Langevin D, and Argillier J-F. Macromolecules 1996; 29:7412.
79. Goddard ED, Hannan, RB. In: Mittal KL, ed. Micellization, Solubilization, and Microemulsions, Vol 2. New York: Plenum Press, 1977:835.
80. Leung PS, Goddard ED, Han C, Glinka CJ. Colloids Surfaces 1985; 13:47.
81. Abuin EB, Scaiano JC. J Am Chem Soc 1984; 106:6274.
82. McCormick CL, Johnson CB. In: Glass JE, ed. Polymers in Aqueous Media. Adv. Chem. Ser. 223. Washington DC: American Chemical Society, 1989:437.
83. Ananthapadmanabhan KP, Leung PS, Goddard ED. Colloids Surfaces 1985; 13:63.
84. Hayakawa K, Shinohara S, Sasawaki S, Satake I, Kwak JCT. Bull Chem Soc Jpn 1995; 68: 2179.
85. Ohbu K, Hiraishi O, Kashiwa I. J Am Oil Chem Soc 1982; 59:108.
86. Hayakawa K, Fukutome T, Satake I. Langmuir 1990; 6:1495.
87. Yui TSTI, Pal'mer VG, Musabekov KB. Izv Akad Nauk Kaz SSR Ser Khim 1984; 19.
88. Almgren M, Hansson P, Mukhtar E, van Stam J. Langmuir 1992; 8:2405.
89. Chu D-Y, Thomas JK. J Am Chem Soc 1986; 108:6270.
90. Magny B, Iliopoulos I, Zana R, Audebert R. Langmuir 1994; 10:3180.
91. Hansson P, Almgren M. Langmuir 1994; 10:2115.
92. Anthony O, Zana R. Langmuir 1996; 12:1967.
93. Strauss UP, In: Goddard ED, Ananthapadmanabhan KP, eds. Interactions of Surfactants with Polymers and Proteins. Boca Raton, FL: CRC Press, 1992.
94. Strauss UP, Jackson EG. J Polym Sci 1951; 6:649.
95. Glass JE, ed. Polymers in Aqueous Media Adv Chem Ser 223. Washington, DC: American Chemical Society, 1989.
96. Landoll LM. J Polym Sci Polym Chem Ed 1982; 20:443.
97. Sau AC, Landoll LM. In: Glass JE, ed. Polymers in Aqueous Media. Adv. Chem. Ser. 223. Washington, DC: American Chemical Society, 1989:343.
98. Goddard ED. J Colloid Interface Sci 1992; 152:578.
99. Tanaka R, Meadows J, Williams PA, Phillips GO. Macromolecules 1992; 25:1304.
100. Dualeh AJ, Steiner CA. Macromolecules 1990; 23:251.
101. Dualeh, AJ, Steiner CA. Macromolecules 1991; 24:112.
102. Goddard ED, Leung PS. Colloids Surfaces 1992; 65:211.

103. Kastner U, Hoffmann H, Donges R, Ehrler R, Colloids Surfaces 1996; 112:209.
104. Sarrazin-Cartalas A, Iliopoulos I, Audebert R, Olsson U. Langmuir 1994; 10:1421.
105. Iliopoulos I, Wang TK, Audebert R. Langmuir 1991; 7:617.
106. Senan C, Meadows J, Shone PT, Williams PA. Langmuir 1994; 10:2471.
107. Petit F, Iliopoulos I, Audebert R, Szönyi S. Langmuir 1997; 13:4229.
108. McGlade MJ, Randall FJ, Tcheurekdjian N. Macromolecules 1987; 20:1782.
109. Winnik FM, Regismond STA, Goddard ED. Colloids Surfaces 1996; 106:243.
110. Winnik FM, Regismond STA, Goddard ED. Langmuir 1997; 13:111.
111. Kevelam J, van Breemen JFL, Blokzijl W, Engberts JBFN. Langmuir 1996; 12:4709.
112. Ananthapadmanabhan KP, Leung PS, Goddard ED. In: El Nokaly MA, ed. Polymer Association Structures. ACS Symposium Series No. 384. New York: American Chemical Society, 1988:297.
113. Guillemet F, Piculell L. J Phys Chem 1995; 99:9201.
114. Magny B, Iliopoulos I, Zana R, Audebert R. Langmuir 1996; 12:2616.
115. Anthony O, Zana R, Langmuir 1996; 12:3590.
116. Chang Y, McCromick CL. Polymer 1994; 35:3503.
117. Sivadasan K, Somasundaran P. Colloids Surfaces 1990; 49:229.
118. Winnik FM, Ringsdorf H, Venzmer J. Langmuir 1991; 7:905.
119. Winnik FM. Langmuir 1990; 6:522.
120. Winnik FM, Ringsdorf H, Venzmer J. Langmuir 1991; 7:912.
121. Hu Y-Z, Zhao C-L, Winnik MA, Sundaran PR. Langmuir 1990; 6:880.
122. Schild HG, Tirrell DA. Langmuir 1991; 7:665.
123. Saunders FL. J Colloid Interface Sci 1969; 31:557.
124. Drummond CJ, Albers S, Furlong DN, Colloids Surfaces 1991; 62:95.
125. Kamenka N, Burgand I, Zana R, Lindman B. J Phys Chem 1994; 98:6785.
126. Zana R, Binana-Limbele W, Kamenka N, Lindman B. J Phys Chem 1992; 96:5461.
127. Pankhurst KGA. In: Surface Chemistry, London: Butterworths, 1949:109.
128. Goddard ED, Pethica BA. J Chem Soc 1953; 269.
129. Ananthapadmanabhan KP. In: Goddard ED, Ananthapadmanabhan KP, eds. Interactions of Surfactants with Polymers and Proteins. Boca Raton, FL: CRC Press, 1992, Chapter 8.
130. Jones MN. In: Magdassi S, ed. Surface Activity of Proteins. New York: Marcel Dekker, 1996, Chapter 8.
131. Jones MN, Brass A. In: Dickinson E, ed. Food Polymers, Gels, and Colloids. Cambridge: Royal Society of Chemistry, 1991:65.
132. Knox WL, Parshall TO. J Colloid Interface Sci 1970; 33:16.
133. Nishikido N, Takahara T, Kobayashi H, Tanaka M. Bull Chem Soc Jpn 1982; 55:3032.
133a. Cockbain EG. Trans Faraday Soc 1953; 49:104.
134. Greener MJ, Contestable BA, Bale MD. Macromolecules 1987; 20:2490.
135. Schwuger MJ, Bartnik FG. In: Gloxhuber C, ed. Anionic Surfactants. New York: Marcel Dekker, 1980:1.
136. Jones MN, Skinner HA, Tipping E. Biochem J 1975; 147:229.
137. Steinhardt J, Scott JR, Birdi KS. Biochemistry 1977; 16:718; Chattoraj DK, Birdi KS. Adsorption and the Gibbs Surface Excess. New York: Plenum Press, 1984: 379.
138. Whitesides TH, Miller DD. Langmuir 1994; 10:2899.
139. Miller DD, Lenhart W, Antalek BJ, Williams AJ, Hewitt JM, Langmuir 1994; 10:68.
140. Cosgrove T, White SJ, Zarbakhsh A, Heenan RK, Howe AM. Langmuir 1995; 11:744.
141. Turro NJ, Lei X-G, Ananthapadmanabhan KP, Aronson MP. Langmuir 1995; 11:2525.
142. Kaneshina S, Tanaka M, Kondo T. Bull Chem Soc Jpn 1973; 46:2735.
143. Jones MN, Manley P. J Chem Soc (Faraday Trans I) 1980; 76:654.
144. Jones MN, Manley P. J Chem Soc (Faraday Trans I) 1981; 77:827.
145. Jones MN, Manley P. J Chem Soc (Faraday Trans I) 1979; 75:1736.

146. Rendall HM. J Chem Soc (Faraday Trans I) 1976; 72:481.
147. Tokiwa F, Tsujii K. Bull Chem Soc Jpn 1973; 46:2684.
148. Gravsholt S. Proc Scand Symp Surface Chem 1965; 2:132.
149. Brackman J, Engberts JBFN. J Colloid Interface Sci 1989; 132:250.
150. Saito S. J Colloid Interface Sci 1960; 15:283.
151. Reynolds JA, Herbert S, Steinhardt J. Biochemistry 1968; 7:1357.
152. Smith ML, Muller N. J Colloid Interface Sci 1975; 52:507.
153. Brackman JC, van Os NM. Engberts JBFN. Langmuir 1988; 4:1266.
154. Thalberg K, Lindman B, Bergfeldt K. Langmuir 1991; 7:2893.
155. Cabane B, Duplessix R. J Phys (Paris) 1982; 43:1529.
156. Hall DG. J Chem Soc (Faraday Trans I) 1985; 81:885.
157. Arai H, Horin S. J Colloid Interface Sci 1969; 30:372.
158. Murai N, Makino S, Sugai S. J Colloid Interface Sci 1972; 41:399.
159. Goddard ED, Leung PS. Langmuir 1992; 8:1499.
160. Goddard ED, Ananthapadmanabhan KP. Interactions of Surfactants with Polymers and Proteins. Boca Raton, FL: CRC Press, 1992:112, 115.
161. Takagi T, Isemura T. Bull Chem Soc Jpn 1960; 33:437.
162. Nagarajan R, Kalpakci B. Polym Prep Am Chem Soc Div Polym Chem 1982; 23:41.
163. Kiefer JJ, Somasundaran P. Ananthapadmanabhan KP. Langmuir 1993; 9:1187.
164. Saito S, Taniguchi T, Kitamura K. J Colloid Interface Sci 1971; 37:154.
165. Saito S. J Polym Sci 1969; A7:1789.
166. Maltesh C, Somasundaran P. J Colloid Interface Sci 1993; 157:14.
167. Dubin PL, Gruber JH, Xia J, Zhang H. J Colloid Interface Sci 1992; 148:35.
168. Zana R, Yiv S, Strazielle C, Lianos P. J Colloid Interface Sci 1981; 80:208.
169. Hayakawa K, Kwak JCT. J Phys Chem 1983; 87:506.
170. Hill AV. J Physiol (Lond) 1910; 40:190.
171. Nagarajan R. Colloids Surfaces 1985; 13:1.
172. Nagarajan R. J Chem Phys 1989; 90:1980.
173. Ruckenstein E, Huber G, Hoffmann H. Langmuir 1987; 3:382.
174. Evans DF, Mitchell DJ, Ninham BW. J Phys Chem 1984; 88:6344.
175. Schwarz G. Eur J Biochem 1970; 12:442.
176. Shirahama K, Yuaza H, Sugimoto S. Bull Chem Soc Jpn 1981; 54:375.
177. Shirahama K, Tashiro M. Bull Chem Soc Jpn 1984; 57:377.
178. Satake I, Yang JT. Biopolymers 1976; 15:2263.
179. Somasaundaran P, Healy TW, Fuerstenau DW. J Phys Chem 1964; 68:3562.
180. Piculell L, Lindman B. Adv Colloid Interface Sci 1992; 41:149.
181. Bungenberg de Jong HG. In: Kruyt HR, ed. Colloid Science. Amsterdam: Elsevier, 1949, Chapters VIII, X.
182. Albertsson PA. Adv Protein Chem 1970; 24:309.
183. Jones MN. Chem Soc Rev 1992; 21:127.
184. Scatchard G. Ann NY Acad Sci 1949; 51:660.
185. Chattoraj DK, Birdi KS. Adsorption and the Gibbs Surface Excess. New York: Plenum Press, 1984:339.
186. Dickinson E. In: Goddard ED, Ananthapadmanabhan KP, eds. Interactions of Sufactants with Polymers and Proteins. Boca Raton, FL: CRC Press, 1992:295.
187. Tanford C. The Hydrophobic Effect: Formation of Micelles and Biological Membranes, 2nd ed., New York: Wiley-Interscience, 1980, Chapter 14.
188. Reynolds JA, Tanford C. Proc Natl Acad Sci USA 1970; 66:1002.
189. Bull HB. Biochim Biophys Acta. 1956; 19:464.
190. Sen M, Mitra SP, Chattoraj DK. Ind J Biochem Biophys 1980; 17:370.
191. Jones MN. In: Magdassi S, ed. Surface Activity of Proteins. New York: Marcel Dekker, 1996:244.

192. Dominguez, JG, Parra JL, Infante RM, Pelejero RM, Balaguer F, Sastra T. J Soc Cosmet Chem 1977; 28:165.
193. Guo XH, Chen SH. Phys Rev Lett 1990; 64(21):2579.
194. Schwuger MJ. In: Rosen MJ, ed. Structure/Performance Relationships in Surfactants. Symposium Series. Washington, DC: American Chemical Society, 1984:253.
195. Manning GS. J Chem Phys 1969; 51:294.

APPENDIX

Index of Polymers

PAAm	Polyacrylamide
PNIPAM	Poly (N-isopropyl) acrylamide
PAA	Polyacrylicacid (acrylate)
PMA	Polymethacrylicacid (methacrylate)
PDMDAAC	Polydimethyldiallylammoniumchloride
PDMAEMA	Polydimethylaminoethylmethacrylate
PDMAPMAAm	Polydimethylaminopropylmethacrylamide
AM-AMPS	Copol.acrylamide-acrylamidesulfonate
PVA	Polyvinylalchol
PVAc	Polyvinylacetate
PVP	Polyvinylpyrrolidone
PVMMA	Copol.vinylmethylether-maleicanhydride
PEO (PEG)	Polyethylene-oxide (-glycol)
PPO	Polpropyleneoxide
PS	Polystyrene
PSS	Polystyrenesulfonate
PEI	Polyethyleneimine
HEC	Hydroxyethylcellulose
HM-HEC	Alkyl modified HEC
HPC	Hydroxypropylcellulose
MeC	Methylcellulose
EHEC	Ethylhydroxyethylcellulose
CMC	Carboxymethylcellulose
DexS	Dextransulfate

Commercial Polymers

Polymers				Polyquaternium No. (INCI)
Polymer JR		Cationic substituted HEC (M.W. increasing in order JR-125, -400, -30M)	(Amerchol)	10
Quatrisoft	LM 200	HM-cationic HEC	(Amerchol)	24
Celquat	L-200	HEC/DMDAAC Copol.	(National Starch)	4

Gafquat	755	P(VP/DMAEMA)	(ISP)	11
Gafquat	HS100	P(VP/DMAPMAAm)	(ISP)	28
Reten	220	P(AAm/β-methacryloxyethyl-TAC)	(Hercules)	5
Merquat	100	P(DMDAAC)	(Calgon)	6
Merquat	550	P(DMDAAC/AAm)	(Calgon)	7
Jaguar	C-14S	Guar Hydroxypropyl-TAC	(Rhone Poulenc)	

Index of Surfactants

R-SO_4	Alkylsulfate
SDS, SLS	Dodecyl (lauryl) sulfate, Na salt
TEALS	Laurylsulfate, triethanolamine salt
$R(EO)_nSO_4$	Alkylethoxysulfate
LAS, ABS	Alkylbenzenesulfonate
R-TAB (TAC)	Alkyltrimethylammoniumbromide (chloride)
DTAB (TAC)	R = dodecyl
TTAB (TAC)	R = tetradecyl
CTAB (TAC)	R = hexadecyl (cetyl)
DPyCl	Dodecylpyridinium chloride
TPyB	Tetradecylpyridinium bromide

Barquat	MB-40	Myristyldimethylbenzylammonium chloride	Lonza
Tergitol	15-S-9	C_{12}-C_{15} sec. alcohol 9EO condensate	Union Carbide
Tergitol	NP-9	Nonylphenol 9 EO condensate	Union Carbide
Triton	X-100	Ter-octylphenol av.9.5EO condensate	Union Carbide
Miranol	C2M	Dicarboxycocoimidazoline derivative	Miranol

5

Polymer/Surfactant Interaction in Applied Systems

E. Desmond Goddard
Union Carbide Corporation, Tarrytown, New York

I. INTRODUCTION

Polymers and surfactants are common components of a number of cosmetic formulations. Polymers, for example, are often used for controlling the rheology of solutions and suspensions and for altering the interfacial properties of solids. Surfactants are used for their wettability, solubilization, emulsification, and general detergency properties. When present together, polymers and surfactants can interact with each other and this can lead to significant alterations in system properties that are sometimes undesirable, but often beneficial. It must be recognized that a knowledge of the interaction characteristics of the particular polymer(s) and surfactant(s) present will greatly aid the understanding and facilitate optimization of the properties of a system, although it is suspected that a great number of commercial products containing such mixtures are still assembled very much on an empirical, trial-and-error basis.

On the other hand, there are now many examples of systems in which interaction between the polymer and the surfactant is exploited (or sometimes circumvented) to provide the beneficial effects sought from the formulation. In Chapter 4 fundamental observations and various aspects of the polymer-surfactant interaction phenomenon were presented and discussed. In this chapter examples of actual or potential application systems in which polymer-surfactant interactions can play a definite role in governing system behavior are presented and discussed. Many opportunities for further exploitation of the phenomenon appear possible.

II. CONDITIONING AND PROTECTION

A. Hair

The term ''conditioning'' is of great significance when applied to a number of domestic cleaning practices, including hair shampooing and body cleaning. In most of these, conditioning is virtually synonymous with the use of cationic adsorption agents. The reason for this is that many surfaces, including hair and skin in contact with water, are negatively charged. Cleaning formulations normally employ anionic surfactants (less often nonionic surfactants) and, without a conditioning component, can leave the substrate in less than optimum condition as a result of high electrostatic charge, high interfiber friction, ''dryness,'' and the like. Experience has taught that the ''right'' conditioning agent can alleviate this deficiency: cationic agents (polyelectrolytes and to a much lesser extent cationic surfactants) enjoy their main use in the personal care industry as hair conditioners, undoubtedly as a result of their high adsorption efficiency and the intrinsic properties of their adsorbed layers. While mechanisms of action are often complex, and can involve several effects, reference to Chapter 12 will show that many of the currently employed evaluation methods are in fact used to assess improvements in hair properties effected by their exposure to cationic polymeric conditioning agents. For the same reason (see Chapter 10) many methods have been developed to measure the adsorption of such materials on keratin substrates.

Today, the traditional method of conditioning hair in a separate step after shampooing has progressively given way to the use of ''2-in-1'' conditioning shampoos. In these, the conditioning polymer, at a relatively low level (~1%), is incorporated directly in the shampoo, which usually contains from 10 to 20% anionic surfactant(s).

In Chapter 10 reference is made to the fact that the adsorption of a typical cationic conditioning agent, Polymer JR 400 (Amerchol), is markedly reduced in the presence of an anionic surfactant SDS in 10-fold excess (1). When present at the same (1) or an even greater excess (1,2), a nonionic surfactant scarcely affected the adsorption. On the other hand, the presence of a cationic surfactant virtually eliminated the adsorption of the polymer (3). (See Fig. 1.) The interpretation in the latter case is that the surfactant itself is strongly adsorbed by the negatively charged fibers and, being of much lower molecular weight and of higher diffusion rate, preempts the negative adsorption sites on the fibers.

The mechanism of adsorption of a polycation from a solution containing an excess of interacting (anionic) surfactant has invited considerable speculation: with this excess of surfactant the overall charge of the ''complex'' will be negative (4) and hence there would be a net repulsion from the negatively charged fiber surface. However, the polymer/surfactant complex will have a dynamic structure and, statistically, there is a finite chance of the disintegration of a polymer bound micelle in the vicinity of the fiber substrate so exposing a segment of the polycation chain to the latter. If adsorption of the segment takes place then, statistically, there is a finite chance of the next segment's adsorbing, and so on.

The above hypothesized mechanism of hair conditioning by cationic polymers in 2-in-1 formulations concerns the breakdown kinetics of the polymer/surfactant complex and the kinetics of adsorption of the ''freed'' polymer. There is, however, a very different and quite widely held hypothesis concerning the utility of 2-in-1 shampoos as (wet) conditioning agents. The mechanism concerns the dilution characteristics of the shampoo concentrate and can be understood by reference to the solubility diagram of the model system, Polymer JR 400/sodium dodecyl sulfate (SDS) (5). As reported and analyzed earlier, the line corresponding to maximum precipitation (stoichiometric charge equivalence) departs from a 45° slope of the log-log plot on sufficient dilution of the system. This means that a composition that was initially clear, containing say 10 times as much surfactant as polymer, could on sufficient dilution yield a turbid system. (See heavy line in Fig. 2.) The hypothesis of conditioning by this mechanism asserts that fine precipitate particles, which are intrinsically slippery, are formed and entrained when the washed hair is rinsed, so facilitating the subsequent wet combing process. Of course, the presence of polymer itself

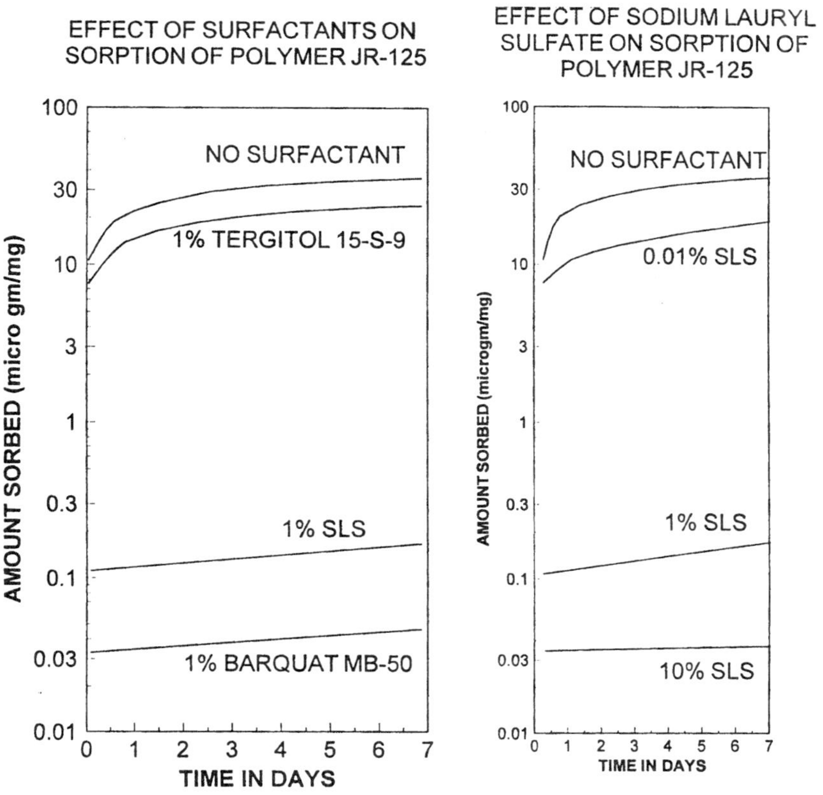

Figure 1 Uptake of Polymer JR 125 from 0.1% solution by bleached hair, in the presence of surfactants. (From Ref. 3.)

on the hair fibers after drying can contribute to conditioning by other postulated mechanisms, such as the reduction in static electrification during combing.

Finally, there is one other general way in which keratin surfaces exposed to polymer/surfactant combinations can be influenced. The deposited polymer or polymer/surfactant combination can favorably influence the receptivity of the surface to a second conditioning species. This effect is claimed, for example, in a patent issued to Colgate-Palmolive Co. (6) in which the presence of a cationic polyelectrolyte in an anionic surfactant shampoo apparently leads to more efficient deposition of a silicone oil conditioner. The mechanism (unspecified) probably concerns heteroflocculation of the silicone droplets onto the hair fibers modified by the adsorption of the first polymer (or complex). A patent on a similar topic has recently been issued to Procter & Gamble (7). Use of cationic polymers for deposition of particulate materials dispersed in anionic surfactant systems has been the subject of several other patents (8–10). In spite of this patent activity, mechanistic understanding of deposition from such surfactant systems is limited. Some fundamental studies on this general subject have, however, been reported by Berthiaume and Jachowicz (11). Employing hair fibers pretreated with a cationic polymer [polymethylacrylamidopropyltrimethyl ammonium chloride], they examined the deposition of silicone oil from surfactant-stabilized emulsions. In this case, the results were unpredictable inasmuch as deposition was higher from the emulsion stabilized with a cationic surfactant than with an anionic

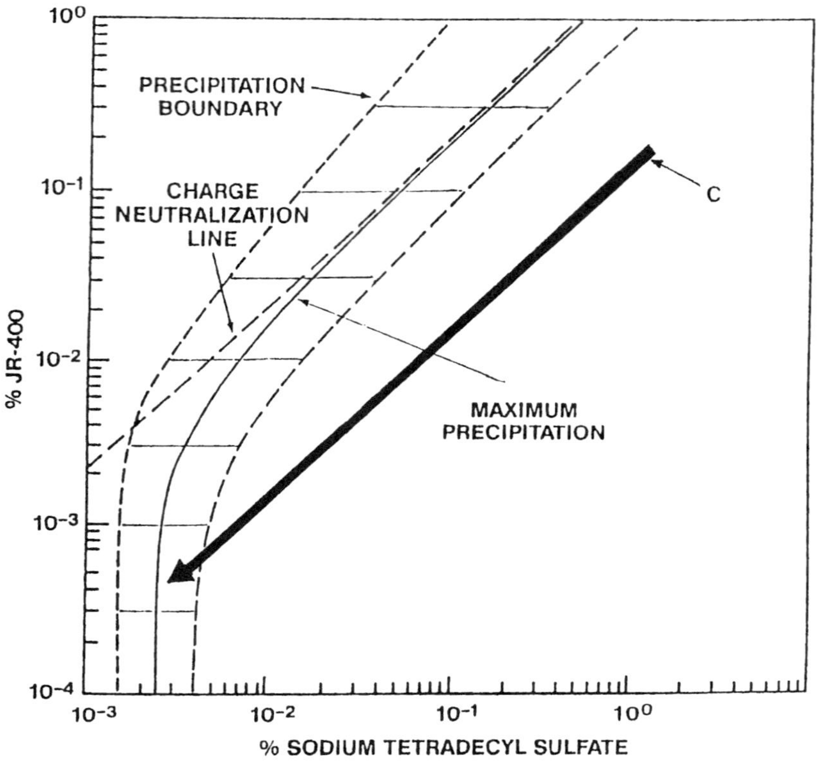

Figure 2 Conditioning via a precipitation mechanism (''Lochhead effect''). An initially clear solution C (shampooing strength) (heavy line) can on dilution (the rinse) pass through a precipitation region. (From Ref. 5.)

surfactant. A tentative explanation was offered in terms of competitive adsorption of the surfactant onto ionic sites on the keratin. Recently Marchioretto and Blakely (12) have presented evidence that the addition of silicone polyethers (which can readily be solubilized or dispersed in surfactant systems) to shampoos containing polycation (Polymer JR 125) can lead to substantial synergistic improvements in the conditioning afforded by the shampoo (essentially of the ethoxysulfate, betaine, nonionic combination type). These included detangling, antistatic, softness, gloss, and ease of combing. These results are obviously very encouraging and of potential importance, but there is as yet no mechanistic information to explain them. Both the adsorption of the polycations on hair and their interaction with the anionic surfactant are expected to be affected by the presence of the silicone polyether. The fundamental interaction and deposition processes involved, as well as the composition of the deposited layer, would clearly be of interest and, once understood, allow further optimization of these interesting systems.

B. Skin

While the discussion above has been restricted to shampoo systems and the keratin substrate, hair, much of the reasoning can be applied to the cleaning and conditioning of the other major keratin substrate, viz., skin, by invoking similar mechanisms. Indeed, there are many parallels between the two and it is not uncommon these days to incorporate "conditioning" cationic polymers into liquid skin cleaning surfactant systems, such as "body shampoos." The patent literature in the personal care area shows significant activity regarding the use of polymers, especially cationic polymers, in skin cleansing formulations. It has been claimed that cationic polymers improve skin feel and mildness (13,14) and provide enhanced moisturization. It has also been claimed that the polymers enhance the tactile properties of lather and of the skin during rinsing (15). The mechanisms of such action have not so far been established. It is, however, instructive to examine the role of polymers in cleansing systems and to speculate on some of the possible mechanisms of action.

While the practice of incorporating polymers in cleansing bars has been rather limited (one possible reason being the processing issues involved), with the rapid growth of liquid skin cleansers, use of polymers in such formulations has become a common practice; the incorporation of cationic polymers in shampoos in many respects has paved the way for this usage. Since cleansing formulations, in general, contain anionic surfactants, interactions of a cationic polymer with the anionic surfactant can be expected. In addition to anionic surfactants, these formulations may contain nonionic or amphoteric surfactants. It has been noted that cationic polymer–anionic surfactant systems can exhibit rather complex phase behavior involving precipitation zones, gel formation zones, and so on (16), and furthermore, that the precipitation behavior can be modulated by choosing appropriate ratios of polymer to surfactant, and adding cosurfactants, electrolytes, and even other polymers (16–19). An understanding of the polymer-surfactant phase diagram, especially in the presence of other relevant additives, is essential for manipulating the processibility and enhancing the delivery of functional benefits from such formulations.

As mentioned earlier, cationic polymers can enhance the mildness of anionic surfactants toward skin. One factor is related to the ability of the polymer to reduce the activity of the surfactant monomer and, in turn, to lower its binding to the corneum. (See below.) It is not, however, possible to isolate this effect from other mechanisms involving the ability of the polymer to bind to the skin surface itself and influence its properties directly.

The presence of the cationic polymer in a typical cleansing system can be expected to affect the lather characteristics of the system. While the polymer can stabilize and enhance the lather under nonprecipitation conditions by increasing the surface viscosity in the liquid film lamellae, it may reduce/destroy the lather under precipitation conditions by lowering the levels of surfactant available in the solution phase. (See Section III.)

Yet another function of the polymer in a cleansing system, as noted above, is to enhance the deposition of agents such as emollient oils, feel enhancers such as silicone oils, and other skin benefit agents (6–10). One mechanism is by classic polymer bridging, even though the dynamics needed to promote such deposition may be rather involved.

Direct evidence of the adsorption of cationic polymers on skin from an anionic surfactant system has been reported by Goddard and Leung (20). The authors determined the uptake of Polymer JR 125, on stratum corneum (SC) in the presence of three anionic surfactants [SDS, alfa olefin sulfonate (AOS), and alkyl 2EO sulfate] and a coco-betaine surfactant. Even though the conditions involved 30 min of exposure to the substrate, the results obtained are indicative of the trends that can be expected under normal conditions. The results reproduced in Figure 3 show that the uptake of the polymer is initially reduced markedly by the surfactants. Interestingly, at surfactant concentrations above about 10%, the polymer uptake in fact increases and at 20% the extent of uptake is in fact higher than that obtained in the absence of the surfactant. Note that the surfactant concentrations are

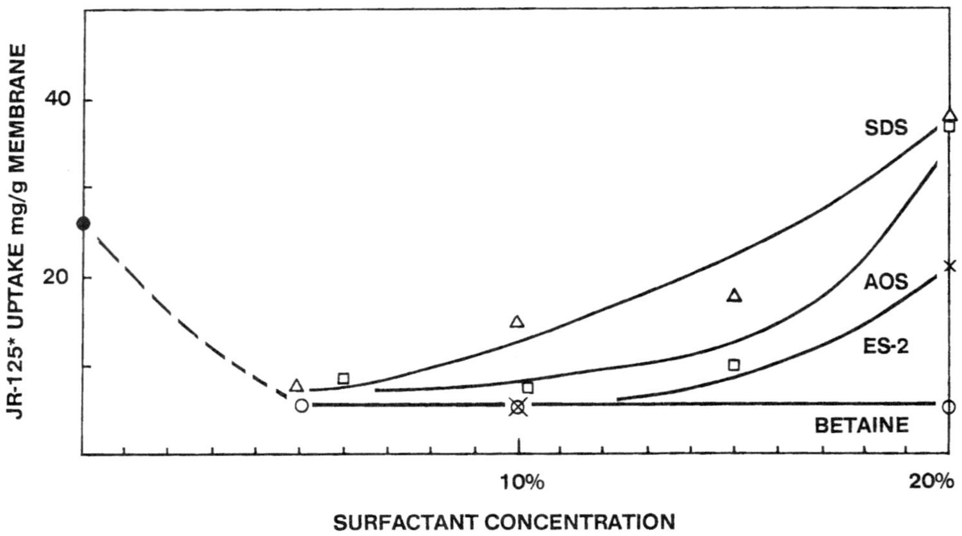

Figure 3 Uptake of Polymer JR 125 from 1% solution onto SC membranes as a function of concentration of added surfactants. Exposure: 0.5 hr at room temperature. (From Ref. 20.)

similar to the levels present in liquid cleansers and shampoos. Essentially, these results show that in spite of the presence of an anionic surfactant, a cationic polymer can bind to skin under conditions of high surfactant concentration. The reduction in the polymer uptake in the presence of the anionic surfactant can be attributed to competition for the polymer between the micelles and the substrate. The observation that alkyl EO sulfates depress the uptake more than that by SDS is also interesting. The reasons for the increase in the polymer uptake at extremely high levels of the anionic surfactant, on the other hand, are not clear. A possible explanation is that at such high surfactant levels, because of the correspondingly high ionic strength of the contacting solution, the interaction of the polymer with the surfactant micelles is likely to be partially inhibited. Also, the high ionic strength may cause some salting out of the polymer. Both of these effects should enhance the binding of the polymer to the substrate. From a practical point of view, the fact that it is possible for a cationic polymer to adsorb from an anionic surfactant solution onto a negatively charged substrate is important for surface conditioning as well as for enhancing the deposition of other materials on the surface.

In contrast to personal care systems, much information exists for the mineral/solid surface as regards details of adsorption and competitive adsorption effects, as will be discussed later.

It is generally agreed that the "barrier," i.e., the stratum corneum layer, of skin serves to protect the sensitive lower regions of the epidermis and the dermis itself from various insults, including exposure to harsh surfactants. Several tests, including that referred to above, have been carried out on SC membranes to assess the mitigation of harsh surfactant effects by the addition of complexing polymers. Here we refer to four such tests.

The first is concerned with the mitigation of moisture vapor transmission (MVT) rate increases brought about by exposure of the membranes to harsh surfactants, like soap. An isolated (yet intact) SC membrane is remarkably efficient as a moisture barrier: values measured in a suitably designed cell (21) of MVT are in the range 0.1–0.2 $mg/cm^2/hr$.

Prolonged exposure to water alone at elevated temperature causes a deterioration of barrier performance (21). If this elevated temperature includes exposure to soap, the deterioration is more serious. However, the latter is reduced if the exposed membrane is then immersed in Polymer JR solution before execution of the MVT test (at room temperature). A possible explanation is the formation of a polymer/surfactant complex in the membrane.

The second method is concerned with the reduction of permeation rate of SDS through SC membranes (22). Measurements were done using a cell based on a design by Loveday [see below (78)] of a SC diffusion membrane and SDS that was radiotagged. The results show that the diffusion rate becomes faster with time, presumably as a result of progressive deterioration of the membrane. Pretreatment of the membrane with 1% Polymer JR 400 was found (Fig. 4) to substantially reduce the diffusion of SDS probably owing to "holdup" of the latter by polymer present in the membrane.

The third test (20) concerns the fact that exposure of SC membranes to water at elevated temperature, especially in the presence of an aggressive anionic surfactant, can lead to substantial swelling of the membrane, by more than 100% in a few minutes at 60°C. By using a standardized technique involving (1) exposure of the membrane, (2)

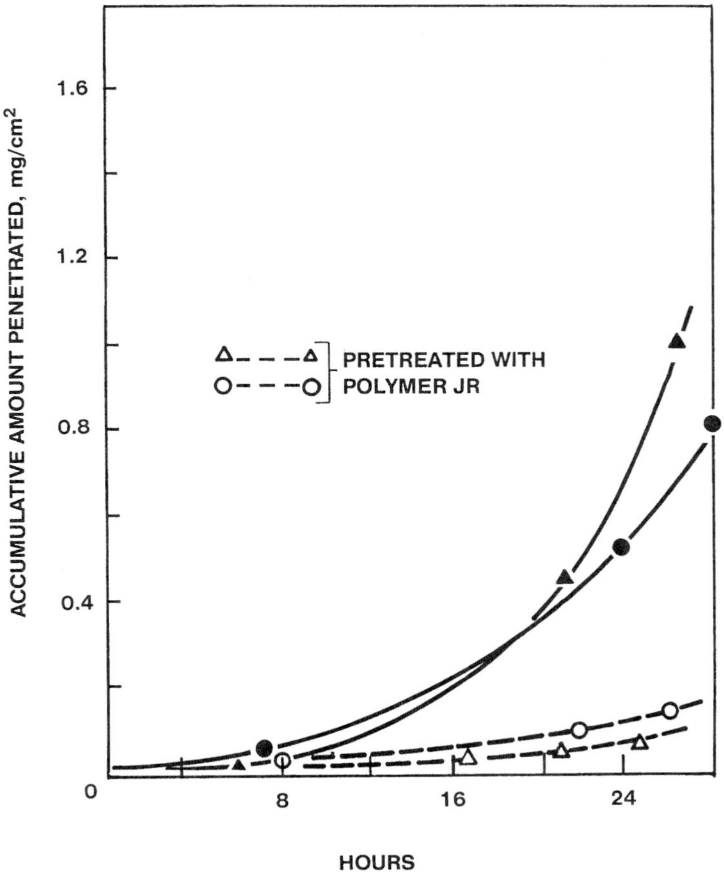

Figure 4 Effect of pretreatment of SC membranes with 1% Polymer JR 400 solution on their subsequent permeability to radiolabeled SDS (10% solution). (From Ref. 22.)

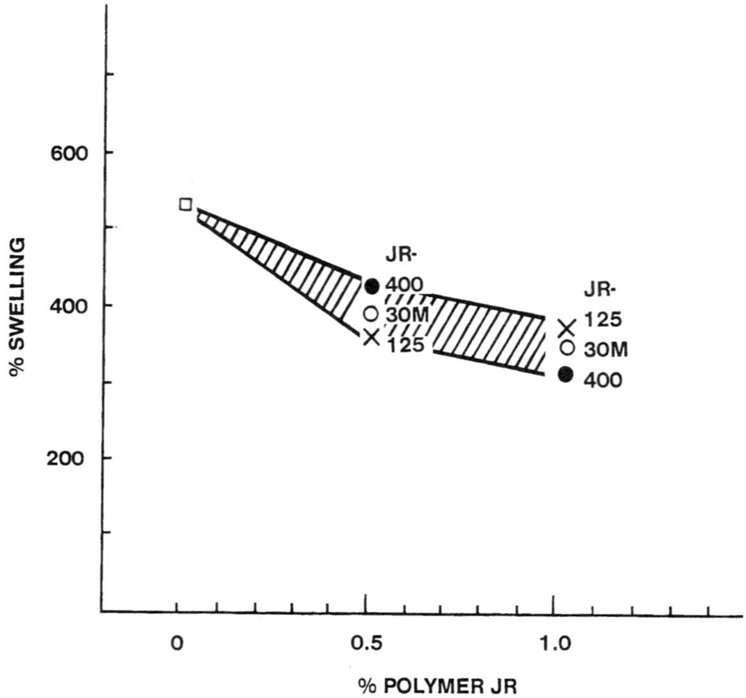

Figure 5 Influence of Polymer JR in reducing the swelling of SC membranes exposed to 20% SDS solutions at 50°C. (From Ref. 20.)

rinsing, (3) padding away excess water, and (4) weighing, it is possible to obtain trends showing the mitigating effects of incorporating protective polymers in the surfactant solution. (See Fig. 5, which presents data for SDS/Polymer JR systems.) Although the trends with polymer molecular weight and concentration are unusual, a reduction in swelling was reported consistently for a wide range of exposure conditions when the polymer was present (20). The fourth test attempts to assess the irreversible damage brought about by elevated temperature/surfactant exposure of the SC membranes, referred to above. In this case, the damage is assessed by the permanent weight loss of the membrane, measured after rigorous drying following exposure and rinsing. The data in Figure 6 show that a SC membrane can lose about 40% of its weight after exposure to 20% SDS solution at 50°C for 4 min; incorporation of Polymer JR 400 at 1% can reduce this weight loss by close to 60% (20).

The above data summarize in vitro information concerning protective effects associated with polymer/surfactant combinations. Reference is made finally to similar results from in vivo (''patch'') tests on skin using 5% SDS solutions (21). While Polymer JR 400 in concentrations of 0.1, 0.25, and 0.5% is barely effective, a 1% solution reduced the inflammatory reaction by about 50% and a 2% solution virtually eliminated it (21).

C. Suspensions

Many cosmetic formulations contain functional solids in finely divided form. Examples are sunscreening pigments (e.g., TiO_2), biologically active materials (e.g., ZnPTO), thick-

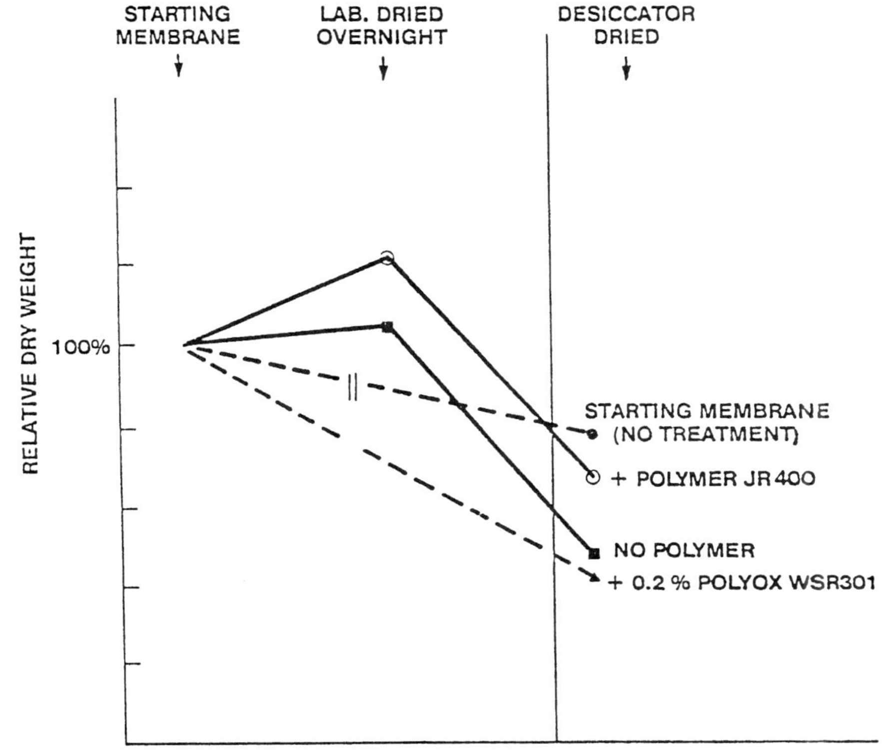

Figure 6 Reduction in weight loss of SC membranes exposed to 20% SDS solution at 50°C with added Polymer JR 400 (1%). (From Ref. 20.)

eners (like clays), pearlescent additives, opacifying materials, and so on. While little is written on the effect of polymer/surfactant combinations upon such systems themselves, one can cite many examples from the growing literature on a variety of solid suspensions of this kind that can be regarded as models. The effects observed (such as stabilization, destabilization, flocculation) can depend not only on the specific composition of the system (the solid itself, the polymer, and the surfactant), but also on the absolute and relative concentrations (23) of the polymer and the surfactant and the sequence of their addition. All these factors are potentially important in formulating any given system.

Following are selected examples of ''conditioning'' of finely divided solids by polymer/surfactant combinations to achieve the desired ''state'' of the suspended solid.

1. Hydrophobic Solids: Wetting

Kilau and Voltz (24) found synergistic wetting of the surface of finely divided carbon (actually coal) using a combination of a high-molecular-weight PEO and an anionic (sulfonate) surfactant. The authors argue that a ''tails down–heads up'' configuration of adsorbed surfactant is required, which allows ready interaction with polymer molecules and, in turn, stabilization of the array of surfactant molecules. In fact, their depiction in Figure 7 is similar to that of a draining foam lamella (Fig. 12) and to that of a polymer-stabilized micelle (Chapter 4, Fig. 11): the driving force for formation of the covered ''hemimicelles'' of Figure 7 and that of the regular polymer-wrapped micelle is evidently much the same.

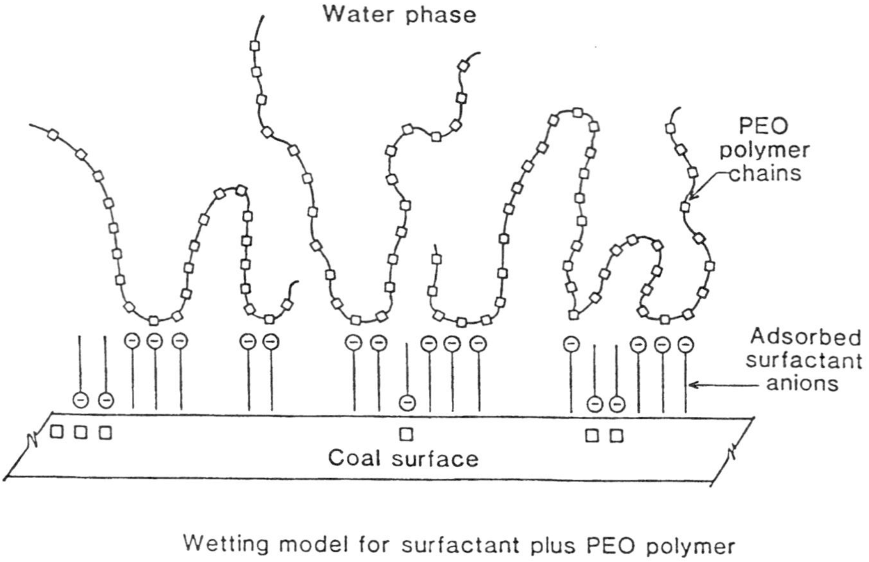

Figure 7 Synergistic wetting of coal by aqueous solutions of anionic surfactant and polyethyleneoxide polymer. (From Ref. 24.)

2. *Hydrophilic Solids: Dewetting*

In seeking to "dewet" particles of quartz/silica Somasundaran and co-workers have found interesting effects with combinations of cationic polymers and surfactants. Although such polymers did not reduce the adsorption of cationic surfactants, they were found to be able to reduce the resulting hydrophobicity of the particles through coadsorption (25). On the other hand, adsorption of anionic surfactants could be induced onto the negatively charged particles by the presence of the polycation and in this way lead to very effective hydrophobization (25,26). (See Fig. 8.) This depiction may well be a reasonable reflection of conditions on a keratin surface exposed to a 2-in-1 shampoo, particularly during some stage of the rinsing process. [Although not concerned with "wettability" evaluations, a study by Shubin (27) has underlined the great importance of relative and absolute concentrations of polymer and surfactant on the adsorption behavior observed. Examining the adsorption of hydrophobically modified cationic HEC (Quatrisoft LM 200, Amerchol) onto silica, he found that, whereas low levels of SDS increase the adsorption of this polymer, at higher concentration levels there is a significant reduction because of competitive binding of polymer by micelles in solution.] A similar reduction observed (28) on another substrate (hair) in the presence of a nonionic surfactant can be similarly explained.

3. *Flocculation*

Traditionally, flocculation of aqueous suspensions has been achieved by addition of electrolyte (in which case the effect would currently be termed "coagulation") or, recently and more often, by addition of a suitable polymer. A "controlled" level of flocculation is sometimes a desired target to develop "structure" within a particular system. Flocculation by a polymer generally allows much more flexibility in this respect than does partial coagulation with an added electrolyte. In flocculation the process usually entails the adsorption of segments of one polymer molecule onto several different particles, so it is

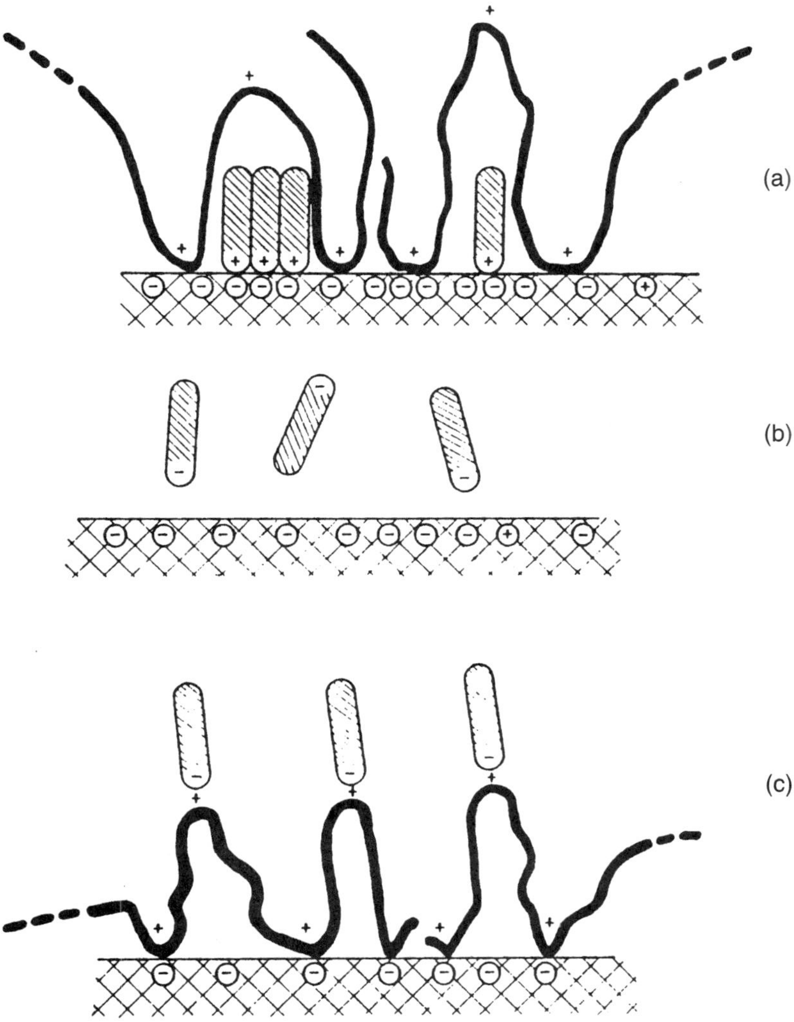

Figure 8 (a) Reduction of hydrophobicity, conferred by an adsorbed cationic surfactant, by a coadsorbing polycation; (b) lack of adsorption of an anionic surfactant on a negatively charged surface (e.g., quartz, silica); (c) a cationic polymer can ''prime'' the adsorption of an anionic surfactant, thus conferring hydrophobicity to the surface. (From Ref. 26.)

easy to envisage the incipient creation of a network structure and to understand why very-high-molecular-weight polymers are usually employed. It is also easy to understand, a priori, that employing the ''right'' combination of a polymer with a surfactant can provide even more flexibility in achieving the desired level of flocculation in a particular system. Here we give one example: Magdassi and Rodel (29) have shown that polymer/surfactant interactions at the solid/liquid interface can be effectively used to flocculate clay (montmorillonite) suspensions. In this case, the clay was treated initially with a cationic polymer and then exposed to SDS solution. Optimal flocculation was obtained when the molar ratio of cationic charge (total) to anionic charge was 1:1. The mechanism of flocculation proposed by the authors involves hydrophobic interactions among SDS molecules bound to the cationic sites of the polymer that is already attached to the clay surface. (See Fig. 9.)

As mentioned previously, a considerably body of literature exists on the interaction (and its consequences) of polymers and surfactants with finely divided particulate suspensions. A representative list of the systems includes: silica/quartz (23,25–27,30–32); calcium carbonate (33,34); clay (29,35); iron oxide (36,37); titanium dioxide (38); alumina (39); graphite (40); PS latex (41). Polymers employed include PEO, PVP, PAAm, starch, several polycations and polyanions, all in mixture with a variety of surfactants. Although the systems studied may not be of immediate relevance to cosmetic formulations, many of the reported effects may well be.

Reference was made above to the conditioning of keratin surfaces by mechanisms involving precipitation of a polymer/surfactant complex. However, precipitation of the polymer/surfactant complex is apparently not a requirement for polymers to enhance the deposition of other active ingredients onto substrates such as hair. For example, Sime (9), using polymer/surfactant combinations in which the systems do not exhibit any precipitation tendency during dilution, has shown that the deposition of zinc pyridinethione (ZnPTO) onto hair can be enhanced markedly by using Jaguar C 13 S (Rhone Poulenc) as the cationic polymer in a lauryl ether sulfate–containing shampoo system. According to Sime, the low charge density of the polymers—in this case less than 0.0017 (charge density = number of charges per monomer unit divided by the molecular weight of the monomer unit)—reduces the precipitation region and therefore does not influence the deposition. Specifically, Sime has shown that the extent of deposition depends on the type of surfactant as well as the relative concentration of the surfactant and the polymer. Thus, for a given polymer concentration, the deposition shows a maximum with increase in the surfactant concentration. Similarly, for a given surfactant concentration, the deposition shows a maximum as a function of the polymer concentration. The reduction in the deposition at high polymer concentration may be similar to the stabilization effect in classical

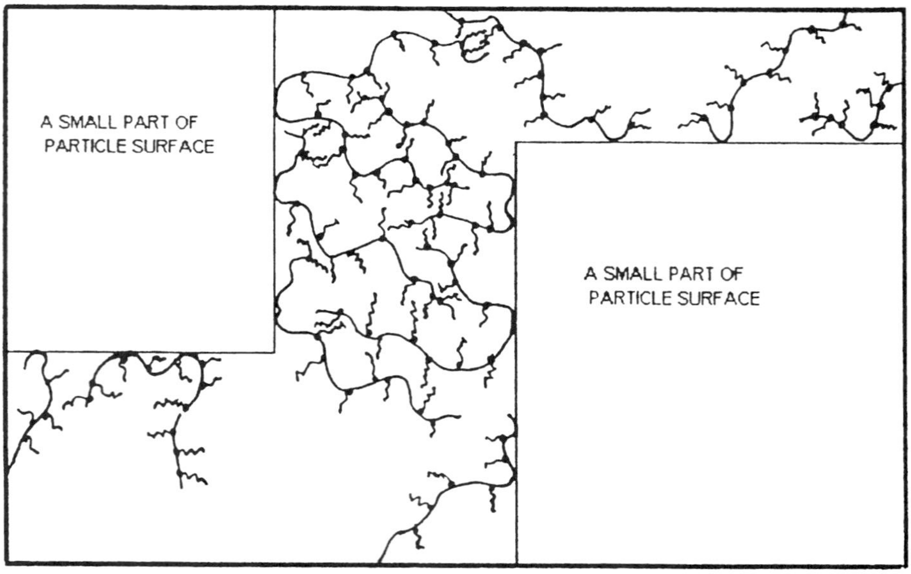

Figure 9 Flocculation based on particle-polymer-surfactant interactions. See text. (From Ref. 29.)

bridging systems at high flocculant levels and this is due to the adsorption of the polymer onto both the surfaces, resulting in repulsion between the surfaces, rather than bridging. The effect of surfactant concentration may be due to the following. At very low surfactant level, there is excess polymer to adsorb on the particles as well as on the surface, resulting in repulsion between the two. With increase in the surfactant level, the polymer is likely to be partitioned among the surface, the particle, and the micelle, leading to a reduction in the binding to the particle and the surface, and consequently, to a decrease in the repulsion between the particle and the surface. At very high surfactant levels, however, the polymer is predominantly adsorbed on the micelle surface and is not available for bridging.

D. Controlled Release

Concepts of controlled, or "slow," release are now well established in the pharmaceutical industry, but they are not yet practiced widely in the personal care field where, in principle, they should be equally applicable. Ingredients such as flavors, colorants, perfumes, biologically active ingredients, and so on are potential candidates for controlled release. While the literature on such systems is extremely limited, it is appropriate to cite one or two references from the pharmaceutical field to illustrate possibilities. In particular, one can cite the work of Alli et al. (42), who employed a combination of rheological and other methods, including DSC, to study the relevant polymer/surfactant "release" systems.

The presence of SDS and other anionic surfactants in the medium was found, in most cases, to prolong the time of release of drug from a tablet containing HPC. The mechanism of prolongation is attributed to increased viscosity of a gel layer that forms on the surface of the tablet when it contacts an aqueous medium. The drugs tested were chloropheniramine maleate and sodium salicylate; the anionic surfactants, in addition to SDS, were sodium hexadecane sulfonate and sodium stearate, and the experiments were carried out at several pH values of the bathing aqueous solution. Gelling systems appear to offer considerable opportunities as regards controlled release of active ingredients. In particular, systems based on polymer/surfactant systems offer much promise. Such ideas have, for example, been advanced by Carlsson and co-workers (43) based on studies of EHEC/ionic surfactant combinations that form gels in the temperature range 20°–60°C, i.e., including the "physiological" range.

To date, the classical gelling polymers have been the main types employed to provide the delayed diffusion characteristics associated with these media. Newer hydrophobe-modified polymers (see below) would also seem to have promise in this respect. These are discussed later.

One method ripe for (further?) exploration is the controlled formation of polymer-treated dispersed systems, such as emulsions or multilamellar vesicles containing the desired "active" ingredient, in which the dispersed particles are stabilized by a surfactant. The formation of a "microgel" stabilizing layer around the dispersed particles by treatment with a suitable polymer has the potential of reducing/controlling the release rate of the active ingredient. Of course, great care would be needed in preparation to avoid the formation of a cross-linked network and potential flocculation. In some respects these structures would bear a (crude) resemblance to biological membranes.

III. FOAMS

Although scientific interest in foams is quite old, it can be said that the "modern" era of research on foams was ushered in about a half-century ago by the advent of highly purified, single-component surfactants, specifically SDS. Both foam stability and single lamella drainage studies of SDS solutions showed unusual sensitivity to a "third component," subsequently identified as parent dodecanol: as little as 1% dodecanol in the SDS specimen sufficed to completely change (improve) the stability of foam and to alter the drainage kinetics of single lamellae, often changing the latter from "fast draining" to "slow draining." Accompanying studies showed that this small amount of dodecanol could, by mixed film formation, dramatically decrease the surface tension and increase the surface viscosity of SDS solutions (44–47). In the case of fatty acid soaps the third component is recognized to be free fatty acid.

History may now be repeating itself in the sense that a "new" type of third component is becoming recognized that can influence the filming and foaming behavior of surfactant solutions. In this case instead of a monomeric species, like dodecanol, of high surface activity, we are speaking of water-soluble polymers, usually of moderate or low intrinsic surface activity. The role of water-soluble polymers in improving the stability of foams has traditionally been viewed as a bulk phase thickening phenomenon to reduce the rate of film drainage unless, of course, the polymer by itself is appreciably surface active (48). In the case of mixed polymer/surfactant systems, while interactions in bulk will have to be considered, it is clear that a full understanding of foaming behavior will also have to take into account the properties of mixed films that may be present at the air/water interfaces. Here, we will be concerned with selected studies of surfactant/polymer pairs in which the polymer either is charged, i.e., a polyion, or carries no charge. A short section is included on polymers that are themselves surface active. In general, it is hoped that the discussion, although restricted to model systems, will help to encourage wider investigation of actual foams.

A. Charged Polymers

Our starting point concerns the polycation Polymer JR 400, whose surface and bulk properties in mixed aqueous solution with various surfactants were first reported about 20 years ago (4,49). A notable point is that this polymer itself is very weakly surface active at the air/water interface. On the other hand, in the presence of an anionic surfactant like SDS, marked synergistic lowering of surface tension was observed. Obviously, strong electrostatic interaction is involved since this polycation showed no interaction with either a nonionic surfactant or a betaine surfactant of net zero charge and no interaction with cationic surfactants can be confidently assumed. Nor did the uncharged parent polymer, hydroxyethylcellulose, show any interaction with SDS. (See Chapter 4, Section II.B.3.) These results are illustrated in Figure 10. The strong synergistic lowering of surface tension observed in the Polymer JR/SDS system led the authors of this work to propose the existence of a surface complex (or a series of surface complexes) comparable to those that form in bulk phase. It was also proposed that beyond the region of precipitation in bulk, i.e., in the resolubilization zone, the growing micellar interface competed with the air/water surface for polymer and eventually denuded it of the latter (see Fig. 11).

Both bulk phase viscosity (50) and, especially, surface phase viscosity effects would be expected to influence the foaming properties of these mixed systems. Surface "phase mapping" of the Polymer JR 400/SDS system, using a qualitative test of surface viscoelasticity, has recently been reported (51). A considerable portion of the diagram (Chapter 4, Fig. 16) reveals the existence of surface viscoelasticity, suggesting that even the smallest levels of polymer could affect the foam properties of SDS. Only cursory testing of the

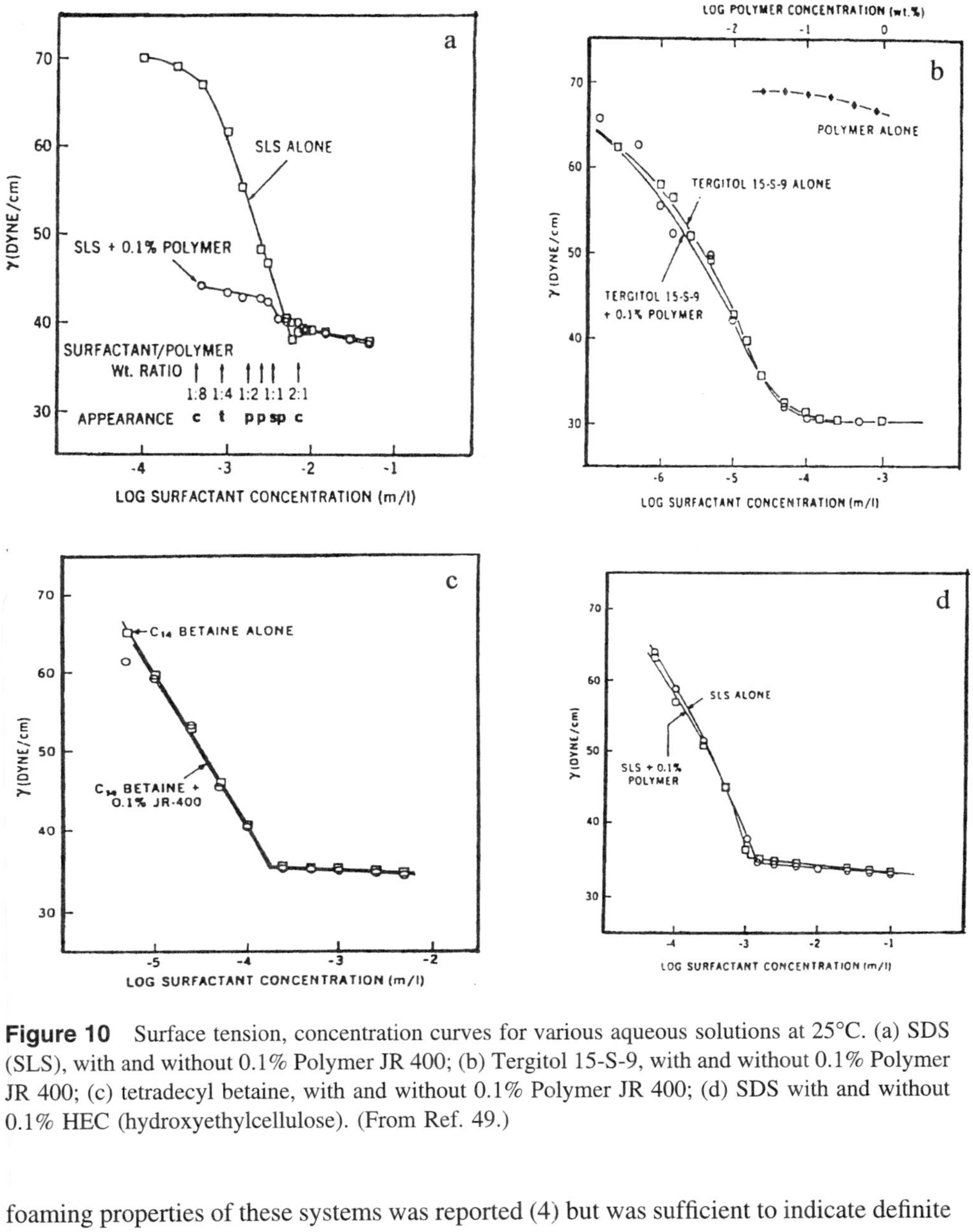

Figure 10 Surface tension, concentration curves for various aqueous solutions at 25°C. (a) SDS (SLS), with and without 0.1% Polymer JR 400; (b) Tergitol 15-S-9, with and without 0.1% Polymer JR 400; (c) tetradecyl betaine, with and without 0.1% Polymer JR 400; (d) SDS with and without 0.1% HEC (hydroxyethylcellulose). (From Ref. 49.)

foaming properties of these systems was reported (4) but was sufficient to indicate definite enhancement effects.

In this connection, work on related model systems, involving film and foam properties of a series of sodium alkysulfates (C_8, C_{10}, and C_{12}) in combination with Polymer 400, has recently been reported by Regismond et al. (52). Substantial foam enhancement effects were found in all cases; in fact, foaming with the lower homologs surpassed that of the C_{12} system. The results indicate adsorption of highly surface active complexes and suggest that the range of enhanced foaming is limited eventually by the intrusion of bulk phase precipitation, which occurs at lower concentrations in the C_{12} system, and/or by stripping of polycation from the surface by bulk phase micelles.

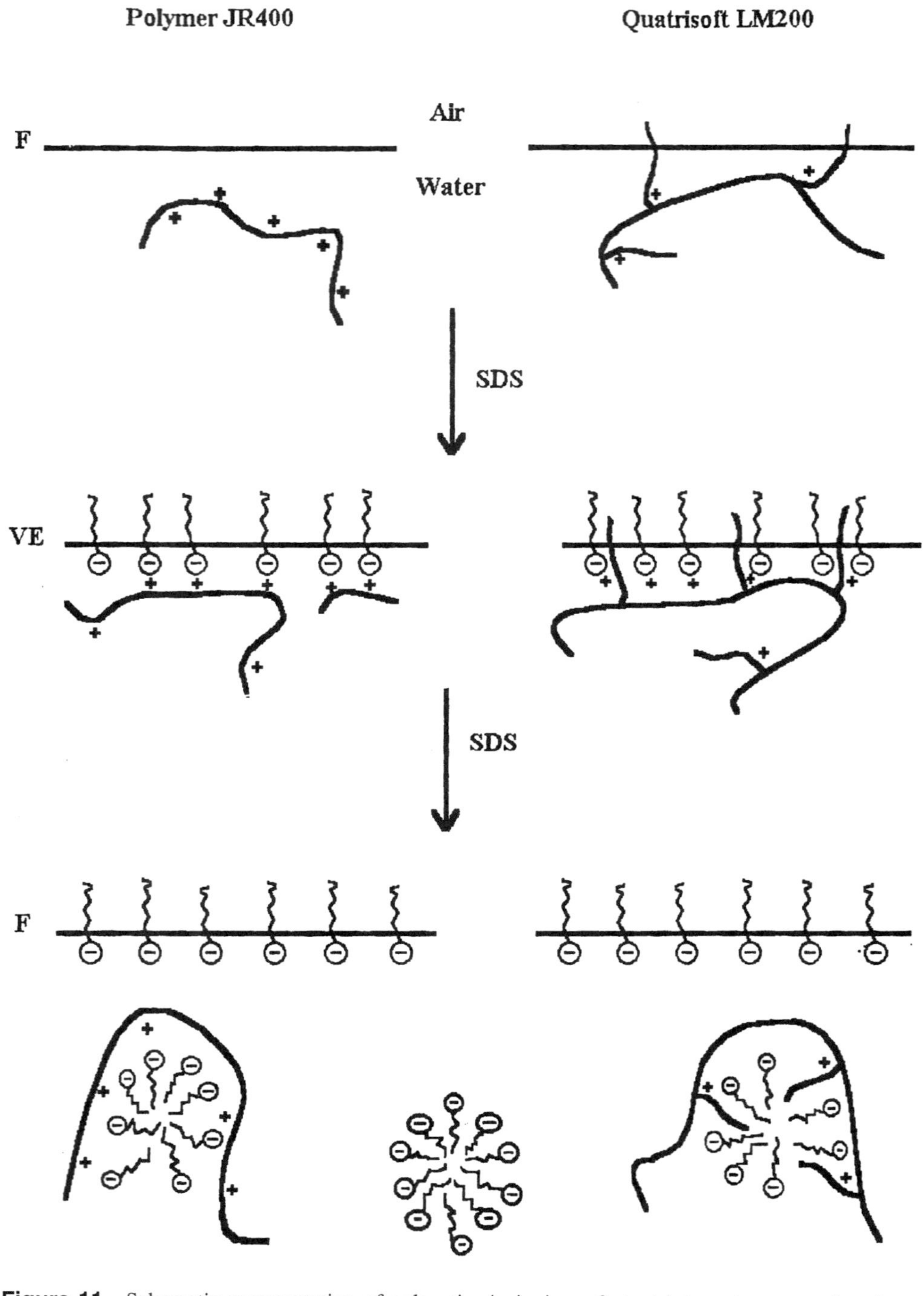

Figure 11 Schematic representation of polycation/anionic surfactant interactions, as a function of surfactant concentration, in bulk phase and at the air/water interface: Polymer JR 400/SDS (left); Quatrisoft LM 200/SDS (right). (From Ref 51.)

Mixed polyion/surfactant films appear to be ripe for further investigation. Parameters such as polyion molecular weight, structure, and charge density are obvious candidates for investigation, as well as variation in the surfactants themselves. It is to be hoped that such studies will include properties of actual foams.

B. Uncharged Polymers

In Chapter 4, Section III, attention was drawn to the Breuer-Robb (53) ''reactivity'' series of uncharged water-soluble polymers: with anionic surfactants the ''reactivity'' followed the sequence PVA $<$ PEO $<$ MeC $<$ PVAc $<$ PPO $\sim$ PVP. Reactivity seemed to increase with increasing hydrophobic nature, and hence surface activity (19), of the polymer. An important implication is that those polymers that are reactive form mixed films at the surface of water when mixed with surfactants. Note that even though Jones (54), the pioneer of the surface tension method to assess interaction between polymer and surfactant in aqueous solution, utilized such measurements as an indicator of interaction in solution, he does not seem to have drawn any inferences of mixed film formation at the air/water interface—or its implications—at least in his early work.

The case of adsorption in a mixed surfactant, uncharged polymer system has been analyzed thermodynamically by deGennes (55). If the polymer adsorbs, one can expect a change in adsorption of the surfactant. This effect has been demonstrated experimentally for the system SDS/PVP by use of specular neutron reflection (56) and by a radiotracer method (57). DeGennes draws attention to the consequences of coadsorption of surfactant and polymer on colloid stability, in general, and on the drainage of ''soap'' films, in particular: drainage rate should be decreased (1) when the layers of adsorbed polymer overlap and (2) by increased viscosity of the surface. The consequences anticipated in both cases would be more stable films and more stable foams generated from these mixed systems. A depiction of possible molecular configurations is presented in Figure 12.

To date, testing of these ideas has been rather limited. For example, Cohen-Addad et al. (58,59) carried out film drainage tests on a series of polymer/surfactant systems and found rather small specific effects of the added polymer, even in the case of the ''strongly interacting'' pair PEO/SDS. Black films were ultimately formed in all cases. All concentrations of SDS were well above the cmc. Other work, using X-ray reflectivity, led this group to conclude that a layer of PEO is adsorbed under the SDS polar heads in the black films (60), at least when the PEO was of high molecular weight.

As with the polyelectrolyte category discussed above, we can expect much more work on film formation on these mixed systems, which, hopefully, will include work on actual foams.

C. "Hydrophobic" Polymers

This is the final category considered: when the polymer is itself markedly surface active, the situation becomes very different; in many cases the polymer alone will be able to sustain a foam generated from its aqueous solution. An example (61) of this is the hydrophobically substituted cationic cellulose polymer Quatrisoft LM 200. Many other examples can be found in the literature, including proteins themselves and their derivatives. On addition of a surfactant, mixed adsorbed films will form and the film and foaming characteristics will depend very much on the specifics of the components themselves, the nature of their interaction, and their relative concentration. (See Fig. 11.)

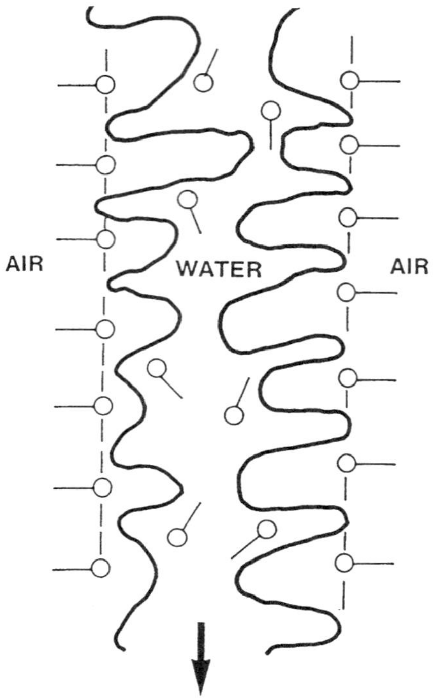

Figure 12 Schematic representation of a draining lamella in a foam prepared from a mixed solution of a polymer and a surfactant.

IV. EMULSIONS

Much of what has been written above for foams is, in principle, applicable to emulsions, in the latter systems the nonpolar disperse phase being a second liquid (oil) rather than a gas (air). However, published work on the stabilization/destabilization of emulsions using combinations of polymer and surfactant has been limited. Therefore, it is appropriate again to consider hypothetical simplistic models to depict possible interfacial structures. Normally, as in foaming, one would anticipate that the faster-diffusing surfactant, by lowering the interfacial tension, would facilitate dispersion of the oil droplets in water (or vice versa) and the polymer reinforce the interfacial structure (Fig. 13).

As in the case of foams, it is expected that the absolute and relative concentration of the polymer and the surfactant could play a critical role in determining the ease of formation and the stability of the emulsion. Simple measurements of interfacial tension, as a function of these parameters, would provide guidelines on how to approach the required condition of low (or very low) interfacial energy. Second, by the well-known mechanism of steric stabilization, the polymer would improve the quality of the suspension. Third, any mechanical strength provided to the extended oil/water interface by formation of viscous, viscoelastic, or ''rigid'' films could also contribute substantially to the stability of the emulsion. Here, although quantitative and qualitative determination of such interfacial effects is more difficult than for the air/water interface it seems logical, using the analogy of the latter to foaming, again to link their existence to an important role in the stabilization of emulsions. Indeed, Th. F. Tadros in Chapter 3 has provided a compilation of

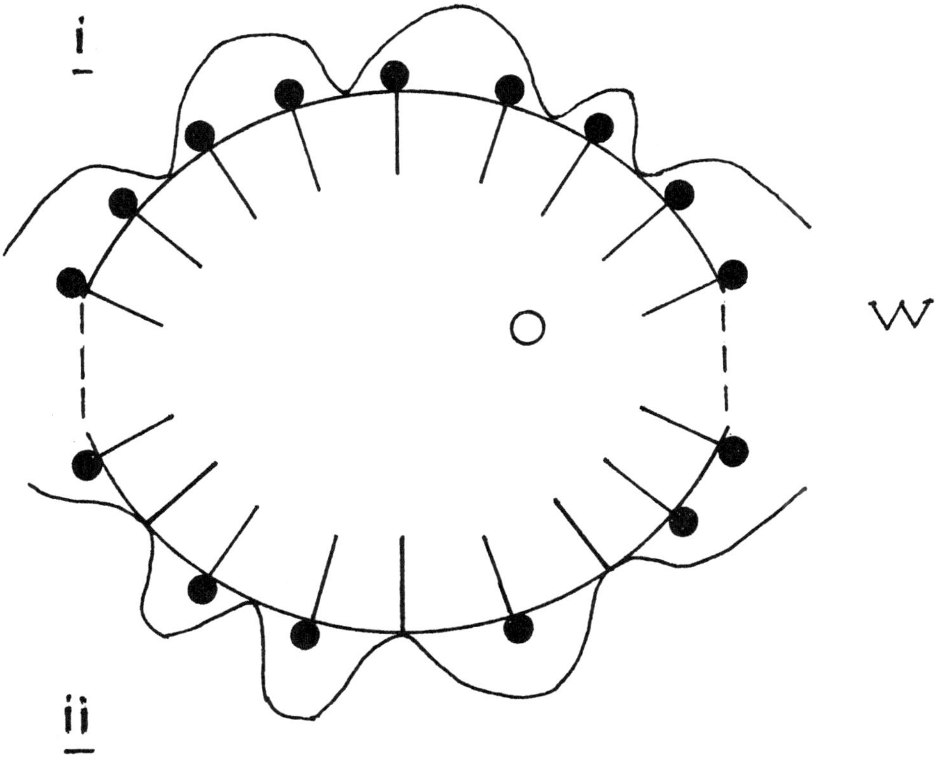

Figure 13 Schematic representation of an oil/water emulsion stabilized by an interacting combination of polymer and surfactant at the interface: (i) conventional polymer, (ii) HM-polymer.

methods of measuring interfacial rheology and has assembled data showing its correlation with emulsion stability.

Polymers that themselves have substantial interfacial activity, such as synthetic hydrophobically modified water-soluble polymers (HM-P) or natural proteins, acting alone (see Chapter 3) or, more especially, in concert with conventional surfactants, constitute a much more complicated, if very interesting, case. (See Chapter 4.) Although instances of such combined use may be found in the literature, this branch of emulsion science must still be regarded as relatively new and often empirical in the case of HM-P. On the other hand, as proteins, in combination with selected surfactants, have been a traditional emulsifier system for edible emulsions, their behavior at the oil/water interface with selected surfactants has been extensively studied. This area is rather specialized and the interested reader is referred to published treatises on the subject (62,63), and also to general technical literature in the field of latex paints.

V. DETERGENCY

In personal care practice, cleaning or ''detergency'' is equated with the removal of certain soiling materials from hair and skin. More specifically, it is usually equated with the removal of materials such as accumulated sebum and dirt particles by the surfactant, and in some respects it can thus be likened to ordinary (cloth) detergency. However, in most cases the processes are more complicated than this and can include removal of proteins, for example from food or blood stains. In the latter event removal can clearly involve the interaction of polymer (protein) and surfactant, and indeed it is still a practice in the detergent industry to include protein in standard test soils. Protein components also accumulate naturally on the skin from ''sloughing off'' of epidermal cells and to a lesser extent on hair from abrasion of the cuticle. It can be anticipated that these insoluble fragments can be conventionally removed as ''dirt'' particles and held in stable suspension by adsorbed surfactant molecules.

Proteins and protein hydrolyzates are still employed as conditioning agents and, as such, can be considered to be part of the ''soil'' makeup. See below. It is well known that such proteins generally react with the surfactant types in personal care cleansing formulations, and under washing conditions (i.e., excess surfactant) will generally form water-soluble protein/surfactant complexes.

Despite the apparent paradox, it is probably true to say of today's consumer that use of a conditioning shampoo or bodywash carries the expectation that the ''old'' conditioning layer (of polymer, oil, etc.) will be removed with the undesired soil and a ''new'' layer be deposited on the freshly cleaned and thus ''conditioned'' surface. A more rational description might be that repeated use of a conditioning cleanser should not lead to undesirable ''buildup'' of the conditioning agent. This expectation is certainly compatible with the (reasonable) hypothesis that deposition of the conditioner takes place mainly during the rinse cycle. On the basis, if the ''old'' conditioner is a polymer, it is probably removed by a polymer/surfactant interaction mechanism during the cleaning cycle. Thus it is important to establish whether or not, or to what extent, a layer of preadsorbed conditioning polymer can be removed by exposure to a surfactant solution. Work on this aspect has been reported: thus, hair previously exposed (in a model experiment) to a 0.1% solution of ^{13}C-tagged Polymer JR 400 for 30 min, rinsed, and dried was contacted with 0.1 M SDS solution and then removed for radioassay (64). After a ''rinse'' time of 30 min it was found that up to 70% of the previously sorbed polymer could be removed, presumably by a polymer/surfactant interaction mechanism. In similar work, on PEI (MW 60,000), a longer period (24 hr) of exposure led to a much lower level (30%) of removal by a 10% shampoo solution (65). [Removal of a low-molecular-weight PEI specimen (65,66) was found to be more complete.] While this level of ''detergency'' may appear modest, as pointed out in Chapter 10 a considerable fraction of the polymer taken up in the initial exposure cycle is apparently sorbed into the fibers, and as such would be difficult to dislodge.

On the other hand, when evaluation techniques that are essentially surface sensitive were used, a different picture emerged. The strong deposition of negatively charged colloidal particles observed on exposing hair pretreated with various polycations is eliminated if these pretreated hair fibers are ''washed'' in SDS solution prior to the colloidal particle exposure (28). Similar evidence of removal of a preadsorbed layer on hair by SDS is also provided by ESCA measurements (67). (See Chapter 10.) By analogy with their generally facile removal from fabrics during detergency, one can assume that the removal of adsorbed protein from natural keratin substrates by cleansing surfactants will be efficient. Another analogy is the ready displacement of protein monolayers at the oil/water interface by sufficiently high concentrations of surfactant (62).

VI. MILDNESS: REDUCTION OF MONOMER CONCENTRATION

Polymers that reduce the effective c.m.c. of the surfactant, by promoting aggregation at lower concentrations than the formal surfactant c.m.c., in effect reduce the surfactant monomer concentration to lower levels than that in polymer-free solutions. As a consequence, interactions that depend solely on monomer activity, and that are not influenced by the polymer-surfactant complex, can be modulated by the presence of the polymer. As can be expected, the stronger the interaction, the lower the monomer activity. Thus, the monomer activity of a charged surfactant can be more effectively lowered by an oppositely charged polymer than by an uncharged polymer. Introduction of hydrophobic groups on the polymer will lead to a further lowering in activity compared to what can be achieved using the unmodified polymer (68). For example, the results given in Figure 28 of Chapter 4, show that the introduction of hydrophobic groups on a cationic HEC (Quatrisoft LM 200) can lower the critical aggregation concentration (c.a.c) to considerably lower values than seen with the unsubstituted Polymer JR.

The practical implications of the modulation of monomer activity by polymers can be significant. For example, even though the mechanisms of skin irritation by surfactants are not fully understood, the irritation potential of surfactants has been related to their monomer activity in solution by several investigators (69). Reduction in monomer activity by adding polymers may result in reduced surfactant binding and possibly in reduced irritation. In support of this argument, evidence in the literature clearly shows that the addition of polymer reduces the irritation caused by a surfactant (70,71). Incorporation of hydrated cationic polymers in toilet bars (13,14) and cationic proteins in surfactant solutions (72) has also been reported to enhance the mildness of surfactant toward skin. Note, however, that other mechanisms could also be contributing to the observed reduction in irritation (21,73,74). The effect of the polymer also can be viewed as the polymer/protein providing an alternate substrate for surfactant binding and thus competing with the substrate for the surfactant molecules. Normally, for the polymer to have a positive effect, the c.a.c. in its presence should be lower than the critical concentration required for the binding of the surfactant to the protein substrate.

From a practical point of view, obtaining information on monomer activity may not be simple. One approach is to use predictive models such as the one developed by Nikas and Blankschtein (75) using a phenomenological-cum-thermodynamic model for calculating the activity of surfactant (SDS) monomers in the presence of different levels of a polymer like PEG (PEO). Typical results, given in Figure 14, show the relative levels of polymer needed to maintain a certain level of monomer activity at different levels of SDS. Thus, in principle, it is possible to estimate the amount of polymer needed to maintain a particular monomer concentration. Interestingly, the activity versus concentration plots reported by these authors (75) are, in fact, mirror images of the surface tension versus log concentration plots, suggesting that from a practical point of view the surface tension plots may be a simple way to predict the activity profiles (75,76). This approach may not, however, provide information in cases in which the polymer-surfactant complex itself is significantly surface active, as in the case of oppositely charged polymer/surfactant systems (16). In such cases, surfactant binding data would allow the construction of such diagrams.

As mentioned earlier, the penetration of an aggressive surfactant like SDS through (and below) the SC can be equated with severe irritation. Accordingly, methods to measure (and reduce) such transport are of great potential interest. Faucher et al. (22,77) have reported such a study using the Loveday (78) diffusion cell with a neonatal rat SC membrane, and radiotagged SDS as the diffusant, in the presence of a series of c.m.c. reducing (54) ''PEGs.'' Results in Figure 15 show that the addition of 1% polyethyleneglycol (PEG 6000–400,000) to the SDS solutions results in a substantial reduction in the rate of diffusion of the SDS. While a reduction in monomer concentration occasioned by the presence

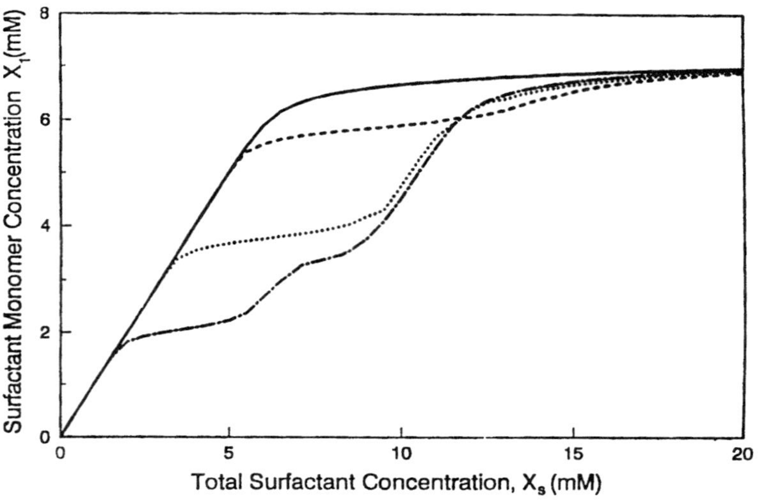

Figure 14 Predicted surfactant concentration X_1 versus total surfactant concentration X_s at 25°C, for a model anionic surfactant, such as SDS, and a model polymer, such as PEO. Solid line corresponds to surfactant solution in the absence of polymer. (From Ref. 75.)

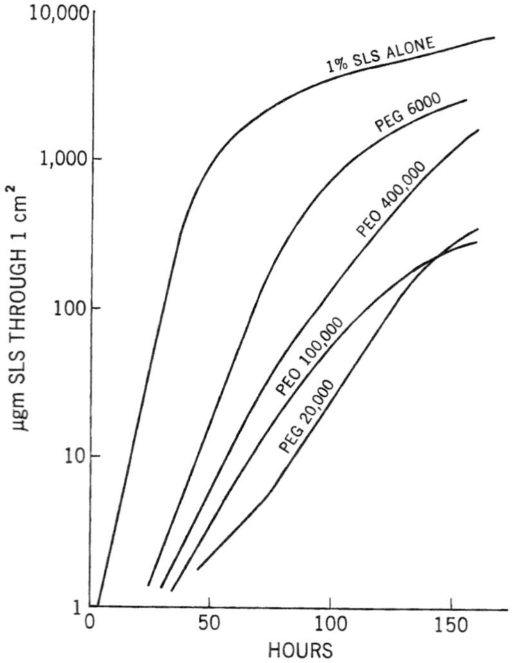

Figure 15 Permeation curves for 1% SLS (SDS) solutions containing 1% of various PEG (PEO) polymers: SC membranes. (From Ref. 77.)

of the PEG is clearly a feasible mechanism, the maximal effect realized with PEG 20,000 is less easy to explain. The falling off of the effect at higher molecular weight may have to do with slower dynamics of complex formation and at lower molecular weight with less effective complexation (79). [Pretreatment of the membranes with Polymer JR 400 had previously been shown to markedly reduce the diffusion rate of SDS (22).]

VII. RHEOLOGY: VISCOSITY ENHANCEMENT AND GELATION

A. Unmodified Polymers

The general effects observed in mixed polymer/surfactant systems have already been described in Chapter 4. Here only brief summaries and some "special" effects will be presented.

It is well established that the interaction of a nonionic polymer such as polyethyleneoxide (PEO) or polyvinylpyrrolidone (PVP) with an anionic surfactant such as SDS can impart polyelectrolyte-like properties to the nonionic polymer (54,80–82). This effect manifests as a significant increase in viscosity at a certain concentration (T_1 or "c.a.c.") of the surfactant, which is independent of molecular weight, and this increase can be as high as fivefold. In addition to an increase in viscosity, these systems can exhibit considerable viscoelastic (82) effects, especially if the molecular weight of the polymer itself is already high.

Viscosity increases resulting from the addition of cationic surfactants to a nonionic polymer are less common because of their relatively weaker interaction. On the other hand, if the hydrophobicity of the polymer is relatively high, the interaction can be enhanced and significantly modify the rheological properties. For example, polymers such as ethylhydroxyethylcellulose (EHEC) exhibiting a lower consolute temperature will phase-separate at higher temperatures indicating their higher hydrophobicity at such temperatures. A substantial increase in viscosity and gel formation reported by Carlsson et al. (43) for the EHEC-CTAB system in a certain temperature-surfactant concentration window may be a manifestation of the increased hydrophobicity of the polymer leading to increased interaction with the cationic surfactant (see Section VIII.B). The gelation itself probably involves network formation and entanglement brought about by the surfactant micelles.

In Chapter 4 it was reported that even larger increases in viscosity can be observed in oppositely charged polyelectrolye-surfactant systems (83–85). In one case, involving the cationic cellulosic Polymer JR 400, at 1% concentration, relatively low levels of SDS led to substantial viscosity increases (as large as 200-fold) or even weak gel formation in the immediate preprecipitation zone. (See Fig. 16.) It should again be emphasized that these manifestations are dependent on both the concentration of the polyelectroylyte and its structure; thus, no such viscosity increase (indeed a decrease) was observed under similar conditions when the concentration of Polymer JR 400 was reduced to 0.1%; nor was a viscosity increase evident with 1% Reten, a polycation based on vinyl chemistry (83). Combination of SDS with the highest available molecular weight grade of the Polymer JR series (30 M) resulted in *strong gels* at polymer levels as low as 1% and surfactant levels around 0.1% (84,85). (See Fig. 17.) In this figure the storage modulus, G', is the measure of the elasticity. The viscosity of the system at the lowest shear rate (0.001 Hz) is 10 kPas, equivalent to 10 million centipoise in the old unit system! Several other anionic surfactants, such as benzene sulfonates, alkyl ether sulfates, and sulfosuccinates, were also found to form such gels. Gel formation in these systems is likely to be due to the increased

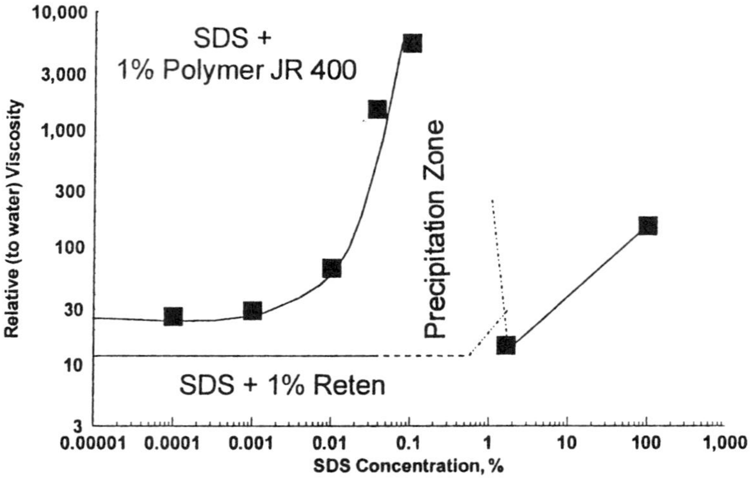

Figure 16 Relative viscosity of 1% Polymer JR 400 and of 1% Reten 220 solutions as a function of added SDS concentration. (From Ref. 83.)

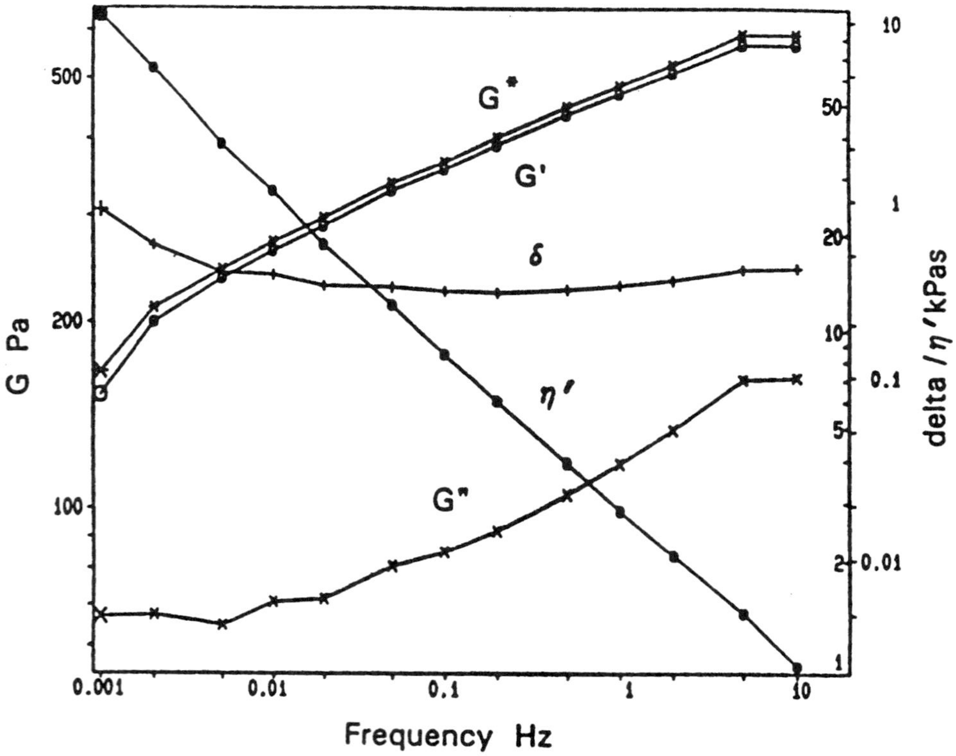

Figure 17 Viscoelastic parameters versus oscillation frequency for 1% Polymer JR 30 M/0.15% SDS mixture. The parameters are elastic modulus, G'; loss modulus, G''; complex modulus, G^*; phase angle, δ; and dynamic viscosity, η'. (From Ref. 84.)

chain entanglement resulting from the cross-linking of bound surfactant clusters and the naturally high entanglement of the higher-molecular-weight polymer.

Viscosity increases and gel formation in polyanion-cationic surfactant systems have also been reported, for example by Thalberg and Lindman (86) for hyaluronan and polyacrylate polymers in combination with alkyltrimethylammononium bromide surfactants. Similarly, viscosity increases and gel formation with polymers such as carboxymethyl cellulose (CMC) and CTAB at relatively low polymer-surfactant levels have been observed (87).

With the current increase in interest in the gel state, a growing need exists to be able to control the extent of gelling and strength of gels. Indeed, increases in viscosity and gel formation may not be desirable in all cases and may have to be modulated to obtain an optimum balance between stability and flow. There are, in fact, several approaches to thinning polymer-surfactant systems. The most obvious approach is to alter the polymer-surfactant ratio to move away from the optimum gelling ratio (85). Addition of competing polymers, surfactants, or salts can also lead to viscosity reduction. Brackman and Engberts (88) have reported an interesting case of viscosity reduction on adding a water-soluble polymer, polypropyleneoxide (PPO) or polyvinylmethylether, to the solution of a cationic surfactant (CTAB) in which the surfactant micelles are rod-like due to the presence of strongly bound salicylate anion. Competition between the polymer and the salicylate is evidently responsible for the pronounced structural reorganization of the system, which is degelled in the thinning process (88). Polymer-surfactant interaction can be expected to influence the swelling-deswelling characteristics of polymer gels. It is well known, for example, that polyelectrolyte gels that are used as superabsorbents for water under physiological conditions (e.g., saline, urine, blood) can lose their absorbing capacity because of electrolyte effects. In a recent study Zhang et al. (89,90) have shown that insensitivity effects can be achieved by using a nonionic polymer gel of poly(*N*-isopropylacrylamide) (PNIPAM) in combination with a surfactant such as SDS. Results from Ref. 89 show that the swelling characteristics in the presence of high levels of salt do not change for the PNIPAM-SDS gel, unlike the case of the SDS-free gel. On the basis of SANS results, the authors suggest that the initial swelling power is due to the ''polyelectrolyte'' character of the SDS micelle-bound gel and the lack of swelling sensitivity to salt is associated with the formation of cylindrical micelles around the polymer at higher salt levels. It appears that the reduced electrostatic effects are to some extent compensated by the increased hydrophobic interactions at higher salt levels and the consequent increase in size of the polymer-bound micelles. The result is increased tolerance to electrolytes. Such effects again offer opportunities to the formulation chemist.

Interaction of nonionic surfactants with most polymers is relatively weak and therefore significant increases in viscosity resulting from polymer-surfactant interactions do not occur unless the polymer has been suitably hydrophically modified (see below). However, interaction of the EO groups of nonionic surfactants with polyacrylic acid–based polymers and copolymers is known and this can lead to substantial alterations in viscosity (91,92). This behavior is associated with the specific interaction of polyethers and polycarboxylic acids (92).

B. ''Hydrophobic'' Polymers

As has already been pointed out and discussed (Chapter 4), hydrophobic modification of the polymer can dramatically increase the level of interaction and can lead to a substantial influence on the rheology of the system, even for mixtures of polymer and nonionic surfactants. As an example, Sarrazin-Cartalas et al. (93) report a marked increase in viscosity of hydrophobe-modified polyacrylate polymers in the presence of model nonionic surfactants (see Fig. 18). An important consequence, since the size and shape of nonionic micelles can be appreciably influenced by temperature, is that these types of nonionic system can be used to bring about thermally induced viscosity enhancement and gelation. These authors have attributed the observed increase in the gelation at higher temperatures, in the case of a hydrophobe-modified polyacrylate-$C_{12}E_4$ system, to network formation mediated by giant surfactant vesicles and the hydrophobic groups of the polymer.

As surfactants will ''compete'' for hydrophobic sites in an aqueous solution (or interface), it can be expected that many properties of hydrophobically modified polymers will change, depending on the exact conditions of the solution. These can include increases, or decreases, in viscosity and such properties as foaming, emulsification, and wetting. For example, Danino et al. (94) report a rather complete study, using several techniques, of the polyamphiphile poly(disodium maleate-coalkylvinylether) and its mixtures with anionic or nonionic surfactants that have a disruptive effect on the association of this polymer.

In general, the scope and opportunities offered for rheology control in such systems are considerable if one bears in mind all the available surfactants and the number of possible structural variations of the polymers. Indeed, today there are many examples of the use of hydrophobe-modified polymers in commercial products, e.g., emollients, cleansers, and other types of products, especially latex paints. Possible association structures in these polymer systems (alone and with surfactant micelles) are depicted in Figure 19. One can predict that this area will continue to be profitable for basic research, and also further commercial development.

Finally, by way of illustration, we mention a polymer type currently receiving much attention. The polymer is referred to as hydrophobically modified ethoxylated urethane (HEUR), the reaction product of a PEG and a diisocyanate, end-capped with a long chain alcohol or amine. HEURs are already recognized as having much potential as ''associative thickeners'' in coating formulations. Their structure suggests they will show pronounced interaction with surfactants in solution and this is indeed the case. Here we refer to two recent studies. The first by Hulden (95) included surface tension studies of the polymer

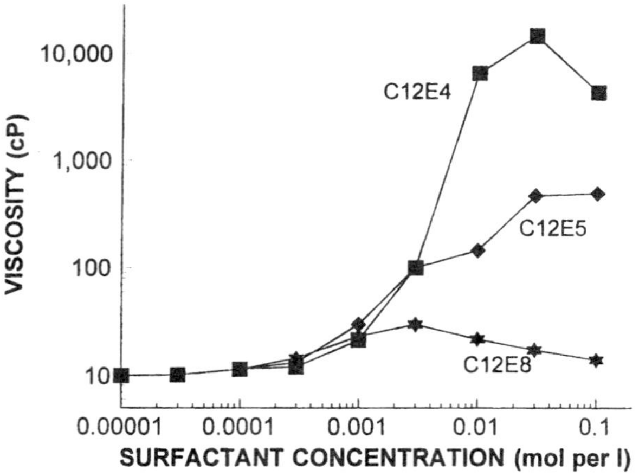

Figure 18 Variation in viscosity of a hydrophobically (3% C_{12}) modified polyacrylate polymer with concentration of added nonionic surfactant: polymer concentration 1%, 25°C. (From Ref. 93.)

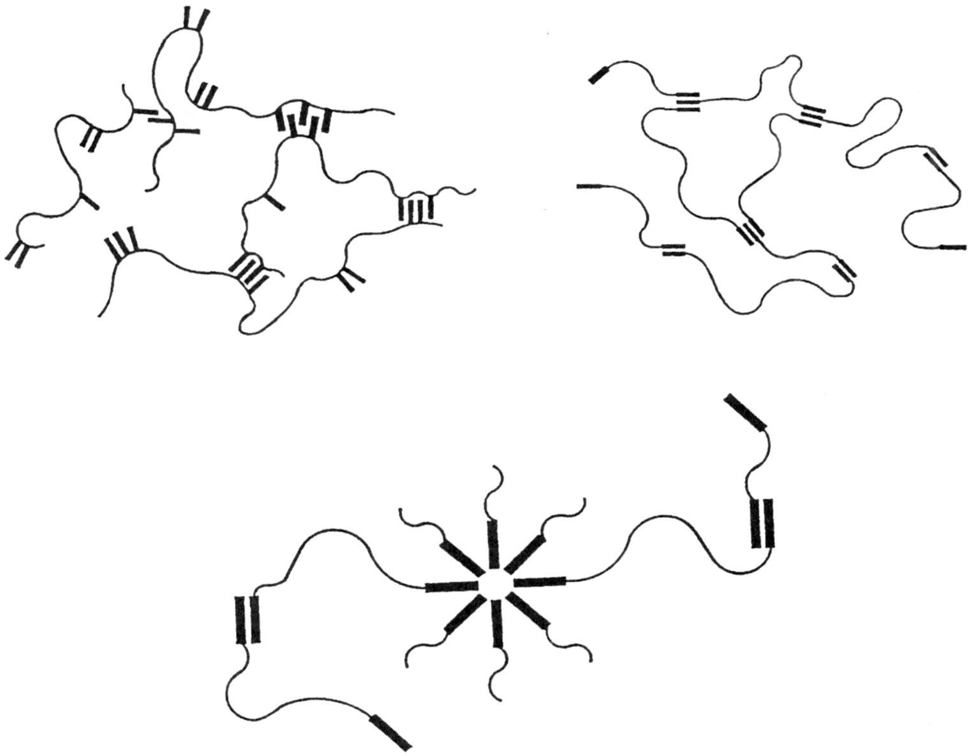

Figure 19 Association structures of hydrophobically substituted polymers: (clockwise from left) "comb," end-substituted, end-substituted associating via a surfactant micellar bridge. (Courtesy D. R. Bassett.)

with both anionic (SDS) and nonionic (NPE10) added surfactants. Clear indications of critical association concentrations (T_1 and T_2) in the former case, and T_2 in the latter case, were found. Furthermore, characteristic viscosity increases (actually maxima) when surfactants were added to solutions of HEUR polymer (i.e., boosting of thickening) were generally observed—a clear indication of association in solution. The second study, by Annable et al. (96), essentially confirms the interaction patterns and presents an in-depth mechanical analysis of the flow properties of these systems. One additional finding was that, at higher polymer concentrations, additions of surfactant no longer led to rheological maxima.

VIII. SOLUBILIZATION

A. General

A well-known feature of surfactant solutions is their ability to dissolve a variety of oil-soluble materials, e.g., hydrocarbons, esters, perfumes, dyes, and so on. This property is utilized in the compounding of many formulations, the process involving the dissolution of the solubilizate in the surfactant micelles. Formation of polymer/surfactant complexes is currently regarded as a depression of the critical aggregation concentration of the surfactant. According to this picture, superior solubilization in such systems can be anticipated over that provided by the surfactant alone. There is, in fact, abundant evidence of this enhancement, e.g., in the solubilization of dyes (97–99), hydrocarbons (100), and sparingly soluble fluorescers (101), as has been observed with combinations of uncharged polymers and charged surfactants. In combinations of polyelectroylyte and oppositely charged surfactants the effect can be much larger, as shown in a model study for the oil-soluble dye Orange OT in the cationic cellulosic Polymer JR/SDS system (102). An important discovery of this work was that solubilization can occur at extremely low concentrations, indicating a c.a.c over two orders of magnitude lower than the c.m.c. of SDS (83,102). While the degree of solubilization fell as the concentration of SDS approached the precipitation zone, it was reestablished at higher concentration and the principal solubilization zone was wider (shifted to lower concentration) than was observed for the micellar region of SDS by itself. (See Chapter 4, Fig. 19.) A practical way to reduce or avoid the above-mentioned ''precipitation'' zone of ionic surfactant/oppositely charged polyion pairs is to incorporate a suitable nonionic surfactant into the system (17,18).

Because of their proclivity to associate in solution, it is to be expected that surfactants and polymers can influence *each other's* solubility. There is abundant evidence of the ability of a surfactant to increase the range of solubility of polymers in water (see the next section). Less well known is the ability of a water-soluble polymer to increase the solubility range of a surfactant: Schwuger and Lange (103), for example, reported that polyvinylpyrrolidone can reduce the Krafft point of sodium hexadecyl sulfate by close to 10°C—an effect evidently linked to a lowering of the monomer concentration required for aggregation in the presence of this polymer.

In some cases, polymers that are normally considered to be insoluble can be solubilized in surfactant solutions, as was demonstrated by Isemura and Imanishi (104) for the polymer polyvinylacetate and the surfactant SDS. This confirmed work carried out earlier by Sata and Saito (105). Similar, but less strong solubilization of certain insoluble polymers by cationic surfactants has also been demonstrated by Saito and Mizuta (106). These types of solubilization make it possible to regenerate the original polymer in a different state, e.g., as a fiber or a film. Work related to this approach was reported by Lundgren (107), in which concentrated equiweight mixtures of protein and anionic surfactant in water were extruded as continuous fiber into a magnesium sulfate coagulating bath prior to final drawing, washing, and drying. Although not directly related to the cosmetics field, this result does draw attention to the wide range and potential offered by mixed polymer/surfactant systems.

B. Cloud Point Elevation

It is well known that many soluble polymers have an inverse solubility/temperature relationship, and their solutions exhibit a ''cloud point'' or lower consolute temperature. Examples are polymers based on polyalkylene oxides and those with multiple amide groups, or multiple ether/hydroxyl groups—as in several water-soluble, cellulose-based materials. While the phenomenon, in general terms, is explained as being due to ''dehydration'' of polar groups such as ether, amide, hydroxyl, and so forth, it is well known that it can often be offset by the addition of ionic surfactants, which can result in increases in cloud point of several degrees. This phenomenon seems to be a clear case of polymer/surfactant interaction with the formation of complexes of increased intrinsic solubility. Practically speaking, prevention of clouding in formulations can be important for maintaining viscosity and the stability of matter in suspension.

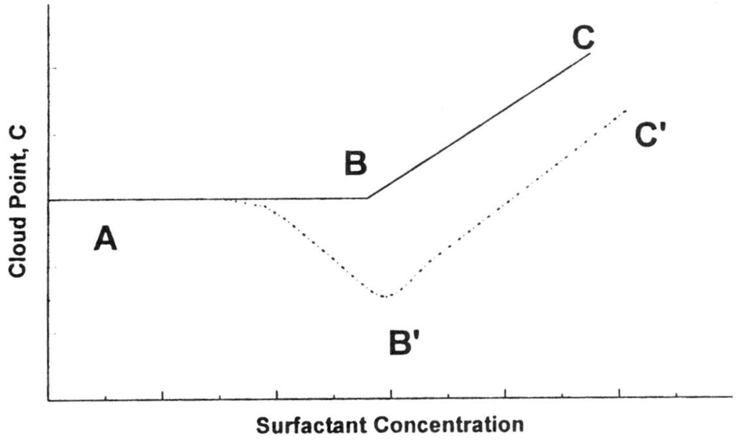

Figure 20 Schematic representation of the effect of ionic surfactants on the cloud point of a nonionic polymer.

A simple representation of the phenomenon is given in Figure 20. In the "ideal" case the cloud point of the polymer is unaffected (AB) by the addition of surfactant until a critical concentration (the c.a.c.?) is reached; thereafter there is a linear increase (BC) of cloud point with increase of surfactant concentration. Whereas many polymer/surfactant systems follow this pattern, it is now known that the response is often more complicated following, for example, the pattern AB′C′, in which a depression of the cloud point precedes the increase observed at higher surfactant concentrations. This behavior is encountered in certain cellulose based polymers (108,109). In particular, the behavior of the polymer ethylhydroxyethylcellulose has been extensively studied by Karlstrom et al. (110–112) and modeled on the basis of Flory-Huggins concepts. At present it can be said that the response of the cloud point of a polymer to added surfactant can be quite complicated and is influenced by (1) the structure of the polymer, (2) its molecular weight and molecular weight distribution, (3) its tendency to self-aggregate, (4) the presence of salt, (5) the type of salt, and (6) the nature of the added surfactant, including the sign of its charge. More work in this (practically interesting) area would be desirable.

The raising of the cloud point of a nonionic surfactant by an anionic surfactant can be considered to be a special case of polymer/surfactant interaction. Here the "polymer" is a hydrophobically substituted species in which the hydrophilic moiety with repeating units (most often ethylene oxide) is an oligomer rather than a true polymer. This phenomenon has been of much importance, and has long been known, to formulation chemists and involves the close association of the two species in mixed micelles—the "complexes" in this case.

IX. SEPARATION AND PURIFICATION OF POLYMERS

Early work by protein chemists referred to in earlier chapters had revealed that the properties of proteins in solution can be substantially changed by addition of ionic surfactants (see also Ref. 113). In outline: (1) Below their isoelectric point, proteins complex strongly with anionic surfactants, generally forming precipitates that can usually be solubilized on adding excess surfactant or salt. The analogous reactions above the isoelectric point take place with cationic surfactants. (2) Even above (below) their isoelectric point, proteins will interact with anionic (cationic) surfactants, which interaction will alter their net charge and, hence, electrophoretic behavior but usually without precipitate formation.

These phenomena obviously provide means of separating proteins based on the addition of appropriate surfactants, at the appropriate pH, with control of electrolyte concentration, and so on, and will not be elaborated upon here (see, however, Chapter 4, Section II.D and III.E). Subsequent to the above work by protein chemists it was found that similar precipitation reactions occur between cationic surfactants and a variety of anionic polyelectrolytes, those investigated being generally anionic polysaccharides (114–116). Scott (115), for example, found for anionic polysaccharides with weak acidic groups (hyaluronic acid, alginic acid, etc.) that precipitation with CTAB could be inhibited as a result of deionization of their carboxyl groups. With carbohydrate monoester sulfates, such as dextran sulfate, no such inhibition was observed. He also reported that the "flocculation end-point" observed for this polyelectrolyte with CTAB corresponds to the formation of a stoichiometric salt.

The above dependence on pH of the precipitation of acidic polyelectrolytes with cationic surfactant clearly affords means of separating mixtures of such polymers based on their acid strength. In an interesting development, it was shown (115) that the method can be applied to the separation of neutral polysaccharides by working at sufficiently high pH to ionize their hydroxyl groups. A more convenient method, however, to develop polyanionic character and hence precipitability with added cationic surfactants is to form the borate complex of the polysaccharide by simple addition of borate ion (116).

Another fractionation method for polyanions came from the finding (117) that, like protein/oppositely charged surfactant complexes (113), polyanion/cationic surfactant precipitates can be solubilized by addition of inorganic salt. Furthermore, solubility occurs at a critical electrolyte concentration (c.e.c.), which was found to depend both on the surfactant itself and on the particular polyanion (its chemical structure, its anionic groups, and its molecular weight, with higher-molecular-weight analogs having a higher c.e.c. than lower analogs). This means, for example, that polyanions can be fractionated according to molecular weight, or, if prefractionated, can have the molecular weight of their fractions determined form their c.e.c. values and a calibration graph. Laurent and Scott (117) applied this method to fractions of the polymers polylacrylate, chondroitin sulfate, and keratan sulfate.

A simple explanation of the c.e.c. effect is based on electrical shielding by the added salt. In a more general context one can refer to the phase diagrams of Piculell and Lindman (118) showing that the progressive addition of salt to precipitating polyanion/cationic surfactant mixtures changes the characteristics from those displaying associative segregation ("coacervates"), through a zone of no precipitation, and eventually to dissociative separation at sufficiently high salt concentration. (See Chapter 4, Figs. 41 and 42.)

X. MISCELLANEOUS INTERACTIONS

A. Polymer Activation by Deionization: pH "Switches"

There are many illustrations of the interaction of charged surfactants with oppositely charged polyelectrolytes, and there are several examples in this chapter of applications that depend on this combination. An implication is that, if the polyelectrolyte is of limited acid (or base) strength, the pH conditions have to be appropriate to achieve its ionization and develop a charge opposite to that of the surfactant to promote interaction. By the same token, no interaction is anticipated if ionization of the polymers leads to the formation of a polyelectrolyte with charges of the same sign as that of the surfactant (119–121) (unless the polyelectrolyte is hydrophobically modified). An interesting finding has, however, recently been made of a polyelectrolyte's being activated for interaction by its *de*ionization. Thus, using fluorescence techniques, Maltesh and Somasundaran (122) have developed evidence that, when polyacrylic acid is ionized, it does not interact with SDS, but under acidic conditions it does. Two potential applications of this effect are the elevation of the viscosity of solutions of the unionized form of this polymer by addition of SDS (123), and the enhancement of the flotation activity of SDS for hematite fines on addition of polyacrylic acid (124). Opportunities thus exist for ''on-off switching'' of effects such as the above by simple alteration of the pH of the solutions, and the effect may involve not only the generation of the ionized form of the polymer but, indeed, sometimes its deionization. It has been found recently (125) that unionized polyacrylic acid also shows marked interaction with the cationic surfactant TTAB. This means that on the Breuer-Robb (53) reactivity scale it must be regarded as being quite hydrophobic.

B. Dendrimer/Surfactant Complexes

Dendrimers are a relatively novel class of macromolecules synthesized from various initiator cores to which radially branched layers, referred to as ''generations,'' are covalently attached (126). The exterior layer of the dendrimer can be modified to provide terminal funtionalities. Tomalia and co-workers have pioneered the work on the polyamidoamine dendrimers, often referred to as ''starburst dendrimers'' (127). Because of the precise nature of synthesis of these compounds, their composition and constitution, including the molecular weight and number of terminal groups, are well defined. The synthesis of starburst dendrimers leads to either carboxylate groups (half-generation) or amine groups (full generation) as terminal functionalities. The molecular weight of dendrimers varies from 924 (half-generation, diameter about 24 A) to as high as 639,247 for the 9.5 generation (diameter about 140 A). The number of terminal groups for the half-generation is only nine whereas that for the 9.5 generation is 3072. Interestingly, the lowest-molecular-weight dendrimer is smaller than a surfactant micelle, but the higher-generation dendrimers can be significantly larger than a conventional spherical micelle. Using molecular probes and photophysical measurements, Turro et al. (128,129) have shown that the interior of the starburst dendrimer is hydrophilic. They have also shown that dendrimers and surfactant micelles exhibit similar abilities to mediate electron-transfer processes conducted on their surface. Interaction of dendrimers with oppositely charged surfactants has also been examined by Turro et al. (129). As can be expected, surfactants do interact strongly with dendrimers, forming inverse micelle-like structures with a hydrophilic interior and a hydrophobic exterior. Interesting schemes representing supramicellar dendrimer/surfactant structures have recently been offered by Ottaviani et al. (130). (See Fig. 21.) The potential utility of these complexes has not been fully exploited and is clearly an area for further research.

See Chapter 4 Appendix for index of polymers and surfactants.

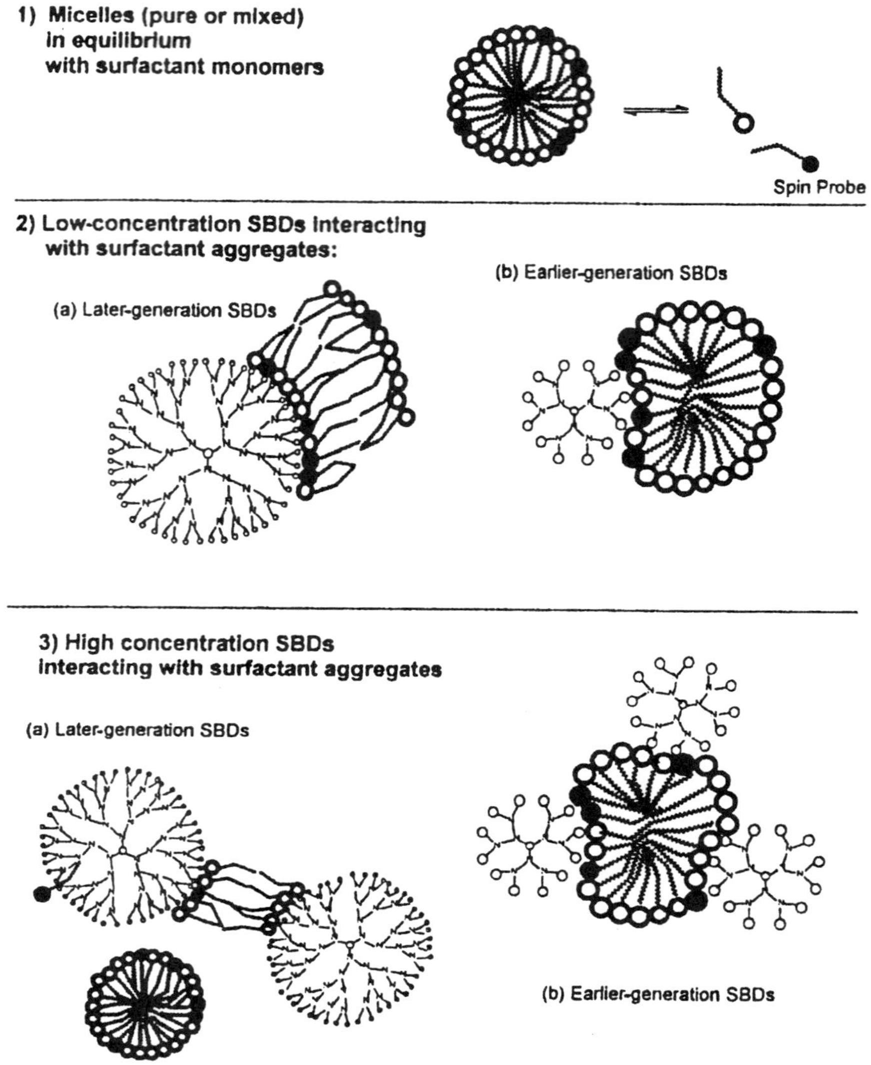

Figure 21 A scheme, in bidimensional projection, of the suggested structures formed by adding increasing concentrations of SBD-C00$^-$ (starburst dendrimers–early generations, G < 4, left side) to mixed micellar solutions of CAT 16 (cationic ESR probe) and CTAB. (From Ref. 130.)

REFERENCES

1. Goddard ED, Hannan RB, Faucher JA. Proc. VII Int'l Congress Surface Active Agents, Moscow 1997; 2:834.
2. Goddard ED, Faucher JA, Scott RJ, Turney ME. J Soc Cosmet Chem 1975; 26:539.
3. Faucher JA, Goddard ED. J Colloid Interface Sci 1976; 55:313.
4. Goddard ED, Hannan RB. J Colloid Interface Sci 1976; 55:73.
5. Goddard ED, Hannan RB. J Am Oil Chem Soc 1977; 54:561.
6. Sukhvinder S, Robbins CR, Cheng WM. WO 94/06409 A1, 1994.
7. Wells RL. US Patent 5,573,709, 1996.

8. Parran JJ. US Patent 3,761,418, 1973; 3,723,325, 1973.
9. Sime J, EP 0 093 601, 1983.
10. Somasundaran P, Ananthapadmanabhan KP, Fujiwara M, Tsaur L. US Patent 5,476,660, 1995.
11. Berthiaume MD, Jachowicz J. J Colloid Interface Sci 1991; 141:299.
12. Marchioretto S, Blakely J. Paper presented at In-Cosmetics Meeting, Dusseldorf, May 12–14, 1997.
13. Medcaliff RF, Jr, Visscher MO, Knochel JR, Dahlgren RM. US Patent 4,820,447, 1989.
14. Jordan NW, Winkler WM, Visscher MO, Seaman SA, McGuffey O. US Patent 3,076,953, 1991.
15. Saud A. U.S. Patent 4,704,224, 1987.
16. Goddard ED. Colloids Surfaces 1986; 19:301.
17. Dubin PL, Davis D. Colloids Surfaces 1985; 13:113.
18. Dubin PL, Vea MEY, Fallon MA, The SS, Rigsbea DR, Gan LM. Langmuir 1990; 6:1422.
19. Goddard ED, Ananthapadmanabhan KP. Interactions of Surfactants with Polymers and Proteins. Boca Raton FL: CRC Press, 1993.
20. Goddard ED, Leung PS. Cosmet Toilet 1982; 97:55.
21. Faucher JA, Goddard ED, Hannan RB, Kligman AM. Cosmet Toilet 1977; 92:39.
22. Faucher JA, Goddard ED. J Colloid Interface Sci 1978; 65:444.
23. Cosgrove T, Mears SJ, Thompson L, Howell I. In: Sharma R, ed. Surfactant Adsorption and Surface Solubilization. ACS Symp Series 615. Washington, DC: American Chemical Society, 1995:196.
24. Kilau HW, Voltz JI. Colloids Surfaces 1991; 57:17.
25. Somasundaran P, Lee LT. Sep Sci Technol 1981; 16:1475.
26. Somasundaran P, Cleverdon J. Colloids Surfaces 1985; 13:73.
27. Shubin V. Langmuir 1994; 10:1093.
28. Goddard ED, Schadt RL. Proc XV Congress IFSCC, London, 1988:197.
29. Magdassi S, Rodel B. Colloids Surfaces 1996; 119:51.
30. Otsuka H, Esumi K, Ring TA, Li JT, Caldwell KD. Colloids Surfaces 1996; 116:161.
31. Tadros Th. F. J Colloid Interface Sci 1974; 46:428.
32. Musabekov KB, Omarawa KL, Izimov AI. Acta Phys Chem 1983; 29:89.
33. Somasundaran P. J Colloid Interface Sci 1969; 31:557.
34. Chibowski S. J Colloid Interface Sci 1980; 76:371.
35. Bocquenet Y, Siffert B. Colloids Surfaces 1984; 9:147.
36. Mougdil B, Somasundaran P. Colloids Surfaces 1985; 13:87.
37. Gebhardt JE, Fuerstenau DW. Am Chem Soc Symp Ser 253, 291. Washington, DC: American Chemical Society, 1984.
38. Ma C. Colloids Surfaces 1985; 16:185.
39. Arnold GB, Breuer MM. Colloids Surfaces 1985; 13:103.
40. Gabrielli G, Cantale F, Guarini G. Colloids Surfaces 1996; 119:163.
41. Zhu PW, Napper DH. Langmuir 1996; 12:5992.
42. Alli D, Bolton S, Gaylord NS. J Appl Polym Sci 1991; 42:947.
43. Carlsson A, Karlstrom G, Lindman B. Colloids Surfaces 1990; 47:147.
44. Mysels KJ, Shinoda K, Frankel S. Soap Films—Studies of Their Thinning. New York: Pergamon Press, 1959.
45. Mysels KJ. J Phys Chem 1964; 68:3441.
46. Miles TD. J Phys Chem 1944; 49:71.
47. Shedlovsky L. Ann NY Acad Sci 1948; 49:279.
48. Kirk-Othmer. Encyclopedia of Chemical Technology, 3rd ed. New York: Wiley, 1980.
49. Goddard ED, Phillips TS, Hannan RB. J Soc Cosmet Chem 1975; 26:461.
50. Leung PS, Goddard ED. Colloids Surfaces 1985; 13:47.
51. Regismond STA, Winnik FM, Goddard ED. Colloids Surfaces 1996; 119:221.

52. Regismond STA, Winnik FM, Goddard ED. Colloids Surfaces, 1998; 141:165.
53. Breuer MM, Robb ID. Chem Ind 1972; 530.
54. Jones MN. J Colloid Interface Sci 1967; 23:36.
55. deGennes PG. J Phys Chem 1990; 94:8407.
56. Purcell IP, Thomas RK, Penfold J, Howe AM. Colloids Surfaces 1995; 94:125.
57. Chari K, Hussain TZ. J Phys Chem 1991; 95:3302.
58. Lionti-Addad S, diMeglio JM. Langmuir 1992; 8:324.
59. Cohen-Addad S, diMeglio JM. Langmuir 1994; 10:773.
60. Cohen-Addad S, diMeglio JM, Ober R. C R Acad Sci Ser 2 1992; 315:39.
61. Goddard ED, Braun DB. Cosmet Toilet 1985; 100:41.
62. Dickinson E, Enston SR, Woskett CM. Prog Colloid Polym Sci 1990; 82:65.
63. Dickinson E. In: Goddard ED, Ananthapadmanabhan KP, eds. Interaction of Surfactants with Polymers and Proteins. Boca Raton, FL: CRC Press, 1992:295.
64. Hannan RB, Goddard ED, Faucher JA. Textile Res 1978; 48:57.
65. Woodard J. J Soc Cosmet Chem 1972; 23:593.
66. Da Chow C. Textile Res J 1971; 41:444.
67. Goddard ED, Harris WC. J Soc Cosmet Chem 1987; 38:233.
68. Ananthapadmanabhan KP, Leung PS, Goddard ED. In: El Nokaly M, ed. Polymer Association Structures: Microemulsions and Liquid Crystals. Symposium Series No. 384. Washington, DC: American Chemical Society, 1988:297.
69. Rhein LD, Robbins CR, Fernee K, Cantore R. J Soc Cosmet Chem 1986; 37:125.
70. Prescott FJ, Hahnel E, Day D. Drug Cosmet Ind 1963; 93:443.
71. Ward JB, Sperandio GJ. J Soc Cosmet Chem 1964; 15:32.
72. Tavss EA, Eigen E, Temnikow V, Kligman AM. J Am Oil Chem Soc 1986; 63:574.
73. Misra M, Anathapadmanabhan KP, Hoyberg K, Gursky RP, Prowell S. Aronson M. J Soc Cosmet Chem 1997; 48:219.
74. Rhein LD. J Soc Cosmet Chem 1997; 48:253.
75. Nikas YJ, Blankschtein D. Langmuir 1994; 10:3512.
76. Goddard ED. Colloids Surfaces 1986; 19:255.
77. Faucher JA, Goddard ED, Kulkarni RD. J Am Oil Chem Soc 1979; 56:776.
78. Loveday DE. J Soc Cosmet Chem 1961; 12:224.
79. Goddard ED. In: Goddard ED, Ananthanpadmanathan KP, eds. Interactions of Surfactants with Polymers and Surfactants. Boca Raton, FL: CRC Press 1992:156.
80. Kresheck GC, Constantinidis I. Anal Chem 1984; 56:152.
81. Francois J, Dayantis J, Sabbadin J. Eur Polym J 1985; 21:165.
82. Brackman JC. Langmuir 1991; 7:469.
83. Leung PS, Goddard ED, Han C, Glinka C. Colloids Surfaces 1985; 13:47.
84. Goddard ED, Leung PS. Langmuir 1991; 7:608.
85. Goddard ED, Padmanabhan KPA, Leung PS. J Soc Cosmet Chem, 1991; 42:19.
86. Thalberg K, Lindman B. Colloids Surfaces 1990; 47:147.
87. Ananthapadmanabhan KP, Goddard ED. Unpubished results, 1988.
88. Brackman JC, Engberts JBFN. J Am Chem Soc 1990; 112:872.
89. Zhang YQ, Tanaka T, Shibayama M. Nature 1992; 360:142.
90. Kokufuta E, Zhang YQ, Tanaka T, Mamada M. Macromolecules 1993; 26(5):1053.
91. Saito S, Taniguchi TJ. J Colloid Interface Sci. 1973; 44:114.
92. Saito S. In: Schick MJ, ed. Nonionic Surfactants: Physical Chemistry. New York: Marcel Dekker, 1987:881.
93. Sarrazin-Cartalas A, Iliopoulos I, Audebert R, Olsson U. Langmuir 1994; 10:1421.
94. Danino D, Kaplan A, Talmon Y, Zana RA. Structure and Flow in Surfactant Solutions. ACS Symp Ser 578. Washington, DC: American Chemical Society, 1994:105.
95. Hulden M. Colloids Surfaces 1994; 82:263.
96. Annable T, Buscall R, Ettelaie R. Colloids Surfaces 1996; 112:97.

97. Lange H. Kolloid Z Z Polym 1971; 243:102.
98. Saito S. Kolloid Z. 1957; 154:19.
99. Jones MN. J Colloid Interface Sci 1968; 26:532.
100. Saito S. J Colloid Interface Sci 1967; 24:227.
101. Turro NJ, Baretz BH, Kuo PL. Macromolecules 1984; 17:321.
102. Goddard ED, Hannan RB, Matteson GH. J Colloid Interface Sci 1977; 60:214.
103. Schwuger MJ, Lange H. Proc 5th Int Congr Deterg Vol 2, Barcelona, 1968 Barcelona: Ediciones Unidas SA, 1969:955.
104. Isemura T, Imanishi A. J Polym Sci 1958; 33:337.
105. Sata N, Saito S. Kolloid Z. 1952; 128:154.
106. Saito S, Mizuta Y. J Colloid Interface Sci 1967; 23:604.
107. Lundgren HP. USP, 2,459,708, 1949.
108. Goddard ED. Unpublished results, 1975.
109. Drummond CJ, Albers S, Furlong DN. Colloids Surfaces 1991; 62:95.
110. Karlstrom G, Carlsson A, Lindman B. J Phys Chem 1990; 94:5005.
111. Carlsson A, Karlstrom G, Lindman B. Langmuir 1986; 2:536.
112. Carlsson A, Karlstrom G, Lindman B, Stenberg O. Colloid Polym Sci 1988; 226:1031.
113. Dervichian DG. In: Lipo-Proteins, Discussions Faraday Soc No. 6, 1949, 7.
114. Jones AS. Biochem Biophys Acta 1953; 10:607.
115. Scott JE. Chem Ind 1955; 168.
116. Palmstierna F, Scott JE, Gardell S. Acta Chem Scand 1957; 11:1792.
117. Laurent TC, Scott JE. Nature 1964; 202:661.
118. Piculell L, Lindman B. Adv Colloid Interface Sci 1992; 41:149.
119. Iliopoulos I, Wang TK, Audebert R. Langmuir 1991; 7:617.
120. Schwuger MJ, Lange H. Tenside 1968; 5:257.
121. Binana-Limbele W, Zana R. Colloids Surfaces 1986; 21:483.
122. Maltesh C, Somasundaran P. Colloids Surfaces 1992; 69:167.
123. Eilassaf J. J Appl Polym Sci 1963; 7:S3.
124. Gebhardt JE, Fuerstenau DW. Min Metal Proc 1986; 3:164.
125. Kiefer J, Somasundaran P, Ananthapadmanabhan KP. Langmuir 1993; 9:1187.
126. Tomalia DA, Naylor AM, Goddard WA. III. Angew Chem Int Ed Engl 1990; 29:138.
127. Tomalia DA, Baker H, Dewald J, Hall M, Kallos G, Martin S, Rock J, Ryder J, Smith P. Macromolecules 1986; 19:2466.
128. Caminati G, Turro NJ, Tomalia DA. J Am Chem Soc 1990; 112:8515.
129. Ottaviani MF, Cossu E, Turro NJ, Tomalia DA. J Am Chem Soc 1995; 117:4387.
130. Ottaviani MF, Turro NJ, Jockusch S. Tomalia DA. Colloids Surfaces A Physiochem Eng Aspects 1996; 115:9.

6

Synthetic Polymers in Cosmetics

James V. Gruber
Amerchol Corporation, Edison, New Jersey

I. INTRODUCTION

A. A Paradigm Shift

Thomas Kuhn stated in his treatise on the progress of scientific discovery that a revolutionary thought or idea that changes people's perception is a paradigm shift (1). More precisely, Kuhn stated: "When, in the development of a natural science, an individual or group first produces a synthesis able to attract most of the next generations practitioners, the older schools gradually disappear." Kuhn intended that his paradigm shift address the way people perceive a prior idea in light of new scientific findings. All older ideas must adjust accordingly when such a shift occurs.

The personal care industry is facing a paradigm shift. Increasingly, the use of once favorably acceptable synthetic polymers, comfortably soluble in organic solvents such as methylene chloride (CH_2Cl_2), ethanol (CH_3CH_2OH), isopropyl alcohol ($CH_3CH(CH_3)OH$), and toluene ($C_6H_5CH_3$), is rapidly finding disfavor. The reason for the paradigm shift lies not in the polymers, but in the solvents, which appear to be creating undo environmental hardships. The shift is pushing the cosmetic industry (as well as others) toward the use of greater amounts of ubiquitous and more benign solvents such as water. Polymers that once worked well in their organic broths must now be made to function in the rigors of aqueous mediums. The changeover presents many challenges and has not been easy.

This chapter will begin by examining briefly the monomer building blocks of many of the key synthetic polymers used in the personal care industry. Chapter 1 addresses, in a more formal and fundamental fashion, the basic elements of polymer science. The functional properties of the synthetic polymers are dictated, in part, by the monomers from which the polymers are comprised. In addition, the architectural arrangement of the monomers will be critical to understanding the functional roles the polymers play in the personal care formulations.

B. Synthetic Monomers

The majority of cosmetically relevant polymers are the product of some type of carbon-carbon bond-forming addition reaction, which typically requires petroleum-based monomers. These workhorse polymers will find applications in personal care long after the last oil wells run dry. The synthetic polymers have grown with the cosmetic industry, and if one considers the multitude of plastic containers used to house the many cosmetic products sold today, the list of unique petroleum-based polymers used in personal care grows even larger. We will, however, ignore containers in this chapter.

When considering the many cosmetically useful synthetic polymers, it is interesting to find that very few condensation polymers, that is, polyesters and polyamides, have found widespread cosmetic utility (we will see a few examples of condensation polymers in the sections on hair fixative and encapsulating polymers). The reason for this lies in the nature of the chemical bonds that hold these condensation polymers together. These polymers, in most cases, are the result of a condensation reaction that itself expels a molecule of water or a low-molecular-weight alcohol. Consequently, these polymers tend to be unstable in the aqueous environments of most cosmetic formulations. Also, if a cosmetic is applied to the hair or skin, it must be removed later. The polyesters and polyamides typically have low water solubility and are, consequently, not readily removed in the washing process.

Recent polymer developments, which include the synthesis of biologically derived polyesters, biodegradable poly(caprolactones), and development of mulitfunctional silicone polymers (Chapter 7), as well as the increasing use of plant proteins (Chapter 9) and polyamides such as poly(caprolactam), demonstrates that the use of these functionally unique condensation materials will, however, continue to grow (2). Regardless of the improved availability of these interesting biological and biodegradable polymers, use of polymers derived from petroleum-based raw materials will continue.

Generic structures of most of the relevant petroleum-based cosmetic monomers used today are shown in Table 1. All of them are based on some type of carbon-carbon unsaturated (olefinic) double bond. Even the oxyalkylene monomers are simply activated olefinic materials. Understanding the nature of the polymerization reaction is not essential to understanding polymer functionality. However, most cosmetically relevant polymers are produced by some type of addition polymerization reactions, which are carbon-carbon bond-forming reactions occurring across the unsaturated double bond of the monomers. These reactions can be initiated by free radicals, anions, or cations and can be run in bulk, in solution, as suspensions, or even as emulsions.

If a single monomer is used to create a polymer, the resulting chain is known as a homopolymer. Homopolymers can be straight-chained or branched (Fig. 1) (3). Polymer characteristics are greatly affected by the architecture of the chains. If one imagines that a linear homopolymer is like a wooden two-by-four, and a branched polymer is like a pine tree, one can further imagine that a certain mass of two-by-fours occupies much less space than a similar mass of pine trees. Branching polymers occupy greater molecular space than their linear cousins. Likewise, the linear polymers, like the linear two-by-fours, are able to pack much more closely. This creates regions of high crystallinity (i.e., high order), which provide the polymers with increased strength and higher melting temperatures.

The thermal transitions that help define a polymer include its melting temperature, T_m (the temperature at which a polymer becomes a liquid), and its glass transition temperature, T_g (the temperature at which a polymer passes from a glassy state to a rubbery state) (4). Generally, the higher the melting and glass transition temperature of a polymer, the tougher its films. However, polymers with high glass transition temperatures can become

Table 1 Cosmetically Useful Monomers

Structure	R^1	R^2	R^3	R^4	Common name
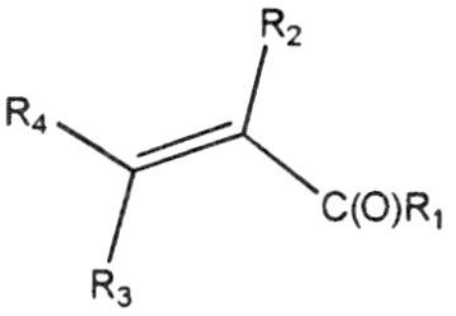	OH	H	H	H	*Acrylic* acid
	O—alkyl	H	H	H	*Acrylic* ester
	OH	CH_3	H	H	Meth*acryl*ic acid
	O—alkyl	CH_3	H	H	Meth*acryl*ate ester
	OH	H	C(O)OH	H	Maleic acid
	O—R^3	H	R^1—C(O)	H	Maleic anhydride
	NH_2	H	H	H	*Acryl*amide
-acryl-	NH—alkyl	H	H	H	Alkyl*acryl*amide
	NH_2	CH_3	H	H	Meth*acryl*amide
	NH—alkyl	CH_3	H	H	Alkylmeth*acryl*amide
		R^5			
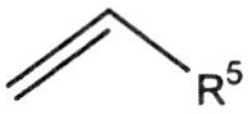		—H			Ethylene
		—CH_3			Propylene
		—Alkyl			Alkylene
		—Aryl			Styrene
		—OCH_3			Methyl*vinyl*ether
		—$OC(O)CH_3$			Methyl*vinyl*acetate
		—$OC(O)CH_2CH_3$			Ethyl*vinyl*acetate
		—NC(O)H			*N-Vinyl*formamide
		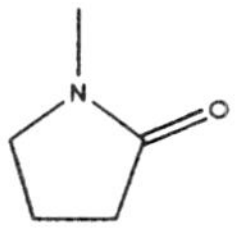			*N-Vinyl*pyrrolidone
-vinyl-		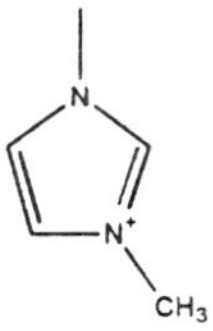			*N-Vinyl*imidazole
		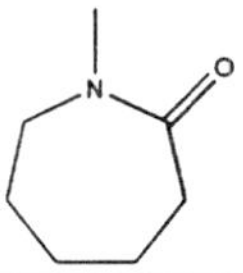			*N-Vinyl*caprolactam
		R^6			
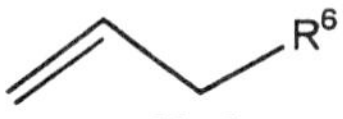		—NH_2			*Allyl*amine
-allyl-		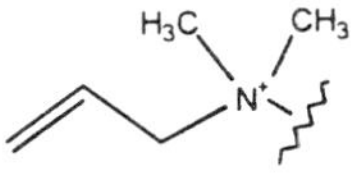			Dimethyldi*allyl*ammonium
		R^7			
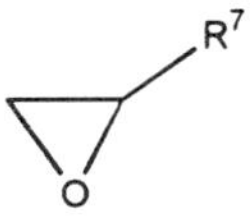		—H			Ethylene *oxide*
		—CH_3			Propylene *oxide*
-oxide		—alkyl			Alkylene *oxide*

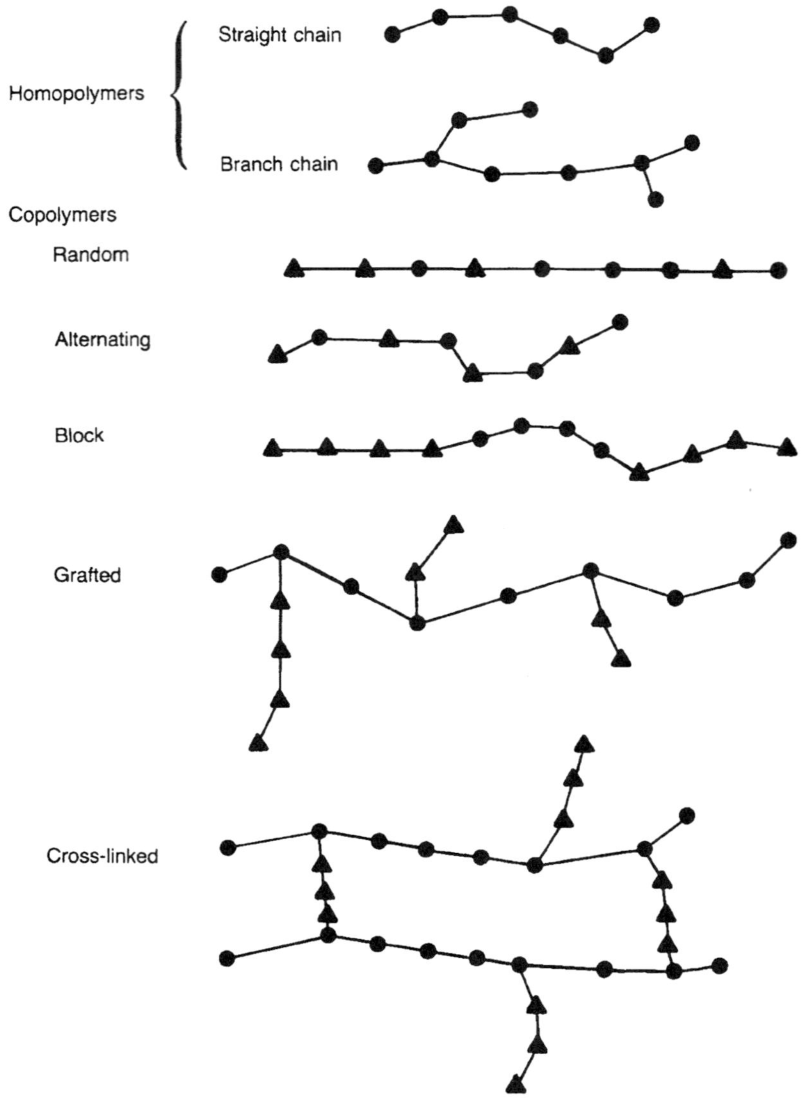

Figure 1 Homopolymer and copolymer architectures. (Reprinted with permission from Burdick DL, Leffler WL. Petrochemicals in Nontechnical Language, 2nd ed. Copyright Penn Well Books, 1990.)

too brittle, which is undesirable in cosmetic applications. Also, polymers with high glass transition and melting temperatures tend to be more difficult to process and dissolve.

The pinnacle of synthetic polymer branching must reside in a new generation of polymers known as dendrimers (Fig. 2) (5,6). Dendrimers are typically branched condensation polymers in which the branching is so well controlled that the polymers grow in well-defined rows described in the dendrimer nomenclature as ''generations.'' The use of dendrimers in cosmetics is only beginning as these polymers are currently costly and not readily available in commercial quantities.

The most unique aspect of dendrimer technology is the extraordinary control that can

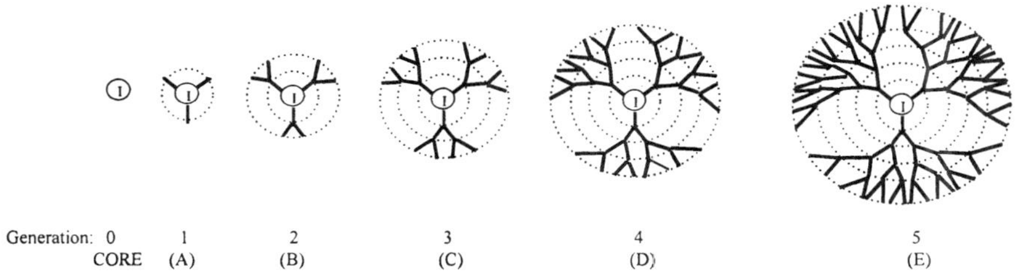

Figure 2 Dendrimer structure.

be exerted on the polymer's weight-average molecular weight, M_w, its number average molecular weight, M_n and its polydispersity, n (7). The weight-average molecular weight (which is biased toward the lower-weight fraction of the polymer sample) defines the weight fraction, w_x, of molecules whose weight is M_x, that is, $M_w = \Sigma(w_x M_x)$. The number-average molecular weight (which is biased toward the higher-molecular-weight fraction of the polymer) defines the total weight of all molecules, w, in a polymer sample divided by the total number of molecules present, that is, $M_n = w/\Sigma(N_x)$. Polydispersity defines the consistency with which a total number of polymer chains occur at a specific molecular weight. That is, n is the ratio of the polymer's molecular weight divided by its molecular number, M_w/M_n. The minimum value is a polydispersity of 1.0, which indicates that every polymer chain in the group has the same molecular mass.

Dendrimers typically have polydispersities of 1–1.08, as can be seen in Figure 3, which shows a gel permeation chromatogram (GPC) tracing of eight generations of den-

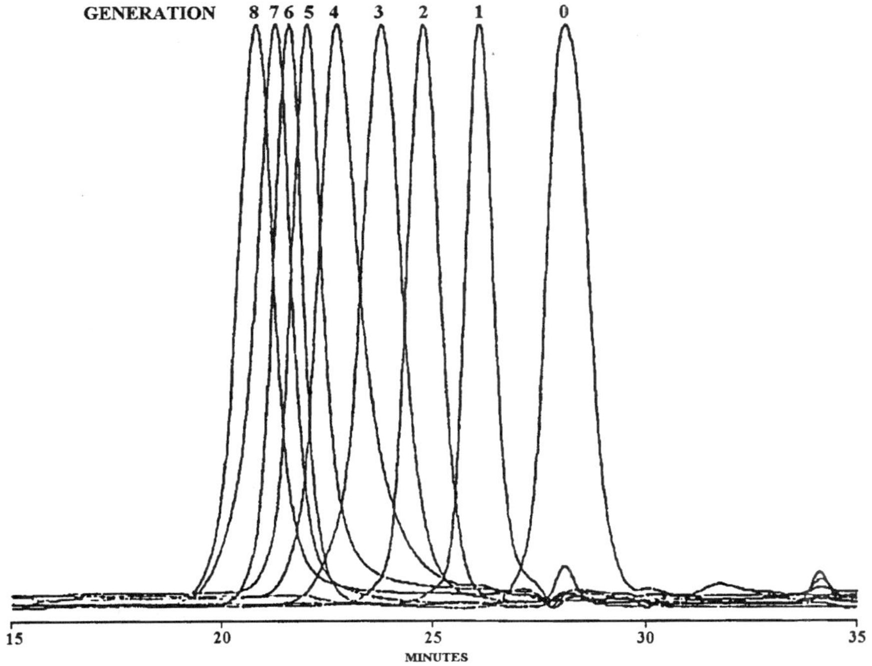

Figure 3 GPC tracing of generation 0–8 dendrimers. (Reprinted with permission from Ref. 6.)

drimers. The sharpness of each peak demonstrates the low polydispersity of each dendrimer generation. Polymers with large polydispersities will have much broader GPC tracings. In fact, dendrimer architecture is so predictable it is mathematically calculable. Most polymer compositions, however, do not have such well-defined polydispersities and occur as a distribution of molecular weights that is typically Gaussian, or bell-shaped. Anionic, cationic, and neutral dendrimers have been synthesized, and recent dendrimer technology has been developed with silane-containing materials and glycodendrimers (8,9). The cosmetic attributes of most of these various dendrimer species remain to be discovered.

If a polymer is comprised of more than one monomer, it is called a copolymer (although the term terpolymer is frequently used when a copolymer comprises more than two monomers). Copolymers can be made to assume a number of unique architectures including random, alternating, block, and grafted copolymers, as shown in Figure 1. The additional category of cross-linked copolymers is particularly important as cross-linking is a useful method for increasing a polymer's molecular weight and radically altering its solution behavior. We will see this, in particular, when we examine the poly(acrylates) used as cosmetic thickeners (Section II.A.2).

The commercial synthesis of homopolymers and copolymers is restricted by little more than the availability of monomers and the chemist's imagination, although the incompatibility of one monomer with another might cause problems. If every monomer listed in Table 1 could be made to react in some fashion with any other one, two, or three monomers listed, in any of the copolymer configurations shown in Figure 1, the magnitude in variations of chemical possibilities begins to emerge. Synthetic polymers, unlike their natural counterparts (Chapters 8 and 9) can have anionic, cationic, neutral, amphoteric, hydrophobic, and hydrophilic groups all on the same polymer chain. Fortunately, restrictions placed on the synthetic polymers by their intended applications, thickening, fixative, conditioning, and encapsulation, help to categorize the vast number of possibilities. This chapter will approach this broad topic from the point of view of these four application areas.

C. Influences of the Surrounding Formulation

Polymer architecture alone does not fully characterize the behavior of a polymer in a formulation. Many other factors influence the behavior of a specific polymer as well. These factors include the nature of the formulation solvent, the presence of additional formulating ingredients, and the temperature and pH of the formulation, among others.

Polymers are defined as hydrophobic if they are repelled by water, lipophobic if they are repelled by oils and hydrocarbons, hydrophilic if they are attracted to water, and lipophilic if they are attracted to oils and nonpolar solvents. Some polymers are repelled by both polar and nonpolar solvents and are called oleaginous. Others are known to contain both hydrophilic and hydrophobic components on the same polymer and are often referred to as polyampholytes. Polymers can be ionic or nonionic and, as a rule of thumb, polymers that are nonionic will be more comfortable in nonionic surroundings and ionic polymers will be more comfortable in polar surroundings.

Unfortunately, this rule of thumb is not universal and additional formulating influences such as salts, surfactants, emulsifiers, and other cosmetically important components change the rules. Additionally, factors such as pH, temperature, and the sequence of formulating can drastically affect the behavior of a particular polymer. One typically finds that cationic polymers favor acidic mediums and anionic polymers basic mediums, while amphoteric polymers are complex and not readily characterized. Some polymers possess a cloud point; that is, they precipitate from solution at high temperatures. Some require high temperature to promote dissolution and do not function until cooled. Critical factors that affect a polymer's functionality will be addressed as they are examined in their characteristic formulation roles.

II. SYNTHETIC POLYMER APPLICATIONS

A. Thickening Polymers

1. *Thickening by Chain Entanglement*

The simplest and most straightforward mechanism of polymeric thickening occurs through chain entanglement. Polymer chains dissolved in a solvent, which, in cosmetic applications, is typically water, one of the lower-molecular-weight alcohols, or combinations of water and alcohol, entangle much the same way soft, cooked spaghetti noodles wrap around each other. Solution viscosity increases as the polymer concentration increases simply because more and more chains are trying to occupy a limited space. As the polymer concentration increases, it becomes more difficult to separate individual polymer chains by the application of force over a given area (known in rheological terms as ''shear''). In addition, increasing molecular weight is also very important in chain entanglement. Considering the analogy of spaghetti noodles further, long noodles tend to clump together much better than short noodles, which manifests itself, for example, in the quantity of long noodles that can be ''picked up'' by a fork.

One interesting aspect of chain entanglement emerges when the log of zero shear viscosity (viscosity measured independent of shear rate) is plotted against the concentration of various polymeric solutions. When the data are normalized for the various polymer molecular weights, the graph shows a clear bimodal zero shear viscosity distribution (Fig. 4) (10). The break in the zero shear viscosity occurs at approximately the same polymer concentration regardless of polymer type. The point of change is known as the critical concentration, c_η, the concentration at which chain entanglement begins. The area on the graph to the left of c_η is known as the dilute regime and the area to the right of c_η the concentrated regime. A similar graph for polysaccharides can be found in Chapter 8 (Fig. 6). The clear effect of chain entanglement on viscosity is evident from these graphs.

The behavior of polymers is also affected by their chemical identities. For instance, if the polymer is actually a copolymer, or if it is cross-linked or hydrophobically modified, variations from typical solution behavior occur. These examples are addressed in this chapter when they become relevant. Simple linear polymers include poly[(meth)acrylic acid], poly(acrylamide), poly(ethylene oxide), polymers and random copolymers of poly(ethylene oxide) and (propylene oxide), poly(vinyl alcohol), and poly(vinylpyrrolidone). Such polymers primarily influence solution viscosity through random chain entanglement. However, all of these polymers possess functional sites, which allows them to bind interpolymerically and aids in chain entanglement. These functional sites also allow all of these polymers to dissolve in highly polar aqueous mediums under the right conditions. We will focus on these polymers initially.

a. Poly[(meth)acrylic] Acid. Poly(acrylic acid) (PAA) is a workhorse polymer for cosmetic thickening (11,12). However, in cosmetic applications this polymer is typically either cross-linked or hydrophobically modified; these altered forms of PAA will be addressed in later sections. Poly(methacrylic acid) (PMA) has found significantly fewer ap-

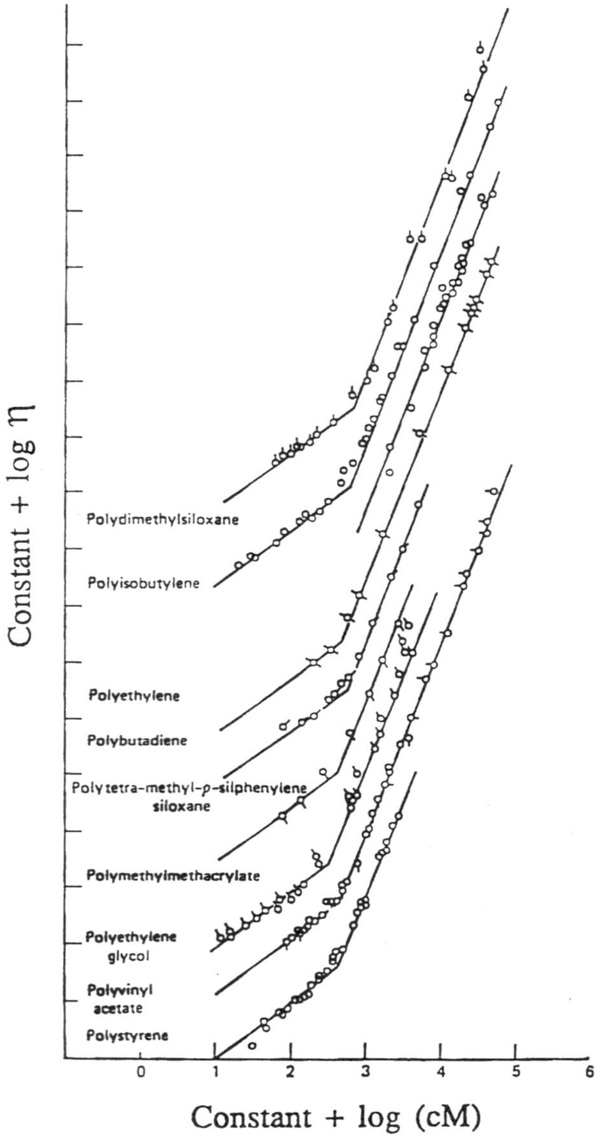

Figure 4 Plot of log of zero-shear-viscosity verses log of polymer concentration times molecular weight for various polymers. (Reprinted with permission from Ref. 10. Copyright 1991 American Chemical Society.)

plications in the cosmetic industry (13). Both polymers, PAA and PMA, are manufactured by free-radical polymerization of their corresponding acrylate or methacrylate monomers, **1** and **2**, respectively (Fig. 5). Usually, the polymerization is performed in a solvent in which the monomers are soluble but the polymers are not beyond a certain molecular weight, making isolation and purification of the resulting polymers easier.

The carboxylic acid groups that occur on every other carbon of the backbones of both PAA and PMA impart the characteristic water solubility to these polymers. PMA, how-

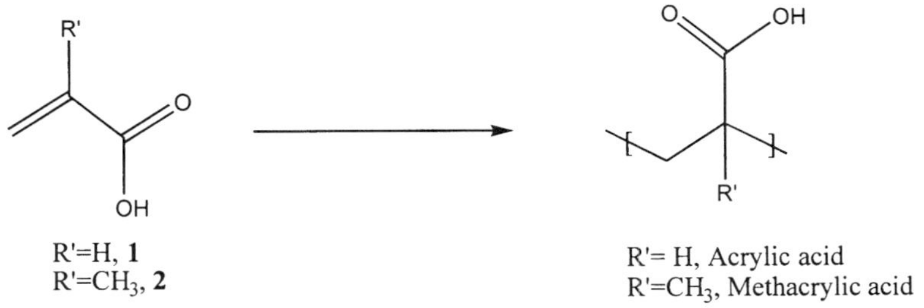

Figure 5 Polymerization of acrylic acid, **1**, and methacrylic acid, **2**, to their respective polymers.

ever, is less water soluble because of the pendent methyl groups residing on every other carbon atom of the backbone. Both polymers exist as collapsed random coils, which interact only marginally with one another when the carboxylic acid moieties are fully protonated as occurs at low pH. Thus, both water solubility and viscosity are low when the polymers are dispersed at low pH. Since viscosity is low at acidic pHs, this allows the formulator to incorporate other ingredients before the neutralization step. Also, there are advantages in hydrating the polymer at low pH without the viscosity buildup. This prevents the formation of ''fish-eyes'' and hydrogels during the subsequent neutralization step. The tight random coils begin to open up, unwind, and tangle with their neighbors as the pH is increased and the carboxylic acid groups are neutralized by the base. The resulting solution viscosity of the polymers increases, as shown in Figure 6.

The nature of the neutralizing agent (i.e., base) affects the polymer solution viscosity. For example, sodium and potassium hydroxide are excellent neutralizing agents, both imparting significant viscosity increases to PAA and PMA solutions. Divalent metal hydroxides such as calcium hydroxide, however, cause precipitation of an insoluble calcium polyacrylate salt. Likewise, low-molecular-weight amines such as triethanolamine or aminomethylpropanol are acceptable neutralizing agents, but higher-molecular-weight

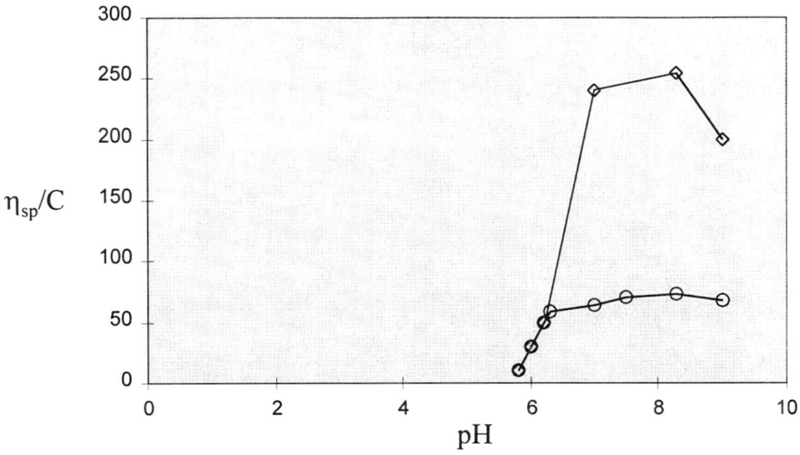

Figure 6 Effect of pH on the specific solution viscosity of poly(methacrylic acid). (○) 0.172 g/100 ml, (◊) 0.011 g/100 ml. (Data taken from Ref. 11.)

polymeric amines, such as poly(ethyleneimine) (Section IV.B.1), produce water-insoluble, cross-linked polyelectrolyte complexes (PEC). Similar instabilities exist when these highly anionic polymers are used in conjunction with high-molecular-weight quaternary cationic polymers or even in the presence of cationic surfactants (14). The influence of pH and neutralizing base type will be addressed in more detail in Section II.A.2.a, covering the cross-linked PAAs.

As the quantity of neutralizing base is increased beyond the amount necessary to fully neutralize the PAAs, further addition of base begins to build excessive positive charge on the polymers (from the neighboring counterion) and the chains begin to repel and untangle from one another. Eventually, when enough excess counterion charge is accumulated, the result manifests itself in an apparent viscosity decrease, as shown in Figure 6.

As mentioned earlier, the newer PAA resins, which incorporate cross-linking and/or hydrophobic modifications, have surpassed the performance attributes of the simple homopolymers, especially in personal care applications. Although very little pure PAA or PMA homopolymer is employed in the industry today, many of the properties discussed above for the homopolymers still apply to these more complex PMAs.

b. Poly(acrylamide). Homopolymeric poly(acrylamide), while having significant commercial and industrial usefulness, has found limited success in personal care applications compared to its acrylic acid cousin (15,16). Commercial poly(acrylamide), **4**, which is a homopolymer made by polymerization of acrylamide, **3**, actually has a finite number of hydrolyzed amide groups, **5**, (Fig. 7). This affords a polymer structurally and chemically not unlike PAA. In fact, it may be the sensitivity of the amide group to hydrolysis that causes formulators to simply develop products using PAA directly. Also, hydrolysis of poly(acrylamide) affords ammonia as a by-product, which imparts an unacceptable and difficult-to-mask ''fishy'' odor.

Because of the strong dipole that occurs between the carbonyl group and the nitrogen in the amide monomers, poly(acrylamide) forms very strong hydrogen bonds to itself, to polar solvents like water, and to multivalent metal cations (Fig. 8). The tenacity with which poly(acrylamide) binds polyvalent metal ions explains its predominant use as a metal flocculant in paper-making and mining applications (17). Combinations of poly(acrylamide) and isoparaffin dispersions have found utility as cosmetic thickeners (18). Many types of chemically modified acrylamide monomers, especially *N*-isopropylacrylamide, are employed in cosmetically useful copolymers, as discussed later when examining associative thickeners and hair fixative polymers.

c. Poly(ethylene oxide) Polymers and Poly(ethylene oxide-propylene oxide) Copolymers. It was mentioned earlier that the carbon-carbon double bond of ethylene, **6**, and propylene, **7**, can be modified by oxidation of these simple monomers to their correspond-

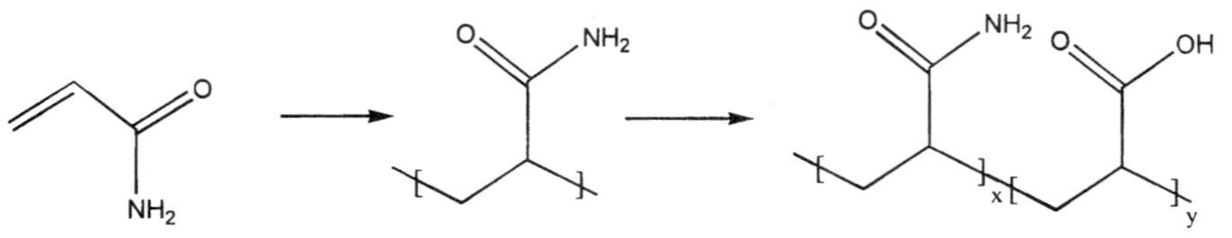

3 **4** **5**

Figure 7 Synthesis and hydrolysis of poly(acrylamide).

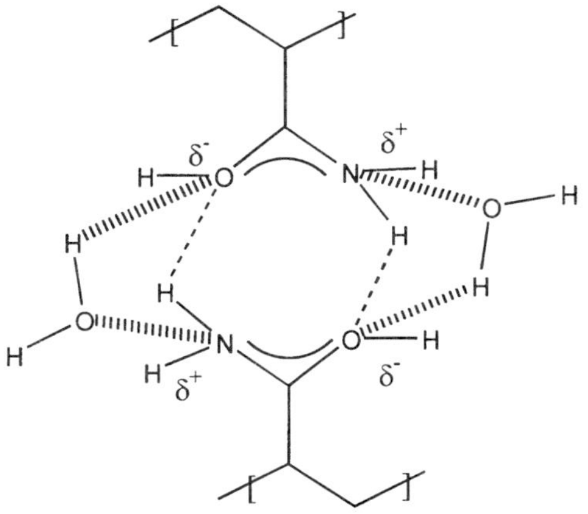

Figure 8 Intermolecular hydrogen bonding between poly(acrylamide) and water.

ing epoxides, ethylene oxide, **8**, and propylene oxide, **9**, respectively (Fig. 9). Homopolymerization of **8**, and **9**, affords the corresponding polyethers, poly(ethylene oxide) (PEO), **10**, and poly(propylene oxide) (PPO), **11**, respectively (Fig. 10) (19–23).

Two categories of nomenclature used to describe the homopolymers of ethylene oxide have developed historically. Ethylene oxide polymers with molecular weights below 20,000 are known as poly(ethylene glycols) and have been assigned the International Nomenclature Cosmetic Ingredient (INCI) designation PEG-N, where N represents the number of ethylene oxide monomer units in the polymer (24). These materials are usually liquids or soft, waxy solids. The nomenclature is further modified if a low-molecular-weight alcohol, like methanol, is used to initiate polymerization. This affords a low-molecular-weight methyl-terminated polyether referred to by the INCI designation PEG-N methyl ether. Polymers with molecular weights greater than 20,000 are referred to as poly(ethylene oxides) and have the INCI designation PEG-#M, where # is a whole number and the M indicates 000, and together, they represent the approximate number of moles of ethylene oxide in the polymer. PEG-2M, for example, is comprised of 2000 moles of ethylene oxide. The high-molecular-weight PEOs are solid materials.

One might expect, considering the similarity in structure of PEO and PPO, that these polymers would have comparable solution characteristics. This could not be further from the truth. The presence of the single alternating methyl group (—CH_3) in PPO lends sufficient hydrophobicity to the homopolymer to make it water-insoluble. Homopolymers of PPO are, in fact, so water-insoluble that they are employed frequently as lubricating metal-

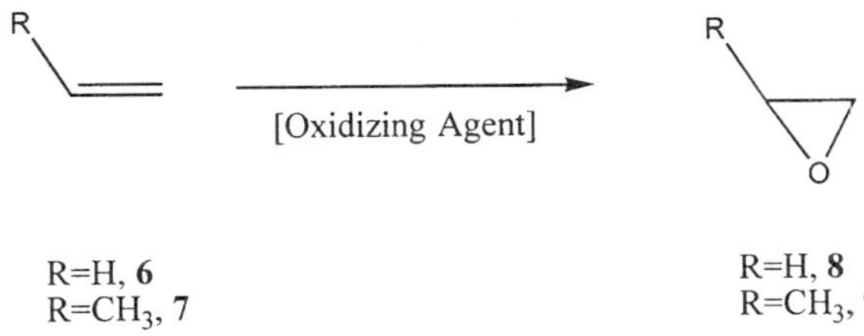

R=H, **6**
R=CH_3, **7**

R=H, **8**
R=CH_3, **9**

Figure 9 Oxidation of ethylene, **6**, and propylene, **7**, to ethylene oxide, **8**, and propylene oxide, **9**.

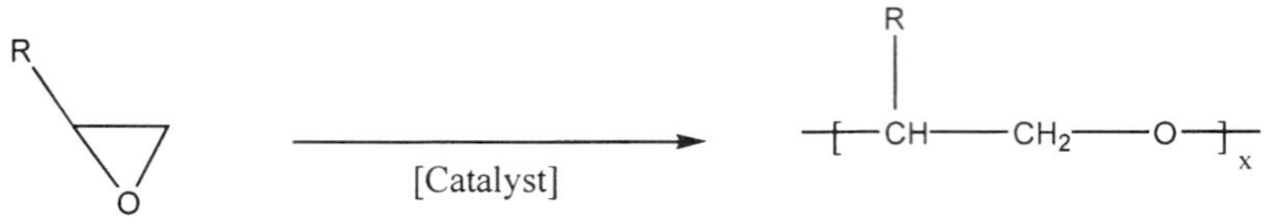

R=H, **8**
R=CH_3, **9**

R=H, **10**
R=CH_3, **11**

Figure 10 Homopolymerization of ethylene oxide and propylene oxide.

working fluids. PPO can only be made to dissolve in water in the presence of a surface-active agent, i.e., a surfactant. PEO, on the other hand, is water-soluble at all molecular weights and in all proportions. The reason for the disparity in the water solubility for these two polymers lies in the ability of the individual polyether monomers to attract and bind water. The polyethers, especially PEO, become water-soluble by surrounding themselves with a sheath of water molecules, which allows the chains to expand and disperse (Fig. 11).

Current research is probing the nature of the hydration sheath around chains of PEO in solution. Molecular dynamic modeling studies of PEO indicate that in its hydrated form, PEO exists as a helical structure with water molecules both outside and inside the helical coil (Fig. 12) (25). The water binds tightly to the ethylene oxide by hydrogen bonding with the electron-rich polyether oxygens. The polyether oxygens will also hydrogen-bond with other polymers, which can create synergistic solution viscosity enhancements. Some of the polymers found to interact with PEO include PAA and PMA. Likewise, electron-deficient metal ions will also bind tightly to the polyether oxygens of PEO forming tight association complexes. Such association complexes manifest their appearance as haze.

Efforts to more fully understand the behavior of both PEO and PPO in the presence of surfactants, especially anionic surfactants, are creating a clearer picture of the behavior of these polymers in solution (26–31). The lipophilic domains of both PEO and PPO bind

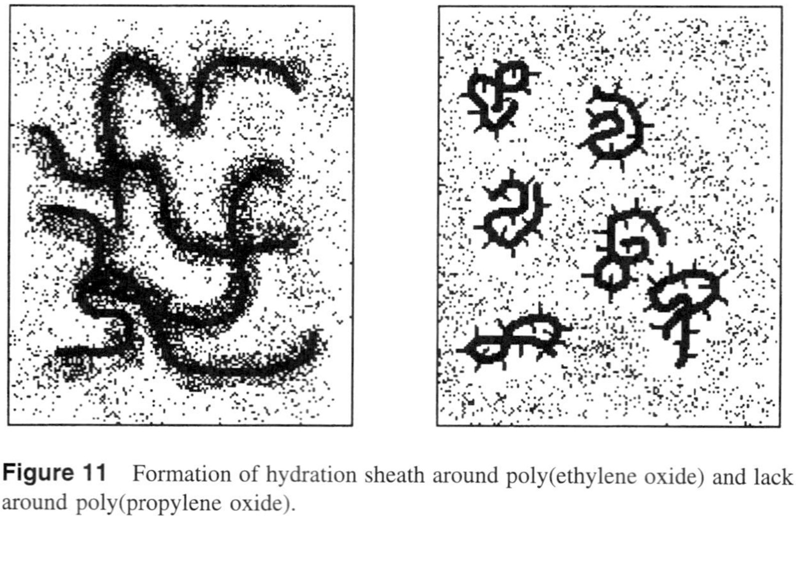

Figure 11 Formation of hydration sheath around poly(ethylene oxide) and lack of such a sheath around poly(propylene oxide).

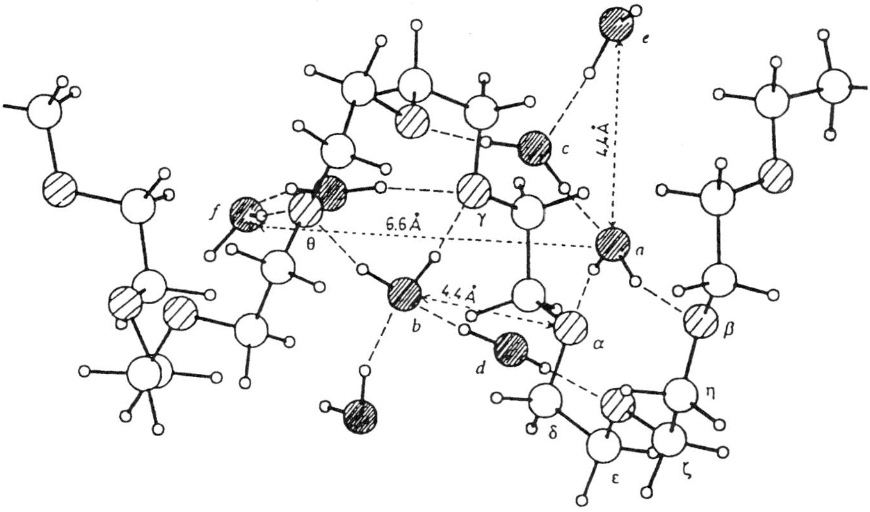

Figure 12 Part of PEO chain with water molecules inside the helix. (Reprinted with permission from Ref. 25. Copyright 1996 American Chemical Society.)

with surfactant micelles, which allows the polymers to fully extend in solution. Extension of the polymer chains permits maximum chain entanglement and results in solution viscosity increases. However, if too much surfactant is added, the polymers begin to collapse on themselves resulting in diminishment in solution viscosity (Fig. 13). These polymers may actually affect the rod-like or spherical morphology of the surfactant micelles in new ways that are just beginning to be understood (32).

Clearly, with two monomers that afford homopolymers having such characteristics, it has been of profound interest to develop copolymers containing their mixtures. The two copolymer combinations possible with these monomers are block, **A**, and random, **B**, copolymers (Fig. 14). Nuclear magnetic resonance spectroscopy has been shown to be a beneficial tool for characterizing these (33,34).

The block copolymers are unique molecular structures that have regions of highly

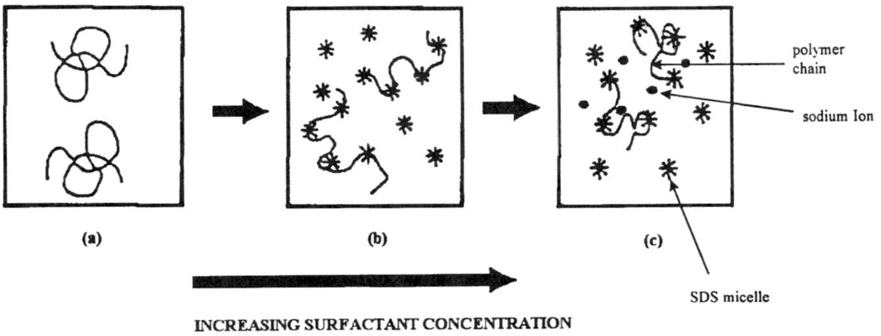

Figure 13 Model of PEO/SDS complex at SDS concentrations of 0 M (a), 0.5 M (maximum coil size) (b), and >0.05 M (reduction in polymer size) (c). (Reprinted with permission from Ref. 26. Copyright 1996 American Chemical Society.)

[A] 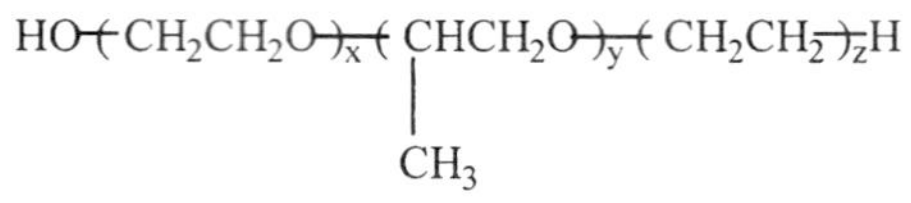

[B] 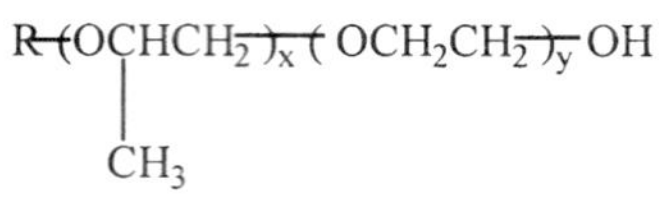

Figure 14 Structure of block (A) and random (B) copolymers of ethylene oxide and propylene oxide.

hydrophilic chains attached to regions of highly lipophilic character. This creates polyampholyte copolymers (copolymers that contain both hydrophilic and hydrophobic groups) capable of lowering the surface tension of water (i.e., they are surface active). The block copolymers have the INCI designation Poloxamer, and their use as ''polysoaps'' is addressed in detail in Chapter 3 (35). Interestingly, when solutions of the block EO-PO copolymers are heated, they cause gelation of their aqueous solutions. This effect is related to a process of micellar packing behavior characteristic of these polymers in heated solutions and has been exploited in commercial applications such as ocular drug delivery (36).

The random copolymers of ethylene oxide and propylene oxide are often initiated by a low-molecular-weight alcohol like butyl alcohol, $CH_3CH_2CH_2CH_2OH$ (37). These alcohol-terminated random copolymers have the INCI designation PPG-N-Buteth-M, where N and M represent the moles of propylene oxide and ethylene oxide in the polymer, respectively. The random copolymers are water-soluble when they contain at least 50% ethylene oxide. Such copolymers possess a cloud point, that temperature at which the water molecules surrounding them no longer adequately sheath the polymer chains. At this temperature, the polymers collapse upon themselves and precipitate from solution. Once the solution has cooled, the polymers will redisperse and redissolve. This solution behavior can have applications in such formulating situations as antifoaming during high-temperature processing of surfactant systems.

These unique linear polymers are extremely lubricious (a characteristic also associated with the high-molecular-weight PEOs) and lend a beneficial slippery feel to a formulation. They are also excellent aids for dispersing sparingly water-soluble components as well as solid materials such as titanium dioxide. One particularly interesting aspect associated with these polymers is their exothermic heat of solution, a thermodynamic phenomenon that causes aqueous solutions in which the polymers are initially dissolved to warm. This quality has found commercial utility in self-heating, hot oil treatments.

d. Poly(vinyl alcohol). Poly(vinyl alcohol) (PVA), **13**, is derived commercially by the catalytic hydrolysis of poly(vinyl acetate), **12**, (Fig. 15) (38,39). The characteristic solution properties of poly(vinyl alcohol) are dictated by the molecular weight of the polymer and by the extent of hydrolysis of the acetate groups on the polymer backbone. The PVA polymer is sparingly water-soluble when hydrolysis is less than 70%. Hydrolysis of the polymer between 70 and 85% affords materials that are readily soluble in cold water and insoluble in hot (i.e., these materials have a cloud point). The optimum level of hydrolysis to obtain complete water solubility in both hot and cold water is above 85%. However, PVA hydrolyzed above 90% is highly crystalline in its solid form and requires

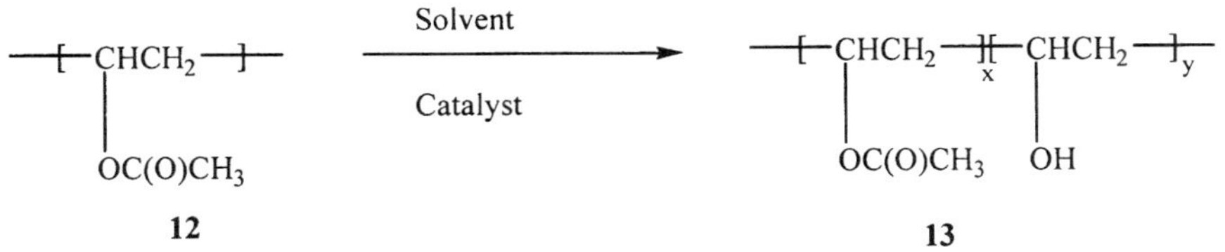

Figure 15 Synthesis of poly(vinyl alcohol) by hydrolysis of poly(vinyl acetate).

vigorous heating to disrupt the strong hydrogen bonds that hold these solid polymers together.

PVA polymers hydrolyzed between 70 and 90% are actually copolymers containing a hydrophobic monomer (vinyl acetate) and a hydrophilic monomer (vinyl alcohol) and are thus polyampholytic. Thus, these polymers lower the surface tension of water (Fig. 16). Consequently, PVA polymers of this type have found commercial usefulness as oil-in-water emulsion stabilizers, particularly in personal care applications. The PVA helps to thicken the continuous phase of these emulsions and aids in suspending the oil droplets in the emulsion.

PVA is generally quite tolerant to different ranges of pH and heat. However, metal ions and certain metal salts, particularly salts of boric acid, cause cross-linking of the polymer chains. This is the mechanism for the development of the well-known commercial product called ''slime'' (Fig. 17) (40,41). The gelation of PVA by borate, a particularly well-known example of this cross-linking effect, is pH dependent and occurs chiefly in alkaline solutions.

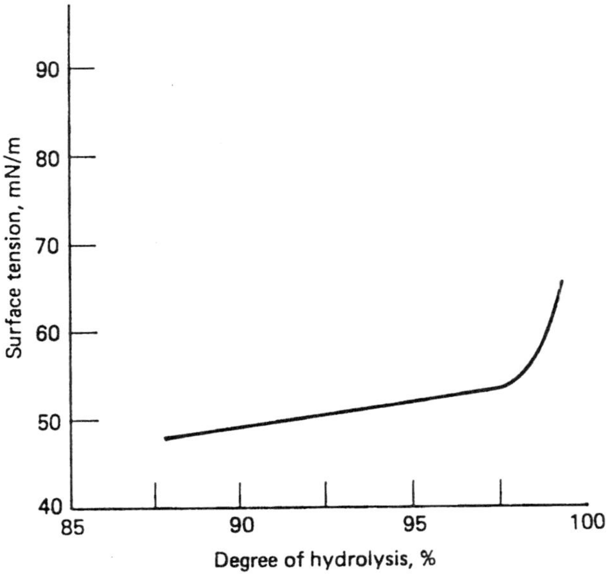

Figure 16 Effect of poly(vinyl alcohol) on water surface tension (From Cincera DL, ed. Kirk-Othmer Encyclopedia of Chemical Technology, Vol 23, 3nd ed. New York: Wiley, 1983. Reprinted with permission of John Wiley & Sons, Inc.)

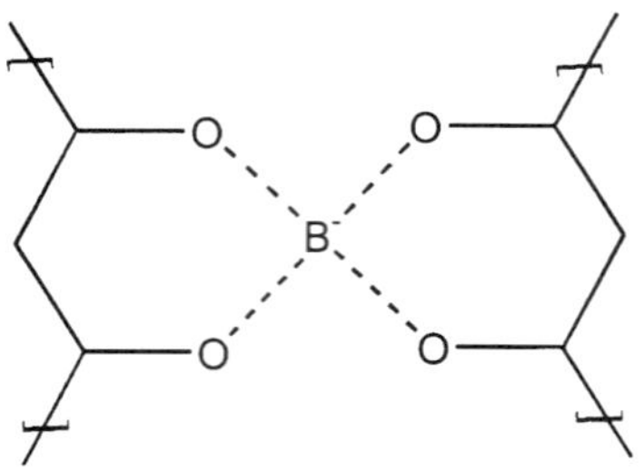

Figure 17 Cross-linking of poly(vinyl alcohol) by tetraborate.

e. Poly(vinylpyrrolidone). Poly(vinylpyrrolidone) (PVP), **15**, is manufactured by the free-radical addition polymerization of *N*-vinyl-2-pyrrolidone, **14**, (Fig. 18) (42,43). The polymer was originally employed as a blood plasma extender and consequently developed a history of extraordinary human compatibility and safety. PVP is a comb-like structure with pendent amide groups on every other carbon of the backbone, and like polyacrylamide (Section II.A.1.b), is resonance-stabilized by delocalization of the carbonyl electrons through the amide bond. This charge delocalization makes the amide carboxyl group quite electronegative and gives PVP its unique viscosifying and complexing abilities. Unlike polyacrylamide, the pyrrolidone ring structure lends stability to the amide functionality, which partially explains the polymer's benign behavior in the human body.

PVP was one of the first successful hair fixative resins (Section III) (44). However, in this application today, it is more frequently present as a copolymer. PVP homopolymer is often employed in solution-based personal care products as a viscosifying and emulsion-stabilizing polymer. Simple emulsions that employ PVP benefit from its stabilizing effects. It has been suggested that, although solutions of PVP display yield stress, the magnitude of this effect is not always sufficient to stabilize emulsions, especially complex multiple ones (45).

The cyclic nature of the PVP amide functionality has attributes similar to the polyamide bonding of proteins, such as collagen and keratin, which occur in human skin and hair. For this reason, emulsions stabilized with PVP have excellent substantivity to these proteins and deliver humectancy and lubriciousness to a formulation that helps to soften and moisturize the skin (42,44).

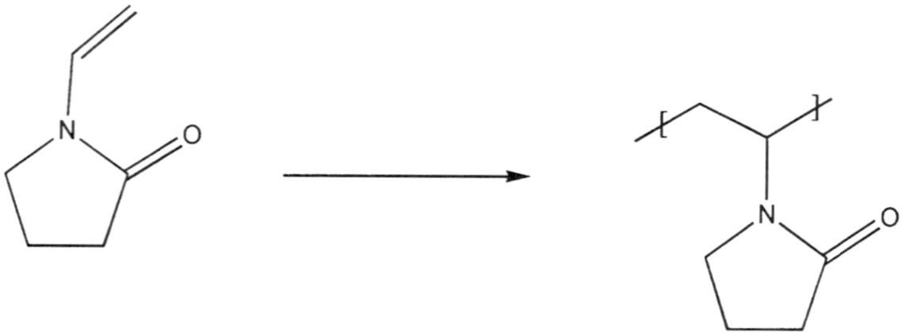

14 **15**

Figure 18 Synthesis of poly(vinylpyrrolidone).

PVP shares many of the solution-binding attributes of PEO (Section II.A.1.c) (29,31). Anionic surfactants bind tightly to PVP by incorporating themselves near the lipophilic portions of the PVP backbone. These surfactants begin binding to the polymer at the critical aggregation concentration (the minimum concentration of surfactant required to begin interaction with the polymer), which is normally below the critical micelle concentration of the anionic surfactant. The presence of anionic surfactants in a formulation that contains PVP builds viscosity as the surfactant micelles cause uncoiling of the polymer and entanglement of the polymer chains. Cationic and nonionic surfactants do not interact to such a strong degree. PVP, like poly(acrylamide), binds multivalent metal ions tightly and interacts with many other solution polymers in a synergistic fashion (42).

2. *Thickening by Covalent Cross-linking*

It is well recognized in polymer science that covalently cross-linking polymers (that is, hooking two polymer chains together by periodic insertion of a difunctional monomer that can react with both chains) radically alters their properties. Perhaps the most well-known instance of functional cross-linking occurs in the vulcanization of rubber. Rubber is a natural gum, which, when harvested from the rubber tree, is a tacky, flowing resin. It was found that by heating the gummy resin with elemental sulfur, a process known as vulcanization, the liquid rubber could be converted via covalent cross-linking into the firm rubber characteristic of automobile tires.

The personal care industry clearly does not typically require such drastic changes in polymer characteristics. But, it has been found that by cross-linking aqueous solution polymers, their usefulness can be extended and improved. However, such effects have been restricted to only a small number of the many useful personal care resins and, as we will see, if cross-linking is not carefully controlled, it can adversely affect the solution properties of a polymer.

The effect of cross-linking density on the standard solution behavior of a cross-linked polymer is schematically represented in Figure 19. An optimum level of cross-linking is required to maximize the polymer's viscosity performance. The reason for this is relatively straightforward. Solution polymers must be able to extend and uncoil in solution so that chain entanglement can occur. If chain entanglement does not occur, the viscosifying effects of the polymer are restricted. Cross-linking assures and enhances the ability of polymers to overlap. At the same time, it effectively increases the molecular weight of the polymers.

With many water-soluble polymers, cross-linking has another effect on their solution characteristics. Light cross-linking in a polymer can decrease its solubility and make it water-dispersible though not completely water-insoluble. The term ''water dispersible'' implies that the cross-linked polymers are incapable of complete dissolution. Instead, they will exist as soft, clear, round, water-logged microscopic sponges known as microgels (Fig. 20) (46). The solution behavior of the cross-linked microgels is a function of the polymer's molecular weight, the monomer type, the type of cross-linking, and the cross-linking density. Careful control and optimization of these parameters gives a polymer peak rheological performance (47,48).

A cross-linked polymer can impart a yield value to a solution in which it is dispersed. When a solution has a yield value, a certain amount of energy or shear force must be applied to initialize flow. Polymers that impart a yield value (sometimes known as yield point) give the solution plastic-like rheology below the yield value and can suspend water-

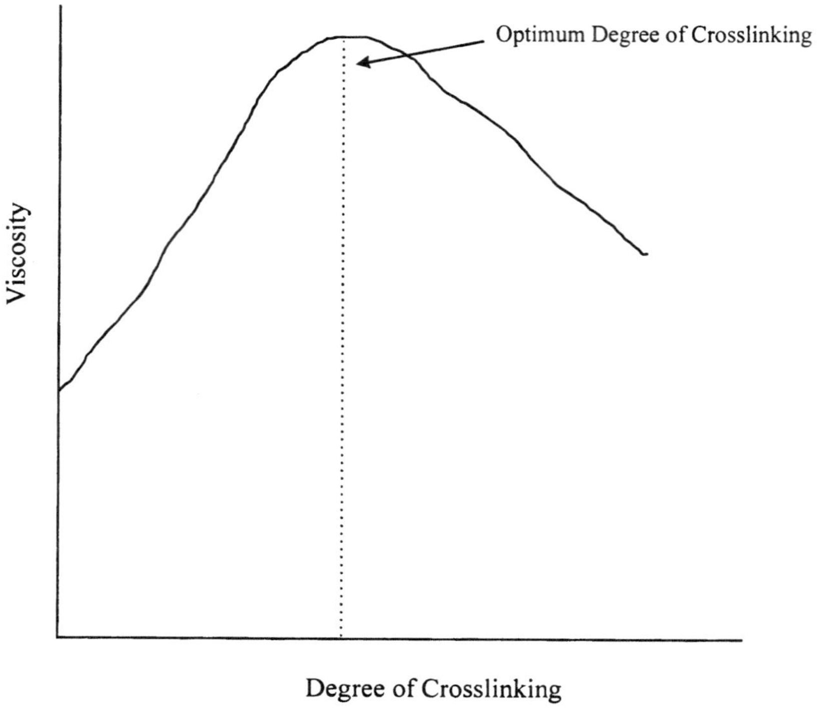

Figure 19 Effect of cross-linking on solution viscosity.

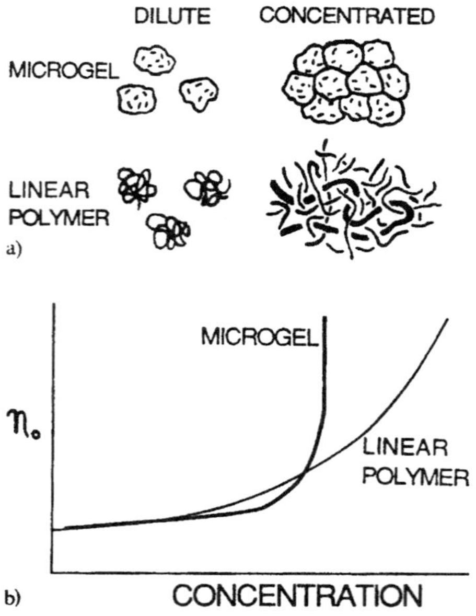

Figure 20 Linear polymers and microgels: (a) qualitative representation of solution conformations; (b) qualitative zero-shear viscosity-concentration behaviors. (Reprinted with permission from Ref. 46.)

insoluble oils and particles. This property helps to stabilize oil-in-water emulsions in personal care applications.

Care must be taken to control the cross-link density (the amount of cross-links per polymer chain) of a polymer for one critical reason: excessive cross-linking can prevent polymers from fully extending in solution. This manifests itself in a reduced solution viscosity, as schematically suggested in Figure 19. Normally water-soluble polymers can even be made insoluble when the cross-linked density is sufficiently high to prevent uncoiling and solvent intrusion.

Fortunately for most formulators, the optimization of cross-linking is usually addressed by the polymer manufacturer. The concerns of the formulator, instead, must be the effects of other ingredients (e.g., surfactants, salts, oils, etc.) on the cross-linked polymer's aqueous solution behavior. We will see that the effects can be significant.

a. Cross-linked, Anionic Acrylate Polymers. It was mentioned earlier that the workhorse of synthetic, aqueous, rheology control polymers is PAA. It is, in fact, the lightly cross-linked, water-dispersible homo-and copolymers of acrylic acid that are the preeminent thickening resins. These polymers are known under a variety of INCI designations that vary depending on the nature of the constituent monomers. They include: acrylates copolymer, PVM/MA decadiene crosspolymer (49–51), carbomer (52–54), and acrylates/VA crosspolymer (47).

Regardless of the monomers from which these various thickeners are made, certain characteristics are common for all. For example, all require neutralization of their carboxylic functionality with base to facilitate effective elongation of the polymer chains. The choice of the neutralizing base can influence the rheology of these polymers in a formulation (Table 2 and Fig. 21) (47,50,55). Because the polymers are optimally cross-linked they will disperse but not fully dissolve.

Cross-linking creates a yield value in solutions containing these copolymers that the non-cross-linked copolymers lack (56). Consequently, their solutions are able to aid in stabilizing the dispersed phase in oil-in-water emulsions, pigments, particles, antidandruff agents, and any other component that requires suspension. The mechanism of suspension is believed to be related to the presence of swollen microgels, which bear an overall

Table 2 Effect of Bases on Viscosity of 0.5 % PVM/MA Decadiene Crosspolymer

Base	Wt. ratio	pH	CPS[a]
10% NaOH	1:2.6	6.84	99,800
10% KOH	1:4.0	6.53	108,000
30% NH_4OH	1:2.0	6.53	107,000
Monoethanolamine	1:0.4	7.05	99,000
Diethanolamine	1:0.7	6.92	103,000
Triethanolamine	1:1.0	6.69	96,500
Aminomethylpropanol	1:0.6	6.95	96,300
Aminomethylpropandiol	1:0.7	6.88	99,000
Tromethamine	1:0.8	6.82	100,000
Sodium hydroxymethylglycinate	1:1.8	6.97	103,500
Tetrahydroxypropylethyleneamine	1:1.8	6.83	111,000

[a] TE spindle, 10 rpm, 25.0°C.
Source: Ref. 49, with permission.

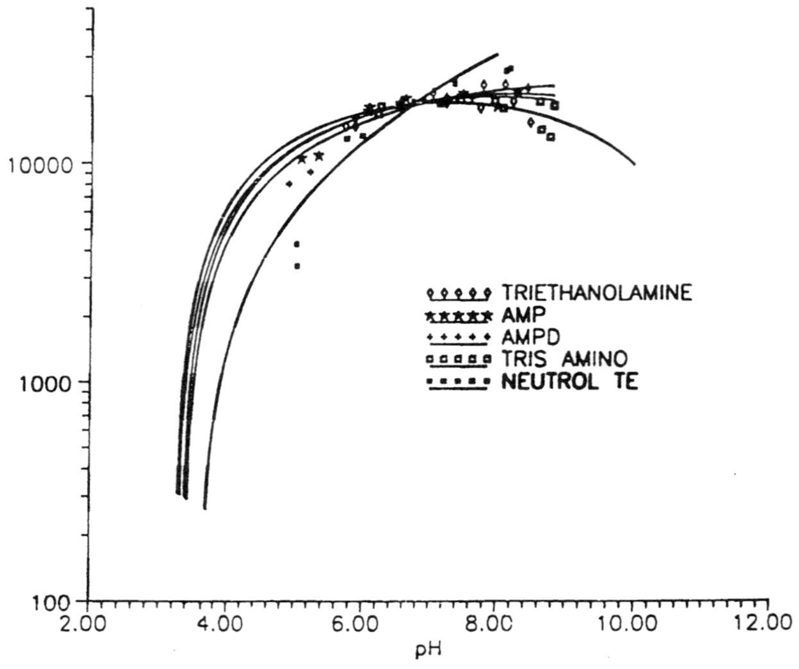

Figure 21 Brookfield viscosity (at 20 rpm) versus pH for 0.2% w/w Carbomer 940 resin. (Reprinted with permission from Ref. 55.)

negative charge. They help the oil droplets, which themselves carry negative charge from their surrounding monolayer of primary emulsifier, repel one another and so prevent coalescence (Fig. 22).

Although they seem simple, the fundamental principles that guide the development of polymer-stabilized emulsions are far from straightforward (57,58). The presence of the cross-linked microgels helps stabilize a dispersion of oil droplets by creating interstitial spaces for the oil droplets to reside. Employing a polymer to help stabilize an emulsion may allow a formulator to decrease the amount of the principal-low-molecular-weight primary emulsifier required to hold the emulsion together. Low-molecular-weight primary emulsifiers are frequently strong surface-active agents that can strip important oils from the body. Removal of the oils may heighten irritation of the skin. Thus, application of these polymers may help to minimize the irritation potential of an emulsion system.

The viscosifying effect of the cross-linked anionic poly(acrylates) depends on the ability of the cross-linked polymer chains to uncoil and extend when neutralized (59). Excessive cross-linking, as mentioned earlier, can impair the polymer's ability to uncoil. Formulating ingredients can have a similar effect on polymer extension and similarly affect the performance. Cationic species, for example, cationic surfactants or cationic polymers, can seriously impede the viscosifying effect of cross-linked, anionic poly(acrylates). Furthermore, cationic molecules may cause precipitation of highly anionic polymers through the formation of electrolyte complexes (60). On the other hand, inorganic smectite clays, popular personal care thickeners and emulsion stabilizers, can interact synergistically with cross-linked poly(acrylates) to produce unusually high solution viscosities (61).

The presence of salts in formulations containing anionic poly(acrylate) thickeners can

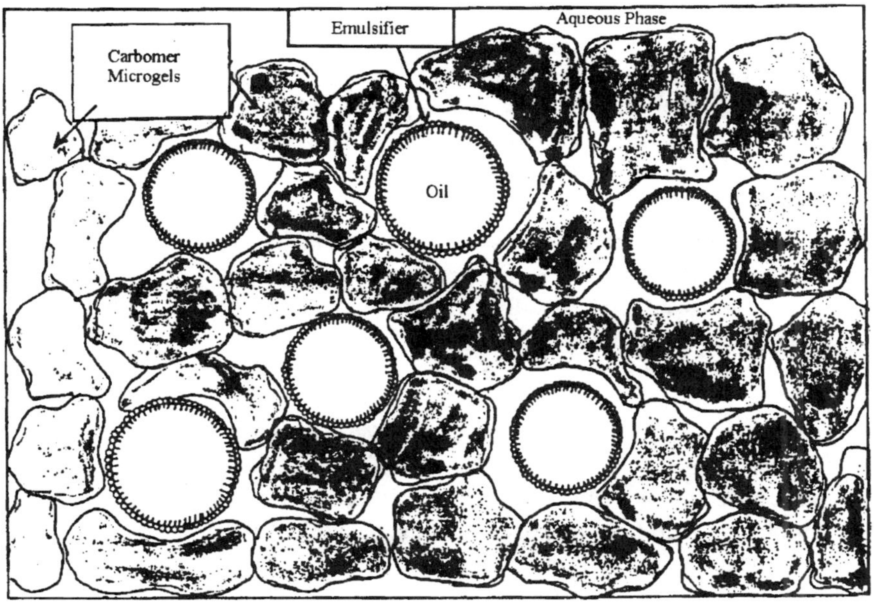

Figure 22 Stabilization of an emulsion of oil droplets surrounded by a primary emulsifier by the presence of swollen microgels. (Reprinted with permission from Ref. 56.)

strongly affect thickener bahavior. Even small amounts of salt, ubiquitous in personal care formulations, can rapidly collapse swollen microgels, destroying their emulsifying ability (50,55). Likewise, ultraviolet radiation and shear are also detrimental. Both can promote polymer chain scission, which reduces the molecular weight. In response to this series of concerns, polymer manufacturers have developed new anionic, polymeric thickeners that operate through an associative thickening mechanism. These fascinating polymers are covered in Section II.A.3.

b. Cross-linked Cationic Acrylate Dispersions. Cationic acrylates have also found practicality as cross-linked thickeners and emulsion stabilizers, although not nearly to the extent of their anionic cousins (62). The cationic acrylates are quaternary-amine-containing copolymers that are sold as dispersions in cosmetically useful solvents, particularly mineral oil, in the personal care industry (Fig. 23). When these hydrophilic, cross-linked dispersion polymers are blended with water, they swell, forming microgels that suspend the oily components of the water-in-oil emulsion.

The cationic copolymers show good stability in the presence of cationic surfactants

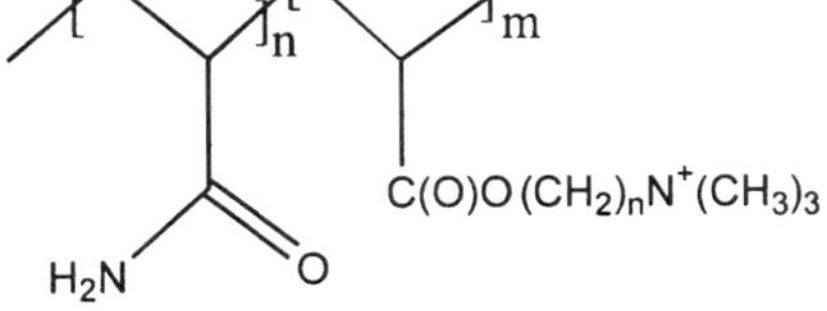

Figure 23 Cationic acrylate dispersion polymers, polyquaternium-32 and polyquaternium-37 ($n = 0$).

and conditioners and are stable at acidic pHs. In this way, they complement the behavior of the cross-linked, anionic thickeners. Because these polymers carry a cationic charge, they will have a strong affinity for the anionic surfaces of the skin and hair. In this way they will also impart conditioning properties as well (see Section IV). Their strong attraction for anionic sites, however, precludes their presence in strongly anionic surfactant systems.

3. *Thickening by an Associative Mechanism*

It is important, in beginning a discussion on associative thickening, to consider how amphiphiles, or surfactants, behave in aqueous solution. A surfactant is classically characterized as a bifunctional entity with a hydrophilic head group, A, attached to a hydrophobic tail, B (Fig. 24). The chemical natures of A and B are the subject of recent reviews as is the behavior of surfactants in aqueous solution (63–66). This chapter will not address these topics. Figure 25 characterizes some of the confirmations adopted by surfactants in solution. Immediately apparent is the desire of the hydrophobic regions, B, of the surfactant (amphiphile) to congregate. They will, in fact, assume a number of unique shapes, depending on the concentration of the surfactant in solution. The presence of hydrophobes in the aqueous phase disrupts the hydrogen-bonding network of the water molecules. The water molecules adapt by creating molecular cavities that exclude the hydrophobes into micelles to minimize the energy of solvation. The process is entropy-driven and is known as the ''hydrophobe effect'' (67).

Surfactants are ubiquitous in industrial applications. Especially in the coatings (i.e., paint) and personal care industries, surfactants play a significant role. These industries share many common concerns since cosmetics are largely coating systems. Often, useful ingredients in coatings applications find their way into personal care formulations. Naturally, the safety considerations are compounded and stricter in the latter application.

The development of associative thickeners has followed a gradual growth from the coatings industry to the personal care industry. Paint formulations, which historically were solvent-based acrylics, rapidly developed into water-based systems, i.e., waterborne latexes, for various regulatory, safety, and application reasons. Principal functional coating polymers, which are not water soluble, are delivered as neat polymer packets that must not coalesce until use. Surfactants are employed to help stabilize these polymer packets in the formulations. The paints are also composed of many different inorganic pigments, fillers, salts, and other peripherally important ingredients. Every ingredient must remain suspended until the product is used.

Unfortunately, simply emulsifying these various components is usually inadequate. The spreading properties of the latex droplets can be adversely affected upon application by the presence of too much low-molecular-weight emulsifier (we will see further repercussions of this difficulty in the section covering fixative polymers, Section III). Therefore,

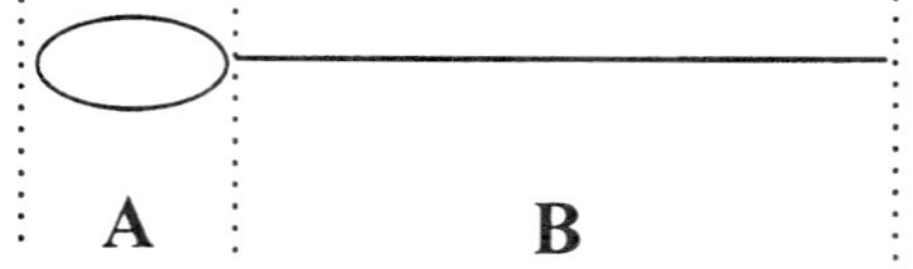

Figure 24 Structure of a surfactant.

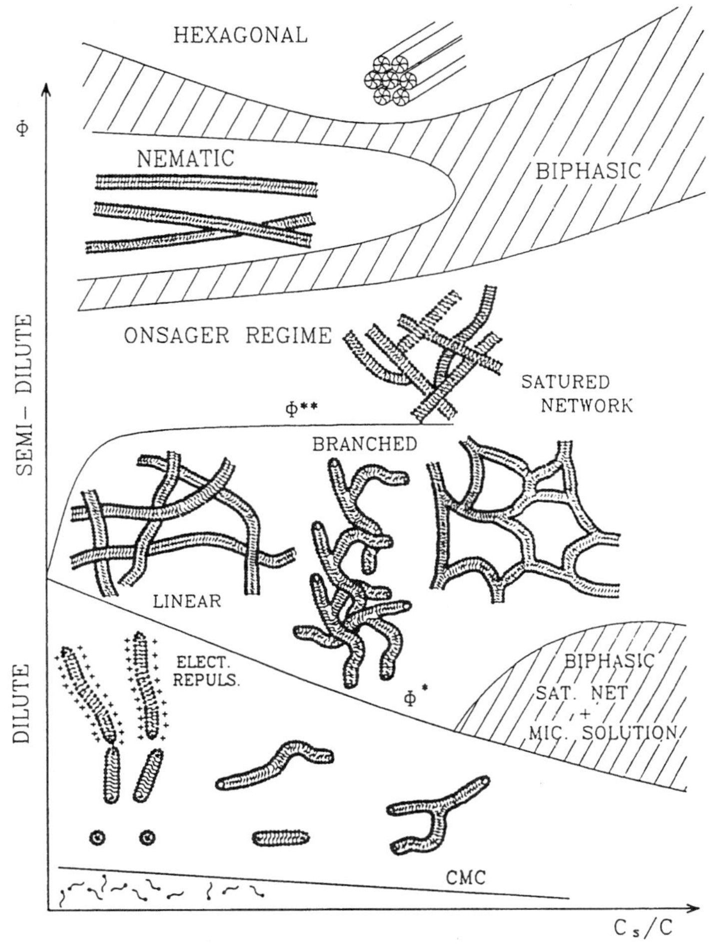

Figure 25 Morphological behavior of surfactant in aqueous solution: surfactant volume fraction Φ verses molar ratio C_s/C of salt over surfactant concentrations. (Reprinted with permission from Ref. 66. Copyright 1994 American Chemical Society).

the use of hydrophobically modified associative thickening polymers has grown into one of the most intensely studied areas of coating technology, and aspects of the topic have been reviewed (28,68,69,70).

The term ''associative thickening polymer'' describes polymers that have been hydrophobically modified to provide them with surfactant-like qualities. This is achieved by grafting the hydrophobe along the length of the hydrophilic backbone of the polymer. The hydrophobic domains of these polymeric thickeners behave like surfactant hydrophobes and find themselves forced together by their unfavorable interactions with water. The associative behavior is concentration dependent, as schematically represented in Figure 26. As the polymer concentration increases, the hydrophobic interactions evolve from intramolecular to intermolecular. These interpolymeric associations create transient, noncovalent, interpolymeric cross-links. Cross-linking, as we saw earlier, can profoundly influence polymer solution rheology. Indeed, what is typically found is that a copolymer

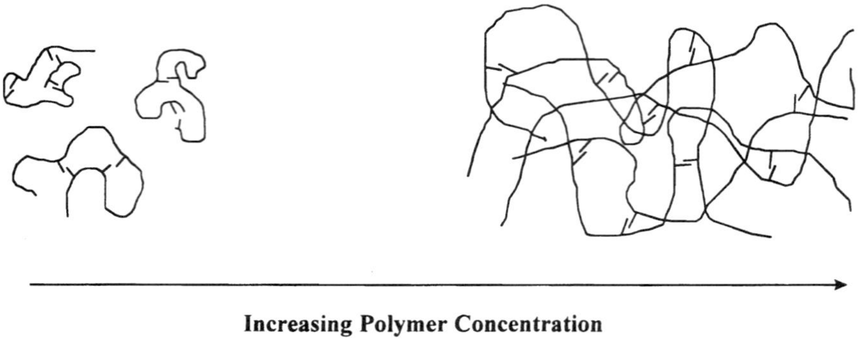

Figure 26 Morphology of associative thickeners in solution at different concentrations.

that has a few hydrophobic groups attached randomly to it can affect significant viscosity increases in solution. However, the hydrophobic monomer density must be kept low enough to avoid making the copolymer water-insoluble or nondispersible.

The associative aggregates in a solution containing hydrophobically modified polymer dramatically affect solution rheology (Fig. 27) (71). As the shearing stress increases, the entangled and associatively interconnected polymers unravel. However, the associated hydrophobic aggregates tend to remain intact even after chain entanglement has broken down. Not until still higher shear has interrupted the hydrophobic aggregates does the viscosity become pseudo-plastic (shear thinning).

In the area of personal care, solution rheology directly affects how a cosmetic product behaves. In this way, associative polymers can influence a cosmetic's aesthetic properties. Perhaps more importantly, they can influence the appearance of the product, the spreading behavior, the film thickness, and the feel of cosmetics from lotions to gels to shampoos. From the consumer's perspective, products that appear stringy (pituitous) or that ball up on application (pilling) are undesirable (72). Good viscosity control can impart a perceived increase in product concentration that the consumer considers beneficial. A low-viscosity product delivered from a bottle or pump is unacceptable, yet low-viscosity products are a necessity for products that are atomized (aerosols). In most cases, the viscosity manipulation is partly the result of appropriate polymer selection.

The behavior of associative thickeners in the presence of surfactants is further influenced by the interaction of the surfactants with the polymer hydrophobes (73–77). The effect of addition of surfactant on an associative polymer can powerfully influence the viscosity of a formulation. The surfactant hydrophobes will further disrupt the hydrogen-bonding network of the water. Consequently, the surfactant hydrophobes are pushed together with the polymer hydrophobes where they become part of the overall mixed surfactant/polymer micelles. The hydrophobe effect can be so pronounced that even when the hydrophobic polymer and surfactant carry the same charge, the surfactant and polymer hydrophobes will reside together in solution. The addition of surfactant to a solution containing hydrophobically modified polymer typically (but not always) demonstrates the aggregation effects shown in Figure 28. The polymer tends to self-associate at low surfactant concentration. This association is predominantly intra- or intermolecular depending on the polymer concentration (Fig. 28a).

The hydrophobe effect occurs at concentrations well below the critical micelle concentration, cmc, of the surfactant. As mentioned earlier, the concentration at which individ-

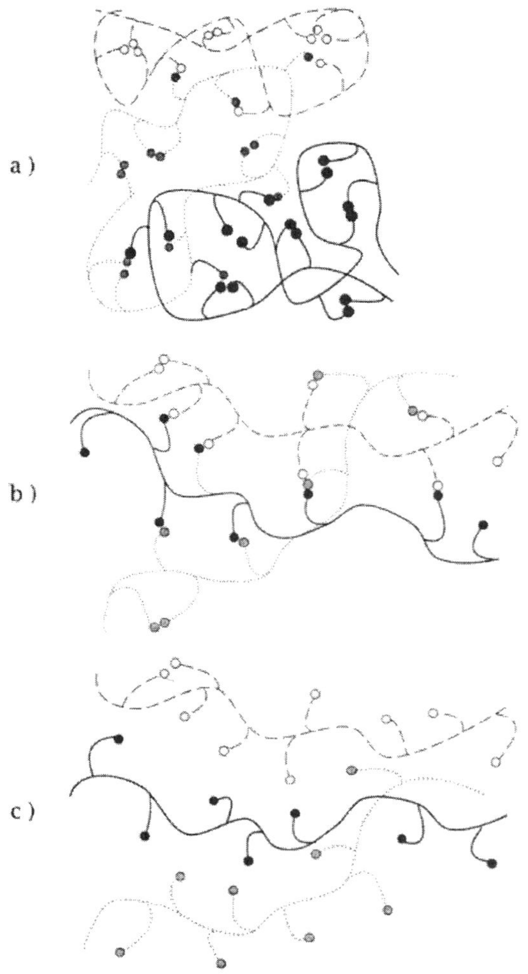

Figure 27 Schematic representation of hydrophilic alkali-swellable polymer network topology. (a) Low-shear regime: dynamic network involving both topological entanglements and hydrophobic associations. Both *intra-* and *intermolecular* associations are envisaged in the nondilute regime. (b) Intermediate-shear regime: deformation of the molecular coils, the more extended conformation promoting *intermolecular* association of the hydrophobes. (c) High-shear regime: possible depletion of the association network leading to pronounced shear thinning. (Reprinted with permission from Ref. 71.)

ual surfactant molecules begin interacting with the polymer hydrophobes is the critical aggregation concentration, cac, and the bundle of polymer hydrophobe and surfactant is termed an ''aggregate'' (28). Increasing the concentration of surfactant forms mixed micelles that contain both surfactant molecules and the polymers hydrophobes (Fig. 28c). This causes an apparent cross-linking of the polymers into a solution-spanning network. The solution viscosity is a maximum for the system, and typically possesses a yield value. Depending on the nature of the surfactant and the hydrophobe polymer, the system can phase-separate (73). This can be manifest as haze or actual separation of polymer and

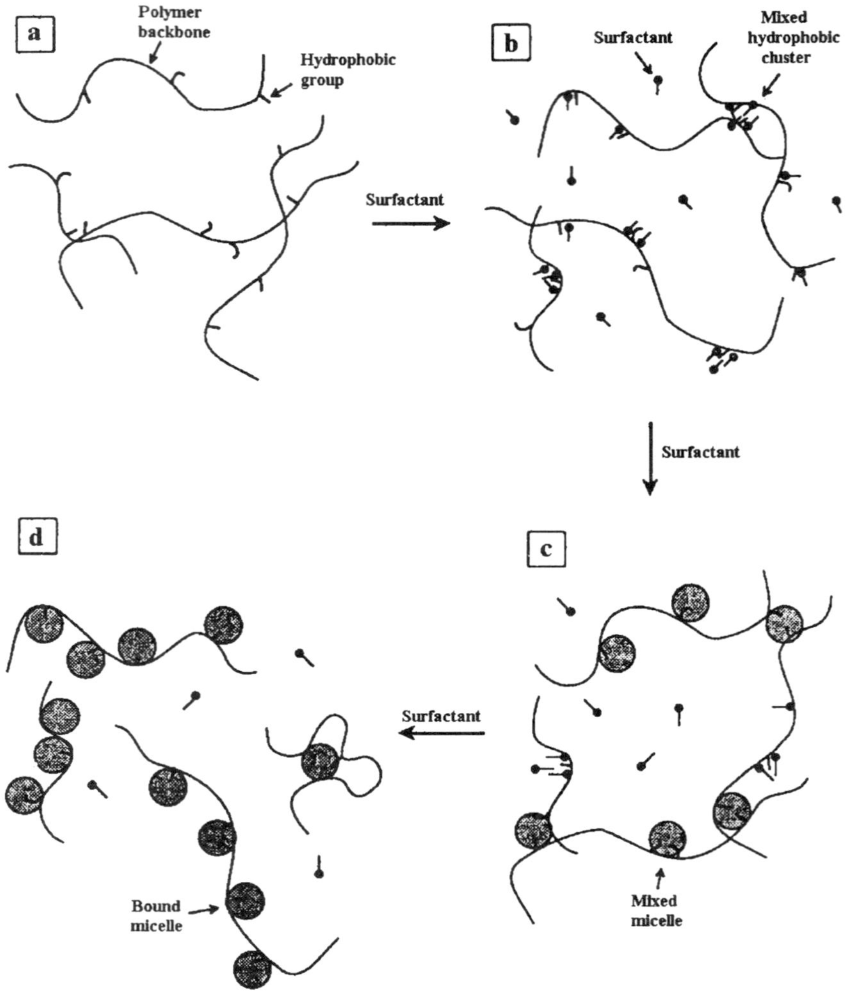

Figure 28 Schematic representation of the association process between HMPA and a cationic surfactant: (a) HMPA solution in the absence of surfactant; (b) the same solution as in (a) but in the presence of a low amount of surfactant, C < cac; (c) more surfactant is added, C > cac. Mixed micelles are formed, leading to the cross-linking of the polymer chains. (d) Further addition of surfactant results in the formation of mixed micelles with a low content of polymer alkyl groups and of micelles free of alkyl groups bound electrostatically onto the polymer backbone. The system approaches the phase separation limit. (Reprinted with permission from Ref. 77. Copyright 1994 American Chemical Society.)

surfactant bundles known as a ''coacervate.'' This is particularly true if the surfactant and the polymer have opposite charges, although formation of coacervates of nonionic polymers and surfactants are not uncommon.

Further addition of surfactant results in each polymer hydrophobe associating with its own surfactant micelle and the solution viscosity diminishing as the cross-linking breaks down (Fig. 28d). Two-phase systems may or may not return to homogeneous mixtures, depending on the nature of the surfactant and polymer. As more surfactant is added, the micelles no longer remain spherical, but will begin to form the branched structures shown in the upper portions of Figure 25. The literature on the interaction of hydrophobic polymers in surfactant solutions containing rod-like and branching micelles is, however, sparse (28,29,32).

The majority of research on associative polymers has been in the coatings area where surfactants are used to stabilize latex particles. Typically, the concentration of surfactant in these systems is low (near the cmc of the surfactant) and surfactant micelles are spherical. Increasing the surfactant concentration drives the micelles to rod-like and branched network configurations where the effect of associative polymers is less clear. Recent work that investigated the effect of non–hydrophobically modified PEO and PPO polymers on oleate surfactant solutions suggests that these polymers cause rod-like surfactant micelles to collapse into spherical micelles (32). The reason for the transition is not understood. Complicating the picture by attaching hydrophobic groups to the polymers makes examination of these systems even more difficult. However, such questions need to be answered if more effective associative thickeners are to be designed.

Figure 29 schematically represents two possible ''associative'' mechanisms that might occur when associative thickener is added to a concentrated surfactant solution containing rod-like or branching micelles. The associative thickener in **A** is intercalated into the rod-like micelles. Here it acts as a cross-linker for the viscoelastic, surfactant micelles. Thickening is provided by both the rod-like micelles and the entangled associa-

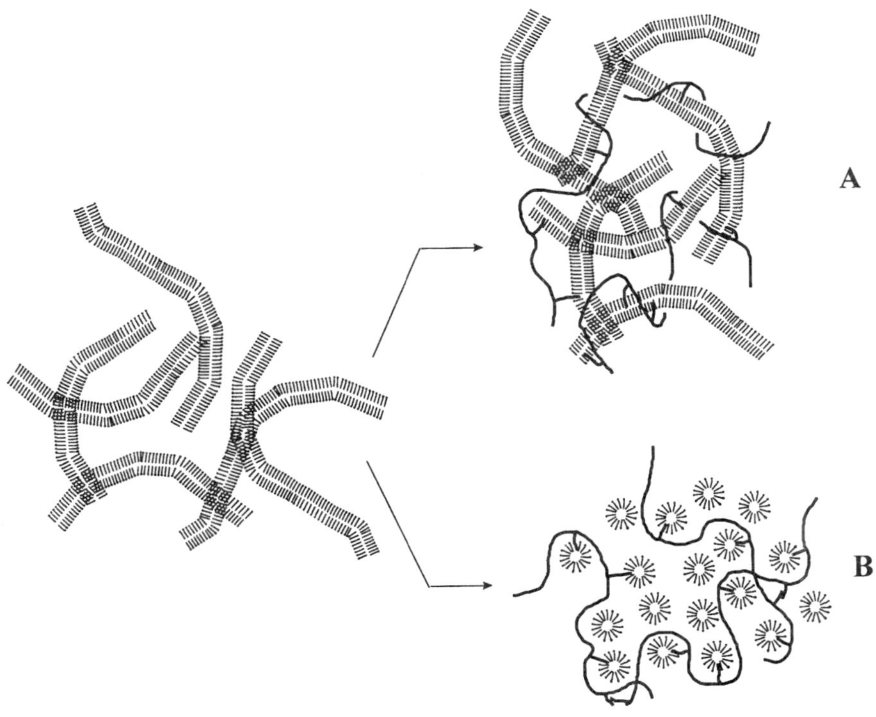

Figure 29 Effect on surfactant micelle morphology by addition of a hydrophobically modified associative polymer.

Table 3 Various Hydrophobically Modified, Acrylate-Based Associative Thickeners

Structure	INCI nomenclature	Ref.
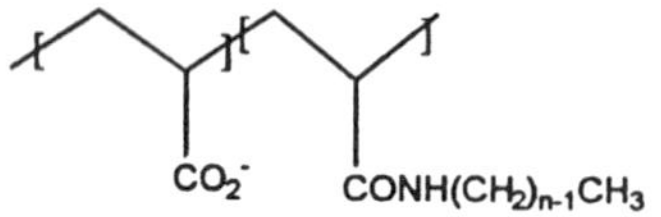		76,77,85–89
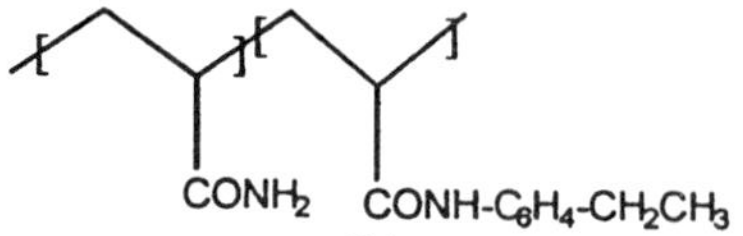		90,91
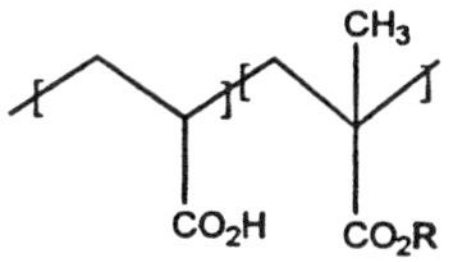	Acrylates/C10–30 alkyl acrylate crosspolymer	52–60,73,75,78–83,92,93

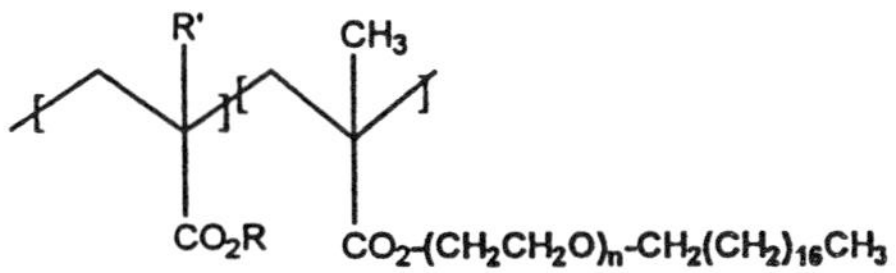	Acrylates/steareth-20 methacrylate copolymer	97
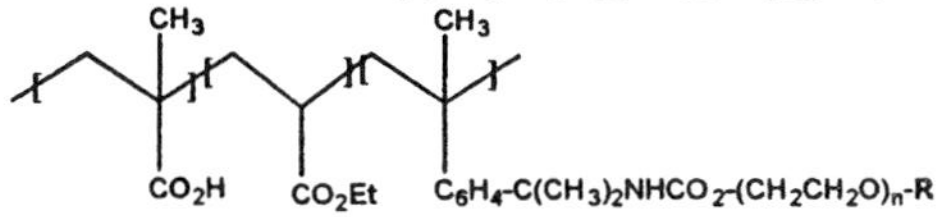		71,84,94,95,98
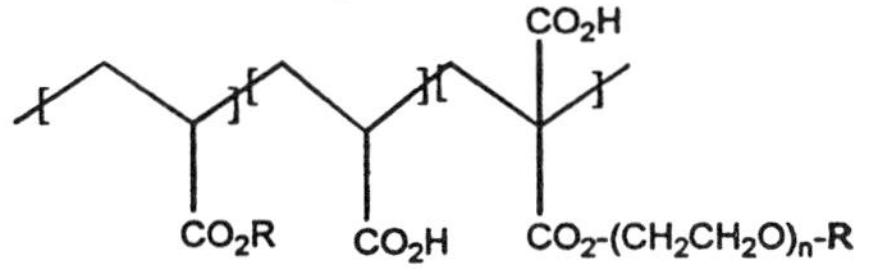	Acrylates/steareth (or ceteth)-20 itaconate copolymer	96
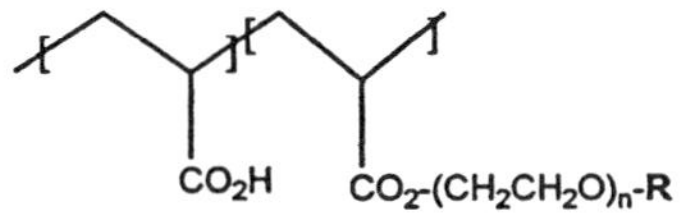	Acrylates/steareth-50 acrylate copolymer	97
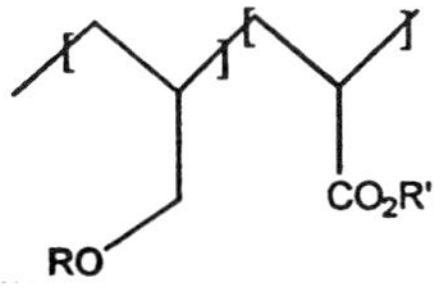	Steareth-10 allyl ether/acrylate copolymer	62

tive polymer, the polymer acting as a polymeric cross-linker for the surfactant micelles. The associative polymer in **B** has caused the rod-like micelles to collapse into spherical micelles (which typically impart Newtonian viscosity) and thickening is provided strictly by the surfactant micelle-cross-linked associative polymers.

The power of such polymers to stabilize emulsions is more easily imagined if each micelle in Figure 28c, surrounds an oily droplet on an emulsion. In this case, the polymer actually becomes part of the emulsion, in contrast to the case of a swollen microgel surrounding emulsified droplets as seen in Figure 22 for cross-linked acrylate thickeners. One might imagine that if a hydrophobically modified polymer were also carefully cross-linked to form microgels, the effects might be synergistic.

a. Hydrophobically Modified Acrylate Associative Thickeners. Professor Robert Lochhead has supplied an extensive encyclopedia of cosmetic polymers used in cosmetics (see Appendix) and has reported extensively on the incorporation of hydrophobically modified, acrylate-based associative thickeners in personal care (55–59,73,75,78–83). The personal care industry has grown to accept the use of acrylate-based associative thickeners and their many functional attributes. However, many research groups are investigating the potential of these types of thickeners.

Table 3 lists several of the hydrophobic acrylate-based polymers currently being investigated. This list can be broken down into two categories, separated by the horizontal line through the table. Hydrophobic acrylates in the upper portion (page 244) have their hydrophobic entity in close proximity to the acrylate backbone. Those in the lower (page 245) portion of the table have their hydrophobic entity separated from the acrylate backbone by a polyether (typically polyethylene oxide) chain. While the presence of the polyether chain is not required for an associative mechanism to operate, it has been demonstrated that its presence can influence viscosity (84). In particular, nonionic surfactants that themselves contain polyether chains seem to have a particular attraction to the polyether chains of the associative thickener.

The nature of the acrylate backbone is controlled by the chemist's imagination and the availability of specific monomers. Some of the polymers are recognized by the cosmetic industry and have INCI designations; others are not recognized. However, all scientific roads must lead to Rome and articles unrelated to personal care cannot be ignored since technology overlap has been a trend.

Recently, it has been found that hydrophobic modification of an acrylate copolymer can help to minimize polyelectrolyte complex formation in the presence of a hydrophobically modified cationic polymer (88). This result is significant: it suggests that stable formulations of anionic and cationic polymers can be made if the powerful, ionic attraction of these polymers is sterically shielded by the hydrophobes. Generally speaking, when cationic and anionic polymers are mixed in solution, regardless of their relative concentrations, a neutral polyelectrolyte complex (PEC) will precipitate. The remaining polymer, whether anionic or cationic, typically resides in the aqueous phase. Hydrophobic modification alleviates this effect. In cosmetic applications, this could have implications where there is a desire to incorporate cationic conditioning polymers (Section IV) into clear gels thickened with an anionic acrylate polymer.

b. Hydrophobically Modified, Cationic Acrylate Associative Thickeners. Recent discussion of a cationic acrylate associative thickener that functions more comfortably in acidic pH has shown the versatility of the associative concept (99,100). This new, lightly cross-linked copolymer is comprised of acrylate esters, tertiary amino acrylates, and a

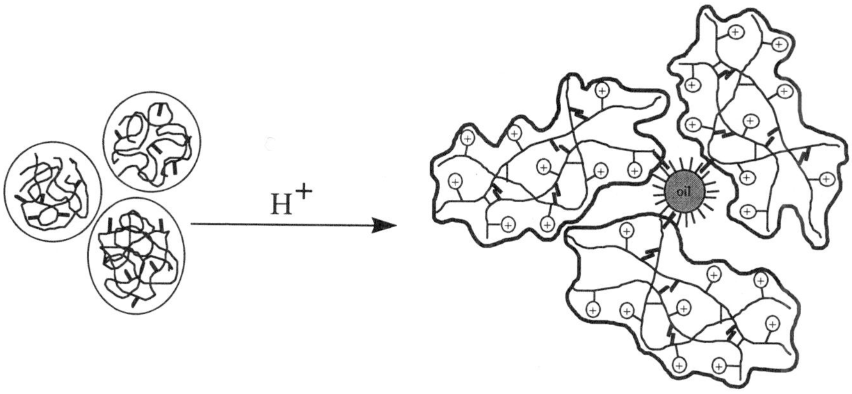

Figure 30 Schematic representation of swollen, cross-linked, hydrophobically modified, cationic acrylate thickener stabilizing an emulsified oil droplet.

small percentage of hydrophobically modified associative monomers. The copolymer is designed to swell and entangle by formation of cationic charges that develop along the copolymer backbone when the tertiary amine groups become protonated as occurs in acidic mediums (Fig. 30). Once swollen, the polymer hydrophobes interact as described above for the anionic associative thickeners. It appears, however, that in the presence of surfactants, the associative effects can cause entanglement to occur even at alkaline pH where the polymer is not specifically designed to uncoil. The associative effects apparently are capable of overcoming the lack of intrapolymeric cationic charge repulsion afforded by the acidic environment.

c. Hydrophobically Modified Polyether Associative Thickeners. One of the first families of hydrophobically modified polyether associative thickeners was the hydrophobically modified ethoxylated urethanes (HEURs) (Fig. 31) (74,101–103). The HEURs are some of the most successful associative thickeners employed in the coatings industry. However, it is interesting that the use of these polymers in personal care has been minimal. This may be the result of their somewhat high cost. It might also be related to potential concerns about residual monomeric isocyanates that might be present in these thickeners. Isocyanates are known to be skin sensitizers.

The cosmetic industry has, instead, embraced hydrophobic polyethers end-capped by fatty acid esters (104–107). These associative thickeners are differentiated by their initiating monomers (Table 4). The initiators include some type of polyhydroxyl-containing molecule (e.g., sorbitan, pentaerythritol, glycols, or methylglucoside). To these multiple hydroxyl groups are attached polyether chains, typically polyethylene oxide, of various lengths some of which are then end-capped with fatty acid ester moieties.

In the presence of dilute surfactant concentrations above their cmc, the hydrophobically modified polyethers complex with the surfactants by intercalating their hydrophobic endgroups into the surfactant micelles (Fig. 32). Some of the remaining hydrophobes

$$\mathbf{R}\text{-HN(O)C-O-}(CH_2CH_2O)_n\text{-C(O)NH-}\mathbf{R}$$

Figure 31 Generalized structure of hydrophobically modified ethoxylated urethanes (HEURs).

Table 4 Hydrophobically Modified Polyether Associative Thickeners

Generalized structure	INCI designation
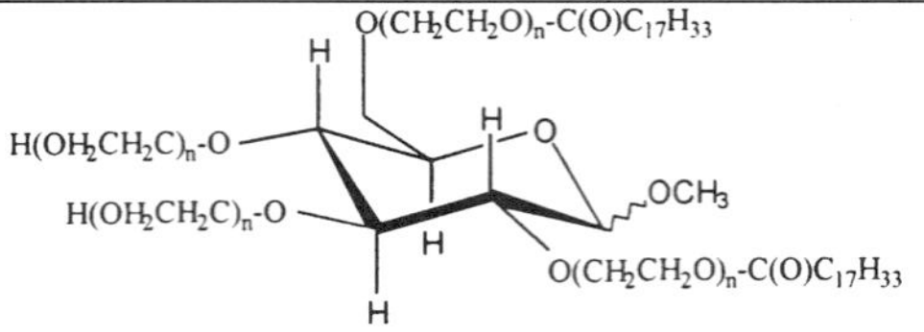	PEG-120-methylglucose dioleate
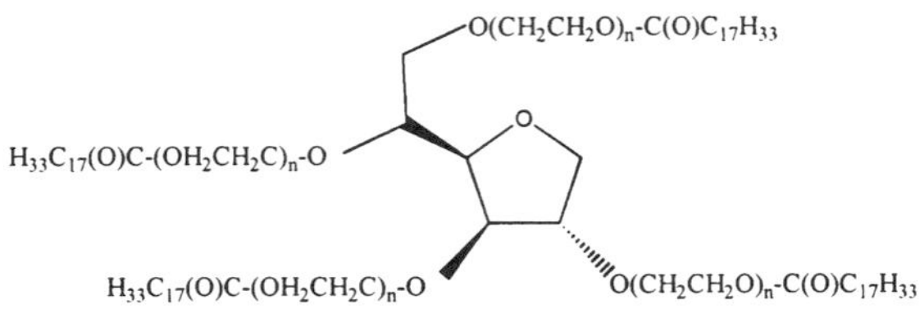	PEG-N(40 or 60) sorbitan tetraoleate
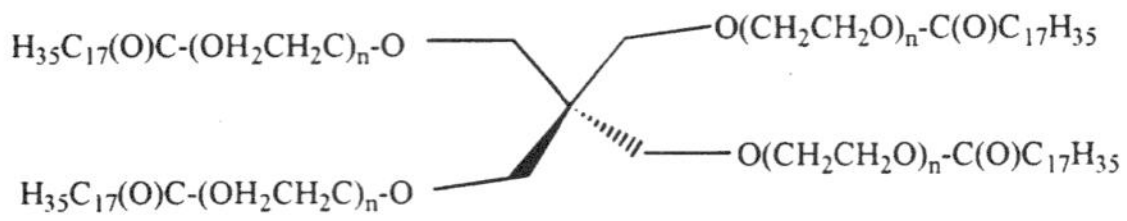	PEG-150 pentaerythrityl tetrastearate
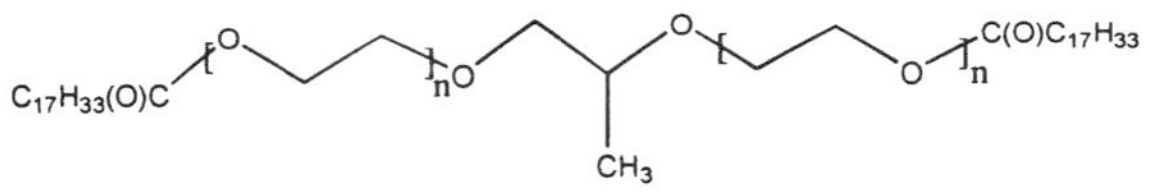	PEG-55 propylene glycol oleate
$H_{35}C_{17}C(O)\text{-}O\text{-}(H_2CH_2CO)_n\text{-}C(O)C_{17}H_{35}$	PEG-150 distearate

self-associate to form an expanded network. This builds viscosity and may confer a yield value to these formulations.

In more concentrated surfactant solutions where rod-like and branched micelles exist, theoretical descriptions of these associative thickeners are lacking. What is clearly understood is that the nature of the surfactants profoundly influences the rheology of personal care formulations (105–107). Factors that influence the electrical environment of the formulation, such as salt and pH, also affect the behavior of these thickeners. Unfortunately, the lack of understanding typically means that formulators must use trial and error to develop stable formulations.

III. FIXATIVE POLYMERS

A. Introduction

Hair fixative polymers do exactly what their name implies: they fix the hair in place. But the science of creating a suitable hair fixative system, simple in statement, is complex in practice. Traditionally, hair fixative polymers have been applied to the hair as liquids (hair sprays, setting lotions), gels, and foams (mousses). Each delivery vehicle has it own unique requirements, and these are addressed only when they place restrictions on the polymers.

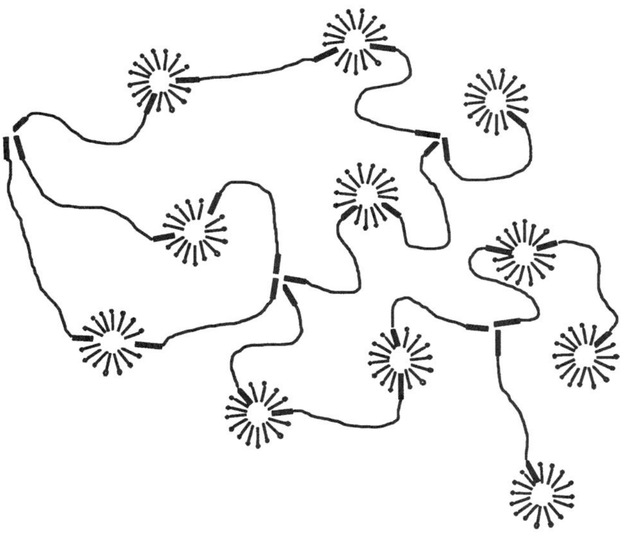

Figure 32 Association of end-capped, hydrophobically modified polyethers with themselves and surfactant micelles.

The polymers that function as hair fixatives have evolved over many years of practical application. Table 5 lists most of the commercially available polymers that have been or are being used in hair fixative products. Most of these resins are addition polymers made by copolymerizing acrylate monomers (Table 1). Very few homopolymers are present. This is not surprising because the development of acceptable hairspray resins is a subtle balance of molecular weight, monomer composition, and functional groups grafted onto the molecule. The solubility and glass transition temperature (T_g) are balanced for the polymer's primary function of coating and fixing the hair with the need to remove it from the hair. The list includes a few condensation polyesters (the Eastman resins).

B. Evolving Aerosol Legislation

Most of the fixative polymers in Table 5 were designed to operate in delivery systems that employ organic solvents to dissolve and apply them. The premiere solvent at one time was methylene chloride, CH_2Cl_2. Because of some toxicological concerns, however, it has disappeared from personal care applications (108). In addition, the use of chlorofluorocarbons (CFCs) as propellants abruptly ceased when they were implicated in the breakdown of the planet's ozone layer (108,109).

These fixative polymers were designed to dissolve in these solvents. The critical performance parameters included polymer/solvent compatibility, polymer tackiness, polymer adhesion to the hairshaft, and the polymer's glass transition temperature (T_g), which influenced the ''feel'' of the resin on the hair as well as its ability to hold the hair in a given style. The history of these fixative systems and polymers is well reviewed (110–117).

In 1973, the Congress of the United States of America passed the Clean Air Act in an attempt to legislate the improvement of air quality around major metropolitan areas of the country. In 1990, it was revised and updated, at which time focus turned toward consumer products as one of the many sources of air-damaging pollutants. Congress also

Table 5 Commercially Available Hair Fixative Polymers

INCI polymer name	Trade name	Company	Form
Acrylates copolymer	*Amerhold DR-25*	Amerchol	ADR-25% solids
VA/crotonates/vinyl neodecanoate	*Resyn 28-2930*	National Starch	Beads
Octylacrylamide/acrylates copolymer	Versacryl-40	National Starch	Powder
Octylacrylamide/acrylates/butylaminoethyl methacrylates copolymer	*Amphomer LV-71*	National Starch	Powder
Octylacrylamide/acrylates/butylaminoethyl methacrylates copolymer	Amphomer 28-4910	National Starch	Powder
Octylacrylamide/acrylates/butylaminoethyl methacrylates copolymer LMW	*Lovocryl 47*	National Starch	Powder
Acrylates/octylacrylamide copolymer	Versatyl-42	National Starch	Powder
VA/Crotonates copolymer	Resyn 28-1310	National Starch	Beads
Acrylates copolymer	*Balance 0/55*	National Starch	ADR-50% solids
VA/butyl maleate/isobornyl acrylate copolymer	*Advantage CP*	ISP	Alcohol soln
VA/butyl maleate/isobornyl acrylate copolymer LMW	*Advantage V*	ISP	Alcohol soln
Butyl ester of PVM/MA copolymer	Gantrez ES-425	ISP	Alcohol soln
Butyl ester of PVM/MA copolymer LMW	*Gantrez V-425*	ISP	Alcohol soln
Butyl ester of PVM/MA copolymer LMW	*Gantrez A-425*	ISP	
Ethyl ester of PVM/MA copolymer	Gantrez ES-225	ISP	Alcohol soln
Ethyl ester of PVM/MA copolymer LMW	*Gantrez V-225*	ISP	Alcohol soln
Ethyl ester of PVM/MA copolymer	Gantrez SP-215	ISP	Alcohol soln
PVP	PVP K series	ISP	Pwd or Aq soln
PVP/dimethylaminoethyl methacrylate copolymer	Copolymer 845	ISP	Alc or Aq soln
PVP/VA	PVP/VA	ISP	Alcohol soln

Vinylcaprolactam/PVP/dimethylaminoethyl methacrylate copolymer	*Gaffix VC-713*	ISP	Alc soln or pwd
Vinylcaprolactam/PVP/dimethylaminoethyl methacrylate copolymer	*H_2OLD EP-1*	ISP	Alc soln or pwd
PCP/DMAPA acrylates copolymer	*Styleze CC-10*	ISP	10% aqueous sol
Acrylates/acrylamide copolymer	*Ultrahold 8*	BASF	Powder
VA/crotonates copolymer	Luviset CA	BASF	Beads
VA/crotonates/vinylpropionate copolymer	Luviset CAP	BASF	Beads
Acrylates copolymer	*Luvimer 100P*	BASF	Powder
Acrylates copolymer	*Luvimer 36D*	BASF	ADR-36% solids
PVP	Luviskol K	BASF	Pwd or aq soln
PVP/acrylates copolymer	Luviflex VBM 35	BASF	Alcohol soln
PVP/VA copolymer	Luviskol VA	BASF	Alcohol soln
PVP/VA/vinyl propionate copolymer	Luviskol VAP	BASF	Alcohol soln
Polyvinylcaprolactam	Luviskol Plus	BASF	Alcohol sol
Polyquaternium-46	*Luviquat Hold*	BASF	20% aqueous sol
Methacryloyl ethyl betaine/methacrylates co-polymer	*Diaformer*	Sandoz	Alcohol soln
AMP-acrylates copolymer	*Diahold A-503*	Sandoz	Alcohol soln
Diglycol/cyclohexanedimethanol/isophthalates/sulfoisophthalates	*AQ- 38S*	Eastman	Pellets
Diglycol/cyclohexanedimethanol/isophthalates/sulfoisophthalates	*AQ-55S*	Eastman	Pellets
Diglycol/cyclohexanedimethanol/isophthalates/sulfoisophthalates	*AQ-48 Ultra*	Eastman	Pellets
Acrylates/hydroxyacrylates copolymer	*Acudyne 255*	Rohm & Haas	ADR-41% solids

Table 6 Current and Pending Aerosol Regulatory Requirements

State	Year	Required regulation
California	*Current* 1993	80% VOC
New York	1994	80% VOC
Connecticut	1996	80% VOC
Rhode Island	1996	15% VOC reduction
Massachusetts	1995	80% VOC
New Jersey	1996	80% VOC
Oregon	1996	80% VOC
California	*Pending* Mid-1999	55% VOC
New York	Mid-1999	55% VOC
Connecticut	Mid-1999	55% VOC
Texas	Mid-1999	55% VOC
New Jersey	Mid-1999	55% VOC

gave individual states more authority to enforce clean air legislation. In response to these revisions, the California Air Resources Board (CARB) began to focus on the problem of volatile organic compounds (VOCs) as a source of ozone-generating species. The legislation controlling VOCs is an evolving document. Information concerning it can be accessed on the Internet at *http://members.aol.com/spraytec/index.htm* (118).

A direct chemical relationship between the level of stratospheric ozone and many types of VOCs has been demonstrated (109,110). Although ozone in the upper atmosphere is necessary for humankind's survival, in the stratosphere above major metropolitan areas it is a primary cause of industrial ''smog.'' The CARB, responding to this concern, mandated in 1991 that any organic compound with a vapor pressure greater than 0.1 mmHg at 20°C or any organic compound whose vapor pressure was unknown and that contained less than 13 carbon atoms was a VOC. This legislation has led to a rapid acceptance of CARB requirements by several densely populated regions. The mandates affect the entire coatings industry of which personal care products are only a very small segment. Especially affected are fixative products delivered from aerosol containers. Table 6 shows many of the existing and pending changes that the aerosol industry faces in the very near future.

The initial response of the aerosol industry was to cull the large list of excluded materials and find solvents and propellants that fit the CARB criteria. In the years since the 1991 California mandates, several select solvents and propellants have risen from the vast collection of undesirables. These popular ingredients are listed in Table 7.

Table 7 Acceptable Low-VOC Solvents and Propellants

Solvents	Propellants
Water	Gases
Alcohol	Air, N_2, CO_2
Ethanol, 2-propanol	Hydrocarbons
Hydrocarbons	Butane, isobutane, propane
Butane, isobutane, propane	Dimethylether
Dimethylether	Hydrofluorocarbon
Dimethoxymethane	

The industry has responded by developing innovative aerosol spray systems that reduce VOC emissions (119–122). All these changes have had a major impact on the primary hair-care ingredient, the fixative polymers (123–125). These had to be made more lipophilic to dissolve in the more hydrocarbon-solvent-based aerosol formulations. Although minor adjustments accommodated the requirement for 80% VOC products, the impending requirement for 55% VOCs by mid-1999 is another matter entirely. Such a drastic change requires similarly profound changes in the way both manufacturers and consumers perceive personal care aerosol products. What effects are these drastic changes having on the nature of the hair-care polymers?

C. Challenges for Low-VOC Fixative Products

The easiest and most cost effective means of reducing VOCs is to remove the organic solvents and replace them with water. Unfortunately, this change creates a new set of challenges. When a solvent-based polymer is applied to the hair, the solvent and polymer quickly spread over the lipophilic hair shaft, coating the hair and creating the spot- and seam-welds that hold the hair in place (106,116,126). The spreading is a function of the surface energy (i.e., measured by the contact angle) of the lipophilic solvent in contact with the lipophilic hair shaft (Fig. 33). This figure also shows the factors that impact the hair fixative polymer as it spreads and dries. The application of mousses and gels is a more mechanical process because the polymers are hand-rubbed into the hair. These systems do not rely as much on the sole ability of the polymers to migrate to the hair junctions by flowing along the hairshaft (116).

Regardless of the application method the development of hold requires solvent evapo-

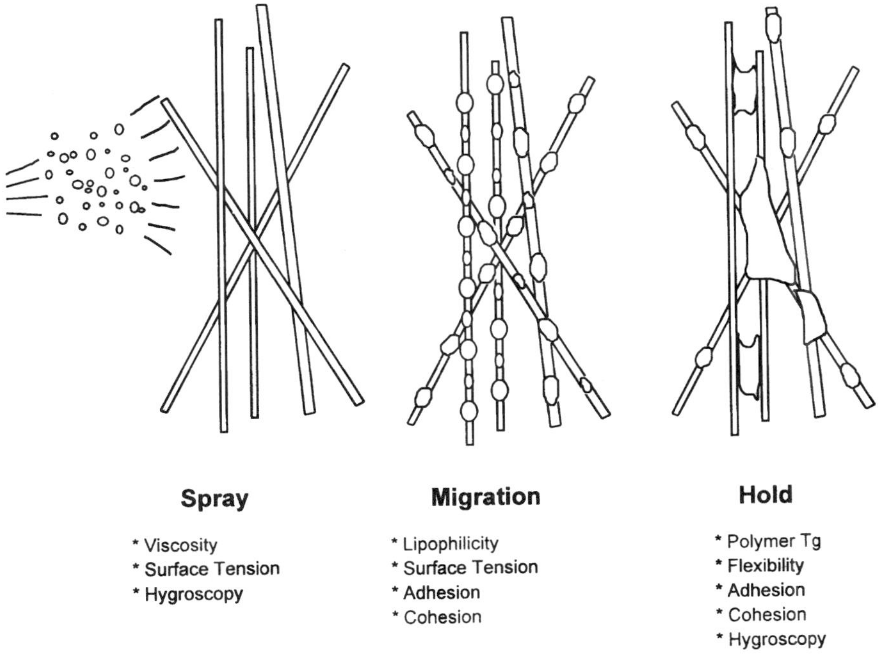

Figure 33 Application of solvent-based hairspray to the hair.

ration, which was a rapid process when hair products were rich in VOCs. As formulations incorporate more water, this is no longer the case. Water evaporates at a rate of 3.6 $\times$ 10^{-5} kg/m^2/sec at room temperature in still air (127). This is considerably slower than the evaporation of any of the solvents in Table 7. In addition, water is an excellent plasticizer for the proteins that comprise hair and will cause hair to soften and droop (128). Also, since water has a higher specific gravity than alcohol, it will weigh the hair down more. These factors are responsible for accentuating a negative attribute termed ''initial curl droop,'' which is defined as the amount of extension that occurs in a curl droop test in the first 6 min.

The presence of even small amounts of water increases the interpolymeric hydrogen bonding in the acrylate-based, solvent-soluble polymers. This leads to improved chain entanglement, which generates higher viscosities in the polymer solutions (126,129–133). One way to minimize these effects is to reduce the polymer's molecular weight. This has been one approach used by a number of polymer manufacturers to improve the water compatibility of their fixative polymers. However, reduced molecular weight adversely affects critically important film-forming properties like tensile modulus or film strength. Another method has been to incorporate oleaginous monomers into polymers that are generally water-soluble, such as the incorporation of silicone-based monomers into acrylate backbones, to help aid in lowering the surface tension of polymers in aqueous solution.

Film strength is influenced by polymer chain entanglement, which is, itself, influenced by the molecular weight of the polymers. Clearly, care must be taken to balance viscosity requirements with film strength when molecular weight reduction is used to address VOC issues. Water can also seriously affect the integrity of the aerosol delivery device. These adverse effects are usually manifest as corrosion of the aerosol can or pump valve assembly (107,134,135).

1. Waterborne Fixatives/Aqueous Dispersion Resins

In the coatings industry, traditional solvent-based paints are being replaced by waterborne coatings, which are one of two types, water-soluble or water-dispersed (136). Figure 34 shows the general relationship of polymer solids level to viscosity for waterborne systems. The horizontal dashed line in the figure shows that, at the critical application viscosity, waterborne emulsions and dispersions can be applied at higher solids levels than the solution polymer of corresponding viscosity.

Waterborne emulsion and dispersion technology is finding its way into the personal care industry (126,133,137–140). The technology is based on the formation of water-insoluble polymer ''packets'' or particles suspended in an aqueous solution. These two-phase heterogeneous mixtures are colloidal suspensions (Fig. 35). Each particle contains millions of high-molecular-weight fixative polymer chains and each particle is surrounded by a monolayer of surfactant molecules. In the case of an anionic surfactant, this layer provides a net negative charge at the surface of all the particles and leads to electrostatic stabilization of the particle suspension. Their small size (usually tenths of a micron) prevents the particles from combining and polymers in neighboring particles from entangling. Several polymer manufacturers have developed aqueous dispersion polymers, also known as latexes, for hair care applications (Table 8). One of the challenges of this technology is elimination of the residual unreacted monomers, which impart an objectionable odor. Also, residual monomer is an important issue from a safety-in-use perspective.

The appearance of a colloidal suspension and its distinction from a homogeneous solution is shown in Figure 36. The polymer solution (A) is comprised of a commercial

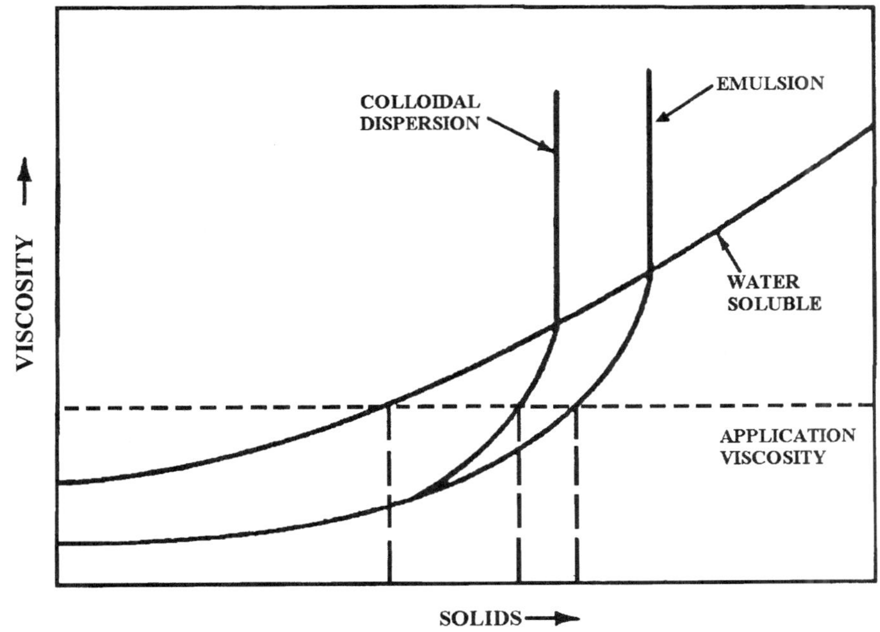

Figure 34 Relationship of viscosity to solids content in waterborne systems. (Reprinted with permission from Ref. 136.)

fixative resin dissolved in a low VOC solvent. The colloid system (B) was made by adding a dispersion hair fixative polymer to a low-VOC solvent. Although clear in diffuse, ambient light conditions, solution B is one of highly swollen polymer particles that still maintain their identity. These particles give rise to Tyndall scattering in the presence of focused light (laser) as seen in Figure 36 (141).

The subject of film formation from waterborne aqueous dispersion resins or latices

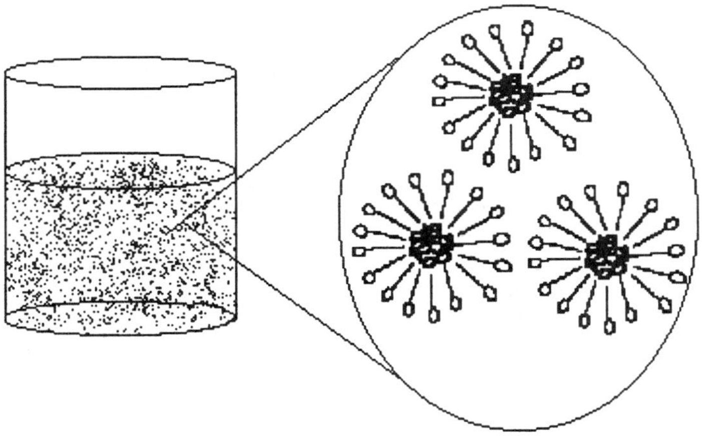

Figure 35 Waterborne aqueous dispersion polymers.

Table 8 Commercial Waterborne Aqueous Dispersion Resins for the Personal Care Industry

INCI polymer name	Trade name	Company	Form
Acrylates copolymer	*Amerhold DR-25*	Amerchol	ADR-25% solids
Acrylates copolymer	*Balance 0/55*	National Starch	ADR-50% solids
Acrylates copolymer	*Luvimer 36D*	BASF	ADR-36% solids
Diglycol/cyclohexanedimethanol/ isophthalates/sulfoisophthalates	*AQ-38S*	Eastman	Pellets
Diglycol/cyclohexanedimethanol/ isophthalates/sulfoisophthalates	*AQ-55S*	Eastman	Pellets
Diglycol/cyclohexanedimethanol/ isophthalates/sulfoisophthalates	*AQ-48 Ultra*	Eastman	Pellets
Acrylates/hydroxyacrylates copolymer	*Acudyne 255*	Rohm & Haas	ADR-41% solids

is a topic of intense recent investigation (142–151). It is generally thought that film formation from a waterborne dispersion passes through several "stages," as shown in Figure 37. Stages I–III involve the evaporation of the surrounding solvent from the intact latex particles. At stage III, evaporation is slowed considerably because of the close packing of the latex particles. Stage IV, the last, represents final film formation.

Stage III is considered to be the most critical. Here, the solids content of the dispersion reaches 60–80% and the polymers coalesce and begin to sinter; i.e., polymer chains in adjoining particles begin to diffuse into one another. From the point of view of hair fixative systems, it is at stage III that the polymer begins to provide fixative effect.

One advantage of a waterborne hair fixative system is the rapid spreading that occurs

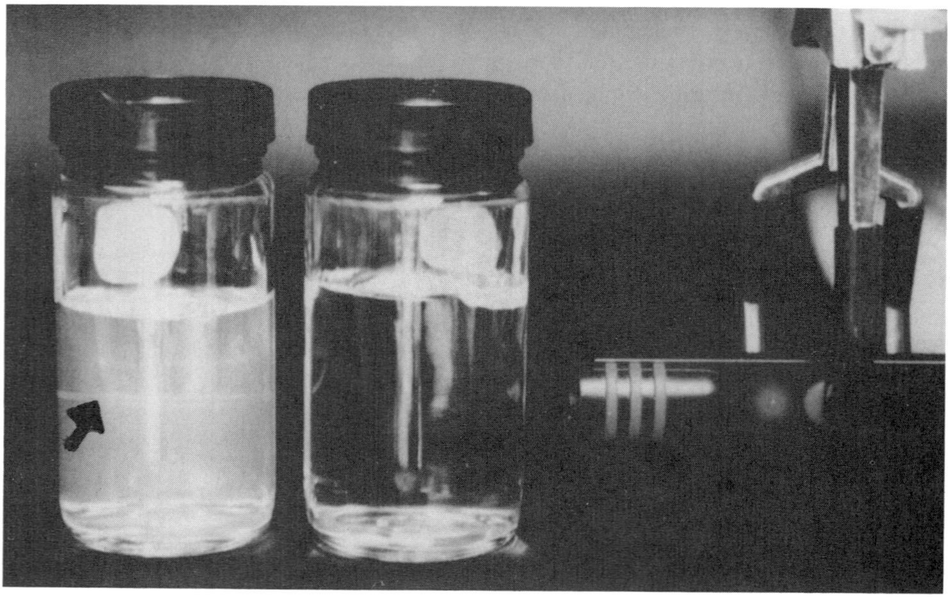

Figure 36 Demonstration of the Tyndall Effect on aqueous polymer dispersion. Arrow indicates faint line of visible laser light in the dispersed formulation (formula (B), left).

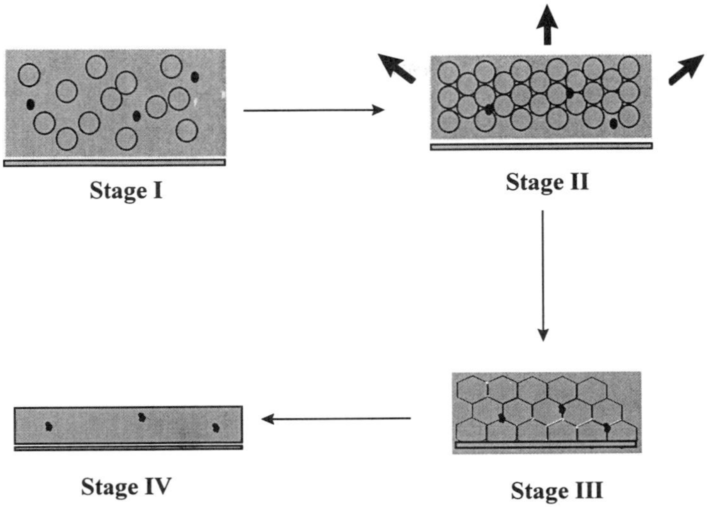

Figure 37 Model stages of polymer latex film drying. (Adapted from Ref. 147. Copyright 1995 American Chemical Society.)

when the water contacts the hair. As mentioned earlier, water plasticizes hair and causes it to droop. Interestingly, it appears that the evaporation rate of water from a latex film is relatively unaffected by the chemical nature of the latex resin. Drying occurs initially at the film/air interface although discussions of exactly how drying occurs are somewhat unresolved. In some cases, it has been suggested that a film forms on the surface of the latex droplets, which the remaining water must pass through to evaporate (147,148). Drying is relatively insensitive to the thickness of the film for this reason as well. However, the possibility of water evaporation occurring more rapidly at the edges of the developing film (especially in the presence of surfactants) has also been observed (149).

The drying mechanism that predominates appears to be dependent on many factors including the presence or absence of surfactant, polymer concentration, and whether or not a blend of a high T_g (good for rapid drying) and a low T_g (good for rapid spreading and film formation) polymer dispersion or only one intermediate T_g dispersion is used. It is speculated that film formation is also affected by the degree of neutralization of acid groups on the polymer chains, although little work has been done in this area (143). Intuitively, one might expect that greater neutralization will create some charge separation of the latex particles, which might slow sintering. At the very least, increasing the hydrophilicity of the polymer chains should make the removal of water more difficult throughout the drying stages.

Proper instrumentation to help understand the phenomena of drying is critical. The atomic force microscope (AFM) and environmental scanning electron microscope (ESEM) have been powerful tools useful in the investigation of latex film formation. Their application in hair fixative studies is overdue.

For waterborne dispersions the ability to deliver polymer particles to the hair near the critical 60–80% solids level will minimize the effects of water plasticization of the hair. As can be seen in Figure 34, however, waterborne dispersions rapidly gain viscosity as their solids level increases. In this regard, the more water evaporation that occurs during application the better. Atomization helps in this regard. The smaller the droplet size that exits the aerosol valve, the more rapidly will evaporation occur while the polymer travels to the hair. But, water, because of its high surface tension, resists the formation of small droplets (126). Addition of surface-active agents (i.e., surfactants and silicones) may help as long as they do not cause foaming at the actuator.

It is not unreasonable to expect that aqueous polymer dispersions will be effective in gels and mousses. Furthermore, the technology of hydrophobically modified acrylate thickeners discussed in Section II.A.3.a, useful for suspending latex particles, fits naturally into fixative gels.

IV. CONDITIONING POLYMERS

A. Introduction

The topic of hair and skin conditioning is complex and not easily covered by a short discussion of the polymers used to condition these surfaces. The very concept of ''conditioning'' is hard to define and describe, yet it is an important aspect to understand if one is to appreciate the benefits of conditioning polymers. Two recent reviews have attempted to summarize what it means when consumers talk about the condition of their hair and skin (152,153). It is generally accepted that conditioning describes the perceived benefits a consumer receives from a personal care product when it is applied to the hair or skin. These benefits manifest themselves in the way the hair and skin feel, look, shine, and so forth after the consumer applies a particular product.

Several chapters in this book address polymers useful as conditioning agents for the hair and skin. These functionally unique materials include the synthetic polymers discussed in this chapter, silicone polymers discussed in Chapter 7, the polysaccharide polymers discussed in Chapter 8, and the proteins discussed in Chapter 9. Most commercially available personal care products contain one or more of these critical ingredients (154,155).

The conditioning polymers discussed in these chapters are effective skin and hair modifiers because they are designed to deposit, adhere, adsorb, or absorb to proteinaceous elements of the hair and skin. In the personal care industry, the term ''substantivity'' describes the binding of a material to these surfaces. To be effective conditioners, however, it is not sufficient for the materials simply to adhere to the skin and hair. They must contribute some attribute that the consumer perceives as beneficial to these surfaces. Indeed, conditioning effects are among the most important characteristics the consumer seeks when purchasing a personal care product.

This chapter covers two types of synthetic conditioning polymers, (1) cationic polymers and (2) nonionic polymers. The literature on cationic polymers is extensive. In addition to the polymers addressed in this section, the reader will find references to cationic polymers in the other chapters mentioned above. The prevalence of cationic conditioning polymers is not surprising. It follows from the fact that proteins that comprise the structural elements of hair and skin, that is collagen, keratin, elastin, and so forth, are anionic at the normal physiological pH of the human body (156). Consequently, the attraction of cationic conditioners to these surfaces is greatly enhanced by powerful electrostatic forces. Other types of attractive forces can stimulate polymer adhesion to these surfaces as well, including hydrogen bonding and van der Waals forces. These two forces help explain why many lipophilic and protein-like polymers can also function as conditioning materials. Examples of both are discussed in this section.

B. Synthetic Conditioning Polymers

1. Cationic Conditioning Polymers

The literature discussing synthetic cationic conditioning polymers and natural or seminatural cationic conditioning polymers typically overlaps. Readers interested in natural or seminatural cationic conditioning polymers are advised to read Chapters 8 and 9. The following discussion focuses on synthetic cationic conditioning polymers (excluding those that incorporate both cationic and silicone moieties). The Cosmetic, Toiletries, and Fragrance Association (CTFA) recognizes most cationic conditioning polymers under the label ''polyquaternium-X'' where ''X'' is simply sequentially chosen.

Table 9 shows the structure and INCI designation for many of the cosmetically useful synthetic, cationic, conditioning polymers. Figure 23 shows the structures of Polyquaternium-32 and 37, both of which can also function in a conditioning capacity. The structures are separated by the nature of the cationic moiety, which distinguishes each class of cationic polymer. It is clear that only a few monomers that carry cationic charge are currently employed in the industry. Most of the polymers are the product of addition polymerization reactions employing unique acrylate or vinyl monomers. However, Polyquaternium-2, -17, and -18 are condensation polymers, and poly(ethyleneimine), a new conditioning polymer currently devoid of an INCI designation, is the product of a ring-opening polymerization of aziridine, the nitrogen equivalent of ethylene oxide (157). The structures of these polymers is determined by the coreactivity of the monomers and the chemist's imagination.

A variety of terms, some of them confusing, are used in the patent and open literature to describe the ''amount'' of cationic charge on the cationic polymer. Table 10 lists three of the most common terms. The distinction of cationic nitrogen from other forms of noncationic nitrogen in these polymers is important. For instance, both Kjeldahl and combustion analysis, which report the combination of cationic nitrogen and other nitrogen, can be applied to Polyquaternium-7. Only the cationic nitrogen is, however, important in these charge calculations.

It is also important to realize that some nitrogen-containing monomers are cationic only if the formulation pH is sufficiently low to protonate the nitrogen group. As an example, Polyquaternium-16 is comprised of a quaternary vinyl imidazole monomer attached to the polymer backbone through a tertiary vinyl amine. Although the quaternary nitrogen is almost always positively charged, the tertiary nitrogen may or may not be, depending on the pH of the formulation. When calculating charge on this polymer, the formulator must consider that the tertiary nitrogen might contribute to the polymer's cationicity.

Cationic substitution (CS) is a dimensionless descriptor that tells the formulator something about the moles of cationic substituent per mole of polymer. Charge density is calculated from CS and defined as milliequivalents per gram (mEq/g). It describes the amount of cationic charge per gram of polymer. A polymer with a charge density in the range of 3–6 is highly charged. Poly(ethyleneimine) is reported to have a charge density of nearly 20 at pH 4.5 (157). Polymers with a charge density below 1.0 are lightly cationic.

There has been very little quantitative study of the deposition of synthetic polymers onto proteinaceous substrates (158–163). The most successful methods for measuring this have been radiolabeling and electrokinetic measurements (158,159,162,163). Radiolabel-

Table 9 Structure and INCI Designation or Chemical Name for Several Synthetic, Cationic, Conditioning Polymers

Structure	INCI designation
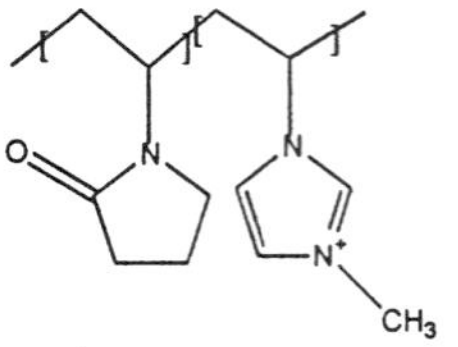	Polyquaternium-16
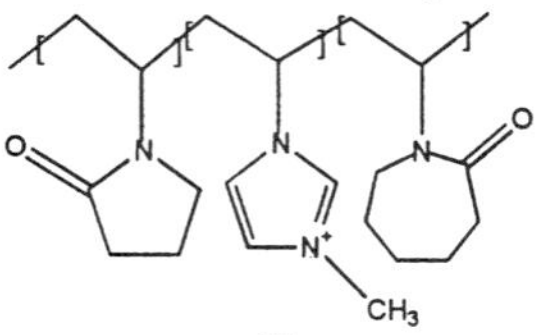	Polyquaternium-46
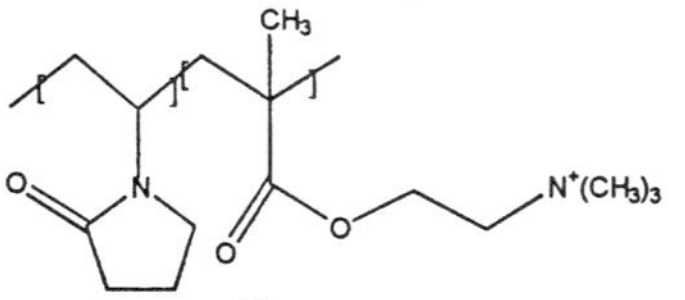	Polyquaternium-11
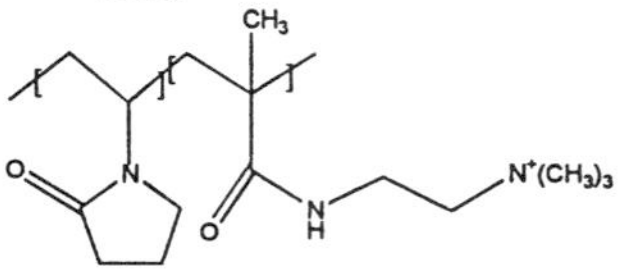	Polyquaternium-28
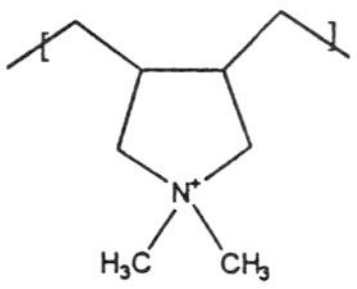	Polyquaternium-6
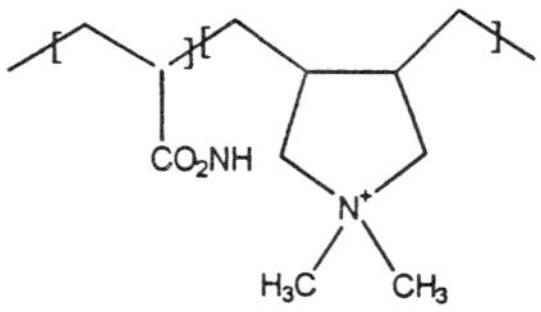	Polyquaternium-7
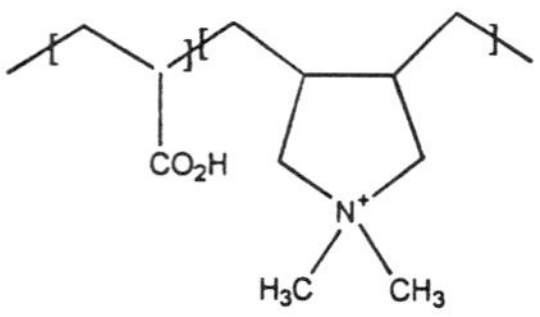	Polyquaternium-22
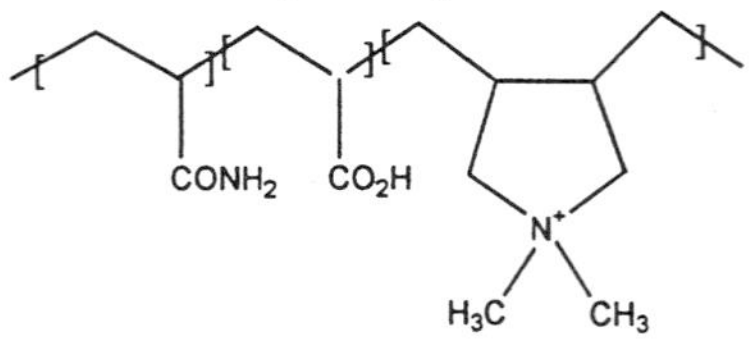	Polyquaternium-39

Table 9 Continued

Structure	INCI designation
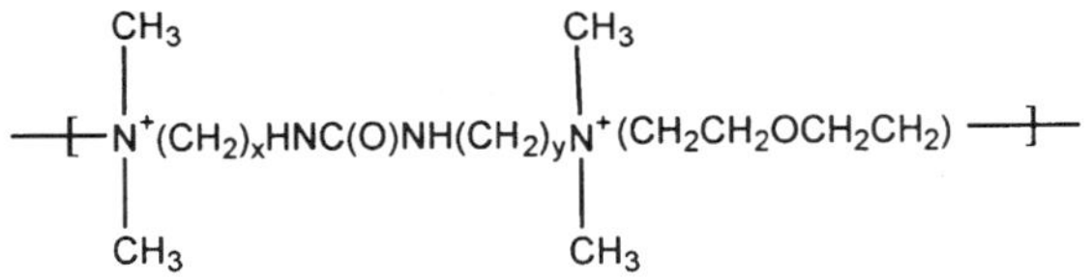	Polyquaternium-2
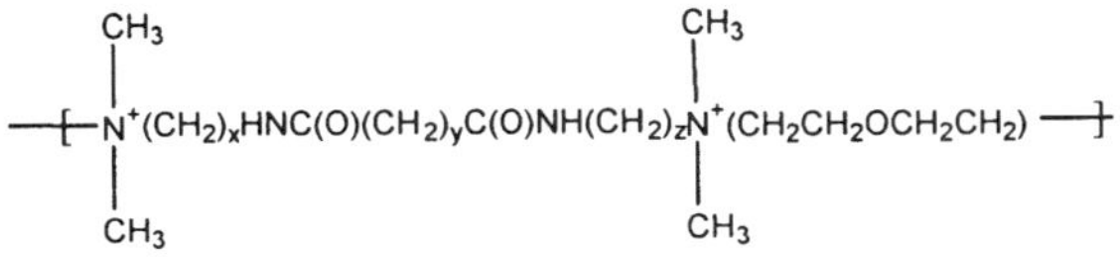	Polyquaternium-17 ($y = 4$)
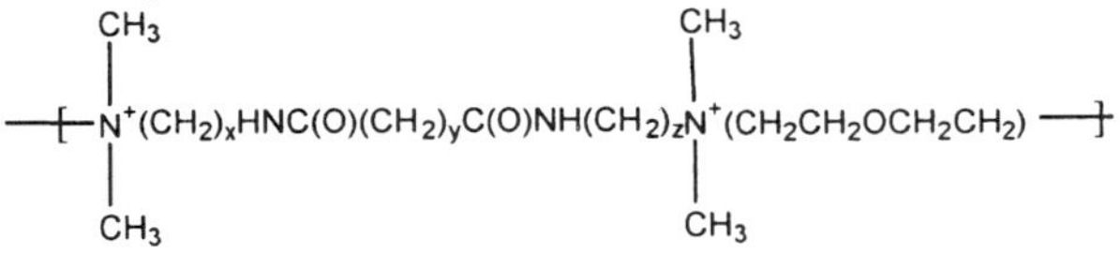	Polyquaternium-18 ($y = 7$)

Structure	Chemical name
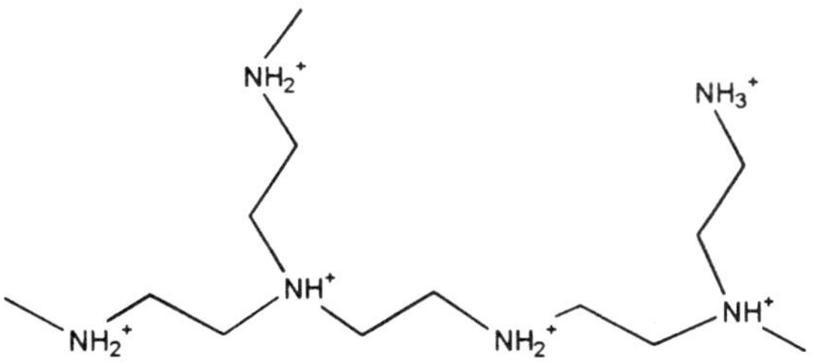	Polyethyleneimine

ing is particularly effective, but the use of radioactive polymers is discouraged in most research institutions. The signal-swamping effect from the amide and primary nitrogens that comprise the polypeptide proteins of hair and skin hinders several spectroscopic methods. Any technique employed to quantitate deposition must be able to exclude the results from these proteinaceous nitrogens. Despite these quantitative challenges, however, there is little question that cationic polymers have a strong affection for skin and hair.

More subjective analyses show that deposition of cationic polymers onto hair and skin elicits improvements in the structure and appearance of these surfaces (160,161,163–166). Such techniques, however, cannot distinguish, for example, the conditioning effect

Table 10 Methods for Describing Level of Cationic Charge on a Polymer

Descriptive term	Units	Mathematical calculation
% Cationic nitrogen	%	Determined by titration, Kjeldahl analysis, combustion analysis, or other analytical techniques
Cationic substitution (CS)	Dimensionless	$\frac{\text{\% Cationic nit} * \text{Mw}_{\text{monomer repeat unit}}}{(100\ \text{Mw}_{\text{cationic nitrogen}} - \text{Mw}_{\text{quat repeat unit}} * \text{\% N})}$
Charge density	mEq/g	$\frac{\text{CS} * 1000}{\text{Mw}_{\text{monomer repeat unit}} + \text{CS} * \text{Mw}_{\text{quat repeat unit}}}$

of a cationic polymer from that of a low-molecular-weight cationic conditioner. Careful control experiments are required to isolate effects from the polymer alone.

The cationic charge on a polymer affects its behavior considerably when surfactants are included in formulations. Cationic polymers (a member of the broader class of polymers termed polyelectrolytes) usually interact strongly with anionic surfactants, weakly with cationic surfactants, and unpredictably with nonionic and amphoteric surfactants (14,167–169). Anionic surfactant binds to cationic polymers at concentrations well below the critical micelle concentration (cmc). The low surfactant concentration where polymer and surfactant begin to interact is known as the critical aggregation concentration (cag).

As the anionic surfactant concentration increases, more of the polymer's cationic sites complex with surfactant. The developing charge forces polymer chains to elongate, which in turn improves chain entanglement. Also the developing surfactant micelles promote interpolymer cross-linking. This, together with the increased chain entanglement, causes an increase in viscosity. This effect is dependent on the concentration of the polymer, which must be in the concentrated regime. With the addition of even more surfactant, neutralization of the available cationic charge occurs and the polymer and surfactant will form a complex phase known as a coacervate. At the extreme, the polymer/surfactant complex may become water-insoluble and precipitate. These precipitates are termed ''polyelectrolyte complexes'' (PEC). The development of a surfactant/polymer coacervate or PEC depends on other factors including, for example, the chain length of surfactant hydrophobes and the presence of electrolytes such as salt.

It is felt that the presence of the polymer/surfactant coacervate is important for deposition of the polymer onto the anionic surfaces of hair and skin (159). It has been demonstrated that when a cationic polymer is deposited onto hair as a coacervate, subsequent rinsing removes the anionic surfactant more quickly than the bound polymer. In these electokinetic measurements, the overall charge of the hair gradually becomes more cationic. It should be kept in mind, also, that coacervate can form when a concentrated anionic surfactant solution containing a solubilized cationic polymer is diluted by the addition of water. This is the typical mode of application of conditioning shampoos to hair and skin during washing. The deposition occurs during the rinsing cycle and is appropriately termed ''dilution deposition.''

Polyelectrolyte complexes have found less practical applications in personal care, principally because they are so water-insoluble. However, they are extremely useful as drug delivery vehicles. Recently, it was demonstrated, for instance, that a PEC formed between polymers like Polyquaternium-6 and retinoic acid (vitamin D), a powerful skin exfoliating agent, helps to stabilize the labile vitamin, prolonging its chemical life and potentially increasing its potency (170).

The development of charge-neutral coacervate is linear in polymer and surfactant concentration (Fig. 38) (167). At surfactant concentrations beyond those required to neutralize the cationic polymer, the coacervate disappears and the surfactant usually, but not always, solubilizes the polymer. Polymers with higher charge density are more difficult to solubilize, and polyelectrolyte complexes will, typically, not redissolve. The behavior of cationic polymers in the presence of highly concentrated surfactant solutions, where the micelles are no longer spherical but instead can exist as rod-like and branching structures, has not been adequately addressed. In such a strongly anionic environment, the rheological influence of the cationic polymers is likely minimal. One possibility is that

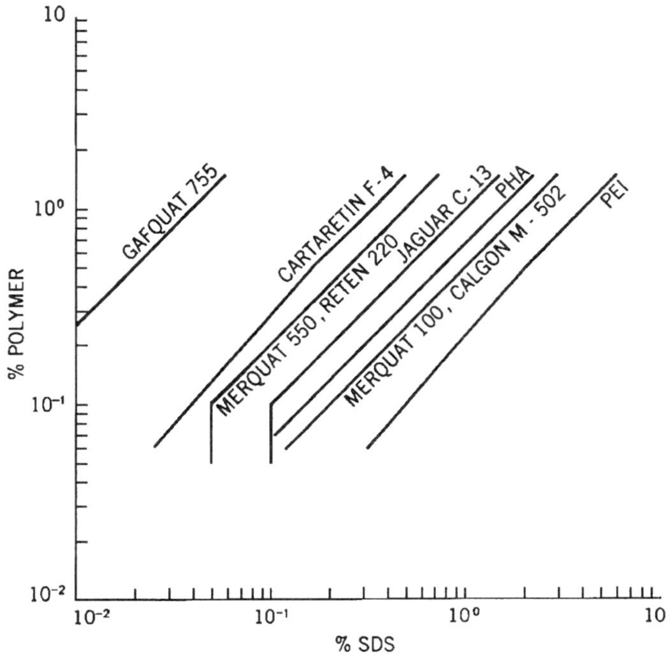

Figure 38 Partial solubility diagram of a series of polycation/sodium dodecyl sulfate systems. The lines correspond to conditions of maximum precipitation. (Reprinted with permission from Ref. 167.)

the cationic polymers adsorb to the rod-like micelles much as was described for the hydrophobically modified poly(acrylates) as seen in Figure 29.

2. *Nonionic Conditioning Polymers*

a. Poly(vinylpyrrolidone). PVP was mentioned previously for its thickening (Section II.A.1.e) and hair fixative (Section III.A) attributes. The cyclic amide functionality of the PVP pyrrolidone ring bears a strong resemblance to the amide polypeptide bonds that hold the proteins of hair and skin together. This similarity suggests that PVP will adsorb to the proteins of the hair and skin. It is generally felt that application of PVP films to the skin, especially, and also hair imparts a soft and silky feeling (42,171). The use of PVP in skin care formulations can allow reduced amounts of the oily conditioners required and leaves a less greasy feel.

b. Hydrogenated Poly(isobutene)s. The proteins that comprise hair and skin are chemically unique polymers. When they are present in a dried state, they are very hydrophobic; when fully wetted, they hydrate and are quite hydrophilic. This dual functionality is characteristic of oleaginous materials. Oleaginous polymers tend to spread quickly over the surface of hair and skin, driven primarily by their low surface tension on these protein substrates. Examples of widely used oleaginous conditioners are the silicone polymers discussed in Chapter 7.

Hydrogenated poly(isobutene)s (Fig. 39) are liquid polymers that possess oleaginous characteristics. Like the silicones, these liquid polymers spread quickly over the surface

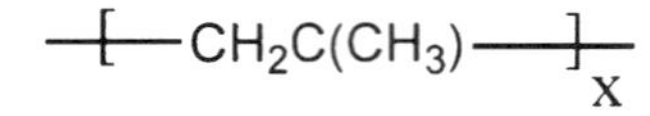

Figure 39 Structure of hydrogenated poly(isobutene)s.

of hair and skin. Once applied they impart softness and shine. They are, however, easily removed by surfactants so that, unlike mineral oil and other oily conditioners, they are easily washed off during shampooing and rinsing. These polymers are not used extensively as conditioners in personal care products.

V. ENCAPSULATION POLYMERS

A. Introduction

A greater understanding of the physiological factors that control the growth of skin and hair has resulted in the development of more powerful agents that manipulate their controlling influences. Particularly in the skin care arena, growth in the number of cosmetic products that affect healing, exfoliation, growth, and coloring has been explosive (172–177). Formulation systems required to deliver active materials to the skin and, in some cases, below it (i.e., transdermal) are complex and this has forced formulators to consider new methods of protecting sensitive molecules from the chemical effects of their surrounding cosmetic vehicles (178,179). Techniques being developed to stabilize active materials employ liposomes and niosomes, multiple emulsions, transdermal patches, and micro- and nanoencapsulation.

Micro- and nanoencapsulation are particularly important methods for protecting bioactive agents. Encapsulation is a process by which active components are surrounded by a polymer shell, the final particle size being as small as a few microns. Polyesters are widely used to create these shells and are examined in more detail below.

B. Encapsulating Polyesters

For a polymer to be effective in a therapeutic encapsulation system, it must meet two criteria: (1) the polymer must be hydrolytically or enzymatically labile, and (2) the resulting hydrolysis by-products must be biocompatible. Many natural polymers are excellent choices for encapsulation polymers, especially the natural polysaccharides discussed in Chapter 8. Synthetic polymers having an all-carbon backbone are generally not hydrolytically labile and are generally not employed as encapsulating polymers, although one does encounter the use of some methacrylate and silicone-based polymers in delivery systems.

Condensation polymers particularly effective as encapsulating materials are listed in Table 11. The six polyesters cited in the table have all demonstrated hydrolytic sensitivity in and on the human body. Equally important, the hydrolysis by-products of these polyesters are biocompatible. This means that as the encapsulated material is released and the encapsulation particle is broken down, the by-products can be processed by the body's waste disposal systems. Research efforts continue to explore new combinations of these esters to create new and more useful polymer properties (180).

The techniques for manufacturing micro- and nanoencapsulation particles have been

Table 11 Synthetic Encapsulation Polyesters, Including Monomer Sources

Structure	Polyester name	Source
—[OCH(CH_3)C(O)]—	Poly(lactic acid) "PLA"	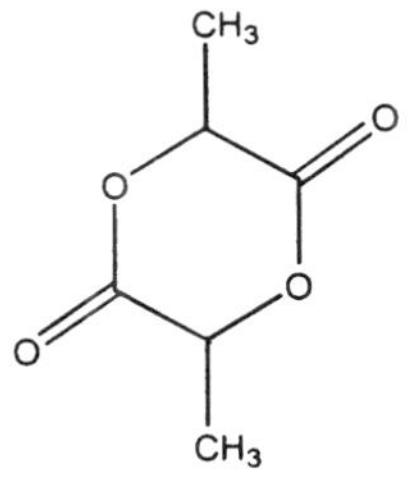 Lactide
—[$OCH_2C(O)$]—	Poly(glycolic acid) "PGA"	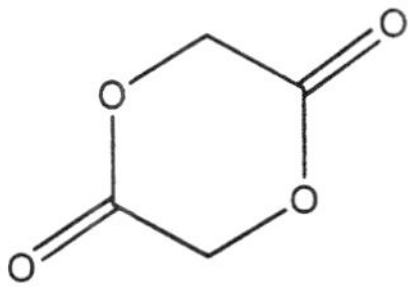 Glycolide
—[OCH(CH_3)$CH_2C(O)$]—	Poly(3-hydroxybutyrate) "PHB"	Fermentation
—[OCH(CH_2CH_3)$CH_2C(O)$]—	Poly(3-hydroxyvalerate) "PHV"	Fermentation
—[OCH(CH_2CH_3)$CH_2C(O)$]—[OCH(CH_3)$CH_2C(O)$]—	Poly (3-hydroxyvalerate-*co*-3-hydroxybutyrate) "PHBV"	Fermentation
—[$O(CH_2)_5C(O)$]—	Poly(caprolactone) "PCL"	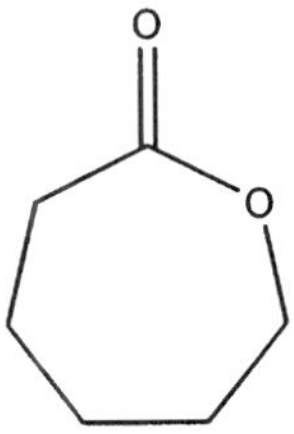 caprolactone

reviewed recently (181). There are many different methods for encapsulating products, but the encapsulated particles often will appear as one of the structures shown in Figure 40. Once an active material has been encapsulated, it can be incorporated into a suspending cosmetic or therapeutic vehicle where it should remain unaffected by the formulation components until application. Other formulation processing steps can present additional challenges to the encapsulating polymer. If the encapsulated particle is to be used, for example, for delivery of an active component to the eye it may also have to withstand the rigors of sterilization (182).

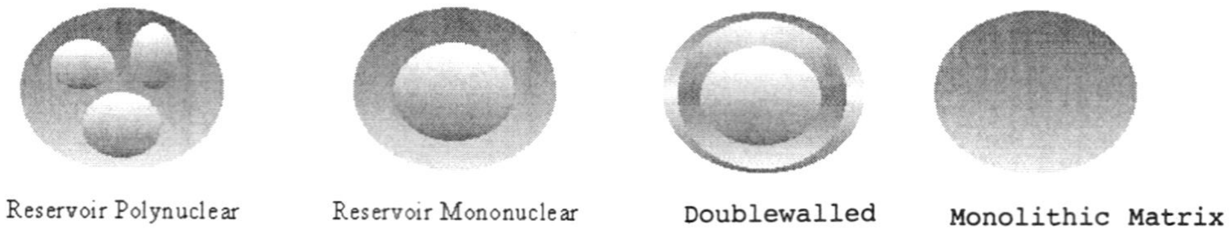

Figure 40 Various structures of encapsulated particles showing active component and surrounding polymer.

ACKNOWLEDGMENTS

The author is indebted to Jim Hatfield, Keith Olesen, Greg Shaw, Mike Philbin, and Ray Rigoletto for their careful review of the manuscript. The author also thanks Cathy Misner and her group for their efforts to locate reference materials and to Leo Walsh and Paul McKeefry for providing the black-and-white photograph (Figure 36). Finally, the author is truly indebted to Freida DeBaro for her kind assistance in preparing the manuscript.

REFERENCES

1. Kuhn T. Structure of Scientific Revolutions, 2nd ed. Chicago: University Press, 1970.
2. Doi Y. Microbial Polyesters. New York: VCH Publishers, 1990.
3. Burdick DL, Leffler WL. Petrochemicals in Nontechnical Language, 2nd ed. Tulsa, OK: PennWell Publishing, 1990.
4. Elias HG. An Introduction to Polymer Science. Weinheim: VCH, 1997:309–310, 315–317.
5. Tomalia DA, Naylor AM, Goddard WA. Starburst dendrimers: molecular-level control of size, shape, surface chemistry, topology, and flexibility from atoms to macroscopic matter. Angew Chem Int Ed Engl 1990; 29:138–175.
6. Tomalia DA, Durst HD. Genealogically directed synthesis: starburst/cascade dendrimers and hyperbranched structures. Topics Curr Chem 1993; 165:193–313.
7. Elias HG. An Introduction to Polymer Science. Weinheim: VCH, 1997: 23–27.
8. Knapen JWJ, Van der Made AW, de Wilde JC, van Leeuwen PWNM, Wijkens P, Grove DM, van Koten G. Homogeneous catalysts based on silane dendrimers functionalized with arylnickel (II) complexes. Nature 1994; 372:659–663.
9. Roy R. Glycodendrimers: a new class of biopolymers. Polym News 1996; 21:226–232.
10. Prud'homme RK. Rheological measurements. In: Shuylz DN, Glass JE, eds. Polymers as Rheology Modifiers. Washington, DC: American Chemical Society, 1991:18–47.
11. Greenwald HL, Luskin LS. Poly(acrylic acid) and its homologs. In: Davidson RL, ed. Handbook of Water-Soluble Gums and Resins. New York: McGraw-Hill, 1980:Chapter 17, 1–19.
12. Novak RW. Acrylic ester polymers. In: Kroschwitz JI, Howe-Grant M, eds. Kirk-Othmer Encyclopedia of Chemical Technology, 4th ed, Vol 1. New York: Wiley, 1993:314–343.
13. Novak RW, Lesko PM. Methacrylic polymers. In: Kroschwitz JI, Howe-Grant M, eds. Kirk-Othmer Encyclopedia of Chemical Technology, 4th ed, Vol 16. New York: Wiley, 1995: 506–537.
14. Antonietti M, Burger C, Thunemann A. Polyelectrolyte-surfactant complexes: a new class of highly ordered polymer materials. Trends Polym Sci 1997; 5:262–267.
15. Volk H, Friedrich RE. Polyacrylamide. In: Davidson RL, ed. Handbook of Water-Soluble Gums and Resins. New York: McGraw-Hill, 1980:Chapter 16, 1–19.

16. Lipp D, Kozakiewicz J. Acrylamide polymers. In: Kroschwitz JI, Howe-Grant M, eds. Kirk-Othmer Encyclopedia of Chemical Technology, 4th ed., Vol 1. New York: Wiley, 1993: 266–286.
17. Kurenkov VF, Myagchenkow VA. Acrylamide (polymerization and applications). In: Salamone JC, ed. The Polymeric Materials Encyclopedia, Vol 1. Boca Raton, FL: CRC Press, 1996:47–54.
18. Clarke MT. Rheological additives. In: Laba D, ed. Rheological Properties of Cosmetics and Toiletries. New York: Marcel Dekker, 1993:109.
19. Powell GM. Polyethylene glycol. In: Davidson RL, ed. Handbook of Water-Soluble Gums and Resins. New York: McGraw-Hill, 1980:Chapter 18, 1–22.
20. Braun DB. Poly(ethylene oxide). In: Davidson RL, ed. Handbook of Water-Soluble Gums and Resins. New York: McGraw-Hill, 1980:Chapter 19, 1–28.
21. Back DM, Clark EM, Ramachandran R. Polyethers, ethylene oxide polymers. In: Kroschwitz JI, Howe-Grant M, eds. Kirk-Othmer Encyclopedia of Chemical Technology, 4th ed, Vol 19. New York: Wiley, 1996:700–722.
22. Kuran W. Poly(propylene oxide). In: Salamone JC, ed. The Polymeric Materials Encyclopedia, Vol 9. Boca Raton, FL: CRC Press, 1996:6656–6662.
23. Koleske JV. Poly(ethylene oxide). In: Salamone JC, ed. The Polymeric Materials Encyclopedia, Vol 8. Boca Raton, FL: CRC Press, 1996:6034–6042.
24. Lochhead RY, Fron WR. Encyclopedia of polymers and thickeners for cosmetics. Cosmet Toilet 1993; 108:122.
25. Tasaki K. Poly(oxyethylene)-water interactions: a molecular dynamics study. J Am Chem Soc 1996; 118:8459–8469.
26. Tam KC. Rheological properties of poly(ethylene oxide) in anionic surfactant solutions. Adv Chem Ser 1996; 248:205–217.
27. Ballerat-Busserolles K, Roux-Desgranges G, Roux AH. Thermodynamics in micellar solutions: confirmation of complex formation between sodium dodecyl sulfate and polyethylene glycol. Langmuir 1997; 13:1946–1951.
28. Li Y, Dubin PL. Polymer-surfactant complexes. In: Herb CA, Prud'homme RK, eds. Structure and Flow in Surfactant Solutions. Washington, DC: American Chemical Society, 1994: 320–336.
29. Goodard ED. Polymer-surfactant interaction. Part I. Uncharged water-soluble polymers and charged surfactants. In: Goddard ED, Ananthapadmanabhan KP, eds. Interactions of Surfactants with Polymers and Proteins. Boca Raton; FL: CRC Press, 1993:123–169.
30. Lindman B, Thalberg K. Polymer-surfactant interactions—recent developments. In: Goddard ED, Ananthapadmanabhan KP, eds. Interactions of Surfactants with Polymers and Proteins. Boca Raton, FL: CRC Press; 1993:203–276.
31. Nikas YJ, Blankschtein D. Complexation of nonionic polymers and surfactants in dilute aqueous solutions. Langmuir 1994; 10:3512–3528.
32. Lin Z, Eads CD. Polymer-induced structural transitions in oleate solutions: microscopy, rheology, and nuclear magnetic resonance studies. Langmuir 1997; 13:2647–2654.
33. Gronski W, Hellmann G, Wilsch-Irrgang A. ^{13}C NMR characterization of ethylene oxide/propylene oxide adducts. Makromol Chem 1991; 192:591–601.
34. Goff LA. Characterization of ethylene oxide propylene oxide copolymers by NMR spectroscopy. J Soc Cosmet Chem 1997; 48:59–60.
35. Alexandridis P. Poly(ethylene oxide)/poly(propylene oxide) block copolymer surfactants. Curr Opin Colloid Interface Sci 1997; 2:478–489.
36. Cabana A, Ait-Kadi A, Juhasz J. Study of the gelation of polyethylene oxide–polypropylene oxide–polyethylene oxide copolymer (Poloxamer 407) aqueous solutions. J Colloid Interface Sci 1997; 190:307–312.
37. Pavlichko JP, Decorte H, Barbeito C, Eng D. Use of ethylene/propylene oxide linear polymers in personal care. Cosmet Toilet Manf Worldwide 1995; 156–160.

38. Modi TW. Polyvinyl alcohol. In: Davidson RL, ed. Handbook of Water-Soluble Gums and Resins. New York: McGraw-Hill, 1980:Chapter 20, 1–24.
39. Cincera DL. Poly(vinyl alcohol). In: Kirk-Othmer Encyclopedia of Chemical Technology, 3rd ed, Vol 23. New York: J Wiley, 1983:848–865.
40. McLaughlin KW, Wyffels NK, Jentz AB, Keenan MV. The gelation of poly(vinyl alcohol) with $Na_2B_4O_7 \cdot 10H_2O$: killing slime. J Chem Educ 1997; 74:97–99.
41. Nijenhuis K. Advances in Polymer Science. Thermoreversible Networks Viscoelastic Properties and Structure of Gels, Vol 130. Berlin: Springer-Verlag, 1997:37–65.
42. Blecher L, Lorenz DH, Lowd HL, Wood AS, Wyman DP. Polyvinylpyrrolidone. In: Davidson RL, ed. Handbook of Water-Soluble Gums and Resins. New York: McGraw-Hill, 1980: Chapter 21, 1–21.
43. Hort EV, Waxman BH. *N*-Vinyl monomers and polymers. In: Mark HF, Othmer DF, Overberger CG, Seaborg GT, eds. Kirk-Othmer Encyclopedia of Chemical Technology, 3rd ed, Vol 23. New York: Wiley, 1983:960–978.
44. Vogel FGM. 50 Years of PVP. Soap Cosmet Chem Spec 1989; 65:42, 46–47, 128.
45. Yazan Y, Aralp U, Seiller M, Grossiord JL. PVP in multiple emulsions. Cosmet Toilet 1995; 110:53–57.
46. Ketz RJ, Prud'homme RK, Graessley WW. Rheology of concentrated microgel solutions. Rheol Acta. 1988; 27:531–539.
47. Reichert WW, Nae HN, Laba D, Dobell K. Lightly cross-linked carboxy copolymers: elegance through rheology. In-Cosmet Conf Proc. Verlag fur Chem. Industrie H. Ziolkowsky GmbH, Augsburg: 1992:53–67.
48. Nae HN, Reichert WW. Rheological properties of lightly crosslinked carboxy copolymers in aqueous solutions. Rheol Acta 1992; 31:351–360.
49. Kopolov SL, Kwak YT, Helioff M. A new thickener/stabilizer technology. Cosmet Toilet 1993; 108:61–67.
50. Kopolov SL, Kwak YT. PVM/MA Decadiene crosspolymer: a new thickener/stabilizer technology. Cosmet Toilet Manf Worldwide 1993; 100, 102, 104–106.
51. Gripp A, Helioff M, Kwak YT. Stabileze® PVM/MA decadiene crosspolymers: versatile thickeners for skin care formulations. Cosmet Toilet Manf Worldwide 1996; 115–118.
52. Amjad Z, Hemker WJ, Maiden CA, Rouse WM, Sauer CE. Carbomer resins: past, present and future. Cosmet Toilet 1992; 107:81–82, 84–86.
53. Lochhead RY. Hair gels. House Person Prod Ind 1990; 27:58–64.
54. Secard DL. Acrylic emulsifying and stabilizing polymers. Cosmet Toilet 1984; 99:73–76.
55. Lochhead RY, Eachus AC, Bremecker KD. The evaluation of alternative neutralizing bases for carbomers. In-Cosmet Conf Proc. Verlag fur Chem. Industrie H. Ziolkowsky GmbH, Augsburg: 1992:302–329.
56. Lochhead RY. Hemker WJ, Castaneda JY. Hydrophobically modified ''carbopol'' resins. Soap Cosmet Chem Spec 1987:28–29, 32–33, 84.
57. Lochhead RY. Water-soluble polymers: solution adsorption and interaction characteristics. Cosmet Toilet. 1992; 107:131–132, 134, 136–138, 140, 142, 146–148, 150, 152–156.
58. Clymans DRJ, Brand HM. Polymeric emulsifiers: an alternative to traditional emulsifiers based on stability of multi-phase systems. Cosmet Toilet Manf Worldwide 1995; 119–125.
59. Fishman HM. Carbopol resins. House Person Prod Ind 1989; 26:26.
60. Castaneda JY, Lochhead RY. Anionic polymeric emulsifiers—a new router to stable and efficacious cationic emulsions. 16th IFSCC Int Cong Preprints. New York: Society Cosmetic Chemists, 1990; 427–436.
61. Braun DB, Ciullo PA. Enhanced stabilization of topical emulsions through interactive synergism of cross-linked acrylic polymers and inorganic clays. 16th IFSCC Int Cong Preprints. New York: Society Cosmetic Chemists, 1990:272–282.
62. Holden C. Formulating hair and skin products more effectively. Spec Chem 1996; 16:21–23.

63. Hoffmann H, Ebert G. Surfactants, micelles and fascinating phenomena. Angew Chem Int Ed Engl 1988; 27:902–912.
64. Rieger MM. Surfactant chemistry and classification. In: Rieger MM, Rhein LD, eds. Surfactants in Cosmetics, 2nd ed. New York: Marcel Dekker, 1997:1–28.
65. Lindman B, Wennerstrom H. Micelles amphiphile aggregation in aqueous solution. Top Curr Chem, 1980;87:1–83.
66. Lequeux F, Candau SJ. Dynamical properties of wormlike micelles: deviations from the ''classical'' picture. In: Herb CA, Prud'homme RK, eds. Structure and Flow in Surfactant Solutions. Washington, DC: American Chemical Society, 1994:51–62.
67. Kronberg B, Costas M, Silveston R. On understanding hydrophobicity. In: Coffey RT, ed. New Horiz: AOCS/CSMA Deterg Ind Conf 3rd 1995. Champaign IL: AOCS Press, 1996: 63–69.
68. Schwab FG. Advantages and disadvantages of associative thickeners in coatings performance. In: Glass JE, ed. Water-Soluble Polymers Beauty with Performance. Adv Chem Ser 213. Washington, DC: American Chemical Society, 1986:369–373.
69. Jenkins RD, Silebi CA, El-Aasser MS. Steady-shear and Linear-viscoelastic material properties of model associative polymer solutions. In: Schulz DN, Glass JE, eds. Polymers as Rheology Modifiers. Washington, DC: American Chemical Society, 1991:222–233.
70. Wetzel WH, Chen M, Glass EJ. Associative Thickeners. An Overview with An Emphasis on Synthetic Procedures. Adv Chem Ser Vol 248. Washington, DC: American Chemical Society, 1996:163–179.
71. English RJ, Gulati HS, Jenkins RD, Khan SA. Solution rheology of a hydrophobically modified alkali-soluble associative polymer. J Rheol 1997; 41:427–444.
72. Balzer D, Varwig S, Weirauch M. Viscoelasticity of personal care products. Colloid Surf A Physicochem Eng Asp 1995; 99:233–246.
73. Lochhead RY, Warfield DS, Gasiewski C. Phase diagrams as a formulation guide in aqueous polymer/surfactant systems. Polym Eng Sci 1985; 25:1110–1117.
74. Lundberg DJ, Ma Z, Alahapperuna K, Glass JE. Surfactant influences on hydrophobically modified thickener rheology. In: Shulz DN, Glass JE. Eds. Polymers as Rheology Modifiers. ACS Symposium Series No. 462. Washington, DC: American Chemical Society, 1991:234–253.
75. Lochhead RY. Electrosteric stabilization of oil-in-water emulsions by hydrophobically modified poly(acrylic acid) thickeners. In: Shulz DN, Glass JE. Eds. Polymers as Rheology Modifiers. ACS Symposium Series No. 462. Washington, DC: American Chemical Society, 1991: 101–120.
76. Iliopoulos I, Wang TK, Audebert R. Viscometric evidence of interactions between hydrophobically modified poly(sodium acrylate) and sodium dodecyl sulfate. Langmuir 1991; 7:617–619.
77. Magny B, Iliopoulos I, Zana R, Audebert R. Mixed micelles formed by cationic surfactants and anionic hydrophobically modified polyelectrolytes. Langmuir 1994; 10:3180–3187.
78. Lochhead RY, Warfield DS. Carbomers as thickeners and suspending agents in shampoos. Soap Cosmet Chem Spec 1985; 614:46, 48, 50, 52, 54.
79. Lochhead RY, Hemker WJ, Castaneda JY, Garlen D. Novel cosmetic emulsions. Cosmet Toilet 1986; 101:125–126, 128–130, 132, 134, 136, 138.
80. Lochhead RY, Castaneda JY, Gasiewski CR. Steric stabilization, associative thickening, amphiphatic carbomers and cosmetic emulsions. Gums, Polymers, Thickeners and Resins Symp., Abstract Paper 10. New York: Society of Cosmetic Scientists, 1986: 1–38.
81. Lochhead RY, Hemker WJ, Castaneda JY. Hydrophobically modified ''carbopol'' resins. Soap Cosmet Chem Spec 1987; 63(5):28–29, 32–33, 84–85.
82. Lochhead RY, Hemker WJ, Castaneda JY. Hydrophob modifizierte Carbopol® polymere. Parfuem Kosmet 1988; 69:218–220, 223–224.
83. Dodwell R, Lochhead R, Hemmker W. Pemulen® polymeric emulsifiers: what they are, how they work. Cosmet Toilet Manf World 1993; 77–80, 83–86.

84. Jenkins RD, Bassett DR. Synergistic interactions among associative polymers and surfactants. In: Asua JM ed. Polymeric Dispersions: Principles and Applications. Netherlands: Kluwer Academic Publishers, 1997:477–495.
85. Iliopoulos I, Olsson U. Polyelectrolyte association to micelles and bilayers. J Phys Chem 1994; 98:1500–1505.
86. Sarrazin-Cartalas A, Iliopoulus I, Audebert R, Olsson U. Association and thermal gelation in mixtures of hydrophobically modified polyelectrolytes and nonionic surfactants. Langmuir 1994; 10:1421–1426.
87. Loyen K. Iliopoulus I, Audebert R, Olsson U. Reversible thermal gelation in polymer/surfactant systems. Control of the gelation temperature. Langmuir 1995; 11:1053–1056.
88. Thuresson K, Nilsson S, Lindman B. Effect of hydrophobic modification on phase behavior and rheology in mixtures of oppositely charged polyelectrolytes. Langmuir 1996; 12:530–537.
89. Perrin P, Lafuma F, Audebert R. Emulsions stabilized with hydrophobically modified poly(acrylic acid). Progr Colloid Polym Sci 1997; 105:228–238.
90. Biggs S, Selb J, Candau F. Effect of surfactant on the solution properties of hydrophobically modified polyacrylamide. Langmuir 1992; 8:838–847.
91. Wang Y, Han B, Yan H. Microcalorimetry study of interaction between ionic surfactants and hydrophobically modified polymers in aqueous solutions. Langmuir 1997; 13:3119–3123.
92. Schumucker-Castner J, Desai DD, Brand HM, Frate DM, Clymans D, Brand-Garnys EE. Novel skin care formulations with optimized sensory parameters using acrylates/C10-30 alkyl acrylates crosspolymers as primary emulsifiers. In: Proceedings In-Cosmetics 1997 Modern Challenges to the Cosmetic Formulation. Augsburg: Verlag fur Chem Industrie H Ziolkowsky GmbH, 1997:274–287.
93. Desai DD, Brand HM, Schuymucker-Castner J, Frate DM, Clymans D, Brand-Garnys EE. Novel skin care formulations. Cosmet Toilet Manf World 1997; 158, 160–166.
94. Kumacheva E, Rharbi Y, Winnik MA, Guo L, Tam KC, Jenkins RD. Fluorescence studies of an alkaline swellable associative polymer in aqueous solution. Langmuir 1997; 13:182–186.
95. Tirtaatmadja V, Tam KC, Jenkins RD. Rheological properties of model alkali-soluble associative (HASE) polymers: effect of varying hydrophobe chain length. Macromolecules 1997; 30:3271–3282.
96. Cardinali S, Pasapane J, Greenburg J. Novel thickeners for hard-to-thicken personal care products. Drug Cosmet Ind 1997; 160(5):42, 44–46, 48.
97. Wenninger JA, McEwen GN, eds. International Cosmetic Ingredient Dictionary, Vol 1. Washington, DC: Cosmetic, Toiletry, and Fragrance Association, 1997: 27.
98. Shay G, Bassett D, Rex JD. A new class of alkali-swellable associative thickeners. J Oil Colour Chem Assoc 1993; 76: 446–453.
99. Cardinali MS, Rothman RH. Novel cationic compatible rheology modifiers and their use in personal care cleansing systems. Abstracts IFSCC International Conference, Acapulco, 1997: 177–189.
100. Cottrell I. Novel rheology modifiers and their use in personal care applications. In: Proceedings In-Cosmetic 1997 Modern Challenges to the Cosmetic Formulation. Augsburg: Verlag fur Chem. Industrie H. Ziolkowsky GmbH, 1997: 324–339.
101. Dersch R. Associative thickeners past, present and future. Surf Coat Aust 1994; 31:18–22.
102. Fonnum G, Bakke J, Hansen FK. Associative thickeners. Part 1. Synthesis, rheology and aggregation behavior. Coll Polym Sci 1993; 271:380–389.
103. Annable T, Buscall R, Ettelaie R, Whittletone D. The rheology of solutions of associating polymers: comparison of experimental behavior with transient network theory. J Rheol 1993; 37:695–725.

104. Clarke MT. Rheological additives. In: Laba D, ed. Rheological Properties of Cosmetics and Toiletries. New York: Marcel Dekker, 1993:114–118.
105. Pavlichko JP. Methyl glucoside derivatives: naturally derived multifunctional ingredients for personal care. Cosmet Toilet Manf World 1994; 38, 40–42, 44–45.
106. Leidreiter HI, Maczkiewitz U. Modern thickening agents for toiletries. Cosmet Toilet Manf World 1995; 162, 164–166.
107. Tadros TF, Dederen C, Taelman MC. A new polymeric emulsifier. Cosmet Toilet 1997; 112: 75–76, 79–80, 82–86.
108. Johnsen MA. The hair spray and the mousse...the mystique and the promise. Spray Tech Mark 1996; 6(5):46.
109. Johnsen MA. US regulations affecting aerosols. Cosmet Toilet Manf World 1991/1992; 255–268.
110. Dallal JA, Rocafort CM. Hair styling/fixative products. In: Johnson DH, ed. Hair and Hair Care. New York: Marcel Dekker, 1997:105–165.
111. Robbins CR. Polymers and polymer chemistry in hair products. In: Chemical and Physical Behavior of Human Hair, 3rd ed. New York: Springer-Verlag, 1994:263–297.
112. Price SNC. Keeping VOCs under control. Cosmet Toilet 1995; 110:42–44, 46, 48–49.
113. Hort EV, Gasman RC. Vinyl ether monomers and polymers. In: Mark HF, Othmer DF, Overberger CG, Seaborg GT. eds. Kirk-Othmer Encyclopedia of Chemical Technology, 3rd ed., Vol. 23. New York: Wiley, 1983:937–960.
114. Petter PJ. Acetylene-derived polymers and their applications in hair and skin care. Gums, Polymers, Thickeners and Resins Symp., Abstract Paper 14. New York: Society of Cosmetic Scientists, 1986:1–19.
115. Beaven RC. Hairspray polymers, formulations and trends. Gums, Polymers, Thickeners and Resins Symp., Abstract Paper 15. New York: Society of Cosmetic Scientists, 1986:1–19.
116. Lochhead RY. The history of polymers in hair care (1940–Present). Cosmet Toilet 1988; 103:23–26, 28–30, 32–34, 36–61.
117. Login RB, Barabas ES. Personal care application polymers (acetylene-derived). In: Salamone JC, ed. The Polymeric Materials Encyclopedia, Vol 7. Boca Raton, FL: CRC Press, 1996: 4950–4965.
118. San Giovanni ML. Sprays under pressure: a compilation of issues of immediate interest to the spray packaging industry. Spray Tech Mark 1996; 6(5):8, 12, 14, 16.
119. Molenaar M. Second generation spray systems. Cosmet Toilet Manf World 1991/1992; 224, 226.
120. The future of the aerosol. Cosmet Toilet Manf World 1991/1992; 249–253.
121. An aerosol spray system using compressed air as a propellant. Cosmet Toilet Manf World 1993; 280, 282.
122. Ganiere J, Laumet A. New technology in pressurized dispensers: compressed gas aerosols. Cosmet Toilet Manf World 1993; 284, 286–287.
123. Guth J, Martino G, Russo J. Addressing the North American trend towards low VOC hair sprays. Seif-Ole-Fette-Wach 1991; 117:464–467.
124. Wekel HU, Sperling-Vietmeier K. Modern hairspray formulations/trends and new polymers. Seif Ole-Fette-Wach 1990; 116:130–137.
125. Rouse WM, Nowak F. The development of hydrocarbon-tolerant hairspray polymers. Aerosol Age 1988; 33:48–50, 56, 58–65.
126. Gormley JL, Martino GT, Pluyter JGL, Tong QK. Using physical measurements to optimise water-containing aerosol hair sprays. Cosmet Toilet Manf World 1997; 209–216.
127. Croll SG. Drying of latex paint. J Coat Tech 1986; 58:41–49.
128. Robbins CR. The physical properties and cosmetic behavior of hair. In: Chemical and Physical Behavior of Human Hair, 3rd ed. New York: Springer-Verlag, 1994:299–370.
129. Schehlmann V. Polyvinylcaprolactam physical and cosmetic properties of a new hair fixative

resin. In: Proceedings In-Cosmetics 1997 Modern Challenges to the Cosmetic Formulation. Augsburg: Verlag fur Chemische Industrie H. Ziolkowsky GmbH, 1997:378–390.
130. Guth J, Russo J, Kay T, King N, Beaven R. Addressing the low VOC hair spray issue: new options. Cosmet Toilet 1993; 108:97–103.
131. Walls E, Krummel HK. Low VOC hairsprays formulation: challenges for a changing industry. Cosmet Toilet 1993; 108:111–117.
132. Martino GT, Russo JV, Morawsky NA, Guth JJ. Investigation of low VOC hair spray alternatives. Spray Tech Mark 1992; 2:34–39.
133. Cook PM, Dobbs SW, Garber DM, Underwood VL. Eastman AQ polymers for low VOC hair spray. Spray Tech Mark 1996; 6(5):44–45.
134. Morawsky N, Martino G, Bushy C. Corrosion study of 80% VOC aerosol hairsprays containing water. Spray Tech Mark 1993; 3(5):57–65.
135. Tazi M. Progress in water based hairspray II. Cosmet Toilet Manf World 1991/1992; 238–245.
136. Martens CR. Types of waterborne coatings. In: Waterborne Coatings Emulsion and Water-Soluble Paints. New York: Van Nostrand Reinhold, 1981:41–51.
137. Pavlichko JP. Novel new hair spray resin utilizing aqueous dispersion technology for 0–80% VOC systems. In-Cosmetics 1995. Augsburg: Verlag fur Chemische Industrie H. Ziolkowsky GmbH, 1995:549–563.
138. Pavlichko JP. Aqueous dispersion hair-spray resin. Cosmet Toilet 1995; 110:63–67.
139. Hatfield J. Dispersion polymers for hair fixatives. Spray Tech Mark 1996; 6(5):32, 34–36.
140. Dorman S. Hair care 1996. Spray Tech Mark 1996; 6(5):18–20, 22, 24, 26, 28.
141. Kerker M. Historical Note: Classics and classicists of colloid and interface science 6. John Tyndall. J Coll Interface Sci 1987; 199:602–604.
142. Wang Y, Juhue D, Winnik MA, Leung OM, Goh MC. Atomic force microscopy study of latex film formation. Langmuir 1992; 8:760–762.
143. Dobler F, Pith T, Lambla M, Holl Y. Coalescene Mechanisms of polymer colloids. 1. Coalescence under the influence of particle-water interfacial tension. J Coll Interface Sci 1992; 152: 1–11.
144. Juhue D, Lang J. Effect of surfactant postadded to latex dispersion on film formation: a study by atomic force microscopy. Langmuir 1993; 9:792–796.
145. Lin F, Meier DJ. A study of latex film formation by atomic force microscopy. 1. A Comparison of Wet and Dry Conditions. Langmuir 1995; 11:2726–2733.
146. Feng J, Winnik MA, Shivers RR, Clubb B. Polymer blend latex films: morphology and transparency. Macromolecules 1995; 28:7671–7682.
147. Keddie JL, Meredith P, Jones RAL, Donald AM. Kinetics of film formation in acrylic latices studied with multiple-angle-of-incidence ellipsometry and environmental SEM. Macromolecules 1995; 28:2673–2682.
148. Keddie JL, Meredith P, Jones RAL, Donald AM. Film formation of acrylic latices with varying concentrations of non-film-forming latex particles. Langmuir 1996; 12:3793–3801.
149. Winnik MA, Feng J. Latex blends: an approach to zero VOC coatings. J Coat Tech 1996; 68:39–50.
150. Dobler F, Holl Y. Mechanism of latex film formation. Trends Polym Sci 1996; 4:145–151.
151. Eckersley ST, Rudin A. Film formation of acrylic copolymer latices: a model of state II film formation. In: Provder T, Winnik MA, Urban MW, eds. Film Formation in Waterborne Coatings ACS Symposium Series No. 648. Washington, DC: American Chemical Society, 1996: 1–21.
152. Robbins CR. Interactions of shampoo and conditioning ingredients with human hair. In: Robbins CR, ed. Chemical and Physical Behavior of Human Hair. New York: Springer-Verlag, 1994:153–232.

153. Hoshowski MA. Conditioning of hair. In: Johnson DH, ed. Hair and Hair Care. New York: Marcel Dekker, 1997:65–104.
154. Midha S, Bolich RE. Hair and skin cosmetics. In: Salamone JC, ed. Polymeric Materials Encyclopedia, Vol 5. Boca Raton, FL: CRC Press, 1996:2910–2916.
155. Gallot BR. Hair and skin care biomaterials (cosmetology and dermatology). In: Salamone JC, ed. Polymeric Materials Encyclopedia, Vol 5. Boca Raton, FL: CRC Press, 1996:2901–2910.
156. Goddard ED. Substantivity through cationic substitution. Cosmet Toilet 1987; 102:71–80.
157. Feigenbaum HN. Polyethylenimine: prospective applications. Cosmet Toilet 1993; 108:73–77.
158. Sykes AR, Hammes PA. The use of merquat polymers in cosmetics. Drug Cosmet Ind 1980; 126:62, 64, 66, 68, 136.
159. Jachowicz J, Williams C. Fingerprinting of cosmetic formulations by dynamic electrokinetic and permeability analysis. I. Shampoos. J Soc Cosmet Chem 1994; 45:309–336.
160. Pfau A, Hossel P, Vogt S, Sander R, Schrepp W. The interaction of cationic polymers with human hair. Macromol. Symp. 1997; 126:241–252.
161. Ishii MK. Objective and instrumental methods for evaluation of hair care product efficacy and substantiation of claims. In: Johnson DH, ed. Hair and Hair Care. New York: Marcel Dekker, 1997:261–302.
162. Franz TJ, Lehman PA, McGuire EL. In vivo methods for the assessment of percutaneous absorption in man. In: Zatz JL, ed. Skin Permeation Fundamentals and Application. Wheaton, IL: Allured Publishing, 1993:73–92.
163. Rigoletto R, Moral L, Pavlichko JP. Differentation of cationic polymers based on modern analytical techniques. Cosmet Toilet Manf World 1996; 131–137.
164. Robbins CR. The physical properties and cosmetic behavior of hair. In: Robbins CR, ed. Chemical and Physical Behavior of Human Hair. New York: Springer-Verlag, 1994:299–370.
165. Gabriel KL, Mark R, Stoudemayer T. Application of new technologies for the evaluation of skin changes. Cosmet Toilet Manf World 1991/1992; 215, 217–219.
166. Hossel P. A new multifunctional polymer. Cosmet Toilet 1996; 111:73–74, 76, 78.
167. Goddard ED, Hannan RB. Polymer/surfactant interactions. J Am Oil Chem Soc 1977; 54: 561–566.
168. Goddard ED. Polymer-surfactant interaction. Part II. Polymer and surfactant of opposite charge. In: Goddard ED, Ananthapadmanabhan KP, eds. Interactions of Surfactants with Polymers and Proteins. Boca Raton, FL: CRC Press, 1993:171–201.
169. Li Y, Xia J, Dubin PL. Complex formation between polyelectrolyte and oppositely charged mixed micelles: static and dynamic light scattering study of the effect of polyelectrolyte molecular weight and concentration. Macromolecules 1994; 27:7049–7055.
170. Thunemann A. Immobilization of retinoic acid by cationic polyelectrolytes. Langmuir 1997; 13:6040–6046.
171. Johnson SC. Acetylene-derived polymers. Cosmet Toilet 1984; 99:77–81.
172. Draelos, ZD. New developments in cosmetics and skin care products. In: James WD, ed. Advances in Dermatology, Vol 12. St. Louis: Mosby-Year Book, 1997:3–18.
173. Fox C. Advances in cosmetic science and technology. IV. Skin care and treatment. Cosmet Toilet 1995; 110:63–66, 68–72, 74–76, 78–79, 81–82, 84, 86–88, 90–93.
174. Rawlings AV, Scott IR, Harding CR, Bowser PA. Stratum corneum moisturization at the molecular level. J Invest Dermatol 1994; 103:731–740.
175. Martin P. Wound healing—aiming for perfect skin regeneration. Science 1997; 276: 75–81.
176. Fox C. Advances in cosmetic science and technology. II. Topical bioactive materials. Cosmet Toilet 1994; 109:83–86, 88–90, 92, 94–96, 98, 100, 102, 104–106, 108–110, 112, 114.

177. Eller MS, Yarr M, Gilchrest BA. DNA damage and melanogenesis. Nature 1994; 372:413–414.
178. Magdassi S. Delivery systems in cosmetics. Colloid Surf A 1997; 123–124: 671–679.
179. Banakar UV. Advances and opportunities in delivery of therapeutic proteins and peptides. J Biomat Appl 1997; 11:377–429.
180. Domb AJ, Amselem S, Maniar M. Biodegradable polymers as drug carrier systems. In: Dumitrui S, ed. Polymeric Biomaterials. New York: Marcel Dekker, 1994:399–433.
181. Nobes GAR, Marchessaoult RH, Maysinger D. Review. Polyhydroxyalkanoates: materials for delivery systems. J Microencap (in press).
182. Masson V, Maurin F, Fessi H, Devissaguet JP. Influence of sterilization process on poly (ϵ-caprolactone) nanospheres. Biomaterials 1997; 18:327–335.

7

Silicones in Cosmetics

Marianne D. Berthiaume
Wacker Silicones Corporation, Adrian, Michigan

I. INTRODUCTION

Silicon, atomic number 14, is the second most abundant element known, composing 28% of the earth's crust. Elemental silicon does not exist in the free state, and is most often found in nature in the form of silica (sand) or silicates (minerals comprising silicon, oxygen, and metals such as aluminum, magnesium, iron, calcium, or mica). Silicones are polymers of silicon, carbon, hydrogen, and oxygen, sometimes also including nitrogen or sulfur. Silicone compounds are chemically referred to by a similar nomenclature system as organic materials. For example, a CH_4 molecule is known as methane, while SiH_4 is referred to as silane; silanols (Si—OH compounds) correspond to organic alcohols (R—OH), and so forth. In fact, the term ''silicone'' was coined by Frederic Kipping in the early 1900s because he thought the basic monomer unit, R_2SiO, resembled the organic ketone R_2CO structure. Silicone chemistry cannot, however, be compared to organic chemistry, and unlike the very stable C═O (and C═C) double bonds, the Si═O (and Si═C) double bonds are generally not stable and do not exist under normal conditions. Indeed, Kipping was never able to isolate such a monomeric structure. A more correct method of representing the silicone structure would be $R_2SiO_{2/2}$ since the silicone atom preferentially forms single bonds with two neighboring oxygen atoms. The reason for this is the much lower energy required for the $\pi \rightarrow \pi^*$ transitions in disilanes than in alkenes (3 eV for the $3\pi \rightarrow 3\pi^*$ for Si, 6 eV for the $2\pi \rightarrow 2\pi^*$ transition in carbon). Thus siloxane polymers, the most commonly utilized in personal care formulations, more closely resemble the organic ester structure ROR.

Although it might be assumed that silicon, lying directly beneath carbon in the periodic table, would react in a similar manner to carbon, there are numerous differences between silicone and carbon chemistry. Silicon, like carbon, does form tetrahedral bonds, but unlike carbon, silicon has available d orbitals. The silicon atom (radius 1.17 Å) is larger than carbon (radius 0.77 Å) and less electronegative (1.8 as compared to 2.5 for carbon), thus the resulting bonds to oxygen and chlorine are more polar. The effect of silicon (electropositive) bonding to oxygen (electronegative) leads to a charge transfer from the lone pair of electrons from oxygen to the Si—O bonding region between the

Table 1 Characteristic Properties of Silicon and Carbon Bonds

	C—C	C—O	Si—O
Bond length (°)	1.54	1.42	1.63
Bond angle (A)	112	111	130
Energy of rotation (kcal/mole)	3.6		0.2
Bond strength (kcal)	83	86	108

bonding atoms. This, in turn, results in electronic depletion from the oxygen's lone pair, altering the sp_3 hybridization at oxygen. The net effect is a very unusual bending flexibility for the Si—O—Si bond (1). Table 1 compares some basic properties of silicone and carbon bonds. Silanols, unlike the very stable alcohols, will typically undergo spontaneous hydrolysis to form siloxanes, and in general, silicon compounds are much more reactive than their carbon analogs as seen in Eq. (1) and (2) below.

$$HSiCl_3 \xrightarrow[H_2O]{\text{Cold}} H_2\uparrow + HCl\uparrow + \text{—Si—O—Si—} \quad (1)$$

$$HCCl_3 \xrightarrow[H_2O]{\text{Cold}} \text{no reaction} \quad (2)$$

II. PHYSICOCHEMICAL PROPERTIES OF SILICONES

The unique structure and flexibility of silicone polymers renders their performance properties quite different from those of organic polymers. Table 2 lists some typical characteristics of polydimethylsiloxane polymers (PDMS) of low and high degrees of polymerization (DP) as compared to their organic counterpart (polyethylene) of corresponding DP. Silicones are generally resistant to the types of substances that attack organic materials (ultraviolet, heat, oxidation, etc.) while they are susceptible to attack from strong acids or bases to which hydrocarbon polymers are generally resistant. As compared to their organic counterparts, dimethylsiloxane polymers display much greater thermal and oxidative stability and are fluid over a much larger range of molecular weights. The high thermal stability characteristic of siloxane polymers stems from the strength of the Si—O—Si bond. On the other side of the scale, siloxane polymers are quite resistant to low temperatures as well, with pour points and glass transition temperatures of approximately -60 and -120°C, respectively. The flash points of silicone fluids with viscosities over ~100 centistokes (cst) lie above 300°C, with spontaneous ignition occurring at about 420°C. The basic physical properties of silicone polymers, such as dielectric strength (~14 kV/mm), resistivity ($\sim 6 \times 10^{15}\ \Omega$ cm), and viscosity, are relatively independent of changes in temperature as opposed to hydrocarbon-based polymers. Table 3 illustrates the differences in viscosity with changes in temperature for a silicone fluid as compared to petroleum-based oil of the same viscosity at skin temperature (2). Accordingly, in contrast to organic polymers, silicone polymers are typically classified on the basis of viscosity as opposed to molecular weight. The two properties may be easily correlated, however, as shown in Table 4, which displays the relationship between viscosity and molecular weight for commonly utilized dimethicone polymers.

The differences between silicone and organic polymers result from the weak intermo-

Table 2 Properties of Silicone Polymers Compared to their Organic Counterparts: Polydimethylsiloxane Versus Polyethylene

	Silicone	Hydrocarbon
	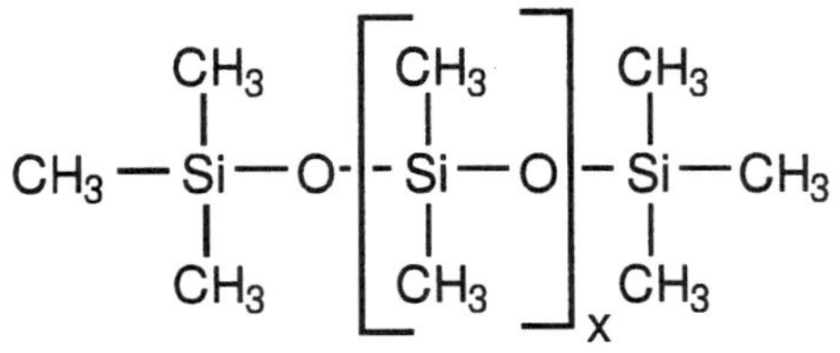	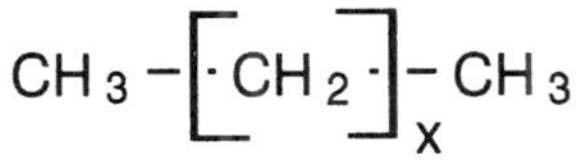
If x equals:	The resulting polymer is characterized as:	
25	Fluid (20 cst)	Paraffin wax
7000	Gum	High-density polyethylene
Resulting polymers are resistant to:		
	O_2	Acid
	O_3	Base
	H_2O	Some solvents
	Heat (500°F)	Electricity
	Cold (−60°F)	
	Electricity	
Resulting polymers are attacked by:		
	HF	O_2
	Strong bases	O_3
	Strong acids	UV
	Solvent (swelling)	Temp. (properties change)
	Fire (somewhat)	Some solvents
	Some metals	Fire (consumed)

lecular attractive forces characteristic of silicone polymers. This is a consequence of: (1) larger (or flatter) Si—O bond angles, (2) longer Si—O—Si bond lengths as compared to C—O—C or C—C bonds, (3) a greater degree of rotation about the Si—O bond as compared to carbon-based compounds, and (4) the freely rotating methyl groups, which swing to the surface and tend to keep the polymer chains more extended, resulting in a large excluded or "free" volume. These characteristic properties are illustrated in Figure 1. Owing to the high coefficients of expansion typical of silicone polymers (expanded polymer chains), polydimethylsiloxanes undergo a very small change in physical proper-

Table 3 Viscosity as a Function of Temperature for Silicone and Hydrocarbon Oils

Temp. (°C)	Silicone oil	Petroleum oil
100	40	11
38	100	100
−18	350	11,000
−37	660	230,000

Table 4 Correlation Between Viscosity and Molecular Weight of Commonly Utilized Polydimethylsiloxane Fluids

Viscosity (cst)	Molecular weight
5	800
20	2,000
50	3,800
100	6,000
200	9,400
350	13,700
500	17,300
1,000	28,000
5,000	49,300
10,000	62,700
12,500	67,700
30,000	91,700
60,000	116,000
100,000	139,000
300,000	204,000
600,000	260,000

ties with either temperature or polymer molecular weight as previously stated. This results in the low modulus and glass transition temperatures (low brittle points) exhibited by dimethicone fluids. Also characteristic of polydimethylsiloxanes is a low surface tension (20.8 N/m^2 at 25°C) and high spreadability and diffusivity coefficients. Therefore, the unmodified silicone polymers will spread into thin uniform films and are highly permeable to gases such as oxygen, carbon dioxide, and water vapor. This is illustrated in Table 5, where the gas permeability of silicone elastomers is compared to that of several other organic compounds. Replacement of one or more of the methyl groups in polydimethylsiloxanes by larger aliphatic or aromatic hydrocarbon substituents, however, markedly decreases both the spreading capacity of the fluids and the permeability of the resulting polymers (3).

The low surface energy characteristic of silicone polymers renders them excellent water-repellent lubricants (contact angles against water droplets ~105°) and good antifoam agents (3). Polydimethylsiloxane fluids have a pronounced antifoaming action and are the basic components of special defoamers. The latter usually contain a small amount of an activating solid such as fumed silica, generally in the range of 3–10 wt%. Unmodified silicones readily satisfy the basic criteria for effective defoaming action; i.e. they are insoluble in the foaming media, they have a very low surface tension, and they rapidly spread out over the foaming media, displacing foam-forming agents from the surface. This gives rise to increased capillary and gravitational drainage, excessive localized thinning of the bubble wall, increased Marongonni flow, and ultimately breakage. Figure 2 illustrates the mechanism of foam collapse resulting from silicone fluids in foaming solutions (20). Incorporation of activating solids such as fumed silica will promote more rapid destruction of foam through a pinholing effect on the bubble lamella. It has been shown that the defoaming action of silicone antifoams is dependent upon the surfactant and electrolyte concentrations in solution and the particular foaming system in question. Adsorption of

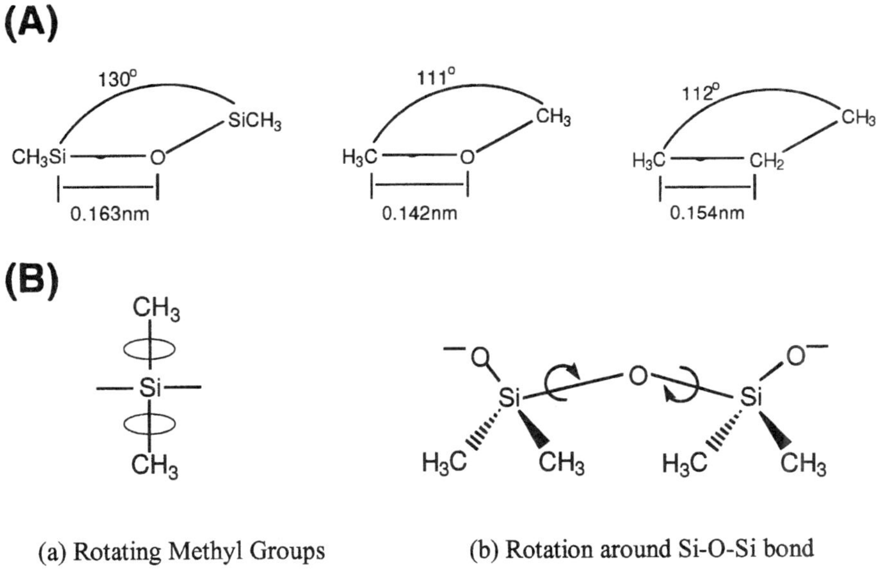

Figure 1 Structure-property relationship of silicone bonds. Silicones have characteristic low-intermolecular attractive forces as a consequence of the following: (A) A flexible polymer backbone. Si—O—Si bond angles vary from 105° to 180° while carbon bond angles are smaller and less variable. Si—O—Si bond lengths are also longer than either C—O—C or C—C bond lengths resulting in a more extended polymer. (B) Freely rotating methyl groups (a) and rotation around Si—O—Si bond (b) maintains separation in the polymer chains, providing a large excluded volume. This results in the small changes in physical properties encountered with large variations in polymer molecular weights or temperature. These properties are also responsible for the low glass transition temperature, low modulus, and high vapor permeability characteristic of siloxane polymers.

an ionically charged surfactant on the silicone droplet in solution (near the critical micelle concentration (CMC) of the surfactant) results in a decrease in antifoam activity owing to the repulsion between the silicone droplet and the similarly charged bubble surface (4). It has also been demonstrated that solution pH, temperature, composition, and concentration of the antifoam will play a role in the activity of the defoaming compound (5).

Polydimethylsiloxanes (dimethicones and dimethiconols) are also characterized by low surface viscosities (10^{-5} surface poise) and low levels of compatibility with aliphatic hydrocarbons and water (soluble to a few hundred ppm only). As a consequence of these

Table 5 Gas Permeability of a Silicone Elastomer as Compared to Organic Polymers

Compound	Gas permeability (10^6 cm^3/sec/cm)
Silicone rubber	60
Natural rubber	2.4
Butyl rubber	0.24
Polyvinyl chloride	0.014
Teflon	0.0004

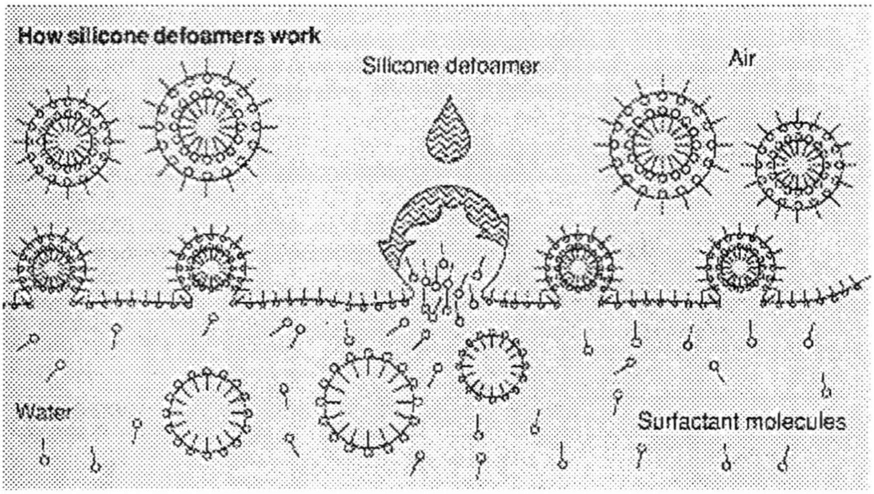

Figure 2 Foam collapse resulting from silicone fluids.

combined properties, the unmodified silicone fluids readily separate from the other ingredients in a formulation when it is spread over the surface of skin or hair. The silicone will then uniformly spread over the surface of the other ingredients forming monomolecular films (6,7). This phenomenon results from the low strength of the intermolecular binding forces as well as the low surface tensions characteristic of the silicone polymers. In general, the work of cohesion, $2\sigma_f$, of the liquid phase having a surface tension σ is smaller than the work of adhesion, ζ_{sf}, to the surface of the substrate, so that the spreading pressure $p_{sp} = \zeta_{sf} - 2\sigma_f$ becomes positive (3). Thus, the aesthetics of the formulation will necessarily be dominated by the silicone, which resides at the surface/air interface of the applied composition (8). The characteristic properties described above are responsible for the unique attributes of silicone polymers, rendering them useful in a large variety of applications in such diverse industries as aerospace, electronics, automotive, construction, and cosmetics.

III. EVOLUTION OF SILICONES IN PERSONAL CARE

The use of silicone materials in hair care and skin care products has been known for over 50 years, with polydimethylsiloxanes (dimethicones) being the first commercially available silicone products offered to the cosmetic industry. Skin care formulations incorporating dimethicone polymers premiered in the marketplace slightly earlier than did hair care products. The first such example dates back to the late 1940s, when Revlon launched a product known as Silicare skin lotion. This formulation contained dimethicone, which provided a protective, breathable barrier on the skin and reduced the whitening or ''soaping'' effect typically encountered during rub-in of the lotion (9). The use of silicones in hair care products debuted a few years later in the early 1950s, with the introduction of a lotion spray product known as Sudden Date. This product, introduced into the marketplace by Lanolin Plus, was designed to be sprayed onto a ''tired hairdo'' to provide ''immediate refreshing.'' The silicone ingredient present in the formulation was claimed to cause the hair to be ''shiny and more spirited'' (10). In 1958 dimethicone polymers for use as conditioning additives in shampoo compositions became known in the art when the first patent detailing this application was issued to the Simonize Co. (11). In antiperspirant applications, silicones entered the market in 1955 in roll-on form, and in 1965 in aerosol products (12). It wasn't until 1973 that the first deodorant stick product containing cyclomethicones was launched, and in 1978 Dry Idea launched a faster drying roll-on, containing 75% cyclomethicone, which was also reported to feel drier during application (13). Following this product introduction, cyclomethicones became the major component in most nonaerosol antiperspirant and deodorant (AP/DO) formulations.

The benefits derived from the incorporation of silicones in hair and skin care products were becoming quite obvious to product development chemists by the late 1950s and early 1960s. Even so, silicone materials were not utilized extensively in the formulation of personal care compositions during this period because of their inherent solubility and compatibility problems. During the last two decades, however, the use of silicones in personal care products has dramatically increased owing to the unique properties and benefits provided by these materials and the introduction of more sophisticated ingredients. This increased use of silicones was made possible by the emergence of new technology in the areas of emulsification, associative thickeners, and suspending agents, and the introduction of a wide variety of organomodified silicone polymers and silicone emulsifiers, which offer increased compatibility with the other ingredients generally contained in cosmetic formulations. The organofunctional silicones have the added advantage of providing multifunctional benefits to the formulations such as shine enhancement from incorporation of phenyl groups, or occlusivity imparted by alkyl modification. The increased use of silicones in personal care compositions becomes obvious when looking at ingredient listings for new products being introduced into the marketplace. For example, well over half of all new personal care products introduced into the U.S. marketplace over the last 2 years contained some type of silicone compound in the composition (14,15).

IV. NOMENCLATURE

The basis of current silicone chemistry nomenclature was established by Alfred Stock in 1916 (16). He referred to silicone hydride compounds as silanes; e.g., SiH_4 was a monosilane, Si_2H_6 a disilane, and so forth. Derivatives were named by adding the appropriate prefixes such as dichlorodisilane for $Si_2H_4Cl_2$. When oxygen joined two silicon atoms, the compound was referred to as a siloxane, and polymeric versions became known as polydimethylsiloxanes. This system was eventually adopted by the International Union of Pure and Applied Chemistry (IUPAC). Although these descriptors are accurate and informative, they are somewhat cumbersome. Silicone chemists thus frequently use an abbreviated notation when referring to the basic groups that comprise typical silicone polymers. According to this system, there are four primary building blocks in silicone chemistry, as illustrated in Table 6. The chainstopper, or end-capping unit, is ''monovalent,'' or reactive through only one bond to the silicone atom, and has been given the shorthand notation of ''M.'' This $Si(CH_3)_3$ group is also commonly known as a ''trimethylsilyl'' unit in cosmetic applications, such as in trimethylsilylamodimethicone. The on-chain repeat unit is referred to as ''D,'' or difunctional, as there are two bonds through which the polymer chain can grow and two unreactive methyl units attached to the silicone atom. Thus, the structure of a linear dimethicone polymer would be represented as MD_xM. Should one or both of the methyl groups in a D unit be replaced with an organic moiety

Table 6 Silicone Shorthand Notation

Notation	Representation	Comment
M	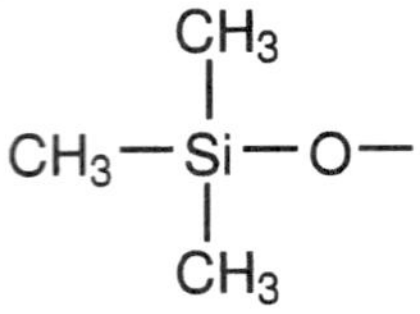	Chain stopper
D	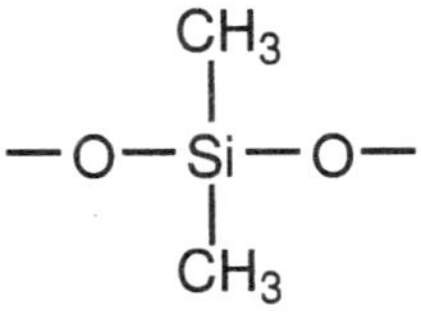	On-chain repeat unit
T	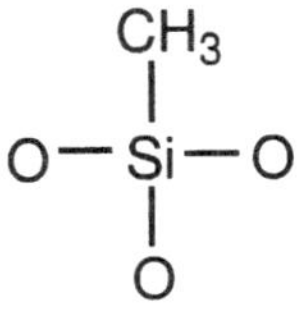	Branching unit
Q	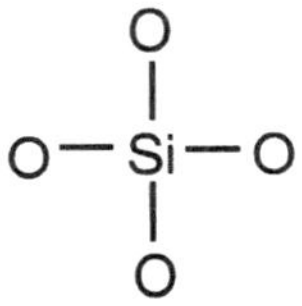	Resinous unit

Thus, in silicone shorthand notation, the structure:

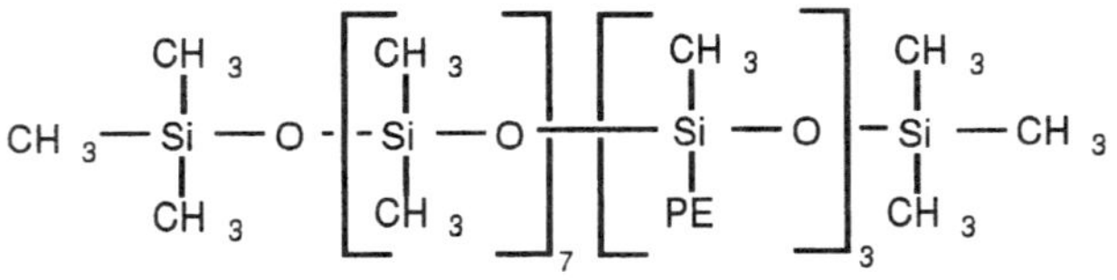

would be represented as $MD_7D'_3M$

such as a polyether unit or an amine group, the notation would become D′. When a silicone copolymer is formed, as in the case of dimethicone copolyol, the compound would be represented as $MD_xD'_yM$, as illustrated in Table 6. Terpolymers containing dimethyl, methylalkyl, and methylpolyether monomer units would be classified as $MD_xD'_yD''_zM$ polymers, and so forth. Trifunctional —$SiO_{3/2}$ groups provide branching characteristics, and since these silicone segments can react through three oxygen linkages on the silicone atom, they are referred to as ''T'' units. These highly branched compounds are referred to in the cosmetic industry as silsesquioxanes, or ''T resins.'' Finally, the second class of silicone resins is composed of quadravalent units, as opposed to tetravalent since the T descriptor was assigned to a trifunctional moiety. These materials are appropriately named ''Q'' groups. A quadravalent silicone resin (Q) containing —$Si(CH_3)_3$ end units (M) is known in the art as an ''MQ,'' or trimethylsiloxysilicate resin. Siloxysilicate resins are similar in structure to fumed or precipitated silica, the primary difference lying in the M:Q ratio, which is much lower in the case of fumed or precipitated silica.

This nomenclature system, while extensively employed by silicone chemists, is rarely encountered in the personal care industry. The more commonly utilized ingredient nomenclature system is that determined by the Cosmetic, Toiletry, and Fragrance Association (CTFA) or International Nomenclature for Cosmetic Ingredients (INCI). This is the system that will be employed throughout this chapter. While this method of nomenclature designation is rather descriptive and detailed for most cosmetic ingredients, silicone compound identification may be somewhat complicated under this system. According to the INCI nomenclature guidelines, the same product name may be representative of numerous and sometimes quite different materials all of which conform to a similar general structure, as will be pointed out below. For this reason, extreme caution must be exercised when evaluating offset products having the same ingredient name. For example, the designation ''dimethicone copolyol'' may be representative of a liquid oil-in-water emulsifier with a low silicone content and low cloud point, a water-in-oil solubilizer containing a low degree of polyether modification, or a high-melting-point wax. ''Dimethicone'' is another example, referring to such varying materials as 1-cst fluids, polymers of several thousand cst, and gums characterized by very low penetration numbers, which appear to be solid under ambient conditions. Since the same INCI designation may be applied to materials of such varying properties, the formulator should carefully evaluate all parameters of a particular silicone compound prior to substituting an ''identical replacement'' into the personal care composition being manufactured.

While there are many types of silicone polymers to choose from when formulating personal care products, the most commonly utilized are PDMS. This class of unmodified silicones comprise approximately 85% of all silicone compounds found in personal care formulations, and include materials under the INCI designations of cyclomethicone, hexamethyl disiloxane, dimethicone, and dimethiconol. PDMS polymers can exist in linear structures with a degree of polymerization ranging from zero (hexamethyl disiloxane) to several thousand. Dimethylsiloxane compounds may also exist in the form of cyclic ring structures known as cyclomethicone. Currently, the term ''cyclomethicone'' is used to refer to all the cyclic dimethylsiloxane compounds employed in personal care formulations; however, there is an expressed desire to specify the individual materials as cyclotrisiloxane, cyclotetrasiloxane, cyclopentasiloxane, and so forth (17). Of the cyclic dimethyl fluids, ring sizes of four (referred to as octamethylcyclotetrasiloxane, D_4, or tetramer), five (referred to as decamethylcyclopentasiloxane, D_5, or pentamer), and six (dodecamethylcyclohexasiloxane, D_6, or hexamer) are most frequently encountered in cosmetic products, but rings containing from three to 10 or more silicone atoms are known to exist.

The term ''volatile silicones'' is often used in the personal care industry to refer to, and interpreted to mean, cyclic PDMS fluids. However, linear fluids characterized by low degrees of polymerization (DP) are also volatile. For example hexamethyl disiloxane (DP $= 0$, $\eta = 0.65$ cst) is completely volatile, evaporating from hair or skin in a shorter period than either D_4 or D_5. Table 7 details the characteristic properties of a number of volatile silicone fluids that may be encountered in personal care formulations, and Figure 3 depicts the kinetic curves of evaporation for several of these fluids. Volatility of the dimethyl silicone polymer decreases as the degree of polymerization increases, approaching a limit around 10-cst fluids (DP $= 15$). As with volatility characteristics, other properties of dimethicone fluids also change with increasing molecular weight or degree of polymeriza-

Table 7 Properties of Volatile Silicones

Compound	MW (g/mole)	Vapor pressure (mmHg, 25°C)	Solubility (mg/L, 25°C)	Density (g/cm^3, 20°C)	Viscosity (cst., 20°C)	Bp (°K)
D3	222	8.6	1.56	0.856	0.5	408.2
D4	297	0.99	0.56	0.953	2.4	448.7
D5	371	0.174	0.017	0.995	4.2	484.2
D6	445	0.03	0.005	0.966	7.7	518.1
MM	162	42.2	0.93	0.765	0.65	373.6
MDM	236	3.88	0.034	0.820	0.9	425.7
MD2M	310	.43	0.006	0.854	1.7	467.1
MD3M	384	.06	7×10^{-5}	0.867	1.4	503.1

tion. For example, low-viscosity fluids are soluble in mineral oil and solvent alcohols such as ethanol or isopropanol, whereas the fluids most commonly employed in personal care applications other than antiperspirant/deodorant formulations (100 cst and higher) are soluble only to a few ppm in these same substances. Table 8 details solubility characteristics of a few selected silicone compounds in several raw materials commonly encountered in personal care formulations. Comparing solubility parameters of typical cosmetic ingredients, it has been shown that most classes of silicones occupy the extreme low end of the scale, while water resides at the opposite end, the exception being certain dimethicone copolyols that contain a large percentage of polyether modification (on average greater than 2 as a ratio of polyether to silicone) (18).

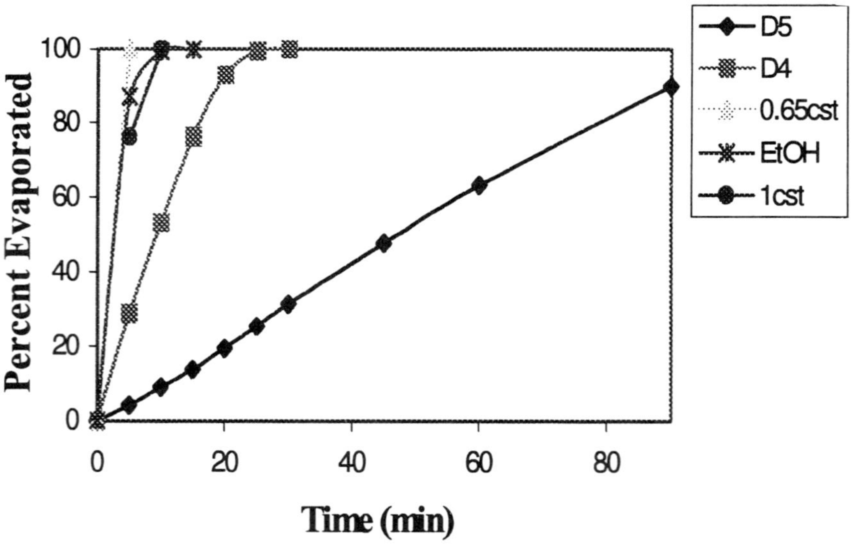

Figure 3 Evaporation rates for several volatile silicone fluids compared to ethanol. (a) Hexamethyl disiloxane; (b) cyclomethicone (D_4); (c) cyclomethicone (D_5); (d) dimethicone (1 cst).

Table 8 Solubility Characteristics of Selected Silicones

Material	100 cst Dimethicone	Cyclomethicone	Phenyltrimethicone
Ethanol	NS	S	S
Isopropanol	NS	S	S
Water	NS	NS	NS
IPP	S	S	S
IPM	S	S	S
Mineral oil	NS	S	S
Beeswax	NS	SH	SH
Carnauba wax	NS	SH	SH
Aromatic solvents	S	S	S
Aliphatic solvents	S	S	S
Octylmethoxycinnamate	PS	S	S
Octyl salicylate	NS	S	S
Lanolin	NS	SH	SH

S = soluble; NS = not soluble; PS = partially soluble; SH = soluble hot.

V. SILICONE CHEMISTRY

A. Formation of Siloxanes

As described in the previous section, there are four fundamental siloxane units, which are most important for the formation of the various silicone polymers utilized in personal care compositions (see Table 6). These are the mono-, di-, tri-, and quadrafunctional siloxanes, which are formed during a hydrolysis (or alcoholysis) reaction of chlorosilanes. Several different processes are utilized on a commercial scale to manufacture silicones. Each production process contains numerous steps, starting with the preparation of silicon metal, followed by formation of chlorosilanes and their subsequent conversion first to silanols and then ultimately to organosiloxanes. The most widely utilized commercial process, referred to as the ''direct process'' or the Rochow synthesis, is illustrated in Figure 4 (2,19). The first step in the process is known as a carbothermic reduction where sand is mixed with coke in an electric furnace to produce silicon metal. Next, the metal is crushed to a particle size range of 45–250 μm and mixed with copper powder. The silicon-copper mixture is put on a septum in a large vertical steel cylinder known as a fluid-bed reactor. A heated stream of methyl chloride gas is passed through the mixture, forcing the powder upward in the column. The temperature of this reaction must be strictly controlled, and is typically kept in the range of 280–290°C. The solid silicon and copper particles are held apart and continuously mixed by the upward-flowing stream of gas, so that this gas-solid reaction is accomplished without mechanical stirring or ''dead spots'' where no gas can penetrate the powder mixture (2). This reaction may be accelerated by addition of up to 0.2% zinc dust (20).

The resulting reaction products are a mixture of chlorosilanes with varying degrees of substitution, as shown in Figure 4. The physical properties of these and other reaction products formed during the production of the basic materials are listed in Table 9 (21,22). The production process is optimized to yield dimethyldichlorosilane, the most important product for the synthesis of silicone polymers. The trifunctional unit is next in commercial importance followed by the mono and quadrafunctional units, respectively (3). The chlo-

1. Carbothermic Reduction:

$$\underset{\text{(sand)}}{SiO_2} + \underset{\text{(coke)}}{2C} \xrightarrow[\text{Furnace}]{\text{Electric}} 2CO_2 \uparrow + \text{Si (metal)}$$

2. Direct Process:

$$Si + CH_3Cl \xrightarrow[300^\circ C]{Cu} \text{Mixture of chlorosilanes}$$

Trimethylchlorosilane	Me_3SiCl
Dimethyldichlorosilane	Me_2SiCl_2
Methyltrichlorosilane	$MeSiCl_3$
Tetrachlorosilane	$SiCl_4$

Chlorosilanes are separated by distillation, process is optimized to yield Me_2SiCl_2

3. Hydrolysis:

$$Me_3SiCl + H_2O \rightarrow Me_3SiOH \rightarrow Me_3SiO_{1/2} + H_2O$$
$$Me_2SiCl_2 + H_2O \rightarrow Me_2Si(OH)_2 \rightarrow Me_2SiO_{2/2} + H_2O$$
$$MeSiCl_3 + H_2O \rightarrow MeSi(OH)_3 \rightarrow MeSiO_{3/2} + H_2O$$
$$SiCl_4 + H_2O \rightarrow Si(OH)_4 \rightarrow SiO_{4/2} + H_2O$$

4. Cracking/distillation:

Siloxanes → Trimer + tetramer + pentamer + hexamer + etc.

5. The equilibrium reaction:

$$(CH_3)_3Si{-}O{-}Si(CH_3)_3 + x[(CH_3)_2Si{-}O]_4 \xleftrightarrow[\Delta]{\text{Catalyst}} \underset{(MD_{4x}M)}{(CH_3)_3Si{-}O{-}[(CH_3)_2SiO]_{4x}{-}Si(CH_3)_3}$$

At equilibrium 12–15% volatiles remain

Figure 4 Preparation of monomeric siloxane units.

Table 9 Products of the Reaction Between Methyl Chloride and Silicon via Direct Synthesis

Compound	Formula	Bp (°C/760 mm)	Vp (mmHg, 25°C)
Dimethyldichlorosilane	$(CH_3)_3SiCl_2$	70.2	143.9
Methyltrichlorosilane	CH_3SiCl_3	66.1	168.3
Trimethylcholrosilane	$(CH_3)_3SiCl$	57.3	231.2
Silicon tetrachloride	$SiCl_4$	57.6	
Tetramethylsilane	$(CH_3)_4Si$	26.2	
Methyldichlorosilane	CH_3SiHCl_2	40.4	422.0
Dimethyldichlorosilane	$(CH_3)_2SiHCl$	35.4	526.3
Trichlorosilane	$SiHCl_3$	31.8	593.4

Also:
α,ω-Dichloropolydimethylsilanes, 2- and 3-Methylhexanes, 2- and 3-Methylpentanes, Hydrogen, methane, ethane, and ethylene

rosilanes generated in the reaction described above are passed through a dust filter at the top of the fluid-bed reactor, and directly into a series of continuous distillation towers. As the silicon powder is depleted by reaction with the methyl chloride, more silicon powder is added continuously to the reactor. A small amount of copper powder is also continuously replaced to make up for that removed in the dust filters. Unreacted methyl chloride (bp 24.2°C) is separated in the first distillation column and returned to the fluid-bed reactor. The remaining chlorosilanes are separated by the subsequent distillation columns (to a purity of ~99.98 mol%) in the order of increasing boiling points, the last one being dimethyldichlorosilane (bp 70°C).

The next step in the Rochow process is known as a hydrolysis reaction in which the various silanol groups are formed. Water and the chlorosilanes are circulated together in a closed loop by a pump, where a mixture of HCl (37% solution) and mixed silanols is formed. Some of the HCl is stripped off and combined with methanol to produce more methyl chloride, which is recycled to the chlorosilane production step. The remaining HCl is returned to the hydrolysis loop to continue the reaction. The silanols undergo spontaneous condensation to form low-molecular-weight siloxanes, or hydrolysates. The monomeric and oligomeric hydrolysates may be utilized in the production of silicone polymers via polycondensation reactions, or may be ''cracked back'' to generate a series of cyclic siloxanes. Both intramolecular and intermolecular condensation can occur, with the former yielding ring structures and the latter, linear polymers (20). The cracking process may be catalyzed by a fourfold excess of sulfuric acid, or it may be base-catalyzed. Polymethylsiloxanes may be formed by reaction of hydrolysate as described above using a phosphorous nitrile chloride ($PNCl_2$) catalyst, or by ring-opening polymerization of cyclic siloxanes in an equilibrium or redistribution reaction, as shown in Figure 4 (23–30).

B. Functionalized Silicones

1. Organofunctional (except Polyether)

Silicon hydrides may be thought of as the first in a series of alkyl-substituted siloxanes. Alkyl (also ester and phenylethyl) functional siloxanes are prepared by a process known as a hydrosilylation reaction, which in part displays the characteristics of both addition and substitution reactions. This synthesis is carried out in a suitable solvent using a platinum catalyst (31) and combining unsaturated α-olefins with silicon hydride compounds according to the mechanism presented in Eq. (3) below.

$$R_3SiH + R'_2C{=}CR'_2 \xrightarrow[\text{Pt, }\Delta T]{} R'CH{-}CR'_2{-}SiR_3 \tag{3}$$

Reactions carried out with alkynes will result in vinyl silanes, which may be further reacted through the unsaturated bond. This synthesis may also be performed using chlorosilanes as opposed to silicon hydrides, but the silicon-chloride bond is stronger than the silicon-hydrogen bond, and thus the reaction with chlorosilanes requires a higher activation energy. These reactions may be catalyzed using ultraviolet light and peroxides in place of platinum (32–34). Under certain conditions alkylfunctional silicones may also be synthesized by condensation reactions or through Grignard syntheses (35). Phenylmodified silanes are generally prepared by a nucleophilic substitution reaction at elevated temperatures ranging from 550 to 650°C with the assistance of Grignard reagents (20).

Alkoxysilanes are prepared by addition reactions of alcohols with organochlorosilanes, by reaction of organometallic reagents with lower alkoxysilanes, or by hydrosilylation using Grignard compounds as catalysts. Organic substitution of chlorosilanes becomes increasingly difficult with increasing size of the organic groups because of steric hindrance effects. The effect of steric hindrance becomes even more difficult with increasing organic substitution, i.e., diorgano, triorgano, and so forth. These reactions are frequently carried out at high temperatures for long periods with a large excess of the Grignard compound, and often with cobalt chloride as a cocatalyst (36–39). Like organic esters, the Si—O—R bond is subject to hydrolytic cleavage; however, its sensitivity to hydrolysis is considerably lower than that of the Si—X bond. The susceptibility to hydrolysis decreases with increasing number of carbon atoms in the substituent chain, and aryloxy groups are less easily split off than lower alkoxy groups, with phenylaryloxysilanes being most resistant because of the size and electronegativity of the phenyl groups (40,41).

The reaction described by Wagner in Eq. (3) concentrated primarily on the modification of linear silicones. It was not until much later that this same mechanism was employed to modify silsesquioxane and siloxysilicate resins with alkyl, ester, polyether, phenyl, and phenethyl groups. The resulting compounds exhibited the highly substantive film-forming properties of the silicone resin, combined with emolliency, shine, occlusivity, and so forth conferred by the various organic groups attached to the resin (42–45). These compounds also displayed increased compatibility with numerous ingredients typically incorporated into personal care formulations.

2. *Amine-Modified Silicones*

Aminosilanes of the general formula $R_nSi(NH_2)_{4-n}$, $R_nSi(NHR)_{4-n}$, $R_nSi(NR_2)_{4-n}$ are prepared by the reaction of silicon hydrides or chlorosilanes with ammonia or other amines in the presence of an inert solvent. These hydrosilylation reactions may be carried out at room temperature, with the reaction products being isolated by simple phase separation (3,46–48). To obtain the $MD_xD'_yM$ type aminofunctional siloxanes typically employed in personal care formulations, aminofunctional silanes (generally aminoethylaminopropyltrimethoxysilane or γ-aminopropyltrimethoxysilane) may be polymerized with linear hydrolysates or with octamethylcyclotetrasiloxane to form aminofunctional silicone fluids. Nucleophilic substitution and redistribution reactions have also been used to prepare one modified silicone from another. For example, aminofunctional siloxanes may be prepared by substitution as illustrated in Eq. (4).

$$\underset{\displaystyle (CH_2)_3Cl}{Me_3SiO(SiMe_2O)_x(SiMeO)_ySiMe_3} + NH_2CH_2CH_2NH_2 \rightarrow \underset{\displaystyle (CH_2)_3NH(CH_2)_2NH}{Me_3SiO(SiMe_2O)_x(SiMeO)_ySiMe_3} \quad (4)$$

The two most extensively utilized aminofunctional silicone polymers in personal care formulations are amodimethicone and trimethylsilylamodimethicone. These compounds are reactive (or uncapped) and nonreactive (or capped), respectively. The amodimethicone polymer may be prepared in emulsion form by ring-opening polymerization of D_4 with aminoethylaminopropyltrimethoxysilane. This emulsion polymerization process is generally carried out in the presence of a cationic/nonionic surfactant pair. Amodimethicone fluids may also be prepared via a linear processing technique starting with the silicone hydrolysates and aminoethylaminopropyltrimethoxysilane. These fluids may then be emulsified with nonionic or ionic surfactants as desired. The trimethylsilylamodimethicone compounds are typically prepared as fluids and then mechanically emulsified, generally utilizing nonionic surfactants, but these systems may incorporate ionic emulsifiers if preferred.

3. *Silicone Surfactants*

Polyether functional silicones (dimethicone copolyols) are usually prepared by the addition of silyl-hydride functional methylsiloxanes to allyl-terminated polyethers. This hydrosilylation reaction is typically carried out in solvent (toluene for industrial grades, isopropyl alcohol for personal care grades) utilizing a platinum catalyst as shown in Eq. (5) (49). Typically, excess polyether is added to the reaction to ensure complete consumption of the Si—H functionality, with increasing amounts of excess polyether being required as polymer molecular weight increases. Upon reaction completion, the solvent is removed by stripping, but the excess polyether usually remains in the product. The siloxanes in these materials may be linear or branched, and the glycol groups may be attached in pendant, terminal, or both positions along the polymer. Terpolymers containing dimethylsiloxane, methylpolyethersiloxane, and methylalkyl functionality may be synthesized by reacting silylhydride functionalized polysiloxanes with long-chain terminal olefins and alkenyl-terminated polyethers. Materials prepared in this manner behave more like conventional surfactants than silicone surfactants, and are characterized by higher surface tensions, lower spreading coefficients, and higher degrees of organic compatibility. Polymers containing Si—O—C linkages are prepared by reacting functionalized polysiloxanes with hydroxy terminated polyalkoxyalkylenes (50,51). The compounds containing Si—O—C linkages are far more susceptible to hydrolysis, and account for a much lower percentage of commercially utilized dimethicone copolyol compounds than do the materials containing Si—C linkages (52).

$$
\begin{array}{l}
Me_3SiO(SiMe_2O)_x(HSiMeO)_y\,SiMe_3 \\
\quad + CH_2{=}CHCH_2O(CH_2CH_2O)_a(CHMeCH_2O)_bR \\
\quad \xrightarrow{Pt} Me3SiO(SiMe2O)x(SiMeO)ySiMe3 \\
\qquad\qquad\qquad | \\
\qquad\qquad (CH_2)_3O(CH_2CH_2O)_a(CHMeCH_2O)_bR
\end{array} \tag{5}
$$

Unlike other substituted polydimethylsiloxanes, which generally contain only a few mole percent modification, the polyether materials may be extensively modified, containing in some cases up to 80–90% polyether, depending on the application and the required HLB. Dimethicone copolyols may be prepared as capped or unreactive polymers, as illustrated above, or they may be synthesized as reactive or uncapped materials, where one of the methyl groups on the end unit (or on the dimethyl repeat unit) would be represented by a reactive group such as —OH, —CH_2OH, and so forth. This is accomplished by not adding a chain-stopper (MM) component to the reaction (or in the case of an on-chain reactive unit, by using a methyltrimethoxysilane rather than a dimethyl moiety in the reaction). Dimethicone copolyol polymers of very low degree of substitution may also be prepared such that the polyether groups are positioned as end-cap units on a polydimethylsiloxane fluid. Depending on the type of polyether moiety employed and the silicone-to-polyether ratio, dimethicone copolyols may be either water-in-oil or oil-in-water emulsifiers. The amount of polyoxyalkylene units required to confer water solubility ranges from 2 to 4 as a ratio to dimethylsiloxane monomer units present.

Dimethicone copolyols, or silicone surfactants, are excellent wetting agents, capable of lowering the surface tension of water to ~21 dynes/cm. These materials are generally characterized by relatively high molecular weights. A special class of dimethicone copolyols exist, however, which contain only a few (in some molecules only one) dimethylsiloxane units. This type of compound may be considered to be an ''inverted surfactant'' and is characterized by a very small hydrophobic head group and a long hydrophilic polyether chain. These special silicone surfactants have been shown to wet out on very-low-energy surfaces such as polyethylene and paraffin to a greater degree than even lower-surface-tension compounds such as fluorocarbon surfactants ($\sim$16.5 N/m^2). For this reason, they have often been referred to as ''superwetters.'' This ability to rapidly wet out on low-energy surfaces results from the compact molecular structure, which promotes a rapid transfer of the surfactant molecules from the liquid-air interface to the solid surface, as opposed to conventional surfactants (and other silicone surfactants) in which the cumbersome hydrophobic groups impede the molecular transfer and spreading process (53,54).

Advances in dimethicone copolyol chemistry have led to incorporation of a variety of other functionalities onto silicone glycol copolymers, including protein hydrolysates. A number of these silicone protein polymers have been prepared from diverse protein sources utilizing either chemical or enzymatic hydrolysis techniques to obtain the desired protein fragments. The silicone protein copolymers may be tailored to deliver various benefits by placing the amino acid groups in either pendant or terminal positions along the chain, by altering the degree of silicone substitution, or by employing secondary, tertiary, or quaternary amines. Other variations include alteration in the glycol content, type, and placement of the glycol moiety along the silicone polymer molecule (55,56). As with the unmodified dimethicone copolyols, the silicone proteins are water soluble up to a certain temperature known as the cloud point, above which they become insoluble and exhibit a greater tendency to deposit onto the hair or skin surface.

To obtain even higher levels of conditioning, the dimethicone copolyols may be reacted with amphoteric materials (e.g., cocamidopropyldimethylamine dimethicone copolyol phosphate copolymer), or with amino functional compounds to produce silicone quaternary materials (e.g., Quaternium 80, Silicone Quaternium-1,-5,-6,-10, etc.). The amphoteric surfactants provide higher levels of denser foam while the cationic surfactants provide higher levels of, and more substantive, conditioning benefits. Silicone surfactants comprising multiple lipophilic moieties have also been developed for use in conditioning shampoos (57–59). These materials are claimed to provide good foam at concentrations well below the critical micelle concentration of organic surfactants containing a lipophilic chain of comparable length. Thus, the silicone surfactants containing multiple lipophilic groups are less aggressive toward the skin and mucous membranes, in particular the mucous membranes of the eye.

Alkylamido silicone quaternary compounds have been synthesized utilizing dimethicone copolyol chemistry with the organoquaternary groups pendant along the polymer backbone. Diquaternary polydimethylsiloxanes have also been synthesized where the alkylamido moieties reside in the terminal positions of the polymer chain (60–66). Silicone quaternary compounds are available in high- and low-molecular-weight versions and are identified by the INCI nomenclature ''Silicone Quaternary-x,'' where the ''x'' in the INCI name identifies the various quaternary groups attached to the silicone polymers. Silicone quaternary compounds are water soluble, and thus easily formulated into aqueous systems, the most common application being in conditioning compositions. The silicone quaternary substances readily deposit onto the hair, providing the combined benefits of the characteristic silicone ''slip'' or lubricity, with the softness and reduction in flyaway associated with the hydrocarbon quat (67).

Dimethicone copolyol chemistry may also be utilized to incorporate low levels of thiosulfate moieties (on average, two to five groups per polymer molecule) onto dimethylsiloxane polymers. The thiosulfate groups, or ''Bunte salts,'' are grafted onto polydimethylsiloxanes via the same method employed in preparation of silicone quaternary compounds. Specific silicone surfactants have been prepared such that the sulfur moiety is attached to the siloxane polymer via a decamethylene group in place of a methyl group in polydimethylsiloxane. As with the quaternary modification, the thiosulfate functionality confers greater hydrophilic properties to the silicone polymer, allowing greater ease of formulation with these materials as compared to the unmodified silicones. These substances adsorb onto keratin substrates via a combination of hydrophobic and electrostatic processes and have proven particularly efficacious in the treatment of badly damaged hair (68,69). Preparation of various other sulfur-containing silicone surfactants has also been reported utilizing this same chemistry. Such materials include aminoalkylsulfonates, sulfonamides, thioethers, and sulfoxides (70–72). In addition to the functional attachment groups specifically discussed, a wide variety of other silicone polymer modifications may be found including siliconized natural waxes, fragrances, vitamins, fatty acids, and amino acids, silicone carboxylates, silicone phosphobetaines, and so forth. Thus, by judicious choice of the substituent, silicone polymers may be modified to provide multifunctional benefits to numerous types of personal care compositions.

The latest class of silicone surfactants to be prepared are the fluorosilicone copolymers (73,74). These compounds combine disiloxane or branched trisiloxane structures modified with fluoroalkyl radicals as the hydrophobic moiety and polyethylene oxide units as the hydrophilic group. Two copolymers containing different fluoroalkyl groups have been reported for use in shampoo systems. The materials containing 3,3,3, trifluoropropyl units were characterized by surface tensions approximately equivalent to dimethicone fluids (~20.1 mN/m), while polymers containing 3,3,4,4,5,5,6,6,6, nonafluorohexyl groups displayed surface tensions as low as 17.6 mN/m (75).

C. Emulsions

Silicone fluids, particularly very-high-viscosity polymers, are often utilized in the form of aqueous emulsions. This promotes rapid dilution in water, homogeneous distribution of small quantities in the formulation, and the ability to process at room temperatures under low shear conditions. Mechanical emulsions of dimethicone fluids ranging in viscosity from 50 to 1,000,000 cst are readily prepared by several methods. Typically, dimethicone emulsions employ nonionic surfactants such as laureth-4, laureth-23, trideceth-10, octoxynol-40, isolaureth-6, and so forth. The required HLB to prepare aqueous emulsions of silicone fluids is approximately 11–12, and combinations of low and high HLB surfactants often produce the most stable systems. Several emulsions may be found, however, that are based on only one surfactant. Macroemulsions of silicone fluids may be prepared using standard techniques. To prepare the emulsions with the smallest particle size distributions (most stable systems), the phase inversion temperature (PIT) method may be utilized. Using this method, the surfactants are combined with the silicone fluid and a small amount of water. The mixture is heated to a temperature at which the surfactants may be equally soluble in water or oil—the phase inversion temperature (~70°C for the system isolaureth-6, octoxynol-40). At this point, the rest of the water (at ambient temperature) is rapidly added with good stirring (76,77). Microemulsions may also be prepared by this method, or they may be produced by first forming an oil concentrate containing the silicone, surfactants, and a small amount of water, and then rapidly dispersing this concentrate in water (78–82).

Emulsions of dimethiconol polymers of even greater molecular weights may be prepared by emulsion polymerization techniques (83–85). These systems most often contain a mixture of anionic and nonionic surfactants in the emulsification system, with the ionic surfactants typically being sodium or triethanolamine salts of dodecylbenzenesulfonic acid. Since dimethiconol polymers are uncapped substances, they will undergo a self-condensation reaction during drying to form an elastomeric film as evidenced near the top of open containers or on the sides of drop tanks. Both dimethicone and dimethiconol emulsions allow cold processing and easy addition to aqueous systems, while providing the same benefits for which high-molecular-weight dimethicone polymers are so well known.

While not strictly considered emulsions, two other systems may be classified in this category, both of which comprise very small particles of silicone fluids in aqueous dispersions. The first method of preparing these microdroplets involves in situ polymerization of a water-soluble vinyl monomer or mixtures of said monomer and acryl comonomers. The silicone fluids are first dispersed into microdroplets in the water phase by means of high-speed agitation and then the vinyl monomers or cationic polymers are added at elevated temperatures in the presence of free-radical catalysts. The resulting aqueous polymer matrix contains stable, discreet microdroplets of the silicone fluids. The second method utilized to prepare such a fine dispersion is very-high-pressure injection of silicone into the aqueous phase. These microdroplets have been referred to as nanoparticles, but they are actually nanometer-sized fluid droplets as opposed to nanometer-sized silicone resin particles, which are referred to by the same term (86). Both of the systems described above have been claimed to readily deposit onto hair and skin, and to increase ease of formulation (87,88).

Emulsions of organofunctional silicone compounds may be prepared by mechanical emulsification techniques in a similar manner to those described for the dimethicone fluids. Amodimethicone emulsions may be formed by emulsion polymerization methods similar to those utilized for the production of dimethiconol emulsions. The main difference between the two methods is that while dimethiconol emulsions typically contain an anionic surfactant, the amodimethicone emulsions are generally prepared with the use of nonionic/cationic surfactant pairs. In this method, the surfactants are dispersed in water, and the aminoethylaminopropyltrimethoxysilane (or other aminofunctional monomer such as γ-aminopropyltrimethoxysilane) is added along with octamethylcyclotetrasiloxane. Regardless of the polymer being synthesized (unmodified or aminofunctional), ring-opening emulsion polymerization is an equilibrium reaction, and therefore there will be a certain amount of residual unreacted cyclomethicone (D_4) in the final products.

VI. STRUCTURE-PROPERTY RELATIONSHIPS AND APPLICATIONS

A. Volatile Silicones

1. Cyclomethicones

Cyclomethicones are clear, colorless, low-viscosity fluids with relatively high volatility and a very slight characteristic odor. Cyclomethicones are characterized by ring structures typically containing 3–10 silicone atoms, the most commonly employed in personal care products containing 3–6 Si—O groups per ring. These products are separated by distillation into the various fractions or ''cuts'' as described in Section V. Cyclomethicone fluids are nonpolar and insoluble in water, but they are completely miscible in mineral oil, lower alcohols, esters, and numerous other typical solvents employed in personal care compositions. They may be supplied as pure fractions or blends of two or more fluids (typically D_4/D_5 and D_5/D_6 blends). In hair care products, cyclomethicones are frequently used as carriers or diluents to help uniformly deliver high-molecular-weight fluids or gums along the hair fiber, as plasticizers in fixative products, as the delivery system in gloss sprays, and to provide wet-combing benefits from conditioning shampoos and conditioners. These products are known to depress foam and viscosity; thus when formulating shampoos containing cyclomethicones, it is advisable to add external thickeners as well as foam boosters/stabilizers. Also, for this reason they are not incorporated into mousse formulations. The use of cyclomethicones has been reported for shine enhancement on hair. The method by which this is accomplished is through enhancement in fiber alignment, resulting in a smoother surface from which to reflect incident light. This effect, however, is transitory at best since these products are volatile and will evaporate from the hair shortly after application. In formulations designed to enhance luster, cyclomethicones are more often employed as the delivery system to provide uniform deposition of other shine-enhancing materials contained in the formulation.

Cyclomethicones are characterized by high vapor pressures and low heats of vaporization. Consequently, they will completely volatilize from the hair or skin over a short period of time; e.g., D_4 will evaporate entirely within 30 min at 25°C, and within 10 min at 37°C. Owing to their low heat of vaporization, these products evaporate from the skin without producing a cooling or stinging effect. For this reason, cyclomethicones have been extensively utilized as the delivery system in antiperspirant and deodorant formulations. Cyclomethicone blends are frequently desirable in these applications to vary the volatility or depress the freezing point of the pure distillates, and to vary the evaporation characteristics. This is particularly advantageous in the preparation of antiperspirants and deodorant products. For example, several major producers of these products are located in a climate where the freezing point of pure D_4 might present a problem in winter; thus a D_4/D_5 blend, characterized by a freezing point of −12°C, would be advantageous as compared to pure D_4, which freezes at 17.6°C. In a product form such as a semisolid or stick, a D_5/D_6 blend might be desirable for the lower volatility rate, which may help to maintain stick integrity. Also, as a result of their low coefficient of friction, they reduce frictional effects on the skin during application of these products. In other skin care applications, cyclomethicones are utilized as carriers to uniformly deliver pigments or other actives (e.g., sunscreens, water-resistant resins, etc.) uniformly over the skin, to improve rub-in properties, as fugitive emollients, to reduce tackiness of acrylic acid thickeners, to improve payout in stick products, to impart lubricity, to improve skin feel, and to reduce dry down times.

2. *Hexamethyl Disiloxane*

Hexamethyl disiloxane, often referred to in silicone nomenclature as "MM," is a clear, colorless, linear volatile dimethylsiloxane fluid characterized by a degree of polymerization equal to zero. This material has a viscosity of 0.65 cst and a heat of vaporization of 46 cal/g, only slightly higher than the cyclomethicones. However, owing to its lower boiling point and higher vapor pressure, this fluid will completely evaporate even more quickly than D_4, as can be seen in Figure 3. Hexamethyl disiloxane is characterized by the same solubility properties and may be used in the same applications as cyclomethicones or may be blended with cyclic compounds to alter drying times for specific product requirements. Typically, hexamethyl disiloxane is not utilized widely in personal care formulations as it is more costly than cyclomethicones, and depending on the source, there may be a residual odor associated with the fluid that would be unacceptable in some applications.

B. Dimethicone Polymers

Dimethicone (or dimethiconol) polymers differ from each other in the nature of the end-group on the polymer chain. The CTFA or INCI designation does not differentiate between linear and branched polymers for either species, nor is polymer viscosity considered in this nomenclature system. Dimethicone is a nonreactive polymer characterized by a trimethylsilyl end-group, and is often referred to as a ''capped'' silicone polymer. Dimethiconol, on the other hand, is a reactive or uncapped polymer, and may undergo a self-condensation reaction during drying through the reactive hydroxyl or methoxyl end-units contained on the polymer chain. Both dimethicone and dimethiconol products may range from low-molecular-weight polydimethylsiloxane fluids (e.g., 1-cst fluids) to high-molecular-weight polymers (up to 1,000,000 cst) or silicone gums (>40,000,000 cst). The most commonly employed dimethyl fluids have viscosities ranging from 100 to 300,000 cst, with the material of choice dependent upon the particular application. Blends of dimethicone gums in dimethicone fluids, or blends of fluids with differing viscosities, would all be classified by INCI designation as ''dimethicone,'' with no regard for the number of species present. The same argument would apply for dimethiconol polymers.

Dimethicone and dimethiconol fluids readily spread into uniform thin films over the surface of hair and skin to form thin hydrophobic films, adding lubricity, shine, and humidity resistance to hair, and providing a protective, breathable barrier on the skin. The high spreading coefficients of unmodified silicones, along with their low interfacial tension toward lipids, results in wetting of proteinaceous substrates and good adhesion of thin cohesive films on the skin surface. These factors are necessary for substantivity. As a result of their high spreading ability, dimethicones improve the rubout of creams and lotions. In O/W emulsions, dimethicones are used as defoamers where they prevent whitening or soaping effects that may occur during rubout, particularly in compositions containing fatty alcohols (89).

Owing to the flexible polymer backbone, dimethicone polymers have high diffusivity factors for gases such as water vapor, oxygen, and carbon dioxide. This permeability allows respiration of the skin, and accordingly, a variety of dimethicone polymers are recognized as skin protectant drugs under both the skin protectant drug and diaper rash monographs (90,91). To be utilized in this application, the polydimethylsiloxane polymers must meet certain criteria specified under USP/NF guidelines, several of which are outlined in Table 10. The durability of this protective film imparted on the skin by dimethicones may be enhanced by incorporation of high-molecular-weight dimethicone gums or silicone resins such as trimethylsiloxysilicate into the formulation (92). Dimethicone fluids are also utilized in skin care compositions to impart lubricity and softness to the skin, as emollients, and to improve payout of antiperspirant salts or pigments in stick products. Very-high-molecular-weight dimethicone gums are often employed to impart water resistance to color cosmetic and sun-care formulations.

Polydimethylsiloxane polymers are the most common conditioning additives employed in 2-in-1 shampoo systems. They are widely utilized in conditioners and cuticle coat formulations (particularly high-molecular-weight fluids or gums) for their ability to

Table 10 Specifications for Dimethicone NF Grade

Viscosity (centistokes)			Specific gravity		% solids	Refractive index	
Min	Nominal	Max	Min	Max	(min)	Min	Max
18	20	22	0.946	0.954	80	1.3980	1.4020
95	100	105	0.962	0.970	98	1.4005	1.4045
190	200	220	0.964	0.972	98	1.4013	1.4053
332.5	350	367.5	0.965	0.973	98	1.4013	1.4053
475	500	525	0.967	0.975	98	1.4013	1.4053
950	1,000	1,050	0.967	0.975	98	1.4013	1.4053
11,250	12,500	13,750	—	—	98	1.4015	1.4055

reduce combing forces and to impart a soft feel to the hair. Dimethicones will provide excellent conditioning benefits to the hair when applied from shampoos or daily use conditioners, but this effect is not durable, being removed in the first wash cycle. It has been shown that modifying the surface charge on the emulsified silicone fluid droplet can increase the amount of dimethicone deposited onto hair. This may be accomplished through addition of cationic surfactants (93,94) including specifically di-long-chain alkyl quaternary compounds (95), tri-long-chain alkyl quaternary compounds (96), and imadazolidinium quaternary compounds (97) or by the use of cationic polymers (98–100). Dimethicone deposition on hair may also be heightened by incorporation of nonionic ''hair bridging agents'' such as wood rosin, siloxysilicate resins, or other resinous materials into the shampoo composition (101,102).

In addition to incorporating a cationic material into the composition, deposition of unmodified silicones onto hair may be influenced by varying the viscosity of the silicone polymer or the particle size of the emulsion droplet (102–110). Quantitatively, the spreading of liquids on solid surfaces was discussed by Dodge, and is given by the following equation, which demonstrates the dependence of spreading rate on the droplet volume and viscosity:

$$d = K[(\sigma V_o^2/\mu)t + (d_i/K)^7]^{1/7}$$

where d is the diameter of the contact area, σ is the liquid surface tension, V_o is the initial volume, μ is the liquid viscosity, K is a nondimensional parameter, and t is time (111).

This suggests, that given identical-size emulsion droplets, for a silicone fluid of 60 cst, surface coverage of the fiber would increase sixfold in 10 min, while it would take 1000 min for a similar-size droplet of 60,000 cst to cover the same area. Also, since the rate of surface coverage is proportional to the term $K(\sigma V_o^2/\mu)^{1/7}$, there is a very strong dependence on the initial volume of the droplet. Thus, if the particle size of the emulsion droplet were increased by a factor of 5, the rate of surface coverage would occur approximately four times as fast as the droplet of smaller particle size.

Dimethicones deposit onto the hair through a hydrophobic process during dilution, as in the rinsing stage of cleansing the hair (112). Once deposited onto the fiber surface, the oil droplets must collapse and spread over the entire surface in a uniform, thin film to prevent removal during rinsing. This process is governed by the work of spreading, which may be estimated from the spreading coefficients of oil onto a solid surface, in this case keratin (113). The spreading coefficient may be calculated from the following equation:

$$S = G_{k/w} - (G_{o/w} + G_{k/o})$$

where $G_{k/w}$, $G_{o/w}$, and $G_{k/o}$ are the interfacial tensions between the keratin-water, oil-water, and keratin-oil interfaces, respectively. It has been shown that the spreading coefficient for silicone on keratin increases with an increase in the zeta potential of the emulsion droplet (114). Other nonionic agents such as oils/waxes deposit via this same process; however, these materials are characterized by higher surface tensions and higher intermolecular cohesive forces. Thus, the droplets of an organic conditioning agent would not collapse and uniformly spread at the hair/water interface into such thin films, as do the silicone compounds. The organic conditioning agents would instead deposit in multilayer spots or patches along the fiber, and tend to weigh down the hair making it appear greasy, without providing the same level of protection. Unmodified silicones, on the other hand, are characterized by low intermolecular cohesive forces, low surface tension, and high spreading coefficients, and thus tend to spread into uniform thin films on the fiber surface, providing a greater level of conditioning.

Dimethyl silicone fluids are frequently incorporated into bleaching or dyeing preparations to impart conditioning benefits to the hair during processing. Hair bleached or colored with preparations containing silicones is characterized by a feel and appearance closer to that of the natural hair, as compared to hair dyed with similar systems without silicones (115–118). In temporary hair color products, incorporation of unmodified or organofunctional silicones has been shown to reduce ruboff tendencies of the direct dyestuffs onto hands or clothing (119). Addition of silicones to direct dye compositions has also been reported to reduce the tendency of the pigments to settle or cake upon standing, particularly formulations containing colored mica (120).

The use of dimethicone fluids or emulsions incorporated into neutralizer compositions is well known in the art of permanently waving or straightening hair (121–127). The neutralizer lotions contain fatty alcohols and nonionic emulsifiers to improve stability of both the emulsion and the peroxide. The silicone is deposited on the hair via a hydrophobic deposition process during the rinsing step, and provides a soft, smooth feel to the dry hair, while reducing combing forces for both wet and dry hair. In fixatives, dimethicones provide both shine and humidity resistance, helping to maintain the curl under conditions of elevated moisture. These properties result from the insolubility of the PDMS polymers in the hair spray resins; therefore, the silicone tends to ''bleed out'' and reside at the resin/air interface, imparting a hydrophobic film over the resin. This also results in an increase in apparent shine or luster of the hair.

C. Dimethicone Copolyol

Dimethicone copolyol is typically a copolymer of a polydimethylsiloxane and a polyoxyalkylene ether. Materials in this category containing a significant amount of polyether are soluble and stable in water and lower alcohols. Compounds containing a low polyether-to-silicone ratio are typically not soluble in polar solvents. The nature of the polyether moiety employed (ethylene oxide only, higher glycols, combinations thereof, etc.), the silicone: polyether ratio, and the degree of polymerization will all influence the performance of the end product. Regardless of changes in these parameters, the INCI designation remains the same as long as it is referring to a neat fluid (dilutions are usually provided in cyclomethicone, and the INCI designation will then list both materials).

As discussed previously, unmodified polydimethylsiloxanes are hydrophobic. Dimethicone copolyols, however, may be hygroscopic depending on the extent of organic glycol modification. The amount of polyether modification required to confer water solubility is typically 2–4 as a ratio of glycol to dimethylsiloxane monomer units. All of the water-soluble dimethicone copolyols, as is characteristic of other ethoxylated surfactants, display inverse temperature solubility. At low temperatures, the polyether groups are fully hydrated, but as temperature increases, the hydrogen bonds between water and polyether groups are broken, and the material becomes insoluble (128). Increasing either the silicone content in the polymer or the molecular weight of the polypropylene oxide chain in a PO or EO/PO modified dimethicone copolyol will result in lower phase separation temperatures (cloud points). There is no such correlation, however, for the compounds modified with only ethylene oxide groups, which become increasingly soluble as the EO content is raised (49). By judicious choice of polyether type and amount, a silicone glycol copolymer may be tailored such that the phase separation temperature permits the dimethicone copolyol to function as a transient defoamer. This application becomes particularly advantageous for foaming compositions that are packaged hot; the antifoaming action of the copolyol in solutions above the cloud point promotes more uniform fill levels and faster packaging times without deaeration of the system.

Dimethicone copolyols provided as neat fluids are typically water-soluble, surface-active silicone polymers, and are the material of choice when formulating clear-aqueous-based compositions. They are generally not utilized as primary surfactants in shampoo or personal cleansing systems as they do not generate foam as efficiently as typical anionic surfactants employed in these product types, and they do not clean exceptionally well. The neat fluids assist in formation of oil-in-water emulsion-type products. They are used in hair and skin care formulations as cosolubilizers for other silicones, some fragrances, and some natural oils, to stabilize foam, and to reduce irritation of primary surfactants as discussed below. In fixatives and styling products, the silicone glycol polymers act as resin plasticizers. In leave-in products, they help improve spreadability of higher-molecular-weight silicones and provide a light conditioning effect to the hair or skin. Typically the dimethicone copolyol materials provided in cyclomethicone are water-insoluble materials, and are utilized as emulsifiers for water-in-oil (or water-in-silicone) systems, particularly antiperspirants and sunscreens.

Dimethicone copolyols are also utilized in cleansing formulations for their ability to reduce eye irritation caused by many of the primary surfactants employed in these systems (129–132). Starch and DeVries studied the eye-irritating effect of sodium lauryl sulfate in the presence of four silicone glycol copolymers. All four dimethicone copolyols were found to decrease the irritation potential, with the effect becoming more dramatic as the degree of ethoxylation, and consequently the HLB of the surfactant, increased. Polymers modified with ethylene oxide moieties only were reported to be less irritating than materials containing EO/PO units. The differences reported in this study, however, were not considered to be statistically significant owing to the small number of rabbits included in these experiments. Finally, owing to their high level of water solubility and emulsification properties, some silicone glycol copolymers aid in the formulation of clear products, acting as cosolubilizers for some fragrances or natural oils (129). For these two reasons, dimethicone copolyols are frequently encountered in mild, geriatric, or ''baby'' shampoo formulations.

Aqueous solutions of dimethicone copolyols will produce foam. The amount and quality of the resulting foam, however, are not sufficient for these materials to be utilized as primary surfactants. Dimethicone copolyols are frequently added to cleansing compositions for their ability to act as ''profoamers.'' This does not mean that they produce a greater volume of foam, but rather that they retard the rate of liquid transport or drainage between the lamellae, effectively reducing the rate of bubble collapse, resulting in a denser, more stable, or ''creamier''-feeling foam consisting of smaller bubbles (133). This phenomenon is ascribed to a maximum in intermolecular cohesive forces in the adsorbed film as the oxyethylene content increases as discussed in further detail below (134). Dimethicone copolyols may act to simultaneously reduce the surface tension of the solution and to adsorb at the surface. These two effects are linked thermodynamically, and both contribute to a reduction in Marangoni flow properties (135).

The relationship of foaming characteristics to structural variation in silicone glycol copolymers is quite complex, with the degree of polymerization and percentage of ethylene oxide units incorporated into the polymer both playing a major role in performance. In a homologous series, foam heights tend to decrease as the degree of polymerization increases to about 20. As the length of the silicone backbone increases further, the decline in foam heights slows, and at sufficiently long chain lengths, it reverses. This phenomenon was explained by Floyd, who observed that the smaller molecules tended to pack more uniformly at the liquid/air interface (136). The more efficient packing results in lower aqueous surface tensions for the smaller molecules, thus smaller differences or surface tension gradients between the small and large bubbles in the foam. This in turn allows for more stable film formation and greater foam production. On the other hand, the higher-molecular-weight copolymers stabilize the foam by means of their ''bulk/size'' effects, i.e., reducing drainage of the films and reducing Marangoni flow characteristics. This results in the observed foam height profiles of initial decrease followed by a leveling off or increase in foam heights with increasing molecular weight of the silicone glycol copolymers. Matalon reported that for the systems in his investigation, 3-mole ethoxylated materials performed best in foam stabilization by addition of dimethicone copolyols (137). Materials characterized by higher degrees of ethoxylation were too hydrophilic, and dramatically decreased the stability of the lamellae, causing more rapid collapse of the foam. At temperatures above their cloud points, silicone glycol copolymers tend to aggregate into dehydrated micelles and will then act as antifoaming agents.

Glycol functionality is useful for increasing compatibility of silicones in polar media, and for increasing interaction with keratinatious substrates. Glycol functional silicones may act as emulsifiers for silicone-in-water or water-in-silicone systems. Alkyl, alkoxy, and ether functional silicones improve compatibility between silicone and organic oils, waxes, fatty alcohols, and so forth. Terpolymers of dimethyl, methylalkyl, methylpolyether functionality, such as cetyl dimethicone copolyol, promote formation of triple-phase emulsions, and improve formulation stability. These materials have been shown to be excellent water-in-oil emulsifiers with low fatting properties. They have been utilized to selectively adjust the rheology of formulations ranging from low-viscosity lotions to thick creams. They are also reported to improve freeze/thaw stability in cosmetic compositions (138). The high stabilizing potential of these terpolymer emulsifiers is likely due to the strong absorption of the phase boundaries resulting from the polymeric character, and the silicone, organic, and water-soluble portions of the molecule. The required HLB values of the coemulsifiers for these materials lie in the 4–7 range (138,139).

It is known in the art that W/O emulsions are more substantive to skin than O/W systems. Typically, W/O cosmetic emulsions containing glycerides of fatty acids are difficult to prepare, require extensive energy input, and are criticized for the reduced spreadibility, tack, and greasy feel characteristic of the waxy emulsifiers employed. The terpolymers described above were utilized in preparing W/O emulsions of various natural oils with an oil:water ratio of 1:3. These systems were prepared by pouring unheated water into 80°C oil phase with vigorous mixing. When the mixture cooled to ambient conditions, the emulsion was homogenized for 2 min at 5.5 m/sec. This procedure utilizes significantly lower energy input than normally associated with rotor stator homogenizers typically used to prepare W/O cosmetic emulsions. The resulting emulsions ranged in viscosity from thin lotions to thick creams, and displayed excellent freeze/thaw and temperature stability as compared to several similar systems comprising organic emulsifiers (138).

Water-in-silicone formulations are also becoming more popular for several reasons. These compositions improve skin substantivity as compared to O/W or silicone-in-water products, they do not leave an ''oily'' or greasy feel on the skin, and they offer enhanced stability and rheological control to the formulator. The use of high-molecular-weight polydimethylsiloxane gums and/or resinous silicones such as trimethylsiloxysilicate in these types of compositions has been shown to improve durability on skin for a number of typical cosmetic ingredients, but not all. For example, PABA and isopropylmyristate demonstrate increased durability to water washoff when applied from W/O emulsions in combination with dimethicone gums or MQ resins while cinnamates and glycerin do not (92). Low-HLB dimethicone copolyols, alkyl dimethicone copolyols, and alkyl dimethicone polyglucosides have all been utilized as efficacious W/O emulsifiers in the formulation of three-phase cosmetic compositions.

D. Amine Functionalized Silicones

1. Amodimethicone

Amodimethicone is typically an emulsion-polymerized polymer; however, utilizing linear processing technology amodimethicone fluids may be prepared as neat fluids, and then emulsified by a mechanical process as desired. The most widely utilized amodimethicone emulsions contain as the surfactant pair either (1) tallowtrimonium chloride (and) nonoxynol-10, or (2) cetrimonium chloride (and) trideceth-10 or -12. These ''uncapped'' amino-functional silicone compounds may be characterized by a linear or branched structure. In either case, amodimethicone polymers will undergo a condensation cure reaction during drying to form a somewhat durable elastomeric film on the hair, providing wet- and dry-combing benefits, lowering triboelectric charging effects, and increasing softness of the dry hair. They are excellent conditioning agents, often found in conditioners, mousses, setting lotions, and less frequently in 2-in-1 shampoos. When formulating shampoos, it is advisable to use the neat amodimethicone fluids or a mechanical emulsion employing nonionic surfactants, the reason for this being that the typical emulsion-polymerized systems may present difficulty with complex formation between the cationic emulsifiers and the anionic surfactants in the shampoo system. It is possible to utilize the cationic emulsion-polymerized amodimethicone systems in formulating shampoo products; however, caution must be exercised relating to order of addition and combinations of ingredients in these compositions.

Amodimethicone polymers may also be utilized to react with other materials instead of undergoing a self-condensation reaction. In this case the coreactant would become substantive to the hair as well through the covalent bond formed with the amodimethicone polymer, which binds through the amine functionality to the keratin surface. Owing to the irritation potential of amines, these materials are generally not incorporated into leave-on skin care compositions. It is possible to use low levels of low-amine-content aminofunctional silicone polymers in rinse-off products such as personal cleaners and liquid soaps, but this is the exception rather than the rule.

2. *Trimethylsilylamodimethicone*

Trimethylsilylamodimethicone is a nonreactive aminofunctional polymer that, as with amodimethicone polymers, may be either linear or branched by addition of trifunctional siloxane units during preparation. The trimethylsilyl or ''capped'' aminofunctional silicone fluids are used to improve wet and dry combing, to reduce triboelectric charging effects, and to impart softness to the hair from a variety of product types including shampoos, conditioners, and nonaerosol styling compositions.

A variety of fluids (and mechanical emulsions prepared from these fluids) are available, which vary in molecular weight, in amine content, and, consequently, in their substantivity to the hair. INCI designations for the mechanical emulsions of these fluids usually include nonionic emulsifiers such as isolaureth-6, octoxynol-40, trideceth-12, pareth-10, and so forth, and sometimes glycerin. Since the emulsions of trimethylsilylamodimethicones are generally nonionic, they are more readily incorporated into anionic systems such as shampoos than are the amodimethicone emulsions, which typically contain a cationic emulsifier. The amodimethicone emulsions may indeed be utilized in shampoo compositions; however, processing is somewhat more complicated to avoid precipitation of insoluble complexes formed with the anionic detergents in these products. Trimethylsilylamodimethicones are generally not incorporated into skin care compositions for the same reasons as amodimethicones.

As is the case with other silicone polymers, the INCI designation ''trimethylsilylamodimethicone'' covers a broad range of diverse materials. It has been shown for trimethylsilylamodimethicone fluids that the level of deposition and durability exhibited toward the hair is dependent upon various structural parameters of the aminofunctional silicone polymer (92,107,108,140). Among the parameters affecting deposition and substantivity of the aminofunctional silicones are: (1) the degree of polymerization (i.e., fluid viscosity), (2) the amine content of the polymer, (3) the polymer structure (linear or branched), (4) the placement of the amine group (pendant or terminal) along the polymer, and (5) if emulsified, the particle size of the emulsion droplets. The results of these investigations revealed that the highest levels of deposition and substantivity were achieved with linear polymers characterized by a high viscosity and a high amine content, with the amine moieties residing in pendant positions along the polymer backbone. Furthermore, when these silicones were applied to the hair from emulsions, it was found that microemulsions (average particle size ranging between 10 and 30 nm) deposited to a greater degree, and remained more substantive than macroemulsions (average particle size ranging between 250 and 400 nm) of the same fluids. In this case, the term ''microemulsion'' refers to small particle sizes ($< \frac{1}{4} \lambda$) of the dispersed phase, resulting in clear or transparent emulsions. This should not be interpreted as the classic definition of a thermodynamically stable system undergoing spontaneous formation and characterized by a negative free energy (ΔG) of formation. Thus, with the above considerations in mind, it becomes important to understand that prior to substituting one material for another, the formulator must carefully evaluate all parameters and performance characteristics of the particular aminofunctional silicone polymer in question.

The parameters discussed above cover only one manner of altering deposition of aminofunctional silicones on hair. While the characteristics of the silicone fluid are important considerations in formulating conditioning compositions, the other ingredients incorporated into the product may also influence the deposition process. This effect was demonstrated using amodimethicone and trimethylsilylamodimethicone emulsions with varying levels of pH and salt concentration (114,141). It was also demonstrated that incorporation of protein derivatives or cationic polymers, specifically polydimethyldiallylammonium chloride, into emulsions of aminofunctional silicones may result in a reduction in the deposition amounts of the aminofunctional silicones on hair with unhindered deposition and increased durability of the cationic polymer or protein derivative. On the other hand, combinations of (1) water-dispersible cationic surfactants, (2) aminofunctional silicones, and (3) either (a) water-soluble quaternized proteins, (b) quaternized ionene polymers, or (c) water-soluble heteropolysaccharides were shown to result in simultaneous deposition of all three components (142–144).

Aminofunctional silicone fluids are widely utilized in standard, emulsion-type conditioning formulations. They are also frequently employed to provide conditioning benefits from other product types as well, such as mousses, styling gels, hair sprays, and so forth. Typically, amodimethicone emulsions contain a fluid of low amine content, while numerous trimethylsilylamodimethicone fluids characterized by varying degrees of amine modification are available, thereby offering greater formulation flexibility. The pendant, highly basic diamine moieties incorporated into amodimethicone and trimethylsilylamodimethicone polymers are fully protonated near neutral pH. Therefore, the polymers possess multiple positively charged sites and readily bind to the available negatively charged sites on the surface of unmodified hair fibers. It has been shown by streaming potential analysis that treatment with aminofunctional silicones will cause a reversal in the surface charge or zeta potential of unmodified hair to positive, and that this modification will resist removal by shampooing (104,145).

Amodimethicone compounds are quite stable in solution or emulsion form, but they will undergo self-condensation reactions during drying, forming a coherent three-dimensionally cross-linked film that will completely surround the hair fiber. The deposition process is self-limiting during typical exposure times with little to no buildup upon subsequent applications as evidenced by ESCA. Fibers treated three times with a 5 wt% emulsion of amodimethicone were characterized by a relative silicone atom percentage of 19.1 as compared to 18.6 for single-treatment fibers (145).

Trimethylsilylamodimethicone polymers, on the other hand, have been shown to undergo a two-step deposition process, with complete solution depletion achieved over extended periods. The first step in this process is monolayer deposition onto the surface of unmodified hair fibers. Complete surface coverage is achieved in very short times, on the order of a few minutes (114). The second step in this process is multilayer deposition with the remaining silicone in solution depositing onto the polymer already residing on the fiber surface. Levels of 25 mg/g hair (representing complete solution depletion) have been observed for trimethylsilylamodimethicone emulsions on untreated hair fibers. It has also been shown that the greater the amine content of the silicone polymer, the faster is the first step in this deposition process, but that regardless of the amount of amine present, trimethylsilylamodimethicones will undergo this characteristic multilayer deposition process (114).

As mentioned above, the use of cationic surfactants and polymers in a shampoo or conditioner formulation to increase deposition of unmodified polydimethylsiloxane fluids on hair fibers is well documented. Though the cationic polymers tend to increase deposition of unmodified silicone fluids, they have not been efficacious in assisting deposition of aminofunctional silicone fluids. In fact, the presence of cationic polymers in the solutions of aminofunctional silicone fluids has been found to interfere with silicone deposition onto hair fibers. It has been shown that in the presence of a cationic polymer (specifically polydimethyldiallylammonium chloride) the deposition of aminofunctional fluids or emulsions decreased, with unhindered deposition of the cationic polymer as determined by titration techniques (114).

Cationic surfactants, on the other hand, appear to increase deposition of aminofunctional as well as unmodified silicones, probably owing to the fact that the cationic surfactant resides at the silicone/water interface, increasing the zeta potential of the emulsion droplet and driving the ionic deposition process. In this manner, cationic surfactants allow for deposition of greater amounts of silicone, both unmodified and aminofunctional, on the surface of the hair fibers. In fact, when hair fibers are placed for a long enough period into an emulsion containing aminofunctional silicone fluids and cationic surfactants, the silicone will continue to deposit on the fiber surface until it is completely exhausted from the solution. The fibers coated to this degree are completely smooth when examined by scanning electron microscopy (104). The kinetics of deposition are slower for multilayer deposition of silicone on silicone as compared to initial deposition kinetics for monolayer deposition of silicone onto the unmodified keratin surface.

The difference in performance between cationic polymers and surfactants in these silicone systems may be better understood through examination of the differences in solution dynamics. While cationic surfactants will incorporate themselves into the micellar structure containing the aminofunctional silicone fluid, cationic polymers will exist separately from the silicone droplets in aqueous systems (146). This arrangement leads the polymers themselves to deposit via an electrostatic attraction with the fiber surface, competing with the aminofunctional silicone droplets for available sites on the fiber surface, thereby reducing the amount of aminofunctional silicone deposited onto the hair. The unmodified silicone fluids, on the other hand, will deposit via hydrophobic instability during dilution onto either the unmodified hair surface or the surface covered by predeposited polymer. Since the polymer does not sit completely on the fiber surface, but rather forms loops protruding from the hair fiber, this creates a greater surface area on which the polydimethylsiloxane fluids may deposit. Aminofunctional silicones will not deposit onto the cationic polymer due to ionic repulsion. Since there exists long-range charge-charge repulsion between the adsorbed polymer and the aminofunctional silicones in the bulk, the latter will not come into close proximity with the cationic polymer (and hence the hair fiber), and consequently will not adsorb onto the surface of the hair from solution (104). Thus, deposition of cationic polymers onto hair will decrease the amount of amine-modified fluids deposited while increasing the deposition amounts of unmodified dimethicone or dimethiconol fluids.

The data presented in Figure 5 are representative of the typical reductions in combing forces obtained for virgin hair treated with emulsions of high-, medium-, and low-amine-content trimethylsilylamodimethicone fluids. Combing forces are displayed for tresses treated with these emulsions immediately after application, and again following eight shampooing cycles (107). Typical values of an untreated shampooed control tress are included in Figure 5 for comparison purposes. The combing forces for untreated hair tend to increase slightly following numerous shampooings. This may be attributed to excess removal of natural oils and mechanical damage to the cuticle structure, particularly near

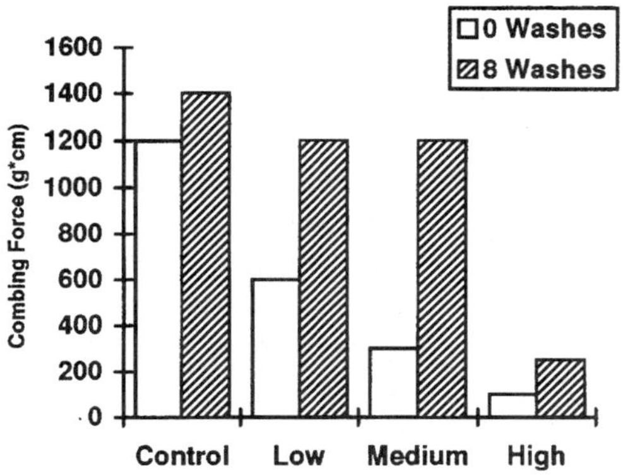

Figure 5 Representative combing forces for wet hair. Measurements were taken following application of aminofunctional silicone fluids and again after eight shampooing cycles. Hair treated with trimethylsilylamodimethicone fluids characterized by low, medium, and high levels of amine modification are compared to an untreated control.

the tip ends. The data illustrate that as the amine level of the silicone polymer is increased, the resulting combing forces following treatment decrease accordingly. This is in accordance with previously published data that demonstrated that silicone uptake on hair during a given period increased as the zeta potential of the emulsion increased (with increasing amine level) (104).

As shown in Figure 5, after eight shampooing cycles, the low- and medium-amine-content fluids are completely removed from the hair, while the tresses treated with the high amine content fluid continue to display a significant reduction in combing forces. These representative data suggest that while the INCI nomenclature remains the same regardless of polymer structure, amine content, degree of polymerization, and so forth, the product development chemist must exercise caution in choosing the appropriate trimethylsilylamodimethicone fluid for the desired application. For example, linear, high-viscosity, high-amine-content fluids may not be a good choice for a daily use conditioner targeted for fine hair, while a low-viscosity, low-amine fluid might not provide enough conditioning for badly damaged or ethnic hair types.

Aside from increasing the amine content of a nonreactive silicone polymer, it was found that the conditioning benefits, specifically reductions in combing work, could be enhanced by incorporating a small amount of a perfluorinated polyether compound into the formulation. The perfluorinated polyether, in and of itself, did not provide any noticeable conditioning benefits; however, this material was found to synergistically enhance the conditioning action of a trimethylsilylamodimethicone fluid contained in the product. The greater reduction in combing forces resulting from such a combination apparently occurred without increasing deposition amounts of the silicone polymer, i.e., without imparting a coated appearance or heavy feel to the hair (147).

Because they are stable under alkaline conditions, amine functional silicones may be employed in conditioning products designed for use with chemical processing of hair. Trimethylsilylamodimethicone materials characterized by a high level of amine modification have proven useful as conditioning pretreatments for hair undergoing bleaching, oxidative dyeing, or permanent waving or relaxing processes. Amine functional silicones and emulsions thereof have been successfully formulated into components of waving and straightening products, as well as into hair dye lotions and the developer or neutralizer portion of hair dye, permanent wave, or bleach treatments (108,117,143,148–153).

In addition to providing conditioning benefits during the dyeing process, aminofunctional silicones have been incorporated into the base of temporary, semipermanent, and demipermanent dye products to enhance depth and/or duration of color on the hair. Several investigations have demonstrated that aminofunctional silicones may influence the durability of certain nonoxidative hair dyes, particularly red shades, when incorporated into the dye lotion or applied to the hair as an afterdye conditioning treatment. It has been reported that the aminofunctional siloxanes react differently according to the dye species present, with the greatest effect on both enhanced depth and duration of color being observed primarily with red shades. Additionally, microemulsions of the aminofunctional silicone fluids were found to display superior performance characteristics in these applications as compared to macroemulsions of the same fluids. It has been shown that by adding a specific aminofunctional silicone to a hair dye base, a greater depth of color may be achieved with lower amounts of dyestuffs. (92,107,108,154–159). This was particularly advantageous with temporary dye systems since deposition of higher amounts of direct dyes on the surface of the hair results in the hair (1) feeling stiffer, (2) being more difficult to comb, and (3) exhibiting undesirable dye rub-off properties. Combinations of hydroxyfunctional silicone derivatives and aminofunctional silicones in semipermanent dye compositions have been shown to provide improved adhesion of the cationic silicone to the hair and to increase resistance to shampoo removal of the dye, which resides on the fiber surface under a silicone coating (157). The longer-lasting color effects reported with the aminofunctional silicones result strictly from reduction of shampoo removal, and do not extend to photoinduced degradation of oxidative dyestuffs.

Aminofunctional silicones possessing a lower degree of amine substitution have been incorporated into the neutralizing lotion for waving/straightening treatments to improve feel, softness, combability, and triboelectric charging characteristics (143,144,149,151, 160). The particular silicone emulsion employed contains a curable amodimethicone polymer characterized by a low amount of amine modification (~0.12 mEq/g). At use levels of 1–2% active, the conditioning benefits imparted during the neutralization step, i.e., reduction in combing forces and triboelectric charging effects, were found to be durable through several shampooing cycles.

It has subsequently been demonstrated that if the amine level of the silicone polymer is increased to 0.8 mEq/g, noncurable, high-viscosity trimethylsilylamodimethicone fluids provide greater conditioning benefits than do the low-amine curable polymers, without the processing complications encountered with amodimethicones. An aqueous microemulsion of this high-amine-content, noncurable fluid was found to provide durable conditioning benefits when applied to the hair prior to the reduction step, while the lower-amine-content silicone polymers did not survive the permanent-waving or straightening treatments (108). This same material has been shown to provide substantive conditioning benefits when incorporated into either the reducing or neutralizing solutions, and to be more stable in such systems as compared to amodimethicone emulsions, demonstrating improvements in both emulsion and peroxide stability (107,108). It has been found that, in these applications, particle size of the emulsion is important, with microemulsions performing better than macroemulsions of the same fluid. Anhydrous formulations containing the high-viscosity, high-amine-content trimethylsilylamodimethicone fluid were shown to provide an increase in moisture retention for relaxed black hair as compared to polymers characterized by a lower degree of amine modification. As it is known that water is an excellent plasticizer for hair, it was suggested that the processed hair treated with the aminofunctional silicone fluid will become more elastic and undergo less breakage during grooming as a result of this treatment (161). Thus, aminofunctional silicones not only provide excellent conditioning benefits to normal and processed hair types, they also act as hair protectant agents, imparting a higher level of elasticity and preventing subsequent damage from occurring.

E. Phenyltrimethicone

Phenyltrimethicone may be a low- or high-molecular-weight phenyl-substituted homopolymer, copolymer (with dimethylsiloxane), or terpolymer (with dimethyl and methylphenylsiloxane units). These compounds (particularly low-molecular-weight homopolymers) are compatible with many organic materials including alcohols, hydrocarbon solvents, mineral oil, and organic esters and waxes. The refractive index of phenyl modified silicone polymers may be custom-tailored by varying the ratio of $x:y:z$, in the case of the terpolymers. It would not be uncommon to encounter terpolymers prepared in this manner with refractive indices in the 1.5–1.6 range. Physical characteristics of several phenyltrimethicone polymers are presented in Table 11. Again, all of these materials are classified as ''phenyltrimethicone'' according to INCI designation, regardless of their viscosity, phenyl content, or number and type of monomer units present. These variations might dramatically affect the interaction of the chosen ''phenyltrimethicone'' with various other ingredients in the cosmetic product being formulated, and might alter the final performance characteristics of the composition.

The most commonly encountered ''phenyltrimethicone'' fluid utilized in personal care formulations is a homopolymer, where $x = 1$–3. This low-viscosity fluid ($\eta = 15$–30 cst) is characterized by a relatively high refractive index ($n_D = 1.46$) as compared to dimethicone fluids (which range in refractive index from 1.3774 to 1.4035 depending on the molecular weight of the polymer). Phenyltrimethicones are frequently used to increase apparent luster or shine on hair, and are typically encountered in finishing products such as gloss sprays and cuticle coats. They may also be used as a detackifying agent in pomades, curl refreshers, and hair-dressing compositions, and as resin plasticizers in hair fixative applications. These low-molecular-weight, phenyl-modified silicone fluids may volatilize slowly from the hair over the course of several hours, eliminating potential buildup concerns. The higher-molecular-weight copolymers and terpolymers are not volatile and will provide longer-lasting benefits on hair. In skin care formulations, phenyltrimethicones are utilized as emollients, to impart shine, and as detackifying agents, particularly for acrylic-acid-thickened systems. Owing to their optical reflective properties, phenyltrimethicones are utilized in color cosmetic formulations, particularly liquid foundations and facial powder products, to improve the appearance of the skin.

F. Alkyl-Modified Silicones

While alkyl modified silicone (AMS) polymers have been known for many years, primarily as metal or textile lubricants, it is only within the past several years that these materials have become desirous in personal care formulations. The reason for this is that in the past, the alkyl groups grafted onto the silicone polymers were long-chain linear moieties resulting in very hard, brittle waxes that were difficult to work with and did not offer significant advantages over organic materials in personal care products. With introduction of branched alkyl moieties into the silicone polymers, the molecular symmetry is disrupted,

Table 11 Physical Characteristics of Several Phenyltrimethicone Polymers

Polymer	A	B	C	D	E	F
Viscosity (cst) (25°C)	20	200	1000	100	1300	40
Refractive Index (n_D^{25})	1.437	1.448	1.460	1.493	1.508	1.504
Average MW	750	1600	1900	1300	2400	1200
Phenyl content (mole%, approx)	14	20	25	47	56	62
Melting point (°C)	−65	−40	−20	−35	−35	−30
Functionality	$PhSiO_{3/2}R$ $Me_2SIO_{2/2}$ $Me_3SiO_{1/2}$	$PhSiO_{3/2}R$ $Me_2SiO_{2/2}$ $Me_3SiO_{1/2}$	$PhSiO_{3/2}R$ $Me_2SiO_{2/2}$ $Me_3SiO_{1/2}$	$PhSiO_{3/2}R$ $PhMeSiO_{2/2}$ $Me_2SiO_{2/2}$ $Me_3SiO_{1/2}$	$PhSiO_{3/2}R$ $PhMeSiO_{2/2}$ $Me_2SiO_{2/2}$ $Me_3SiO_{1/2}$	$PhSiO_{3/2}R$ $PhMeSiO_{2/2}$ $Me_2SiO_{2/2}$ $Me_3SiO_{1/2}$

where, in all cases, R = $Si(CH_3)_3$

and the resulting materials can be custom-tailored to be liquids or soft or hard waxes with varying softening and melting points. This may be accomplished by synthesizing molecules comprising copolymers of linear and branched or long- and short- chain olefin moieties on the siloxane backbone, or they may be prepared as homopolymers of alkyl methicone.

Alkyl-functionalized silicones are notable for their moisturization properties and improved compatibility with other cosmetic raw materials. Alkyl- or alkoxy-modified methicones and dimethicones may be fluids or waxes of varying melting points and varying alkyl content, as illustrated in Table 12. Alkyl-modified silicone polymers help to enhance stability of silicone and oil (or wax) systems in much the same manner as silicone glycol copolymers act as emulsifiers for silicone and water systems. Additionally, these organofunctional polymers provide substantivity, rheology modification, enhanced product stability, and lubricity in personal care products, and have been reported to impart a volumizing benefit in hair care applications (42,162), and to enhance sunscreen efficacy (163–166). Cetyl dimethicone, cetearyl methicone, stearyl methicone, behenoxy dimethicone, and stearoxy dimethicone are just a few of the INCI designations referring to alkyl- or alkoxy-modified silicone polymers utilized in personal care formulations.

In skin care, sun care, and color cosmetic formulations, alkyl-modified silicones are known to form an occlusive barrier on the skin. These materials, often referred to as silicone ''waxes,'' are excellent moisturizing agents, reducing transepidermal water loss (TEWL) values to levels comparable to petrolatum, the extent of this benefit being dependent upon both the degree of substitution and the alkyl chain length, as illustrated in Table 13 (167,168). Silicone alkyl ''waxes'' provide a thickening effect at lower levels than natural waxes such as beeswax, castor wax, or carnauba wax, with the additional aesthetic benefits typically associated with silicones in skin care formulations. Polymers characterized by longer alkyl chain lengths and/or higher degrees of alkyl modification are also noted for their improved water-resistant properties. These compounds are often utilized in color cosmetic products, frequently in combination with silicone resins, to impart moisturization benefits, water-resistant properties, and reduction of pigment transfer (43). In lipstick formulations, silicone waxes improve stick integrity, impart an occlusive barrier providing moisturization, enhance pigment payout, and may reduce pigment transfer depending on the other ingredients in the composition.

Table 12 Physical Properties of Several Alkyl Modified Silicone Polymers

Product	MP°C (approx)	Physical form
Decyl dimethicone	18	Liquid
Lauryl dimethicone	20	Liquid
Cetyl methicone	32	Soft wax
Cetyl dimethicone	28	Soft wax
Cetearyl methicone	35	Soft wax
Stearyl methicone	42	Brittle wax
Stearyl dimethicone	31	Soft wax
Stearoxy dimethicone	35	Hard wax
Behenoxy dimethicone	45	Hard wax
C_{30} + alkyl methicone	73	Brittle wax

Table 13 In Vitro Water Vapor Permeability of Alkylmodified Silicones

Alkyl chain length	Degree of substitution	Silicone: alkyl ratio	Permeability ($g/m^2/hr$)
6	Intermediate	High	121
12	Intermediate	Intermediate	108
16	High	Intermediate	74
18 (branched)	Low	High	112
18 (linear)	High	Low	37
24	Intermediate	Intermediate	14
30	High	Low	1.4
Petrolatum			1.2
Dimethicone (350 cst)			136

Incorporation of alkyl silicone waxes into cream neutralizers, emulsions, or dispersions containing polydimethylsiloxane polymers has been reported to enhance both the stability of the neutralizer composition and the conditioning benefits imparted to the processed hair (72,73,169). Ester silicone waxes and siliconized natural waxes such as dimethiconol hydroxystearate or ''siliconyl beeswax'' are also advantageous in these applications. Alkyl-modified silicone waxes can also be found in cream developer systems designed for use with permanent hair dye systems (170). The high-melting-point silicone waxes have been demonstrated to increase stability of developer creams, and to provide durable conditioning benefits to the hair. These types of silicone polymers have also been utilized in conditioning and fixative formulations for their ability to impart volumizing effects to the hair. This phenomenon has been documented for both alkyl- and ester-modified silicones in daily-use rinse-out and leave-in conditioning formulations and compositions specifically designed for chemically processed hair (42,162,163,171–173).

G. Silicone Resins

1. *Silsesquioxanes*

Silsesquioxanes, or ''T resins,'' are branched structures consisting of $SiO_{3/2}$ units. The most prevalent of the silicone T resins found in personal care applications is the methyl-capped resin known by the INCI designation polymethylsilsesquioxane. This material is generally supplied as perfectly spherical, solid particles of tightly controlled particle sizes in the 2–5 μ range. These substances are frequently utilized as a processing aid for pigment grinding in color cosmetic applications to assist in dispersing and reduce clumping or agglomeration of the pigments. They are also used in talcs and loose powder products to maintain a free-flowing quality. Polymethylsilsesquioxane resins have been reported to provide volumizing benefits when incorporated into hair care compositions, but their use in this area is limited.

This class of silicone resins has also been found to be useful in hair fixative applications as set-holding agents (45,174,175). In contrast to typical organic resins, which tend to lose holding power under extended conditions of high humidity, organomodified nonpolar silsesquioxane resins: (1) are hydroalcoholic compatible without neutralization, (2) provide high humidity resistance, and (3) are capable of being formulated into high-solids products. The particular polymer described in the above references was found to be especially advantageous in hair-holding applications. Owing to the high modulus of the silsesquioxane resin, the resulting film was found to be stiffer than films obtained with conventional organic resins. The film stiffness is also reported to be more uniformly dispersed throughout the film, thereby eliminating localized regions of varying moduli. Another advantage of this polymer is that low-solution viscosities were obtained at high solids levels (up to 15%), thus allowing formulation of a product containing less volatile organic compounds without the associated clogging problems in spray pumps known to arise from high levels of organic resins.

2. *Siloxysilicates*

Siloxysilicates, or ''Q resins,'' are highly cross-linked structures consisting of $SiO_{4/2}$ units. Two siloxysilicate compounds are frequently encountered in cosmetic formulations. These are trimethylsiloxysilicate, which is a methyl-capped quadrafunctional silicone resin and is often referred to as an MQ resin. The second siloxysilicate compound utilized in personal care applications is known by the INCI designation diisostearolytrimethylolpropane siloxysilicate. This is an ester-modified resin prepared by hydrosilylation of an MHQ resin (43). The methyl-capped material is available in powdered form and is often provided as a dilution in either dimethicone or cyclomethicone to provide ease of formulation and improve spreadability of the resin. Trimethylsilylsiloxysilicate is a film-forming material that increases water resistance of pigments, sunscreens, antimicrobial agents, and hair fixatives. This material has also been reported to impart a volumizing effect to the hair, increasing ''body'' or ''volume'' and manageability. Trimethylsiloxysilicate resins have also demonstrated application in systems containing dimethicone polymers to increase deposition and improve substantivity of the dimethicone polymer to the hair (100,176–178). They have been shown to help maintain curl under conditions of elevated humidity in hair fixative applications as well. In skin care formulations, these silicone resins are primarily utilized for their ability to form excellent water-repellent films, and help to hold pigments and other actives in place. Siloxysilicate resins are widely utilized in longer-lasting color cosmetic formulations to reduce pigment transfer or smudging of the applied product (43,44,179–181).

Resinous silicones such as trimethylsiloxysilicates act as effective substantivity additives alone and in combination with other silicones such as high-molecular-weight dimethicone gums. In skin care evaluations, the number of water wash cycles required to remove a silicone barrier was shown to increase markedly with the addition of an MQ or siloxysilicate resin (92). In other studies, it has been demonstrated that modification of the siloxysilicate resin with alkyl and ester functionality increased the resistance to water washoff even further (163). The water-resistant properties of these materials have also been demonstrated to be dependent upon other ingredients in the formulation (182).

Silicone resins, particularly siloxysilicates, are utilized in conditioning formulations for several purposes. These materials have been reported to increase the deposition and substantivity of dimethicone or dimethiconol fluids. Substantivity increases markedly as the proportion of resinous silicone to dimethylsiloxane increases, the improvement being directly related to the decreased solubility of the resin. Multilayer deposition is reported to be limited; thus buildup is not considered to be an issue (92,100,174). Siloxysilicate resins have also been utilized in conditioning formulations to impart mild set retention properties to the hair. In addition to daily use conditioning products, the silicone resins may be incorporated into hairsprays, mousses, gels, and so forth, to provide humidity resistance as well as improved set retention properties, without detracting from dry hair aesthetics. The silicone resins are frequently formulated into these products in conjunction with volatile silicones, which tend to improve application and spreadability characteristics of the siloxysilicate resins (42,171,176).

In general, unmodified siloxysilicate resins are not water soluble and may be quite difficult to incorporate into aqueous systems. New methods of preparing microemulsions of unmodified siloxysilicate resins have been reported in the literature (183). In microemulsion form, the resins are easily formulated into aqueous systems and, in particular, low-VOC hairsprays. The microemulsions of the unmodified siloxysilicate resins were reported to provide curl retention benefits obtained from mousse compositions, and the use of these microemulsions in curl refresher formulations was also disclosed.

In addition to providing set retention benefits, the siloxysilicate resins have also been shown to increase the volume or body of hair tresses. Body is a rather subjective and poorly defined quality, and as such is difficult to measure. It is generally accepted that tress volume is related to or provides a means for quantitatively measuring hair body. Thus, an increase in hair volume is correlated to consumer perception of an improvement in body. Robbins and Crawford have described a technique for evaluating the volume of hair tresses (184). Using this technique, various silicones have been evaluated for their effect on hair volume. Thompson et al. generally found that silicones known to provide conditioning benefits (polydimethylsiloxanes and aminofunctional silicones) also provide a reduction in tress volume corresponding to their reduction in combing forces. In this same study, they report on a nonionic silsesquioxane resin that was found to impart a volumizing effect to the hair. In panel tests, this resin was found to rate favorably as a volumizing additive, receiving very high ratings in the categories of body and overall manageability. In combing evaluations, however, the ratings were significantly less than the controls for both wet and dry hair (185).

In unrelated experiments, a second silicone resin, an alkyl-modified siloxysilicate polymer, was also found to provide a volumizing effect to hair (42,163). This alkyl-modified siloxysilicate resin was further shown to impart a moderate reduction in combing forces when applied to tresses in a standard conditioning base composition. In these experiments, the conditioner base was found to reduce combing forces by 9% and resulted in a corresponding reduction in tress volume of 2.8%. The base composition comprised of the alkyl-modified siloxysilicate material, on the other hand, provided a reduction in combing forces of approximately 20%, while increasing hair volume by 16.7%. Included in this study for comparison purposes was a second siloxysilicate resin, which had been modified with organic ester linkages in place of the alkyl moieties. The ester-modified material was found to perform in a similar manner to other known conditioning agents; i.e., the conditioning base that included the ester-modified resin provided a reduction of combing forces of 14% with a corresponding decrease in maximum tress diameter or hair volume of 6.4%. Thus, while the investigations reported herein indicate that silsesquioxane or siloxysilicate resins may be employed as volume-enhancing agents in hair-finishing products, the specific material of choice must be evaluated in a given composition. It must not be extrapolated from these findings that all silicone resins will provide similar results.

Organomodified siloxysilicate resins have also been shown to provide enhancement of other benefits depending on the organic substituent covalently bonded to the silicone resin. For example, while alkylmodified siloxysilicates provide a greater increase in body/volume than the corresponding unmodified silicone resins, compounds modified with other moieties may not provide the same benefit. In fact, both phenyl functional resins, which provide greater shine enhancement, and polyether functional siloxysilicates, which impart emulsification properties as well as improving set retention attributes, were found to decrease volume of hair tresses. Treatment of hair with these materials also resulted in a decrease in combing work for both wet and dry hair tresses (42,163).

H. Silica

Silica may be supplied as ''fumed'' or ''precipitated'' silica. Both versions are found on cosmetic ingredient labels; however, ''silica'' is the proper INCI designation. This white, fine powdery material is very similar to an MQ resin in empirical formula, but the M:Q ratio is much lower than that characteristic of siloxysilicate resins. Silica may also be provided as a mixture in dimethicone under the INCI designation of ''simethicone'' or as hydrophobically modified material under the designation of silica dimethyl silylate or silica silylate. The most common application for silica-type compounds in personal care applications is as antifoaming agents. However, the various types of silica can provide interesting rheology modification to both aqueous and anhydrous systems. These materials will act as thixotropic additives and alter flow characteristics of the resulting products to produce non-Newtonian behavior. At rest the silanol groups on adjacent silica molecule aggregates associate to form hydrogen bonds between neighboring molecules. Thus, a three-dimensional network of silica particles develops. This restricts the mobility of the particles through the liquid, and also imparts a thixotropic effect to the liquid in the formulation. The tighter the network of silica particles and aggregates, the higher is the resultant viscosity of the composition. Under an applied shear force such as squeezing a tube or shaking a bottle, energy is introduced into the system, resulting in breakage of the established three-dimensional network described above. Some of the hydrogen bonds, which conferred stability, are ruptured and the particles of liquid become more mobile and the product begins to flow, with a resulting decrease in viscosity. The greater the applied force, the more linkages are broken and the more fluid the substance becomes. The most common example of this application is found in toothpaste products, particularly poloxamer-based systems. As a result of hydrogen bonding between neighboring particles, the silica will structure the product, imparting pseudoplastic flow characteristics.

It is important that the correct version be chosen for each application. For example, in systems containing 94% avocado oil and 6% silica, the fumed silica was found to form a clear, yellowish, solid gel. Silica silylate was found to form a soft, turbid gel while silica dimethyl sililyate formed a turbid liquid. Unmodified silica is the material of choice when formulating aqueous products such as toothpastes and clear antiperspirants or deodorants. In addition to structuring the gel or solid, the silica acts as a suspending aid for the AP salts. Because of the small size of the primary particles, clear products may be formulated using these materials. Silica may also be found in shampoo compositions where it acts as a suspending agent for antidandruff actives.

In addition to the commonly encountered silicone compounds listed above, a number of other specialized silicone derivatives may be found in personal care formulations. These substances include siliconized natural waxes, fragrances, sunscreens, pigments, amino acids, minerals, vitamins, botanical extracts, essential oils, fatty acids, fatty alcohols, and the like. The various types of compounds that have been covalently bonded onto silicone polymers are quite extensive and will not be discussed in further detail in this chapter.

I. Summary

In summary, silicone materials can provide numerous benefits in all aspects of personal care product formulation. Dimethicones act as skin protectant drugs, imparting a breathable barrier on the skin. Additionally they act as emollients, providing a velvety soft, lubricious film while reducing the whitening effects during rub-in of various skin care products including antiperspirants. Volatile silicones improve rub-in characteristics and are frequently utilized as diluents in hair and skin care applications. They provide transient conditioning benefits in hair care applications and act as transient emollients as well as detackifying agents in skin care formulations. Phenyl-modified silicones enhance apparent luster or shine of hair and skin and provide a detackifying effect while acting as emollients in skin care and color cosmetic compositions. Aminofunctional silicones provide excellent hair-conditioning benefits and certain substances in this class of compounds have been shown to improve color retention properties of dyed hair. Alkyl modified silicones impart an occlusive barrier to the skin, reducing transepidermal water loss values to levels comparable with petrolatum, while helping to improve formulation stability and acting as rheology modifiers. These materials have also demonstrated applications as hair volumizing agents. Silicone resins of both silsesquioxane and siloxysilicate character are utilized for their ability to form water-resistant films in sun care and color cosmetic applications and to reduce transfer of pigments in color cosmetic products. The silicone resins have also been utilized to increase deposition of dimethicone polymers in hair care formulations, to improve set retention of fixatives, and as volumizing agents for hair. Polyether-modified silicones, including terpolymers containing an alkyl or polyglucoside moiety, are very efficacious emulsifiers for water-in-silicone, silicone-in-water, or three-phase water/oil/silicone systems. These silicone surfactants have been shown to act as either defoaming agents or profoamers, depending on the amount and type of glycol modification and the application temperature. They are also utilized to reduce irritation to skin and mucous membranes caused by primary surfactants in personal cleansing and shampoo compositions. Finally, numerous specialty silicones are available incorporating standard sunscreens, fragrances, proteins, amino acids, quaternary groups, pigments, natural waxes, and the like. There are quite a large number of these specially modified materials found in personal care applications, but none of them are used to a great extent at this time. Tables 14–16 summarize the various benefits obtained from incorporation of the various types of silicones in hair care, skin care, and color cosmetic formulations.

VII. SAFETY AND ENVIRONMENTAL CONSIDERATIONS

As detailed in the preceding sections, silicones exist in a wide variety of forms as utilized in cosmetic compositions. The environmental fate and effect of these various compounds have been extensively investigated and evaluated on an individual basis for the numerous types of materials. The following section details the environmental impact of various types of silicones that may enter the environment through a number of common pathways, as described below.

A. Volatile Silicones

Approximately 13%, or 20,000 metric tons, of volatile polydimethylsiloxanes are used in personal care formulations, of which 92% (mainly D_4 and D_5) partitions to the air (186). Because of their extremely low water solubility, high vapor pressure (see Table 7), and high Henry's law constant (>3), these materials are not found to any appreciable extent in soil or water. Indeed, the aquatic volatilization rate (the rate at which a compound migrates from water to air) of D_4 has been found to be 0.57, corresponding to a half-life

Table 14 Benefits Derived from Silicones in Hair Care Formulations

Material	Benefit
Cyclomethicones	Wet combing, transient shine, no ''buildup,'' carrier/diluent, reduced drying times, prevention of clogging or ''windowing of pumps and valves, resin plasticizer
Dimethicones	Wet/dry combing, shine, improved feel/softness, reduced triboelectric charging, humidity resistance, lubricant for pumps and valves, resin plasticizer
Dimethicone copolyols	Resin plasticizer, emulsification, foam stabilization, reduction in irritation, light conditioning
Aminofunctional silicones	Wet/dry combing, improved feel/softness, reduced triboelectric charging, color protectant
Phenyl-modified silicones	Shine enhancement, improved feel, resin plasticizer
Alkyl-modified silicones	Volume/body, improved combing, improved feel
Silicones resins	Volume/body, set retention, humidity resistance
Silica	Rheology modification, suspending agent

Volatile silicones tend to depress foam and viscosity; thus external thickeners and foam boosters/stabilizers must be added to the formulation. These materials are not used in mousse formulations due to foam depression.

ranging from 3 hr to 6 days for fresh and salt water, respectively (187). In the atmosphere volatile silicones undergo oxidative chemical degradation, and ultimately are converted to SiO_2, H_2O, and CO_2. Volatile silicone compounds do not absorb radiation beyond 190 nm, and thus are not subject to photolytic cleavage (188). The presence of O_3 in the atmosphere leads to formation of OH radicals by photolysis at wavelengths of 290–320, however, and this species will initiate degradation of the dimethylsiloxanes by H-atom abstraction of the—CH_3 groups present (189). The rate constants for gas-phase reaction

Table 15 Benefits Derived from Silicones in Skin Care Formulations

Material	Benefit
Cyclomethicones	Transient emollient, improved rub-in and spreading characteristics, carrier/diluent detackifier, lubricant for valves/roller balls, improved pay-out
Dimethicones	Antiwhitening, antidusting, spreading agent, emollient, lubricant, improved rub-in and spreading characteristics, skin protectant, water-resistant film former, lubricant for valves/roller balls
Dimethicone copolyols	Emulsification, foam stabilization, enhancement in formulation stability and efficacy, improved skin feel
Aminofunctional silicones[a]	Improved feel/softness
Phenyl-modified silicones	Shine enhancement, refractive index match, emollient, spreading agent, detackifier
Alkyl-modified silicones	Occlusive barrier, emulsification, rheology modification, enhanced stability, water resistance
Silicone resins	Water-resistant film formers
Silica	Rheology modification, suspending agent

[a] Aminofunctional silicones are considered to be skin irritants; consequently, only low-amine-content fluids or emulsions may be used in skin care applications, and only in rinse-off products such as personal cleansers.

Table 16 Benefits Derived from Silicones in Color Cosmetics

Material	Benefit
Cyclomethicones	Lubricant, spreading agent, improved rub-in, improved pay-out, emollient, diluent/carrier
Dimethicones	Lubricant, spreading agent, improved rub-in, improved pay-out, emollient, protective barrier, water resistance
Dimethicone copolyols	Emulsification, improved feel
Aminofunctional silicones	Not used
Phenyl-modified silicones	Shine enhancement, enhanced depth of color, improved skin appearance
Alkyl-modified silicones	Moisturization, water resistance, rheology modification, emulsification
Silicone resins	Water resistance, reduction of pigment transfer, prevention of pigment or powder agglomeration
Silica	Rheology modification, suspending agent, alteration in optical properties

of the OH radical with organosilicone compounds at room temperatures range from 5.2×10^{-11} for hexamethylcyclotrisiloxane to 1.6×10^{-12} for decamethylcyclopentasiloxane. This leads to calculated lifetimes of 8 days and 23 days for these two materials, respectively. The calculated lifetimes are inversely proportional to the OH radical concentration in the atmosphere, and hence vary somewhat with changes in season and latitude (190,191).

The formation of ground-level ozone is a serious problem in many areas. Ground-level ozone is formed primarily from the gas-phase reactions of emitted volatile organic compounds (VOCs) and oxides of nitrogen in sunlight and air (187). Mainly, the only significant reaction contributing to the formation of O_3 is photolysis of NO_2 followed by the rapid reaction of the oxygen atoms with atmospheric O_2. Absent other factors, there is a steady-state equilibrium established as O_3 reacts with NO to form NO_2 and O_2. When VOCs are present, however, they will react to form radicals that may consume available NO, shifting the equilibrium in favor of ozone formation. The rate of ozone increase is dependent on the amount of VOCs present, the rate constants for their initial reactions, and the level of OH radicals and other species with which they may react. As previously discussed, when dimethylsiloxanes are present, OH radicals will tend to react with hydrogen atoms present in the methyl groups to form water. Thus, volatile silicones actually have a negative effect on the formation of ground-level ozone due to depletion of the OH radicals in the environment. Several investigations have been carried out with a number of volatile methylsiloxanes and have shown that indeed the rate of ozone formation was significantly reduced under these conditions, even in the presence of other VOC compounds known to contribute to ozone formation (192,193). Another issue with emission of volatile organic compounds is atmospheric particulate formation, or the formation of ''greenhouse gases.'' A series of experiments involving several species of volatile methylsiloxanes have shown that these compounds ''do not significantly enhance or contribute to formation of aerosol formation under typical atmospheric conditions'' (187,194–196). Based on these findings, the US EPA and almost all individual states in the United States have issued formal VOC exemptions for volatile methylsiloxanes, acknowledging that they are not VOC ozone precursors (197).

The effect of volatile siloxanes in water is not an issue of concern because, as stated earlier, the partition coefficient between air and water is sufficiently high to assure virtually no volatile silicones remain in water for any appreciable period. In all acute studies investigating effects on aquatic life, the lethal concentrations were found to be greater than the highest maintained exposure levels, i.e., the functional aqueous solubility of these materials (198–202). Further studies have shown that at exposure levels of 200 ppm, there are no adverse effects to exposed fathead minnows, sheepshead minnows, or mysid shrimp. Some slight effects were observed with daphia magna and rainbow trout, although larger trout species showed no effect (203,204). Again, owing to volatile siloxane characteristics, these tests had to be carried out in completely closed vessels to ensure exposure levels were maintained constant (205,206). Thus, it has been concluded that toxicity of volatile siloxanes to aquatic organisms is limited, and the corresponding risk is low. It has also been proven that the levels required to pose a risk in such systems are unrealistic in natural waters (187,207–209).

B. Polydimethylsiloxanes

Approximately 15%, or 24.9×10^6 million pounds, of the total polydimethylsiloxane polymers produced annually in the United States are used in ''down-the-drain'' applications (210). Assuming a U.S. population of 250×10^6 persons and an average wastewater flow of 500 L/person/day, the predicted influent concentration of PDMS can be calculated to be about 310 μg/L (211–213). Using a partition coefficient of 25,000 (214) and a Henry's law constant of 0 (215), it was determined that ~97% of all silicone in down-the-drain applications is bound to sludge solids (216). The remaining 3% is discharged to surface waters, leading to effluent concentrations of approximately 9 μg/L according to this model (217). The sludge from wastewater treatment plants is disposed of in a number of ways, with approximately 16% being incinerated, i.e., converting the polydimethylsiloxanes back to silicon dioxide and carbon dioxide. The remaining material is almost equally divided between landfills and surface soil treatments. The environmental fate and effect of silicone-containing sludge, soil, and water have been extensively investigated. Studies employing ^{14}C-labeled PDMS in wastewater treatment sludge have shown that after 70 days under both aerobic and anaerobic conditions, no labeled CO_2 or other organic product was formed. At the conclusion of the incubation periods, greater than 90% of the labeled ^{14}C remained in the sludge, indicating no biodegradation of the PDMS polymers (218–220).

In further studies conducted by Spivack employing several organisms that use different extracellular enzyme oxidative metabolisms to hydroxylate terminal methyl groups on hydrocarbons, no evidence was found of PDMS biodegradation under a variety of conditions (221). Sludge loadings of PDMS up to 100 mg/kg showed no effect on the operating parameters (pH, suspended solids, sludge volume index, and specific oxygen uptake) of wastewater treatment processes. Subsequent sludge digestion indicated no change in the polymer profiles of PDMS in the extract as evidenced by gel permeation chromatography (222). Thus, polydimethylsiloxanes are not biodegraded in landfills.

Soil treatments, on the other hand, yield very different results. Experiments involving PDMS on soil demonstrated that the polymer will undergo hydrolysis with a half-life of approximately 30 days. Results of these experiments indicated rearrangement of the PDMS to lower-molecular-weight homologs accompanied by formation of dimethylsilanediol (monomeric hydrolysis product) and a loss of PDMS from the soil (223–224). These studies have been confirmed by other authors who found that the PDMS degradation in soil occurs faster (half-lives of several days) when the soil is kept under conditions of low humidity (3% as compared to 12%) and in soils with high sand or clay contents as compared to rich loam (225,226). Additional investigations involving four different soil types showed a decrease in high-molecular-weight PDMS concentration from 100% on day 0 to less than 25% on day 14, concurrent with an increase in water-extractable products determined to be dimethylsilanediol. The degradation results were similar for all soil types in these studies, regardless of pH, organic matter, and percent clay (227,228). The dimethylsilanediol was found to further degrade first to methylsilanetriol and ultimately to silica and carbon dioxide over the course of 2–30 days for 12 different soil types, with the fastest degradation occurring for sandy soils (191,229,229a).

In wastewater effluents, PDMS was found to deposit in sediments; this behavior being attributed to high K_d values and water insolubility of even the lowest-molecular-weight polydimethylsiloxanes (230). The deposited silicones were not mobile in the sediments, with concentration decreasing with depth in sediment cores (231,232). In freshwater sediments, a slight change in polymer molecular weight was observed over time with approximately 10% of ^{14}C-labeled material degrading to CO_2 within a year (233,234). Since the majority of PDMS in the environment is found in soil and sediment, recent toxicity studies have focused on soil- and sediment-dwelling organisms. Sediment-dwelling organisms such as the midge, marine, and freshwater amphipods, diporeia, hexagenia libata, and other bethnic organisms have shown few toxic effects (204,235–237). Terrestrial organisms and the interaction of macro- and microinvertebrates have been studied as follows: no adverse effects were noted on the reproduction of earthworms; survival of springtails was not affected by PDMS treatment; spring wheat, soybeans, and *Rhizobium* bacteria were not affected by PDMS-amended sludge; avian feeding studies with PDMS have shown no adverse effects on the survivability or growth of ducks, quail, or chickens (238). Aquatic effects testing with microorganisms such as bacteria, fungi, and phytoplankton have demonstrated no effects from high concentrations of PDMS. Testing with invertebrates and mollusks has shown no effect on the mortality of mollusks, and where exposure to a surface film of PDMS is controlled, there have been no adverse effects to daphnia magna. In fish toxicity studies, PDMS has been shown to have a very low toxicity potential (239–242). Furthermore, it has been shown in several studies that PDMS does not bioaccumulate in fish, earthworms, phytoplankton or zooplankton, while annelids had a bioconcentration factor of less than 1. Thus, it has been concluded that polydimethylsiloxanes pose no threat to the environment, nor do they have an adverse effect on terrestrial or benthic organisms (241).

C. Polyether-Modified Silicones

In the United States, approximately 39% of all dimethicone copolyols produced, or 7.2 thousand metric tons, are incinerated or landfilled. An additional 2.7 thousand metric tons (~15%) enter wastewater treatment facilities, and about 340 metric tons (~2%) are applied directly to the soil in the form of agricultural adjuvants for pesticides and fertilizers. The remaining 44% of silicone glycol copolymers manufactured are utilized as intermediates in production of other compounds (120,186). Unlike other organofunctional silicones, which generally contain only a few mole percent organic substituent, dimethicone copolyols may contain up to 80–90% polyether modification. Depending on the silicone-to-glycol ratio and the particular glycol moiety, these materials will demonstrate varying degrees of solubility in water ranging from completely insoluble to levels of several hundred parts per thousand (243). It might be expected that these water-soluble silicones would remain in wastewater following treatment; however, it has been shown that the dimethicone copolyols adsorb to sludge, settle into sediments in rivers, and undergo parallel decomposition reactions as compared to the polydimethylsiloxanes (244–246). On soils, clay-catalyzed hydrolytic degradation of the polyether moieties occurs readily (247). Consequently the polyalkyleneoxide groups contained in the dimethicone copolyols are biodegraded while the dimethylsiloxane chain segments display similar nondegradative characteristics as the polydimethylsiloxane polymers described above (222,224,225,248). The rate and extent of biodegradation of the glycol units have been found to be inversely proportional to the glycol chain length and to the propylene oxide content in the polyether moiety (249–251). Incineration of dimethicone copolyols, as with other types of silicone compounds, leads to generation of carbon dioxide, water, and amorphous silica (252–255).

D. Organofunctional Silicones

As a group excluding polyether-modified silicones, organofunctional silicones constitute only a minor portion of the total environmental loading of organosilicone materials. Collectively, about 742 metric tons enter the environment in wastewater while approximately 294 metric tons of all modified PDMS from all applications, such as mold release agents, paint additives, and personal care products, are dispersed into the environment, and about 3.3 metric tons are disposed in landfills or incinerated (187,256). These compounds, mainly aminoalkyl-and methylalkylsiloxanes, typically contain only a small mole percent functionality, and thus would be expected to behave in a similar manner as the polydimethylsiloxanes in degradation characteristics. Alkoxysilanes, on the other hand, are degraded by hydrolysis reactions to form alcohols and silanols with half-lives on the order of seconds to days (257). The hydrolysis rate is dependent on the pH, temperature, molecular structure, and solubility of the alkoxysilane in water. If the solubility is high and the water-to-silicone ratio is greater than 10, the degradation will follow pseudo-first-order kinetics. At higher silane concentrations, the hydrolysis reaction becomes second order. The alkoxy group also affects the kinetics of degradation, with reaction rates decreasing with increasing alkyl chain length (258–262). Low-molecular-weight silanols resulting from the hydrolysis reactions will further undergo biodegradation to silica and carbon dioxide by photolysis reactions in air and water as described above for dimethylsilanediol and methylsilanetriol (222,263,264).

E. Conclusions

The amount of silicones incorporated into personal care formulations is quite small in comparison to all other applications for silicones. Therefore, the resulting environmental loading of various types of silicones from personal care applications is considered rather low. Environmental exposure of silicones has been extensively studied in laboratory and field investigations in several organisms. Environmental fate studies have shown that silicones degrade and do not contribute to the formation of ozone or greenhouse gases. Accordingly, volatile silicones have been exempted from federal VOC considerations. These studies have also demonstrated that there is a complex mechanism involving a combination of chemical and biological degradation that occurs in soil and sediments. Aquatic, sediment-, and soil-dwelling organisms have been tested for acute, chronic, and reproductive effects. This testing has indicated no adverse effects are expected at the levels of silicones that have been found in the environment. The by-products of silicone incineration are silica, carbon dioxide, and water, all of which are completely harmless to the environment.

REFERENCES

1. Grigoras S, Lane TH. Adv Chem Series Am Chem Soc. 1990; 224:125.
2. Rochow EG. Silicon and Silicones. New York: Springer-Verlag, 1987.
3. Noll W. Chemistry and Technology of Silicones. New York: Academic Press, 1968.
4. Kulkarni RD, Goddard ED, Kanner B. J Coll Interface Sci 1977; 59(3):468.
5. Kulkarni RD, Goddard ED, Rosen MR. J Soc Cosmet Chem 1979; 30(2):105.
6. Solomon EM, Zisman WA. J Phys Chem 1950; 54:723.
7. Ellison AH, Zisman WA. J Phys Chem 1956; 60:414.
8. Wendel SR, DiSapio AJ. Cosmet Toilet 1983; 103(5):98.
9. Klempsch H. In: Smith AL, Ed. The Analytical Chemistry of Silicones, Vol 112. New York: Wiley, 1991: 117–132.
10. Lochhead RY. Cosmet Toilet 1988; 103(12):23–61.
11. US 2,826,551, Geen HC, assignee: Simonize Co, March 11, 1958.
12. Kintish L. Soap Cosmet Chem Spec 1979; 73(7):29.
13. Abrutyn E. Presented at Global HBA, Silicone Technology Section, New York, June 11, 1997.
14. DiSapio A. Presented at the Society of Cosmetic Chemists Annual Meeting, New York, December 1994.
15. Steinberg, D. The Frequency of Use, 1996 Cosmetic Ingredients, report #118, Steinberg & Assoc, Plainsboro, NJ, 1996.
16. Stock A. Berl Dtsch Chem Ges 1916; 49:108.
17. INCI Dictionary and Handbook, 7th ed, Vol 1. Washington, DC: Cosmetic, Toiletry, and Fragrance Association, 1997, p 366.
18. Vaughn C. J Soc Cosmet Chem 1985; 36:319.
19. US 2,380,995, Rochow EG, assignee: General Electric Co, Sept 26, 1941.
20. Tomanek A. Silicones and Industry: A Compendium for Practical Use. Munich: Wacker-Chemie GmbH, 1991.
21. Scheiber WJ Hadsell EM. J Am Chem Soc 1948; 70:4254.
22. Setinek K, Bazant V, Sorm F. Chem Listy 1956; 50:1954.
23. Tyler LJ. J Am Chem Soc 1954; 76:1030.
24. US 2,371,068, Rochow EG, assignee: General Electric Co, April 30, 1940.
25. US 2,472,629, Sprung, MM, assignee: General Electric Co, June 11, 1946.
26. US 2,459,387, McGregor RR, Warrick EI, assignee: Dow Corning Corp, Oct. 5, 1942.
27. US 2,469,883, Marsden J, Rodel GF, assignee: General Electric Co, June 11, 1945.
28. US 2,676,163, Spier JL, assignee: Dow Corning Corp, Sept 3, 1952.
29. US 2,605,274, Tyler LJ, assignee: Dow Corning Corp, Jan 9, 1950.
30. US 2,448,756, Agnes M, assignee: General Electric Co, March 14, 1944.
31. US 2,637,738, Wagner GH, assignee: Union Carbide, Sept 17, 1949.
32. Webster JA. J Org Chem 1956; 21:1044.
33. Barnes GH. J Am Chem Soc 1957; 79:974.
34. Saam JC, Speier JL. J Am Chem Soc 1957; 80:4140.
35. Fessenden RJ, Fessenden JS. J Org Chem 1963; 28:487.
36. US 2,813,887, Ramsen HE, assignee: Metal and Thermit, Nov 20, 1941.
37. DiGeorgio, PA, Strong WA, Sommer LH, Whitmore FC. J Am Chem Soc 1946; 68:1380.
38. Ingram RK. J Am Chem Soc 1955; 77:1680.

39. Schumb WC, Schafer CM. Jr. J Am Chem Soc 1939; 61:363.
40. US 2,674,579, Morgan CR, Olds WF, assignee: California Research, July 16, 1953.
41. Pearlson WH, Brice TJ, Simons JH. J Am Chem Soc 1945; 67:1769.
42. US 5,684,112, Berthiaume MD, Miranda PM, assignee: General Electric Co, Nov 4, 1997.
43. US 4,752,658, Thayer BK, Traver FJ, assignee: General Electric Co, Feb 16, 1988.
44. US 5,051,489, O'Lenick AJ. Jr, Assignee: Siltech Inc, Sept 24, 1991.
45. US 5,075,103, Halloran DJ, Vincent JM, assignee: Dow Corning Corp, Dec 24, 1991.
46. DE 1,163,862, Ruhlmann K, assignee: VEB-Berlin Chemie, March 23, 1962.
47. US 2,381,139, Sauer RO, assignee: General Electric Co, May 14, 1942.
48. Hasek RH. J Am Chem Soc 1946; 68:241.
49. Allport DC, Janes WH. Block Copolymers. New York: Wiley, 1973.
50. Pawlenko S. Organosilicon Chemistry. Berlin: Walter de Gruyter, 1986.
51. Auner N, Weis J. Organosilicon Chemistry II; From Molecules to Materials. New York: Weinheim, 1996.
52. Schmidt GL. In: Karsa DR, ed. Industrial Applications of Surfactants. London: Royal Society of Chemistry, Burlington House, 1987:24.
53. Anathapadmanabhan DP, Goddard ED, Chandar P. Coll Surf 1990; 44:281.
54. Goddard ED, Anathapadamanaghan KP, Chandar P. Langmuir 1995; 11:1415.
55. US 5,100,956, O'Lenick AJ Jr, assignee: Siltech Inc, March 31, 1992.
56. US 5,070,171, O'Lenick AJ Jr, assignee: Siltech Inc, Dec 3, 1991.
57. US 5,149,765, O'Lenick AJ Jr, assignee: Siltech Inc, Sept 22, 1992.
58. Imperante J, O'Lenick AJ. Soap Cosmet Chem Spec 1994; 70(10):32.
59. US 4,523,921, Sebag H, Vanlerberghe G, assignee: L'Oreal, June 18, 1985.
60. US 4,567,039, Stadnick RP, and Schnetzinger RW, assignee: Revlon Inc, Jan 28, 1986.
61. US 4,601,902, Fridd P, Taylor RM, Hill MP, assignee: Dow Corning Ltd, July 22, 1986.
62. US 4,597,964, Ziemelis MJ, Roth CA, assignee: Aplin & Barrett, Ltd, and Dow Corning Corp, July 1, 1986.
63. US 4,749,732, Kohl G, Lane TH, assignee: Dow Corning Corp, June 7, 1988.
64. O'Lenick AJ, Parkinson J. Cosmet Toilet, 1994; 109(5):85.
65. Sacklowski H. Seifen Oele Fette Wasche 1989; 115(17):607.
66. Imperante J, Hannon J, Parkinson JK. Cosmet Toilet 1993; 108(4):79.
67. Alexander P. Manufact Chem 1992; 63:28.
68. US 4,342,742, Sebag H, Vanlerberghe G, assignee: L'Oreal, Aug 3, 1982.
69. Capozzi G, Menichette S, Rosi A. J Chem Soc Perkin Trans 1992; 2(12):2247.
70. Gruening B, Leidreiter H. Seifen Oele Fette Wachse 1992; 118(3):117.
71. Gruening B, Leidreiter H. Parfum Cosmet Arom 1991; 98:55.
72. US 4,423,032, Yoshiaki A, Tsushima R, assignee: Kao Soap Co Ltd, Dec 27, 1983.
73. US 5,063,044, Kohl GS, Giwa-Agbomeirele PA, Vincent JM, assignee: Dow Corning Corp, Nov 5, 1991.
74. Halloran DJ. Soap Cosmet Chem Spec 1992; 86(3):22.
75. Kobayashi H, Owen MJ. J Coll Interface Sci 1993; 156:415.
76. US 5,578,298, Berthiaume MD, Merrifield JH, assignee: General Electric Co, Nov 26, 1996.
77. US 5,683,625, Berthiaume MD, Merrifield JH, assignee: General Electric Co, Nov 4, 1997.
78. US 4,620,878 Gee R, assignee: Dow Corning Corp, Nov 4, 1986.
79. US 4,797,272, Linn EE, West P, assignee: Eli Lilly & Co, Jan 10, 1989.
80. US 4,782,095, Gum ML, assignee: Union Carbide Corp, Nov 1, 1988.
81. US 4,801,447, Gum ML, assignee: Union Carbide Corp, Jan 31, 1989.
82. US 5,057,572, Chrobaczek H, assignee: Ciba-Geigy Corp, Oct 15, 1991.
83. US 4,908,140, Bausch GG, Seelbach EA, Zombeck A, assignee: Dow Corning Corp, March 13, 1990.
84. US 4,943,431, Awamura M, Yamamoto K, Nanjo M, assignee: Sunstar Kabushiki Kaisha, July 24, 1990.

85. US 5,049,377, Lamb JA, Dillon KL, assignee: Dow Corning Corp, Sept 17, 1991.
86. Active Organics. Technology showcase poster at Society of Cosmetic Chemists Annual Meeting, New York, December 1997.
87. US 5,252,325, Bries CD, Kopolow SL, Burlant WJ, Helioff MW, Login RB, Tazi M, assignee: ISP Investments Inc, Oct 12, 1993.
88. US 5,169,623, Kopolow SL, Burlant WJ, Helioff MW, Bries CD, Login RB, Tazi M, assignee: ISP Investments Inc, Dec 8, 1992.
89. Schaefer D. Tenside Surf Det 1990; 27(3):154.
90. Fed Reg 1983; 48(32):6819.
91. Fed Reg 1990; 55(119):25203.
92. Disapio A, Fridd P. Int J Cosmet Sci 1988; 10:75.
93. US 5,198,209, Zhon J, Fochtman DJ, assignee: Amway Corp, March 30, 1993.
94. Nanavati S, Hami A, J Soc Cosmet Chem 1994; 45(3):135.
95. US 5,034,218, Duvel LA, assignee: Helene Curtis, Inc, July 23, 1991.
96. US 4,704,272, Oh YS, Dahlgren RM, Russell GD, assignee: Procter & Gamble Co, Nov 3, 1987.
97. US 5,393,452, Raleigh WJ, Thimineur, RJ, Stoklosa SJ, assignee: General Electric Co, Feb 28, 1995.
98. US 5,246,694, Birthwistle DH, assignee: Chesebrough Ponds USA Co, Sept 21, 1993.
99. EP 432,951A2, Reid ES, Murray AM, assignee: Unilever, June 19, 1991.
100. WO 92/10162, Wells RL, assignee: Procter & Gamble Co, June 25, 1992.
101. US 3,964,500, Drakoff R, assignee: Lever Brothers Co, June 22, 1976.
102. US 4,788,006, Bolich RE Jr, Williams TB, assignee: Procter & Gamble Co, Nov 29, 1988.
103. US 4,741,855, Grode MB, Russell GD, assignee: Procter & Gamble Co, May 3, 1988.
104. Berthiaume MD, Jachowicz J. J Polym Interface Sci 1991; 141:299.
105. Sejpka J. Seifen Oele Fette Wachse 1992; 118(17):1065.
106. US 4,728,457, Fisher GM, Stacy LV, assignee: Procter & Gamble Co, March 1, 1988.
107. Jachowicz J, Berthiaume MD, Cosmet Toilet 1993; 108(3):65.
108. Berthiaume MD, Merrifield JH, Riccio DA. J Soc Cosmet Chem 1995; 46(5):231.
109. US 5,246,694, Birthwistle DH, assignee: Chesebrough Ponds USA Co, Sept 21, 1993.
110. EP 432,951A2, Reid ES, Murray AM, assignee: Unilever, June 19, 1991.
111. Dodge FT. J Collloid Interface Sci 1988; 121(1):154.
112. Robbins CR. Chemical and Physical Behavior of Human Hair, 3rd ed. New York: Springer-Verlag, 1994, Chapter 5.
113. Davies JT, Rideal EK. Interfacial Phenomena. New York: Academic Press, 1961.
114. Jachowicz J, Berthiaume MD. J Coll Interface Sci 1989; 133(1):118.
115. US 5,143,518, Mandrange A, Canivet P, assignee: L'Oreal, Sept 1, 1992.
116. US 5,066,485, Brieva H, Jose N, Tietjen M, assignee: Revlon, Inc, Nov 19, 1991.
117. DE 3,706,053 Al, Fridd PF, Taylor RM, assignee: Dow Corning Ltd, Feb 26, 1986.
118. JP 4,059,721 A, assignee: Kao Corp, Feb 26, 1992.
119. GB 2,198,949 A, Mandrange A, Canivet P, assignee: L'Oreal, Oct 14, 1987.
120. GB 2,149,806 A, Nakamura Y, assignee: Yamahatsu Sangyo Kaisha, Ltd, June 19, 1985.
121. DE 4,232,944 A, Flemming E, Gross P, Hoch D, assignee: Wella AG, April 7, 1994.
122. EP 014,479 A, Wajaroff T, assignee: Wella AG, Aug 20, 1980.
123. EP 0 260,641, Yamamoto H, Ishido H. assignee: Kao Corp, March 23, 1988.
124. US 4,954,335, Janchipraponvej B, assignee: Helene Curtis, Inc, Sept 4, 1990.
125. WO 89/04164, Donkers AC, John VB, assignee: Dow Corning Ltd, May 18, 1989.
126. US 4,770,873, Wolfram LJ, Cohen D, assignee: Clairol Inc, Sept 13, 1988.
127. Sakuta K. Fragrance J 1993; 21(6):73.
128. Gould C. Spec Chem 1991; 11:354.
129. Starch M, DeVries C. Parfuem Kosmet 1986; 67(3):148.
130. Frye CL. Soap Cosmet Chem Spec 1983 (Aug):32.
131. Starch M. Drug Cosmet Ind 1984; 134(6):38.

132. Halloran DJ. Soap Cosmet Chem Spec 1992 (March): 22.
133. Yahage K. J Soc Cosmet Chem 1992; 43:275.
134. Rosen MJ. Surfactants and Interfacial Phenomena. New York: Wiley, 1989.
135. Ross S. In: Grayson M, Eckroth D, eds. Encyclopedia of Chemical Technology, 3rd ed, Vol 11. New York: Wiley, 1980:127–145.
136. Floyd DT. In: Gelelein CE, Cheng TC, and Yang VC, eds. Cosmetic and Pharmaceutical Applications of Polymers. New York; Plenum Press, 1991:49–72.
137. Matalon R. J Soc Cosmet Chem 1952; 3:216.
138. Hameyer P. HAPPI 1991 (April):88.
139. Henderson C, Berthiaume MD. Unpublished results.
140. Thayer BK, Merrifield JH. Presented at the XVI IFSCC Congress, New York, October 1990.
141. Karjala SA, Williamson JE, Karler A. J Soc Cosmet Chem 1967; 18:599.
142. US 4,749,565, Grollier JF, assignee: L'Oreal, June 7, 1988.
143. US 4,597,962, Grollier JF, Dubief C, Cauwet D, assignee: L'Oreal, July 1, 1986.
144. GB 2 164 558 A, Grollier JF, assignee: L'Oreal, March 26, 1986.
145. Wendel SR, DiSapio AJ. Cosmet Toilet 1983; 98(5):103.
146. Jachowicz J, Berthiaume MD, Garcia ML. Coll Polym Sci 1985; 263:847.
147. US 5,160,733, Berthiaume MD, Jachowicz J, assignee: Clairol Inc, Nov 3, 1992.
148. US 4,563,347, Starch MS, assignee: Dow Corning Corp, Jan 7, 1986.
149. US 4,592,586, DeMarco R, Varco J, Wolfram LJ, assignee: Clairol, Inc, July 16, 1985.
150. Starch M. J Soc Cosmet Chem. 1986; 62(4):34.
151. US 4,770,873, Wolfram LJ, Cohen D. assignee: Clairol, Inc, Sept 13, 1988.
152. DE 30 30119 A1, Hauck W, Wehnet W, Schmidt W, Carstens W, Graalfs E, Doring W, assignee: Freidrich-Karl Marcus, Feb 25, 1982.
153. US 4,673,568, Grollier JF, Dubief C, Cauwet D, assignee: L'Oreal, June 16, 1987.
154. GB 2,138,845A, Nomura T, Memoto T, Ikeda Y, assignee: Kao Corp, Oct 31, 1984.
155. GB 2,168,082 B, Houlellebecq TF, Day ME, Wilkins AL, assignee: Beecham Group, plc, Sept 14, 1988.
156. US 4,820,308, Mandrange A, Canivet P, assignee: L'Oreal, April 11, 1989.
157. GB 2,173,515B, Houlellebecq TF, Day ME, Wilkins AL, assignee: Beecham Group plc, Jan 18, 1989.
158. JP 57,192,310, assignee: Kao Corp, Nov 23, 1982.
159. JP 86,055,887, assignee: Kao Corp, Nov 29, 1986.
160. US 4,777,037, Wagman J, assignee: Helene Curtis Ind, Inc, Oct 11, 1988.
161. Berthiaume, MD, Riccio DA, Merrifield JH. Drug Cosmet Ind 1994; 153(6):24.
162. US 5,393,521, Lance-Gomez TE, Husam AA, assignee: DEP Corp, Feb 28, 1995.
163. Berthiaume MD, Baum, AD. J Soc Cosmet Chem 1997; 48(1):1.
164. Glover D. Soap Cosmet Chem Spec 1997 (Nov):54.
165. Floyd DT, Sarnecki BJ, Macpherson BA. SPC, March 1996, pp 26–31.
166. DiSapio A. Cosmet Toilet 1987; 102(3):102.
167. Van Reeth I, Dahman F, Hannington J. Poster session presented at the 19th IFSCC Congress, Sydney Australia, October 1996.
168. Van Reeth I, Wilson A. Cosmet Toilet 1994; 109(7):87.
169. Berthiaume MD, Baum AD. Unpublished results.
170. EP 095 238 A2, Starch MS, assignee: Dow Corning Corp, Nov 30, 1983.
171. DE 3,030,119 A1, Marcus FK, unassigned, Aug 6, 1980.
172. EP 0 313 307 A1, Cobb, DS, Lorincz NM, Smith MM, assignee: Procter & Gamble Co, March 26, 1989.
173. US 5,213,793, Moses RE, Roberto FM, assignee: T Gillette Co, May 25, 1993.
174. US 4,374,825, Bolich RE Jr, Hartsough LB, Cothran PE, assignee: Procter & Gamble Co, Feb 22, 1983.
175. US 5,225,190, Halloran DJ, Vincent JM, assignee: Dow Corning Corp, July 6, 1993.

176. US 5,135,742, Halloran DJ, Vincent JM, assignee: Dow Corning Corp, Aug 4, 1992.
177. EP 240,350 B1, Snyder ME, Bolich RE Jr, Stentz DM, Cobb DS, Kowasniewski VJ, assignee: Procter & Gamble Co, June 28, 1995.
178. US 4,902,499, Bolich RE Jr, Cobb DS, Kwasniewski VJ, Snyder MA, Stentz DM, assignee: Procter & Gamble Co, Feb 20, 1990.
179. US 5,505,937, Castrogiovanni A, Barone S, Krog A, McCulley M, Callelo J, assignee: Revlon Consumer Product Corp, April 9, 1996.
180. EP 602,937, Castrogiovanni A, Barone S, Krog A, McCulley M, Callelo J. assignee: Revlon Consumer Product Corp, June 22, 1994.
181. US 5,334,737, Thimineur R, Traver F, Van Valkenburgh V, assignee: General Electric Co, August 1994.
182. Berthiaume MD, Riccio DA. Unpublished results of substantivity evaluations performed by Consumer Products Testing Corporation on sunscreen formulations prepared by Reinhardt Consultants.
183. Berthiaume MD, Merrifield JH, Riccio DA. Patent pending.
184. Robbins CR, Crawford RJ. J Soc Cosmet Chem 1984; 35:369.
185. Thomson BD, Halloran DJ, Vincent JM, presented at the 17th IFSCC International Congress, Yokohama, October 1992.
186. Allen R. In: Hutzinger O, ed. The Handbook of Environmental Chemistry, Organosilicon Materials, Vol 3, part H. Berlin: Springer-Verlag, 1997, Chapter 1.
187. Hobson JF, Atkinson R, Carter WP. In: Hutzinger O, ed. The Handbook of Environmental Chemistry, Organosilicon Materials, Vol 3, part H. Berlin: Springer-Verlag, 1997.
188. Bell S, Walsh A. Faraday Trans 1966; 62:3005.
189. Atkinson R, Tuazon E, Kwok E, Arey J, Aschmann S, Bridier I. J Chem Soc Faraday Trans 1995; 91:3033.
190. Atkinson R. Environ Sci Technol 1991; 25:863.
191. Sommerlade R, Parlar H, Wrobel D, Kochs P. Environ Sci Technol 1993; 27:2435.
192. Carter WP, Atkinson R. Environ Sci Technol 1990; 23:864.
193. Carter WP. Air Water 1994; 44:881.
194. Pope C, Bates D. Raizenne M, Environ Health Perspect 1995; 103:472.
195. Gartrell G, Friedlander S. Armos Environ 1975; 9:279.
196. Zhang SH, Shaw M, Seinfeld J, Flagan R. Geophys Res 1992; 97:20717.
197. Fed Reg Ref, December 1995.
198. Sousa J, McNamare P, Putt A, Machado M, Supernant D, Hamelink J, Kent D, Hobson E. Environ Toxicol Chem 1995; 14:1639.
199. US EPA Report #EPA/600/4-85/013, Cincinatti, OH, 1985.
200. Grau R. TSCA Docket #OPTS-42071B, Washington, DC, 1991.
201. Annelin R. TSCA Docket #OPTS-42071B, Washington, DC, 1990.
202. Ann Arbor Testing Services. TSCA Docket #OPTS-42071B, Washington, DC, 1989.
203. Annelin R. TSCA Docket #OPTS-42071B, Washington, DC, 1993.
204. Annelin R, Frye CL. Sci Total Environ 1989; 83:1.
205. Fackler P, Dionne E, Hartley D. Hamelink J Environ Sci Technol 1995; 12:1332.
206. Hobson J, Silberhorn E. Environ Toxicol Chem 1995; 14:1667.
207. Kent D, McNamara P, Putt A, Hobson J, Silberhorn E. Ecotoxicol Eviron Safety 1994; 29: 372.
208. Petrasek A, Kugelman I, Austern B, Pressley T, Winslow L, Wise R. J Water Pollut Control Fed 1983; 55:1286.
209. Govind R, Lei L, Dobbs R. J Water Pollut Control Fed 1991; 59:670.
210. Chemical Economics Handbook. Menlo Park, CA: Stanford Research Institute, 1996.
211. Holman WF. Aquatic Toxicology and Hazard Assessment: Fourth Conference, ASTM, STP 737, 1981, p 159.
212. US EPA Report to Congress, EPA 430/9-84-011, 1985.

213. Namkung JE, Rittman BE. J Water Pollut Control Fed 1987; 59:670.
214. Fendinger NJ, Whittington DE. Procter & Gamble Internal Report, Study #E92-026, 1994.
215. Fendinger NJ, Lehmann RG, Mihaich EM. In: Hutzinger O, ed. The Handbook of Environmental Chemistry, Organosilicon Materials, Vol 3, part H. Berlin: Springer-Verlag, 1997.
216. Watts RJ, Kong S, Haling CS, Gerhart L, Frye CL, Vigon BW. Water Res 1995; 29:2405.
217. Cowan CE, Larson RJ, Feijtel TC, Rapaport RA. Water Res 1993; 27:561.
218. Street JR. Dow Corning Internal Report #BL/B2078, 1980.
219. Hobbs EJ, Keplinger ML, Calandra JC. Environ Res 1975; 10:397.
220. Palmer DT. Dow Corning Internal Report, #SC900091, 1992.
221. Spivack J. General Electric. Unpublished results, 1993.
222. Lehman RG, Frye CL, Tolle DA, Zwick TC. Water Air Soil Pollut 1996; 87:231.
223. Spivack J, Dorn B. Environ Sci Technol 1994; 28:2345.
224. Buch RR, N Ingebrigston D. Environ Sci Technol 1979; 13:676.
225. Lehman RG, Varapath S, Frye CL. Environ Toxicol Chem 1994; 13:1061.
226. Carpenter JC, Cella JA, Dorn SB. Environ Sci Technol 1995; 29:864.
227. Lehman RG, Varapath S, Annelin RB. Arndt J, Environ Toxicol Chem 1995; 14:1299.
228. Fendinger NJ, McAvoy DC, Eckhoff WS. Environ Sci Technol 1997; 31:1555.
229. Lehman RG, Miller JR. Environ Toxicol Chem 1996; 15:1455.
229a. Atkinson R. Environ Sci Technol 1991; 28:863.
230. Varapath S, Frye CL, Hamelink JL. Environ Toxicol Chem 1996; 15:1236.
231. Bateley GE, Hayes JW. Aust J Mar Freshwater Res 1991; 42:287.
232. Pellenbarg RE. Environ Sci Technol 1986; 20:743.
233. Christensen K. Silicone Environmental Health and Safety Council Report, Document ID #47, 1994.
234. Carpenter JC, Leib TK, Sabourin CL, Spivack JL. SETAC 17TH Annual Meeting, Washington, DC, 1996, abstract #PO579.
235. Japan EPA, Chemicals Report issued by Japan Environmental Agency, Environmental Health Dept, 1980.
236. Waranabe N, Nagase H, Ose Y. Sci Total Environ 1988; 73:1.
237. Tolle DA, Frye CL, Lehmann RG, Zwick TC. Sci Total Environ 1995; 162:193.
238. Fletcher D, Industrial Bio-Test Laboratories, IBT Report #651-03645 and 651-03646, 1973.
239. Mann H, Ollenschlager B, Reichennnbach-Klinke HH, Fisch Umwelt 1977; 3:19.
240. Aubert M, Aubert J, Augier H, Guillemaut C. Chemosphere 1985; 14:127.
241. Annelin RB, Klein R, Varapath S. Dow Corning Internal Report #1994-I-0000, 1994.
242. Craig NC, Caunter JE. Chemosphere 1990; 21:751.
243. Gruning B, Koerner G, Tenside Surf Det 1989; 26:312.
244. Powell DE, Carpenter JC. In: Hutzinger O, ed. The Handbook of Environmental Chemistry, Organosilicon Materials, Vol 3, part H. Berlin: Springer-Verlag, 1997.
245. Griessbach EF. PhD thesis, Gembloux, Faculte des Sciences Agronomiques, 1995.
246. Ziemelis M. Dow Corning. Unpublished results, 1996.
247. Gonsio SJ, West RJ. Environ Toxicol Chem 1995; 14:1273.
248. Anderson C, Hochgeschwender K, Weidmann H, Wilmes R. Chemosphere 1987; 16:2567.
249. Naylor CG, Castaldi FJ, Hayes BJ. J Am Oil Chem Soc 1988; 65:1669.
250. Bailey RE. Surfactant Sci Ser. 1996; 60:243.
251. Balson T, Felix MS. In: Karsa DR, Porter MR, eds. Biodegradable Surfactants. Glasgow: Blackie, 1995:243.
252. Lipowitz J, Ziemelis MJ. J Fire Flammabil 1976; 7:482.
253. Hilado CJ, Casey CJ, Christensen DF, Lipowitz J. J Comb Toxicol 1985; 5:130.
254. Buch RR. Fire Safety J 1991; 17:1.
255. Lipowitz J, Ziemelis MJ. J Fire Flammabil 1976; 7:504.
256. White JW, Treadgold RC. In: Clarkson SJ, Semlyen JA, eds. Siloxane Polymers. Englewood Cliffs, NJ: PTR Prentice-Hall, 1993:567.

257. Spivak JL, Pohl ER, Kochs P. In: Hutzinger O, ed. The Handbook of Environmental Chemistry, Organosilicon Materials, Vol 3, part H. Berlin: Springer-Verlag, 1997.
258. Osterholtz FD, Pohl ER. J Adhes Sci Technol 1992; 6:127.
259. Deiters JA, Holmes RR, J Am Chem Soc 1987; 109:2211.
260. Chiperfield JR, Gould GE. J Chem Soc Perkin Trans II 1974; 1324.
261. Akerman E. Acta Chem Scand 1956; 10:298.
262. Akerman E. Acta Chem Scand 1957; 11:373.
263. Lehman RG, Varapath S, Frye CL. Environ Toxicol Chem. 1994; 13:1753.
264. Sabourin CL, Carpenter JC, Leib TK, Spivack JL. Appl Environ Microbiol 1996; 62:4352.

8

Polysaccharide-Based Polymers in Cosmetics

James V. Gruber
Amerchol Corporation, Edison, New Jersey

I. INTRODUCTION

The use of polysaccharides (''many sugars'') in cosmetics has been as ubiquitous as the use of cosmetics themselves. Historically, because of their ready availability from common natural sources and their varied and unique multifunctionality, polysaccharides have been included in cosmetics for centuries, for example, the use of β-glucan, derived from yeast extracts, as a natural healing agent (1). Today, polysaccharides play an even larger role in cosmetic formulation technology. The interplay of polysaccharides with other ingredients in a formulation (e.g., actives, surfactants, salts, other polymers, etc.) and their facile chemical modification has allowed their preeminent use in cosmetics. In addition, polysaccharides, of natural origin and polymeric, are renewable and have a safety profile not accorded synthetic-based polymers (2).

When considering the many cosmetically acceptable polysaccharides, one finds that their morphology and functionality span all the territory of polymer technology. Polysaccharides in solution can exist as loose random coils or rigid helices. They can be anionic, cationic, nonionic, or even amphoteric depending on the chemical identity expressed on or pendant to their native backbones. They can be single coils, double coils, and even aggregates of coils the nature of which can be influenced by, among other things, temperature, concentrations, and other species such as salts.

Polysaccharides perform a myriad of cosmetic functions. For example, they act as rheology modifiers, suspending agents, hair conditioners, and wound-healing agents. They moisturize, hydrate, emulsify, and emolliate. Trying to distinguish the influence of a single polysaccharide in a formulation is like trying to understand the action of a finger while ignoring the hand. Does a polysaccharide that conditions do so at the expense of its thickening ability? How will it behave in the presence of surfactants or salts? Does it complex with other components of the formulation? Understanding polysaccharide functionality is both multifaceted and challenging.

Researchers, undaunted, continue to struggle to explore the relationship between polysaccharide solution behavior and its performance, and also how other ingredients interact to create acceptable formulations. An overview of this field requires a two-pronged discussion: (1) polysaccharide structure and (2) polysaccharide functionality. The arduous task of understanding the merits of a particular polysaccharide for a particular application becomes easier with a growing appreciation of these two key features.

II. POLYSACCHARIDE STRUCTURE

A. Defining a Polysaccharide

Polysaccharides, primarily of natural origin, are principally manufactured within living systems. But their natural function in living systems may differ considerably from that in a cosmetic formulation. Potatoes, for example, manufacture starch as a food, an energy storage site, not as a viscosifying or gelling agent. Living biological systems adhere strictly to an organism's genetic guidelines and enzymic control; therefore, the manufacture of polysaccharides is also under the same strict control. This leaves little room for molecular manipulation, but it is the epitomy of polymeric consistency. New polysaccharides continue to be synthesized from basic monosaccharide building blocks in the laboratory. However, few of these new polymers have been useful for cosmetic applications (3). Genetic engineering is offering new and interesting polysaccharides. Nevertheless, at present, the majority of cosmetically interesting polysaccharides remain of natural and seminatural origin. In this chapter these natural and seminatural materials are explored in detail.

1. Monosaccharides

Polysaccharides are sometimes referred to as ''polyglycans'' or ''hydrocolloids.'' In this chapter, the terms ''polysaccharide'' and ''polyglycan'' are used interchangeably. ''Hydrocolloids'' is a term more commonly employed when discussing polysaccharides for food use. Polysaccharides can best be thought of as molecular chains. The molecular links in polymer nomenclature are known generally as monomers and in polysaccharide chemistry as monosaccharides (''one sugar''). Nature has a short shopping list of monosaccharides some of the most common of which are listed in Table 1.

The majority of cosmetically interesting polysaccharides are comprised primarily of six-membered cyclic structures known as pyranose rings, themselves composed of five carbon atoms and one oxygen and numbered as shown in Table 1. Rings of four carbon atoms and one oxygen atom are known as furanose rings and occur less frequently in personal care applications. Although the formal polysaccharide nomenclature employs the term ''pyranose,'' informally this is shortened by dropping ''pyrano'' from the name. Thus, D-glucopyranose becomes D-glucose. The monosaccharides vary primarily in the spatial arrangement of the appendage groups (R_1, R_2, etc.) attached to the pyranose carbon atoms. For instance, D-glucose differs from D-mannose by the arrangement of the hydroxyl group at carbon 2 (see $\mathbf{R_1}$ and $\mathbf{R_2}$); in D-glucose it exists in an axial arrangement and in D-mannose it is equatorial. These structural variations in the monosaccharides confer huge variation to the resulting polysaccharide family.

The essential connection that links monosaccharides to polysaccharides is known as an anhydroglycosidic bond (Fig. 1). Formally, it is an acetal bond, and polysaccharides can be termed polyacetals. The pyranose ring in this figure is capable of ring opening to create linear aldehyde molecules as in Figure 2, and the unique spatial arrangement of the appended groups can change when this happens. It is this ring-opening chemistry, inherent in the acetal structure of the monosaccharide, that nature exploits to create its plethora of polysaccharides.

Table 1 Naturally Occurring Monosaccharides (pyranose carbon numbering system)

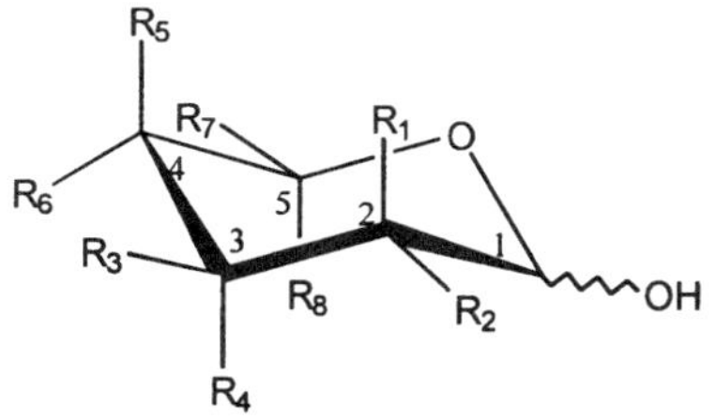

Name	R_1	R_2	R_3	R_4	R_5	R_6	R_7	R_8
D-Glucose	H	OH	OH	H	H	OH	CH_2OH	H
D-Glucuronic acid	H	OH	OH	H	H	OH	CO_2H	H
D-Mannose	OH	H	OH	H	H	OH	CH_2OH	H
D-Mannuronic acid	OH	H	OH	H	H	OH	CO_2H	H
D-Galactose	H	OH	OH	H	OH	H	CH_2OH	H
D-Galacturonic acid	H	OH	OH	H	OH	H	CO_2H	H
L-Guluronic acid	OH	H	OH	H	H	OH	H	CO_2H
3,6-Anhydro-D-galactose	H	OH	O	H	OH	H	CH_2	H
N-Acetyl-D-glucosamine	H	$NHC(O)CH_3$	OH	H	H	OH	CH_2OH	H

Constraining a monosaccharide to a cyclic structure causes the appendage groups to lock into specific arrangements and define the stereochemistry of the pyranose ring. Figure 2, for example, shows the formation of two (1,4)-anhydroglycosidic linkages differing only in the spatial arrangement of the hydroxyl groups at carbons 1 and 4. The change occurred when the pyranose **1a** ring opened and then reclosed to give the new pyranose structure, **1b**. Structure **3a** is referred to as an α-(1,4)-linkage and structure **3b** a β-(1,4)-linkage. Disaccharides **3a** and **3b** are diastereomers of one another, that is, molecules having the same atomic components but different spatial arrangements. Formally, diasteromers are steroisomers that are not mirror images of one another; although **3a** and **3b** have the same number of carbon, hydrogen, and oxygen atoms, they are not the same molecule. As an example, the stereochemical changes seen in **3a** and **3b** can profoundly affect a polysaccharide's solution behavior.

The glycosidic bond shown in Figure 2 formed between carbon 1 of monosaccharides **1a** and **1b** and carbon 4 of monosaccharide **2**. But monosaccharides **1a** and **1b** might just as likely have bonded with carbons 2, 3, 4, or 6 of monosaccharide **2**. Factors that control the construction of anhydroglycosidic linkages in naturally occuring polysaccharides are inherent in the genetic and enzymatic makeup of the polysaccharide source. Examples of each of these monosaccharide linkages, [i.e., (1,2)-, (1,3)-, (1,4)-, and (1-6)-] can be found in all the naturally occurring polysaccharides and examples of many of these will be explored. However, in the polysaccharides discussed below, carbon 1 of at least one monosaccharide, that is the carbon that can ring-open to an aldehyde, is always involved in the formation of the anhydroglycosidic bond.

2. *Structural Influences*

Figure 3 shows examples of a β-(1,4)glycosidic bond **(I)**, a α-(1,4)-glycosidic bond **(II)**, and a (1,6)-glycosidic bond **(III)**. This (1,6)-linkage is common to many branched polysac-

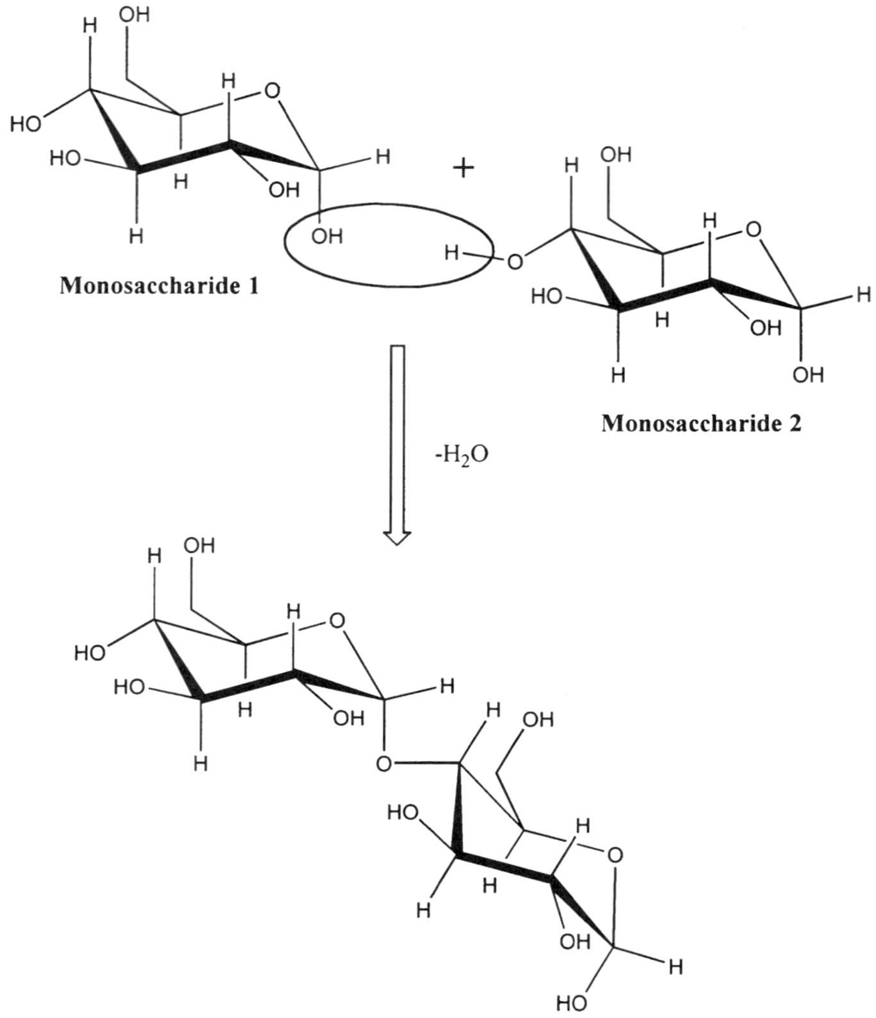

Figure 1 Formation of an anhydroglycosidic bond.

charides (4). Branching can greatly influence the solution behavior of a polysaccharide; it tends to disrupt interpolysaccharide bonds, which otherwise would stack the polymer chains closely one to another. By anology, the effect of branching might be envisioned by comparing the stacking of rows of wooden two-by-fours to the stacking of trees. A given weight of two-by-fours, stacked neatly, occupies considerably less space than the same weight of trees. Likewise, highly branched polymers ''occupy'' greater solution volume when they are dissolved than do linear ones. Highly branched polyglycans entangle more easily and can increase the solution viscosity. Also, highly branched polysaccharides usually dissolve more rapidly, because branching disrupts the crystallinity of the polysaccharide chains. A good example of this will be encountered in the discussion covering starch (Section III.C.1.a).

Glycosidic bonds as seen in Figure 3 can be energetically defined by their dihedral torsional angles, ϕ, ψ, and ω and by the intramolecular hydrogen bonds (indicated by the

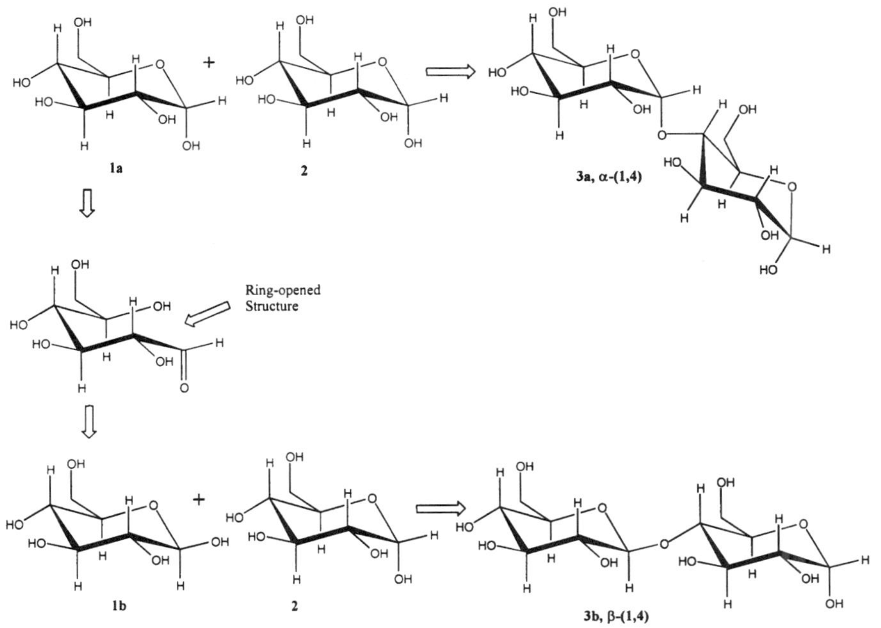

Figure 2 Formation of α-(1,4) and β-(1,4)-anhydroglycosidic bonds.

dashed lines), which restrict the rotation of the monosaccharides around the anhydroglycosidic bond and contribute to their internal energy. The internal energy of a single monosaccharide contained within a polysaccharide is multiplied by the number of monosaccharides, as the sound of a single instrument in a symphony is multiplied by the total number of musicians. Structure **I** in Figure 3 shows, for example, that torsional angles ϕ and ψ and the hydrogen bond between the hydrogen of the carbon 3 hydroxyl group and the acetal oxygen (indicated by the dashed line) would occur between every monosaccharide in the polysaccharide chain. Because of this multiplicity of structural energies, the polysaccharide assumes an overall configuration or shape in which the total energy is minimized over the entire polysaccharide. Typically, the polysaccharide assumes a minimal energy arrangement, one of the most basic being a helicoid (Fig. 4) (5).

Many polysaccharides form helices. This structural behavior is analogous to that of proteins, which are actually members of the family of polypeptides. Examples of these are enzymes and keratin, the protein found in hair. The helical structure is a tertiary (i.e., three dimensional) spatial configuration, arranged to minimize the total energy of the polysaccharide. However, the nature of the helix varies from polysaccharide to polysaccharide. It might be a tight, spring-like coil as found in amylose or a loose, open helix characteristic of cellulose (Fig. 5) (6). It can twist left or right. It is seen that the nature of the helix is predisposed by the monosaccharides that comprise it.

Additional factors that influence the helical structure include the stereochemistry of appendage groups arranged on the monosaccharides and the tendency of monosaccharides to attach linearly or in a branched fashion (Fig. 3, Structure **III**) to one another. The overriding factor that dictates helix shape is the molecular bonding conformations. A polysaccharide that is an open random coil in solution may, by controlling temperature or solvent polarity, assume a much more tightly wound configuration that changes its solution

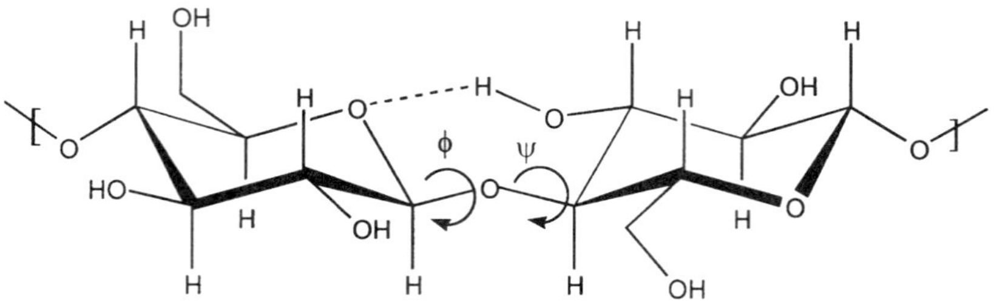

I. Cellulose, β-(1,4)-

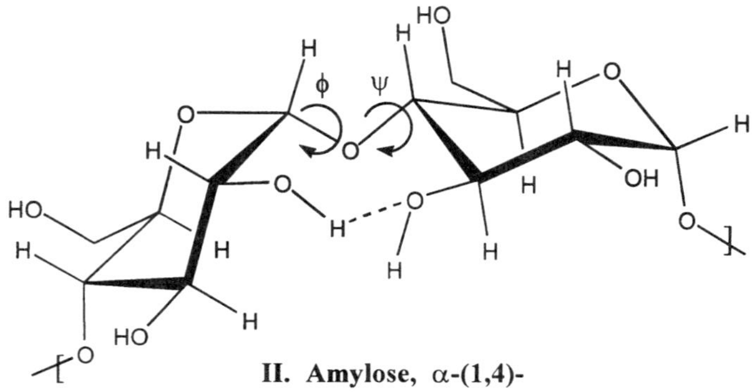

II. Amylose, α-(1,4)-

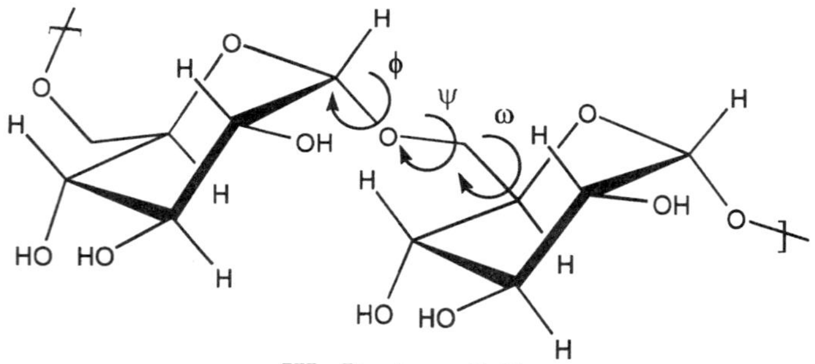

III. Dextran, (1,6)-

Figure 3 Dihedral angles and intramolecular hydrogen bonds in various glycosidic linkages. (Reprinted with permission from Ref. 4.)

properties. The different chain configurations are driven by smaller, more subtle changes in the monosaccharide bonding conformations. The formulator needs to consider these influences when using polysaccharides.

Polypeptides, like polysaccharides, can further minimize their internal molecular energy by wrapping one helical coil around another; a classic example is found in the double helix of deoxyribonucleic acid (DNA) (7). The keratinaceous proteins of hair likewise form double helices. Polysaccharides, too, frequently assume the double-helix conforma-

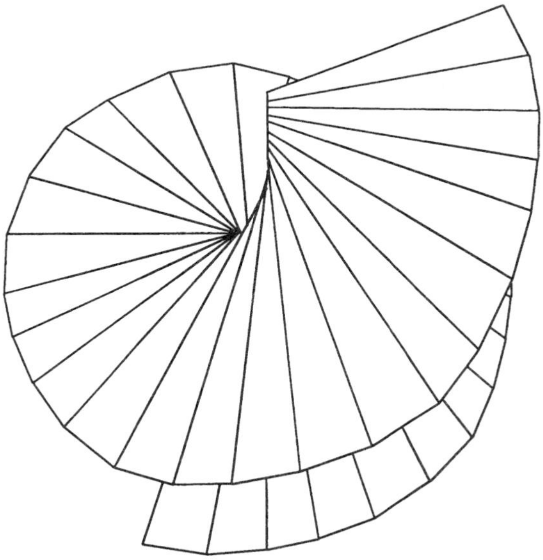

Figure 4 Right-handed helicoid structure.

tion. The molecular energy of a polysaccharide confined in a double helix is further influenced by interpolysaccharide hydrogen bonds, van der Waals forces, steric influences, and the positioning of groups between the polysaccharide chains. These influences, strongly attractive at times, create highly ordered or crystalline segments. When they are weaker or repulsive they create amorphous regions and can even cause chain separation. Understanding the polysaccharide's solution behavior is closely tied to an understanding of these large-scale effects.

Regardless of whether a polysaccharide forms a helix in solution or a random coil, its effect on the viscosity becomes increasingly evident as the concentration increases and individual chains begin interacting with one another. Independent of the "type" of polysaccharide, it is observed that the polyglycan concentration must exceed a critical value before the helices or coils will interact. Usually this interaction is defined by two concentration regimes, dilute and concentrated. The two regimes are represented graphically in plots of zero shear or specific viscosity, η_{sp}, verses the coil overlap parameter, $c[\eta]$ (8,9). As can be seen in Figure 6, at the critical overlap concentration, $c[\eta] \approx 4$, the shape of the viscosity curve changes. The viscosity beyond this point is now influenced by chain entanglement and the polysaccharides are in the concentrated regime.

III. POLYSACCHARIDE FUNCTIONALITY

The behavior of polysaccharides is also critically influenced by the nature of the substituent groups bound to the individual monosaccharides. These substituents can be of natural origin or they may be synthesized and thus of seminatural quality. Whether they are natural or seminatural, the classification of polysaccharides falls into one of five categories, based primarily on the polysaccharide charge. These include: anionic, cationic, nonionic, amphoteric, and hydrophobic.

Some influences, like anionic charge, can occur naturally in the polysaccharide. Oth-

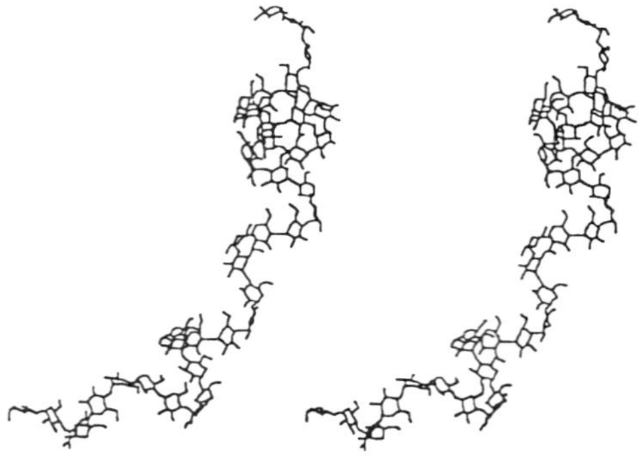

Simulated Structure of (1→4)-α-D-Glucan DP = 40

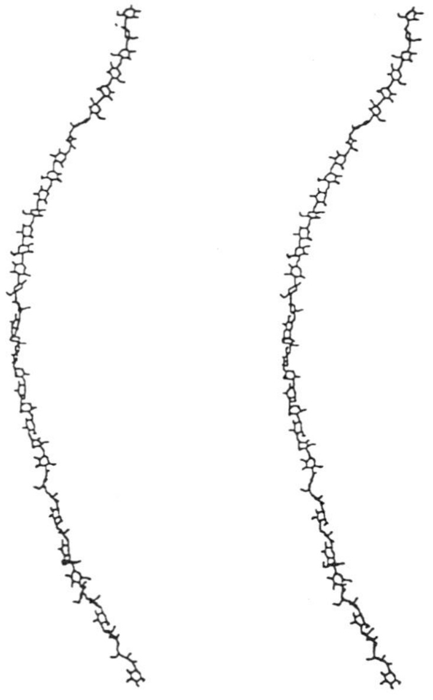

Simulated Structure of (1→4)-β-D-Glucan DP = 40

Figure 5 Simulated stereoview of helical structures of amylose (top) and cellulose (bottom) (Reprinted with permission from Ref. 6.)

ers, like cationicity or hydrophobicity, are primarily the result of human invention. Various cosmetically popular polysaccharides, both natural and seminatural, are explored in this section, and influences of the polysaccharide's structure and functionality on solution behavior are addressed. The effects of additional components (e.g., surfactants, salts, other polysaccharides, or polymers) will be explored in each category with the aim of understanding how these factors modify the principal solution behavior of polysaccharides.

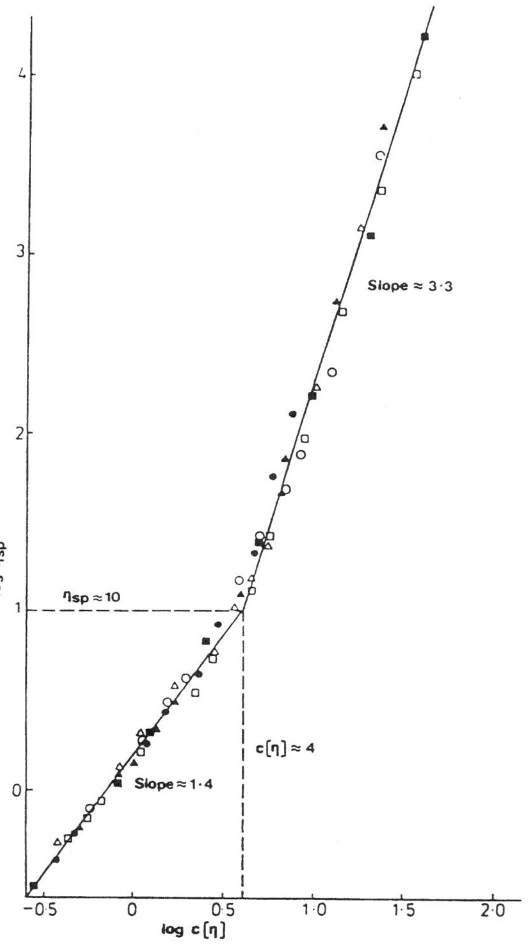

Figure 6 Plot of the log of zero shear viscosity, η_{sp}, versus the coil overlap parameter, c[η], for: (○) dextran; (●) carboxymethylamylose (0.5 M NaCl; pH 7); (△) high mannuronate alginate (0.2 M NaCl; pH 7); (▲) high guluronate alginate (0.2 M NaCl; pH 7); (□) lambda-carrageenan (0.075 M KCl; pH 7); (■) hyaluronate (0.015 M NaCl; pH 7). (Reprinted from Ref. 8 with kind permission from Elsevier Science Ltd, The Boulevard, Langford Lane, Kidlington 0X5 1GB, UK.)

A. Anionic Polysaccharides

The cosmetically interesting anionic polysaccharides are predominantly comprised of a group of naturally occurring materials (10). Indeed, of the available polysaccharides made anionic by human intervention, there are only two commercially interesting derivatives, cellulose gum (carboxymethylcellulose) and carboxymethylchitin (a third, carboxymethylglucan, will be covered in Section III.F.3). These derivatives are anionic as a result of the carboxymethylation of naturally occurring cellulose and chitin, respectively. The list of naturally occurring anionic polysaccharides is more extensive and includes alginic acid, pectin, carrageenans, xanthan gum, hyaluronic acid, and chondroitin sulfate, and the gum exudates including, arabic, karaya, and tragacanth.

1. *Naturally Occurring Anionic Polysaccharides*

a. Alginic acid (Alginates). The alginates, polysaccharides isolated from marine brown algae and from bacterial fermentation, are comprised of two different monosaccharides, β-D-(1,4)-mannuronic acid, **4**, and α-L-(1,4)-guluronic acid, **5** (Fig. 7) (11–16). They function in the algae and bacteria to provide cellular support to the cells, which keeps the cells from collapsing. These two monosaccharides can link glycosidically as polymannuronic acid, as polyguluronic acid, or as combinations. The β-(1,4)-linkage of the D-mannuronic acid, characteristic of many structural polysaccharides, gives the alginates an extended helical structure. The α-(1,4)-linkage of the L-guluronic acid, on the other hand, is more characteristic of the polysaccharides used by plants for energy storage and gives the polysaccharide a tighter helical coil. Alginates comprised primarily of D-mannuronic acid residues tend to be extended coils in solution whereas the presence of L-guluronic acid compresses the coil.

Because the polyglycan in alginates is made up of both D-mannuronic acid and L-guluronic acid residues, both of which have carboxylic acid groups located at carbon 6, they are highly anionic. These acid groups are frequently esterified in bacterially derived alginates. Every monosaccharide, however, has a carboxylic acid group appended to it, which strongly influences solution behavior. For example, polyvalent cations can cause strong intra- and intermolecular bonding with polysaccharides containing L-guluronic acid residues, leading to cross-linked systems.

The cross-linking sites that occur when a polyvalent cation causes interpolysaccharide binding (i.e., between polysaccharide chains) are called ''junction zones'' (Fig. 8) (4,17–21). Furthermore, the ''egg box model'' has been used to describe the relationship between the polyglycan (the box) and the cation (the egg). Calcium ion, Ca^{2+}, in particular, is well known for its ability to form junction zones in alginate solutions. The formation of these zones requires at least two L-guluronic acid residues to be sequential in the chain as shown in Figure 8; this number must be much higher to form strong junction zones. The aqueous solution viscosity increases with concentration of the polyvalent cation until the polysaccharide eventually gels. Further addition of calcium then causes the alginic acid to precipitate from solution. Formulations that employ alginates must control polyvalent metal ion concentrations through the use of sequestrants such as ethylenediaminetetraacetic acid (EDTA), to optimize viscosifying effects of the alginate. Although present in low concentration, even the calcium ions from city water can affect the appearance of an alginate formulation.

The viscosities of aqueous alginate solutions are influenced by pH due to the pendent carboxylic acid groups. Indeed, most of the anionic polysaccharides are affected to some degree by fluctuations in pH, particularly at the higher and lower extremes. The effect of

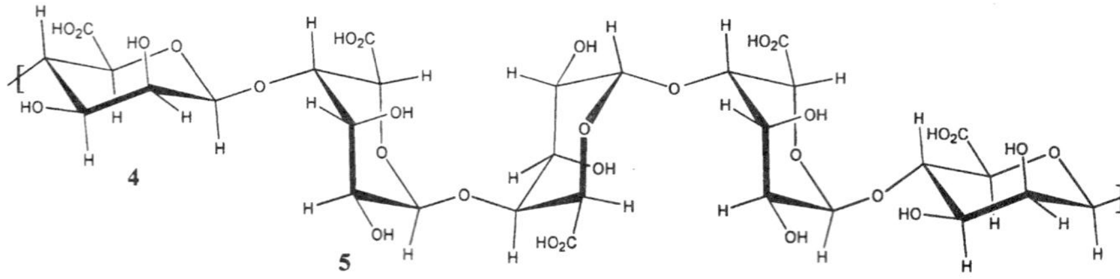

Figure 7 Partial structure of alginic acid showing β-D-(1,4)-mannuronic acid, **4**, and α-L-(1,4)-guluronic acid, **5**, residues.

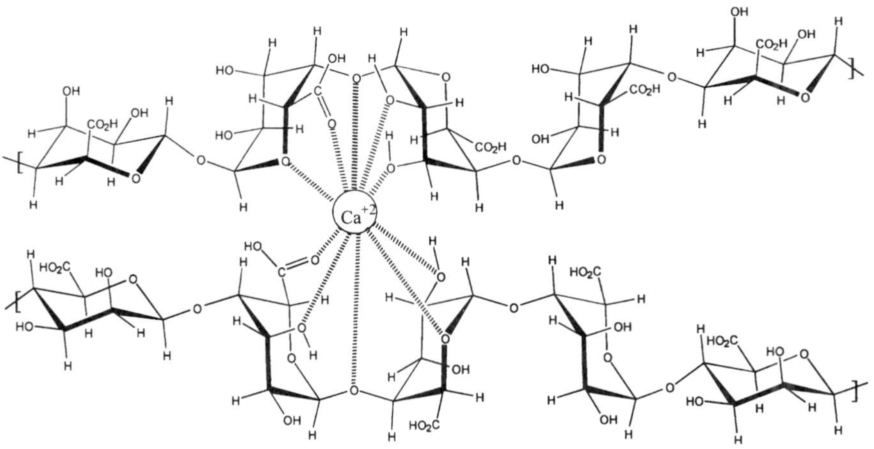

Figure 8 Junction zones formed between alginic acid and Ca^{2+} ions.

pH on alginates is most pronounced near the isoelectric point of the carboxylic acid, near pH 4.0 (Fig. 9). The solution viscosity below this pH rises rapidly as the carboxylic acid salts are protonated. Like most polysaccharides, alginates are not stable at pH < 3.0 owing to hydrolysis of the glycosidic bonds holding the polysaccharides together. They are also unstable at high pH (above 10) and their use is not recommended at either pH extreme.

b. Pectin. Pectin is a cellular support polysaccharide, isolated industrially by extraction from citrus fruit peels. Its structure is similar to that of alginic acid, except pectin is comprised of repeating α-D-(1,4)-galacturonic acid units (**6**), which are interrupted occasionally by an α-L-(1,2)-rhamanose (**7**) as shown in Figure 10 (22–25). Rhamanose is a form of mannose that has been fully reduced to a methyl group at carbon 6. The α-D-(1,4)-linkage of the pectin galacturonic acids affords a shortened chain structure for pectin, and each C6 carbon atom is fully oxidized to a carboxylic acid group. A portion of the carboxylic acid groups of pectin are naturally esterified with O-methyl groups, much like the bacterial-derived alginates. This renders these acidic species partially nonionic and results in gels that behave differently than those formed by nonesterified alginates (26).

The level of methyl ester is monitored by gas chromatography, and pectin is sold in grades designated by this level. Lower levels of ester groups make the pectin more anionic. Pectin behaves much like alginic acid when its methyl ester levels are below 50%; it forms turbid gels in the presence of divalent metal ions, calcium in particular. At high levels, it can form gels without divalent ion, but the concentration of polysaccharide required is typically much higher.

It is not surprising to find that pectin is well suited for low-pH applications considering its source. Pectin functions ideally at pHs near 3.5. Below this pH, it suffers from hydrolysis of both the glycosidic linkage and the ester, and in highly alkaline solutions, hydrolysis of the ester is rapid. Changes in the number of ester groups over time cause unstable viscosities in cosmetic formulations.

c. Carrageenans. The carrageenans are anionic, cellular structural polysaccharides isolated from marine red algae (27–32). At least seven varieties of carrageenans are known, differentiated by Greek letters. They are highly functional owing to the nature

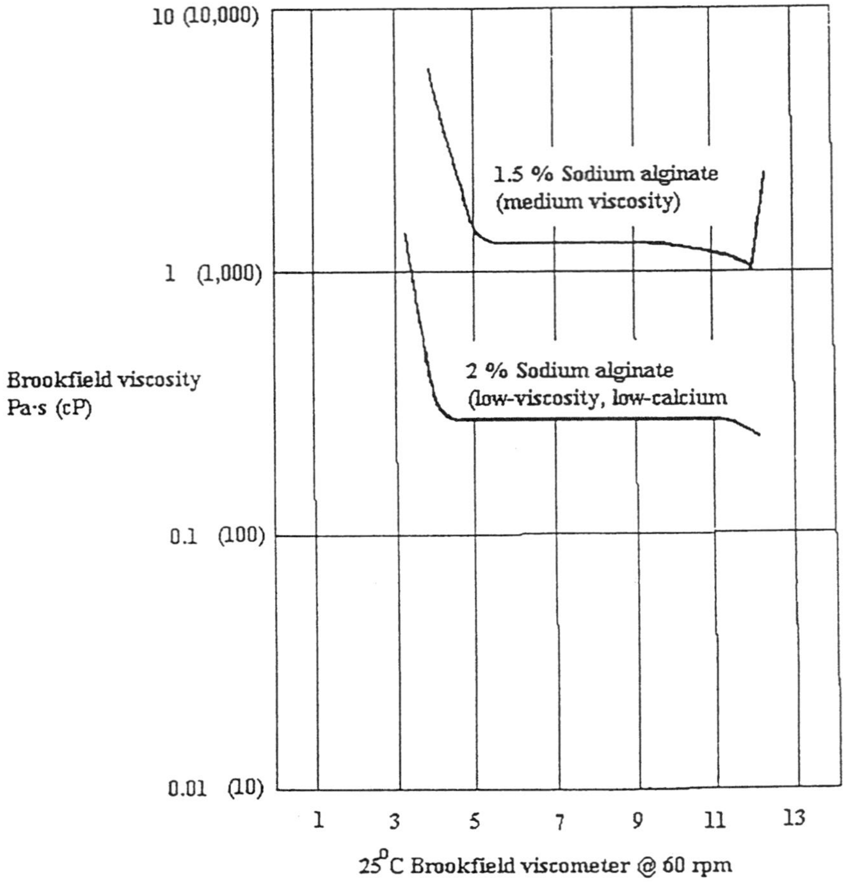

Figure 9 Effect of pH on alginate solution viscosity. (Reprinted with permission from Ref. 11.)

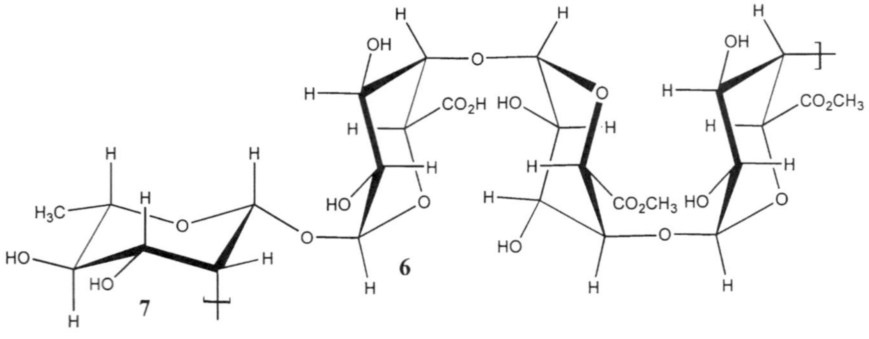

Figure 10 Partial structure of pectin showing α-D-(1,4)-galacturonic acid, **6**, and α-L-rhamanose, **7**. Note methylated esters of two galacturonic acid residues.

of the anionic substituents, and quite diverse structurally. The carrageenans of greatest commercial interest are primarily comprised of two repeating monosaccharides shown in Table 2, including β-D-(1,3)-galactose (**8**) and α-D-(1,4)-galactose (**9**). The most commercially accessible varieties include kappa (κ)-, iota (ι)-, and lambda (λ)-carrageenan.

Kappa- and iota-carrageenans are structurally similar in that the (1,4)-linked D-galactose (**9**) is made more rigid by formation of a five-membered cyclic anhydride ether group between the C6 (**R**$_5$) and C3 (**R**$_3$) carbon atoms. The presence of the 3,6-anhydride ether causes the chains of these carrageenans to more fully extend in solution by making the monosaccharides more rigid. Lambda-carrageenan, lacking this structural rigidity, assumes a more crimped α-(1,4)-linkage like that already seen in the L-guluronic acid portion of the alginates (Section III.A.1.a). The anhydride also creates a more hydrophobic (water-avoiding) environment in this portion of the monosaccharide. To minimize interaction of the anhydride ether with water, these two polysaccharides form tightly wound double helices when dissolved, the interiors of which house the anhydride ether functionality. The lambda-carrageenan does not form double-helical coils and, as discussed below, cannot form aqueous solution gels.

The carrageenans are anionic because some of the pyranose hydroxyl groups are substituted with sulfate half-esters. The sulfate groups are highly acidic (similar to the acidity of sulfuric acid) and hydrophilic (''water-loving''). As a result, the double helices of kappa- and iota-carrageenan are peppered on their exteriors with anionic sulfate groups making their exterior very hydrophilic.

Formation of the carrageenan double helix is temperature sensitive; no polysaccharides spontaneously form double helices without a thermal stimulus. Because of this, following initial dissolution of the polysaccharide in hot water, the polymer chains exist as random coils (Fig. 11) (27). Cooling causes the hydrophobic domains of the kappa- and iota-carrageenans to unfavorably interact with the aqueous environment, causing these region of the polysaccharide chains to group and form, initially, a single helix and, eventually, the resultant double helix (Gel I). Lambda-carrageenan, by contrast, does not form single helices. Even so, it builds significant aqueous viscosities through random chain entanglement. In addition to being temperature dependent, the rheological effect of kappa-

Table 2 Structure of Kappa-, Iota-, and Lambda-Carrageenan (β-D-(1,3)-galactose, **8**, and α-D-(1,4)-galactose, **9**, monosaccharides)

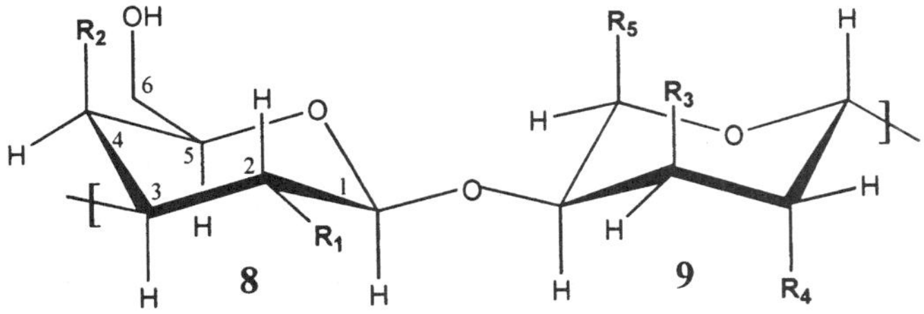

8 **9**

Carrageenan type	R_1	R_2	R_3	R_4	R_5
Kappa	OH	OSO_3^-	O ⌊	OH	CH_2 ⌋
Iota	OH	OSO_3^-	O ⌊	OSO_3^-	CH_2 ⌋
Lambda	OSO_3^-	OH	OH	OSO_3^-	$CH_2OSO_3^-$

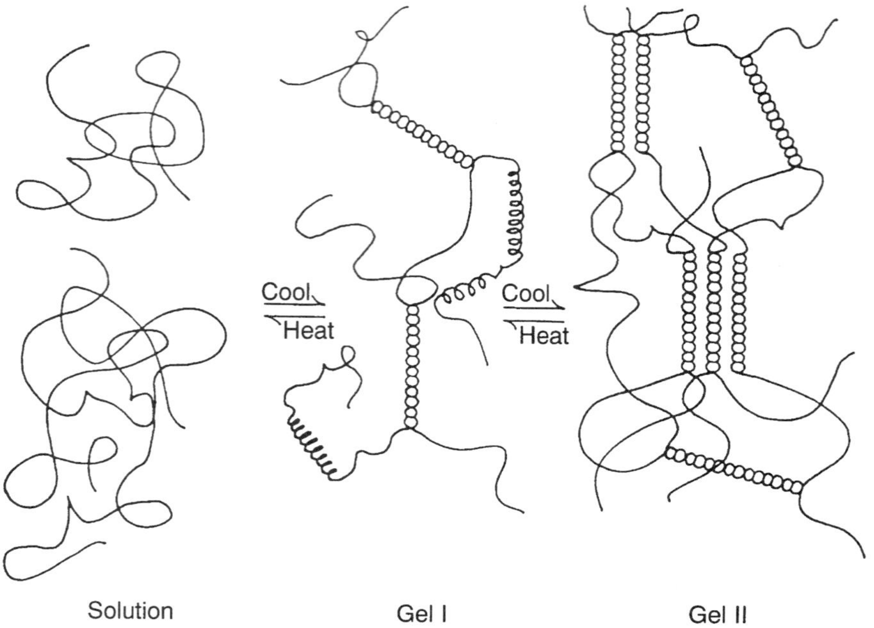

Figure 11 Coil to helix to aggregate transitions for gelling carrageenans. (Reprinted with permission from Ref. 27.)

carrageenan is molecular weight dependent. As its molecular weight increases, so does its solution viscosity (33).

Formation of the double helix creates a unique environment that can, in the presence of various cations, especially K^+ and Ca^{2+}, result in further aggregation or junction-zone formation through the influence of the anionic sulfate groups (34–39). Kappa- and iota-carrageenans require the presence of cationic salts to form the strong gels they are capable of making. Formation of the junction zones creates interhelical cross-links that cause still higher solution viscosities and, eventually, gelation (Gel II).

Another rheologically interesting feature of kappa-carrageenan is the unique and synergistic viscosifying effect seen in blends with either a galactomannan (e.g., konjac mannan) or a glucomannan (e.g., locust bean gum) (Fig. 12) (29,40–44). (The structure of the gluco- and galactomannans will be discussed in more detail later in this chapter.) Details of the interaction are still being debated. The synergy manifests itself in higher solution viscosities and elastic modulii as shown in Figure 13 for blends of κ-carrageenan and galactomannan. The prevailing concept is that gluco- and galactomannans bind to the kappa-carrageenan double helix, interrupting the salt-induced large-scale aggregations of the double helices, increasing the number and strength of the junction zones, and causing stronger gels. Regardless of the mechanism, formulators find that adding one of the abovementioned gluco- or galactomannans to a solution containing kappa-carrageenan further increases its viscosity. Mixing of the two synergistic polysaccharides and the salts of the formulation, however, must be carefully controlled to achieve maximum performance.

d. Xanthan. Xanthan gum is an anionic polysaccharide made commercially by bacterial fermentation. It occurs as an exocellular coating on the bacterial cell walls and is isolated after the fermentation process by precipitation from the broth (45–50). Structur-

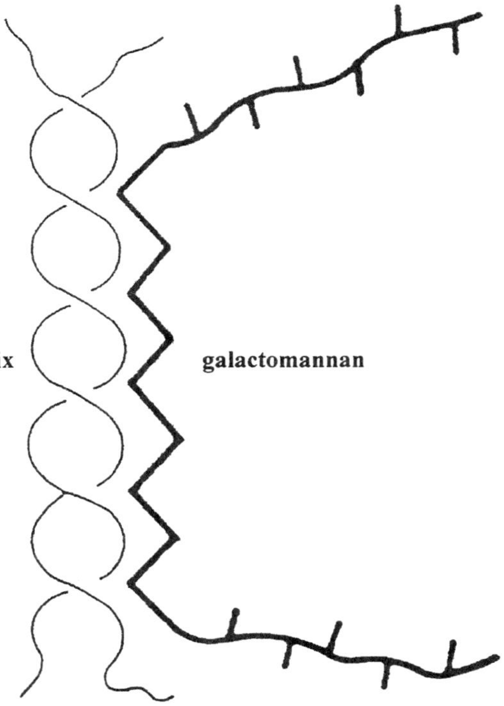

Figure 12 Proposed model for the interaction between kappa-carrageenan and gluco- or galacto-mannan. (Reprinted with permission from Ref. 29.)

ally, xanthan is a complex polysaccharide comprised of a primary chain of β-D-(1,4)-glucose (**10**), which has, on alternating glucose moieties, a branching trisaccharide side chain comprised of β-D-(1,2)-mannose (**11**), attached to β-D-(1,4)-glucuronic acid (**12**), which terminates in a final β-D-mannose (**13**) (Fig. 14).

The hydroxyl group at the C6 carbon in the first D-mannose group is frequently acetylated and the final mannose sugar is frequently derivatized by pyruvic acid. The β-(1,4)-glycosidic bond that connects the β-D-glucose of the xanthan backbone is characteristic of the structural cell wall polysaccharides found in most plants (i.e., cellulose). The backbone is an extended structure in solution; comb-like trisaccharide side chains rendered it water-soluble. Xanthan is anionic by virtue of carboxylic acid residues on the D-glucuronic acid and the pyruvic acid moiety on the terminal D-mannose.

It is generally accepted that xanthan forms helical coils in the presence of cationic salts, but the need for salts to build solution viscosity, as seen, for example, with kappa-carrageenan, is minimized by the rigid xanthan backbone. Whether or not xanthan forms double helices in solution is still being debated (51,52). In any case, the mechanism of thickening and gelation still requires the formation of junction zones, which are thought to occur through the interaction of hydrophobic sites on the xanthan helix. Cations tend to ''salt out'' these sites, improve the strength of the junctions, and produce a slight increase in solution viscosity. These solutions also show remarkable viscosity stability at increasing temperatures because the viscosity is generated by hydrophobic interactions in the polysaccharide. This can be useful when developing thermally stable formulations.

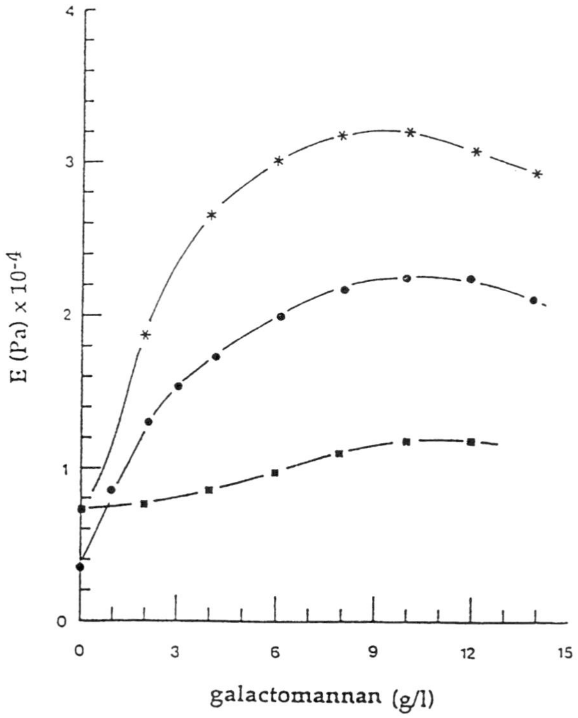

Figure 13 Elastic modulus of kappa-carrageenan (4 g/L)-galactomannan blends as a function of galactomannan concentration. (*) Carob in 0.1 M KCl; (●) carob in 0.05 M KCl; (■) guar in 0.1 M KCl. (Reprinted from Ref. 43 with kind permission from Elsevier Sciences, Ltd, The Boulevard, Langford Lane, Kidlington 0X5 1GB, UK.)

Xanthan forms lyotropic and isotropic liquid crystals in water at appropriate concentrations (53). The formation of solvent-based liquid crystals is an area of expanding interest in personal care because of their unique ability to form emulsifier-free suspensions, which is discussed in the section describing hydroxypropylcellulose (Section III.C.2.a.ii). Specifically, xanthan forms cholesteric mesophase lyotropic liquid crystals in water at concentrations as low as 3.5 wt%. Formation of the liquid crystal phase is influenced by salt concentration: the higher the salt concentration, the lower the xanthan concentration required to form the liquid crystal phase.

When a shear stress below a critical value is applied to a xanthan solution, the solution resists deformation (Fig. 15) (54). That is, a finite amount of force is required to initialize flow. This appears as an inflection point at low shear rates in Figure 15 and is known as the ''yield value.'' Such solutions can stabilize or suspend water-insoluble materials like solids or oily droplets. Xanthan solutions are pseudoplastic, i.e., shear-thinning, and their viscosity recovers rapidly once the shear force is removed. One use of this behavior might occur in a pump spray application. The viscous xanthan solution will thin when pumped through the high shear aerosol valve, but thickens immediately upon exiting the nozzle. Xanthan's rheological effects can also improve the effectiveness of other typical emulsifiers (55–58). The effects are generally seen as stabilization of the formulation, which prolongs its lifetime and might also reduce the quantity of primary emulsifier required.

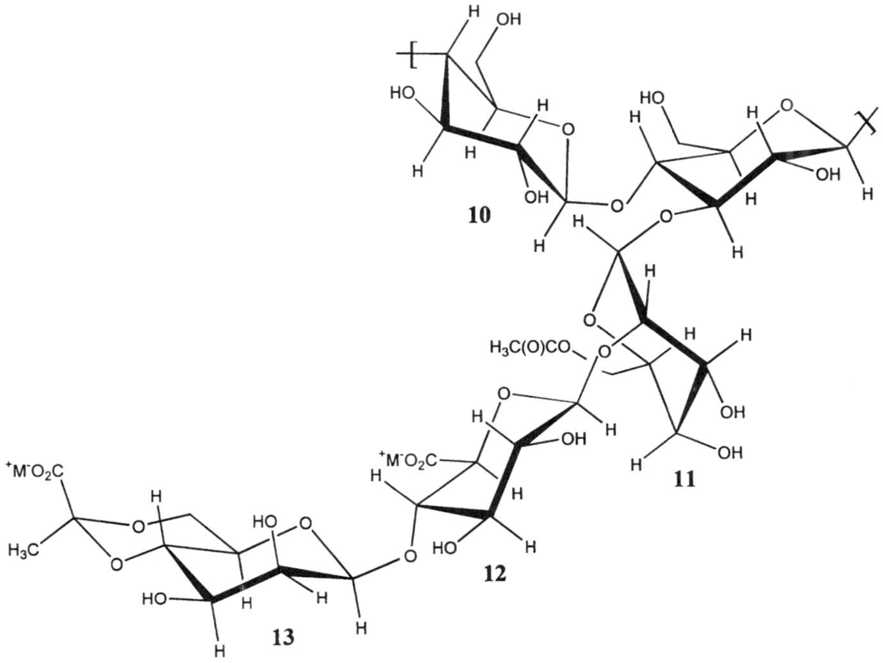

Figure 14 Partial structure of xanthan gum showing β-D-(1,4)-glucose, **10**, acetylated β-D-(1,2)-mannose, **11**, β-D-(1,4)-glucuronic acid, **12**, and pyruvic acid terminated β-D-mannose, **13**.

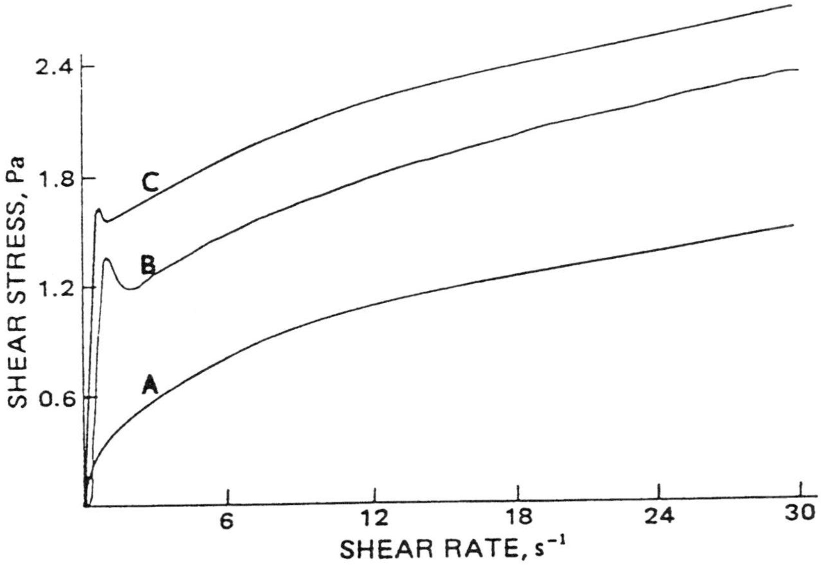

Figure 15 Shear stress verses shear rate for various xanthan gum concentrations: (A) 0.133%; (B) 0.3%; (C) 0.5%. Yield value is indicated by a small increase in shear stress at low shear rate seen in B and C. (Reprinted with permission from Ref. 54.)

Because primary emulsifiers are sometimes skin irritants, this can help to minimize their deleterious impact.

Xanthan exhibits rheological synergism in the presence of gluco- or galactomannans much like kappa-carrageenan. Here too, the mechanism is debated, but it might occur by interaction of the hydrophobic domains of the xanthan helices (or double helicles) with those of the gluco- or galactomannan (Fig. 16) (59). Recent molecular modeling studies suggest an alternative mechanism of gelation may involve commingling of the xanthan helix and that of the gluco- or galactomannan (Fig. 17) (60). The presence of the gluco- or galactomannan likely increases the number and strength of the junction zones that cause higher solution viscosities.

Xanthan, because of its anionic character, is incompatible with most cationic surfactants. In the presence of nonionic surfactants, xanthan solution viscosities are relatively unaffected regardless of surfactant concentration (61). Anionic surfactants at levels greater than 1 wt% increase viscosity, particularly at low shear rates (Fig. 18). This further improves the suspending capability of xanthan gum. In addition, xanthan's thickening efficiency is synergistically enhanced by the addition of colloidal magnesium aluminum silicate (Veegum), an inorganic clay frequently employed to thicken cosmetic formulations (62).

e. Hyaluronic Acid and Chondroitin Sulfate. Hyaluronic acid and chondroitin sulfate are anionic polysaccharides isolated from various animal tissues. Hyaluronic acid, important in many cosmetic formulations, is also commercially manufactured by bacterial fermentation (63,64,65). Characteristically, hyaluronic acid and chondroitin sulfate are covalently bound with various proteins in the animal tissue where the coupled polysaccharide/protein macromolecules are referred to as "proteoglycans." Both hyaluronic acid and chondroitin sulfate (Table 3), of which there are principally two, chondroitin-4-sulfate and chondroitin-6-sulfate, are comprised of two repeating monosaccharides, β-D-(1,4)-glucuronic acid (**14**) and *N*-acetyl-β-D-(1,3)-glucosamine (**15**). The latter unique acetylated-amine-containing monosaccharide classified these polysaccharides as gluco-

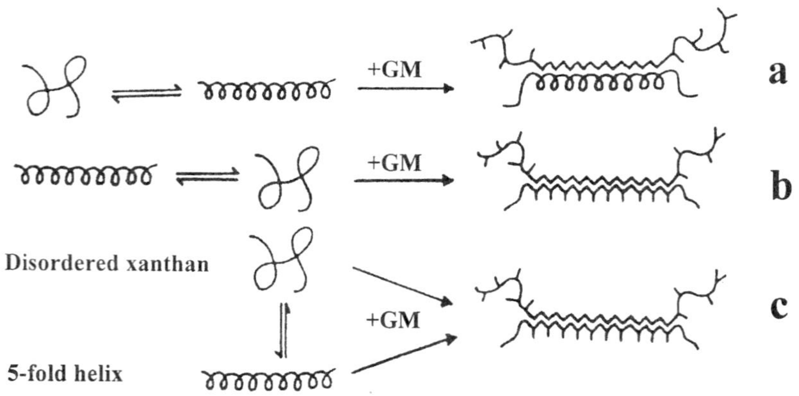

Figure 16 Proposed interactions of xanthan and gluco- or galactomannan. (a) Attachment of unsubstituted regions of mannan backbone to xanthan helix. (b) Attachment of mannan backbone through heterotypic junction zones to extended disordered xanthan chain. (c) Attachment of mannan backbone through heterotypic junction zones on xanthan helix, which uncoils to an extended disordered chain. (Reprinted with permission from Ref. 59. Copyright 1995 American Chemical Society.)

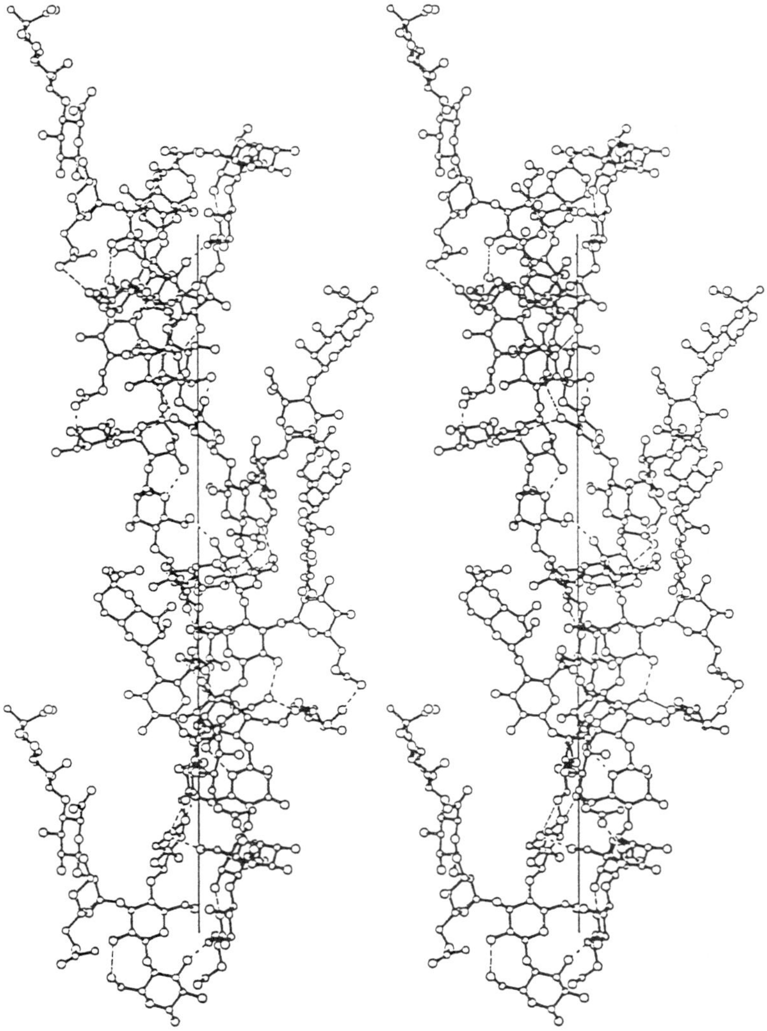

Figure 17 Stereoview of the antiparallel intertwining of xanthan and galactomannan. (Reprinted from Ref. 60 with kind permission from Elsevier Science Ltd, The Boulevard, Langford Lane, Kidlington 0X5 1GB, UK.)

saminoglycans (amino-containing sugars). The glucuronic acid residues give these polysaccharides their primary anionic charge. The chondroitin sulfates have additional anionic charge available from the sulfate half-ester groups bound to the glucosamine pyranose hydroxyl groups (66).

These polyglycans have important and varied psychological roles in animal tissue. Hyaluronic acid, for instance, is known to occur in the dermis of the skin, in the vitreous fluids of the eye, and in the body's synovial fluids (67). It has many functions, the most significant being cellular turgidity (because of its water-binding capacity) and lubrication. It has also been shown to play a key role in wound healing, which will be discussed in Section III.F.1.

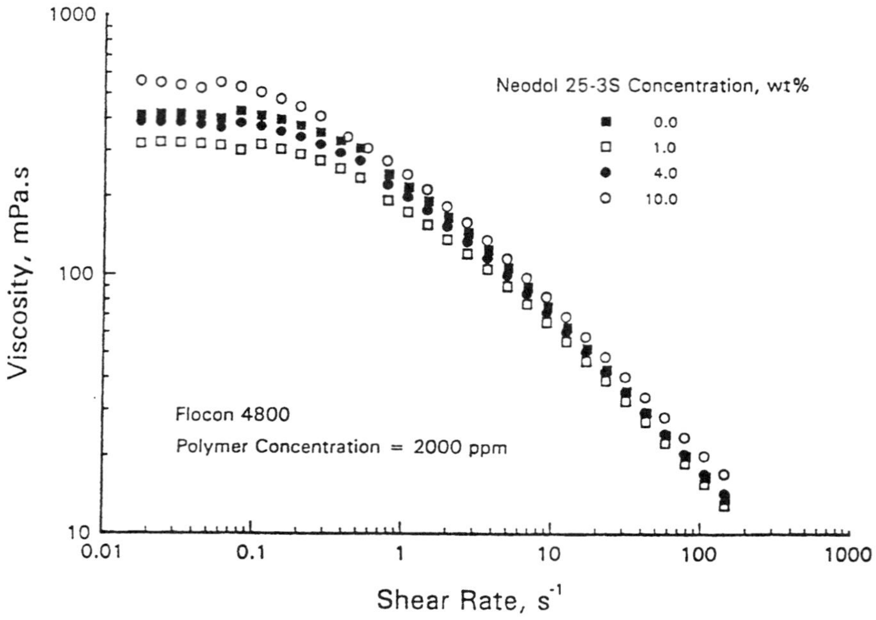

Figure 18 Effect of various concentrations of anionic surfactant, neodol 25-3S, on xanthan solution viscosity (2000 ppm flocon 4800). (Reprinted with permission from Ref. 61.)

The glycosaminoglycans form loose random coils in solution. The presence of diavalent metal ions, like Ca^{2+}, is not required to attain significant solution viscosities and, in fact, may cause the polysaccharides to precipitate. The high solution viscosities generated by hyaluronic acid, even at low concentrations, are primarily the result of chain entanglement of the high-molecular-weight polysaccharides (68). Furthermore, strong intra- and intermolecular hydrogen bonding interactions allow hyaluronic acid to bind several times its weight in free water.

Table 3 Structure of the Glycosaminoglycans, Hyaluronic Acid, and Chondroitin Sulfate (β-D-(1,4)-glucuronic acid, **14**, and *N*-acetyl-β-D-(1,3)-glucosamine, **15**, monosaccharides)

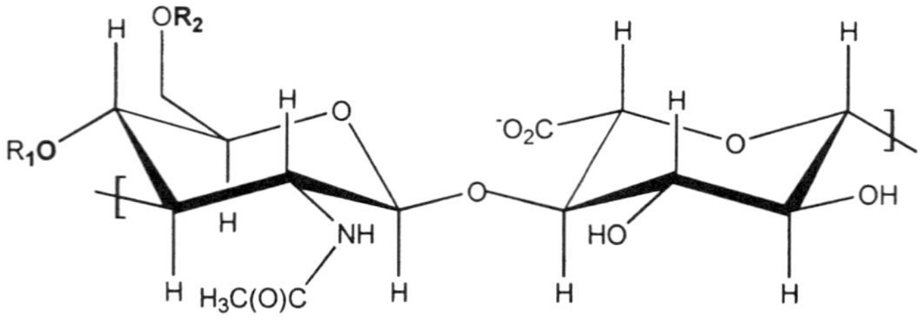

15 **14**

Polysaccharide	R_1	R_2
Hyaluronic acid	H	H
Chondroitin-4-sulfate	SO_3^-	H
Chondroitin-6-sulfate	H	SO_3^-

It is not surprising to find that hyaluronic acid and, to a lesser extent, chondroitin sulfate, because they are significant components of the extracellular fluids of human dermis, are important ingredients for improving the appearance of skin (69,70). Hyaluronic acid is completely biocompatible with human tissue. However, because of their inherent anionic charge, the glycosaminoglycans are not substantive, i.e., electrostatically attracted, to the anionic surfaces of skin and hair (71–73). It has been demonstrated, on the other hand, that combinations of hyaluronic acid and cationically charged polymers can improve its binding to keratinized surfaces like skin (Fig. 19) (74,75). Care must be taken in developing such polyelectrolyte complexes because the interaction of anionic and cationic polymers frequently forms water-insoluble complexes.

f. Arabic, Karaya, and Tragacanth Gum. Arabic, karaya, and tragacanth gums are some of the oldest and most commercially well-established anionic polysaccharides, yet their complex molecular identities are still only superficially known (76). It is difficult to establish their chemical identity because, instead of being a single polysaccharide, they are a group of many having different molecular weights and structures.

The exudate gums are isolated from the sap of specific trees and bushes that use each particular sap for protection, fluid transport, and energy storage. The isolation process usually involves injuring the tree bark and collecting the sticky gum fluids as they leak out, much like maple syrup is collected from the maple tree. Usually, the "harvest" of exudates is seasonal and the quality of the gums affected by weather fluctuations. All of the gum exudates are nontoxic and are generally recognized as safe (GRAS) for use in cosmetics.

Arabic gum is comprised of a neutral backbone of β-D-(1,3)-galactose residues that have multiple branching glycans, some of which impart anionic charge to the gum (77). Arabic gum, because of its relatively low molecular weight, is used in applications where high levels of polysaccharide solids are desired without significant viscosity buildup. Arabic gum dissolves in water at greater than 50 wt% solids while remaining flowable. It is, however, surface active and lowers the surface tension of water. Thus it can be classified

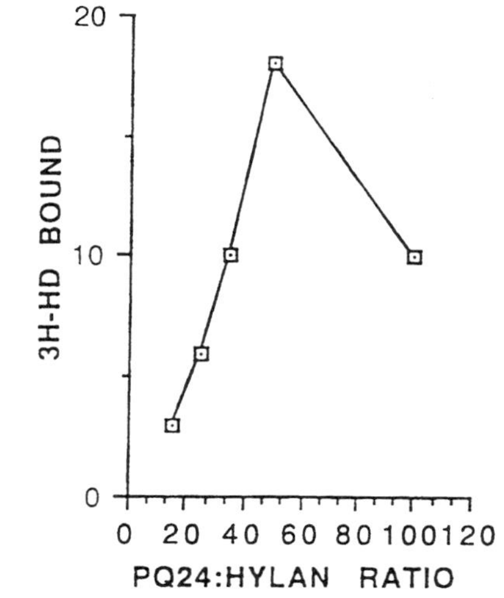

Figure 19 Improvement in binding of tritiated (3H[1]) hyaluronic acid onto neonatal rat skin at various hylan to cationic polymer (PQ24) ratios. (Reprinted with permission from Ref. 74.)

an emulsifier. Arabic gum solutions are influenced by pH and by the presence of salts. The gum has its maximum viscosifying effect near pH 6.0; the viscosity drops quickly when the solution pH becomes higher or lower. Multivalent cations reduce the viscosity of solutions of arabic gum, but the gum will not precipitate in the same way many anionic polysaccharides are salted out.

Gum karaya is not a truly water-soluble material (78,79). It is composed primarily of a highly branched D-galacturonic acid backbone. Many of the acidic monosaccharides are acetylated, which causes the water insolubility. Instead of dissolving, gum karaya swells in water and develops significant viscosity even at low concentration. Stickiness accompanies the swelling, which explains its popularity in denture adhesives.

Gum karaya has many acetylated acid groups, which allow its stability and viscosity to be strongly influenced by pH. Karaya performs best at pH values between 7 and 9 where it is also least susceptible to hydrolysis. Interestingly, the viscosity of gum karaya solutions depends on the order of hydration and pH adjustment. If gum karaya is hydrated first and then the solution pH raised, the viscosity is higher than if dried polysaccharide is added directly to an alkaline solution. This suggests that hydration in alkaline mediums might accelerate the ester hydrolysis.

Gum tragacanth is, perhaps, the best characterized of the these commercial gums (80,81). It is not a single gum, but is comprised of two, complex, highly branched polysaccharides: arabinogalactin, a water-soluble, neutral polysaccharide having a D-(1,6)-galactose backbone, and tragacanthic acid, an anionic polysaccharide polyglycan based on α-D-(1,6)-galacturonic acid. The tragacanthic acid backbone resembles the pectin polysaccharide backbone discussed in Section III.A.1.b.

Gum tragacanth shares many of the functional properties found in xanthan gum (Section III.A.1.d.). At low concentrations it produces high solution viscosities. Its solutions also have a yield stress and make it suitable for suspending water-insoluble components. Tragacanth has high pH stability, but its viscosity, unlike that of xanthan, thins as the temperature increases. Tragacanth's thickening effects are not influenced by gluco- or galactomannans as is the case for xanthan gum. In the presence of arabic gum, however, the viscosity of gum tragacanth solutions will diminish but without detriment to its suspending abilities. The reason for this synergistic effect is still unclear. Tragacanth strongly binds multivalent cations. Many, including calcium, precipitate the polysaccharide from solution.

2. *Seminatural Anionic Polysaccharides*

a. Cellulose Gum (Sodium Carboxymethylcellulose). The functional characteristics of many natural polysaccharides can be dramatically improved by chemical modification of the native polysaccharide. Cellulose gum, more precisely termed sodium carboxymethylcellulose (CMC), is a chemically altered derivative of cellulose (82–87). Cellulose is a naturally occurring, structural polysaccharide found in all plants (88). It is isolated commercially from cotton linters and also from wood after removal of various other components such as lignin and hemicellulose.

Cellulose (Fig. 20) is composed of one repeating monosaccharide, β-D-(1,4)-glucose (**16**). The β-(1,4)-linkage gives cellulose an extended helical structure (see Fig 5) and, because of the strength of the intermolecular hydrogen bonding, renders the polysaccharide highly crystalline and, consequently, water-insoluble. To make cellulose water-soluble, it is necessary to disrupt the highly ordered cellulose chains. There are many ways to do this, several of which are discussed in the next section. As one example, cellulose, can

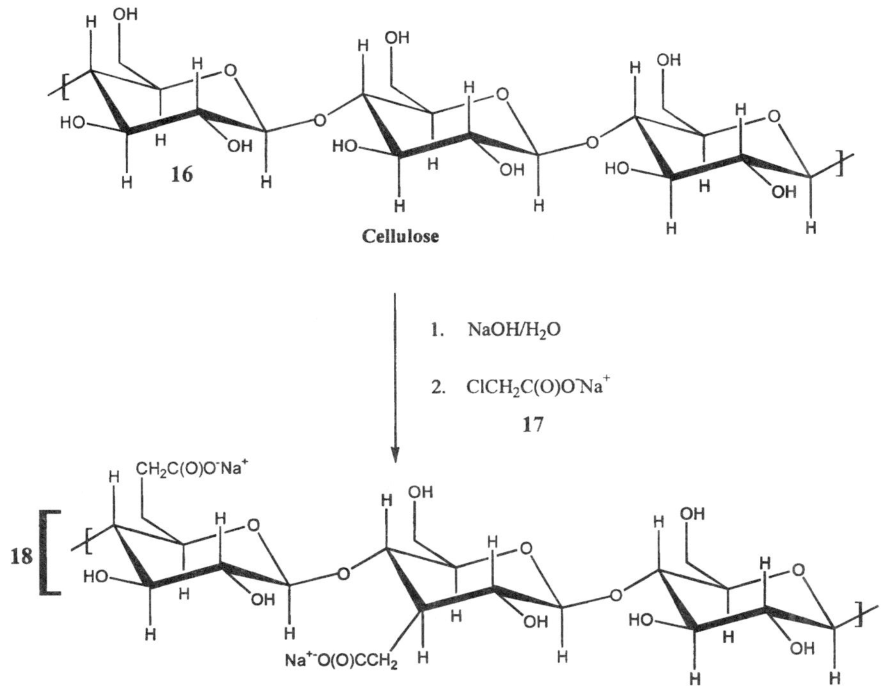

Figure 20 Partial structure and synthesis of cellulose gum, **18**, showing repeating β-D-(1,4)-glucose, **16**, in cellulose backbone.

be derivatized with sodium chloroacetate (**17**) to produce sodium carboxymethylcellulose (**18**).

It is necessary to swell the cellulose fibers prior to treatment with sodium chloroacetate; this is done with aqueous caustic. Sodium chloroacetate reacts with the hydroxyl groups on cellulose, of which theoretically there are three per glucose monosaccharide. The reaction is usually run in aqueous organic diluent in which both the cellulose and the carboxymethylcellulose are swellable, but insoluble. The term ''degree of substitution (DS)'' describes the average number of carboxymethyl groups attached to each glucose monosaccharide.

The presence of the substituted carboxymethyl groups makes the cellulose highly anionic because their acidity is similar to that of acetic acid. Thus, at a pH above 4.5, the majority of acid groups are deprotonated and are in the salt form. The acid groups protonate below pH 4.5, making CMC water-insoluble. The insolubility appears first as an increase in viscosity as chain entanglement increases and phase separation occurs. Eventually, as the CMC continues to phase separate, the solution becomes hazy and precipitation occurs. It has been shown that solutions of CMC as high as 5 wt% are shear-thinning. Even at high gum concentrations, aqueous solutions of CMC do not possess a yield point (Fig. 21). Recently, two studies of the aqueous solution rheology of CMC were conducted (89,90). Cellulose gum also dissolves in and thickens glycerin solutions. Frequently, a small amount of water added to glycerin improves its solubility

Carboxymethylcellulose, like the majority of anionic polysaccharides, strongly binds certain multivalent cations; even small amounts of Ca^{2+} or other multivalent metal ion

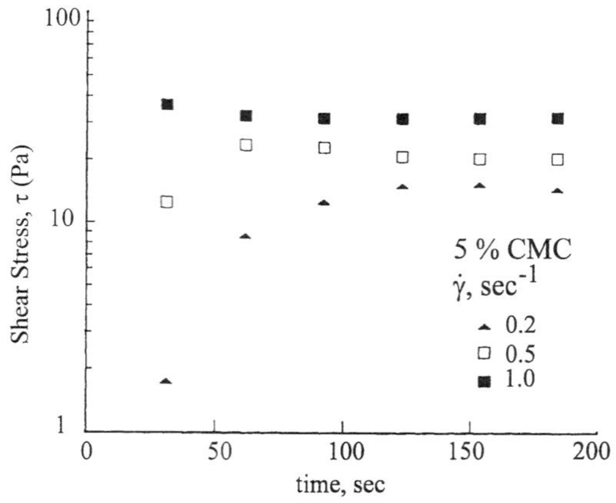

Figure 21 Shear-stress versus time at various constant shear rates for a 5% CMC solution in water: (▲) 0.2 sec; (□) 0.5 sec; (■) 1.0 sec. (Reprinted with permission from Ref. 89.)

cause it to gel. Simple monovalent salts, too, can lower aqueous solution viscosities (90). Carboxymethylcellulose increases solution viscosity through entanglement of its high-molecular-weight chains. It does not rely on the presence of divalent-metal-ion-induced cross-linked junction zones to impart viscosity. Recent investigations suggest that incompletely derivatized CMC forms more viscous aqueous solutions than fully substituted CMC. This suggests that, although the partially substituted CMC is still water-soluble, underivatized crystalline regions form interpolysaccharide junction zones through hydrogen bonding of the pyranose rings.

Carboxymethylcellulose, interestingly, forms association complexes with strongly anionic surfactants; addition of sodium dodecyl sulfate to a solution of dissolved CMC, for example, forms gels. Cationic surfactants, or polyelectrolytes, also have strong ionic interaction with CMC, similar to the behavior of the natural anionic polysaccharides in the presence of cationic species (86). Generally, as the cationic species neutralize the charge of CMC, a polyelectrolyte complex (PEC) appears as a hazy flocculation. Although it may be possible to partially minimize this effect with the addition of other electrolytes, the strength of the anionic/cationic attraction eventually predominates.

While CMC will interact strongly with cationic surfactants, the rheological effects of this interaction are strangely different than the opposite situation where an anionic surfactant is in the presence of a cationic cellulose derivative (90). Figure 22 shows a flat viscosity profile as a cationic surfactant is added to a solution of CMC. At the point of charge neutralization, phase separation occurs. This behavior is quite different from the effect of adding the anionic surfactant, SDS, to a solution of a water-soluble, cationic cellulose ether (Section III.B.2.a). In the presence of cationic surfactants, CMC does not appear to form strong interpolymeric cross-links via the cationic surfactant micelles. Such behavior, as discussed later, is responsible for significant viscosity increases for cationic cellulose derivatives, one example of which is shown in Figure 22.

b. Carboxymethylchitin. Carboxymethylchitin (**20**) (CMCh), is a less widely used anionic polysaccharide that has found greatest acceptance in Japan where it is frequently called ''chitin liquid'' (Fig. 23) (91). It is manufactured by the carboxymethylation of chitin, itself derived from the carapaces of various crustaceans (e.g., shrimp, krill, crab,

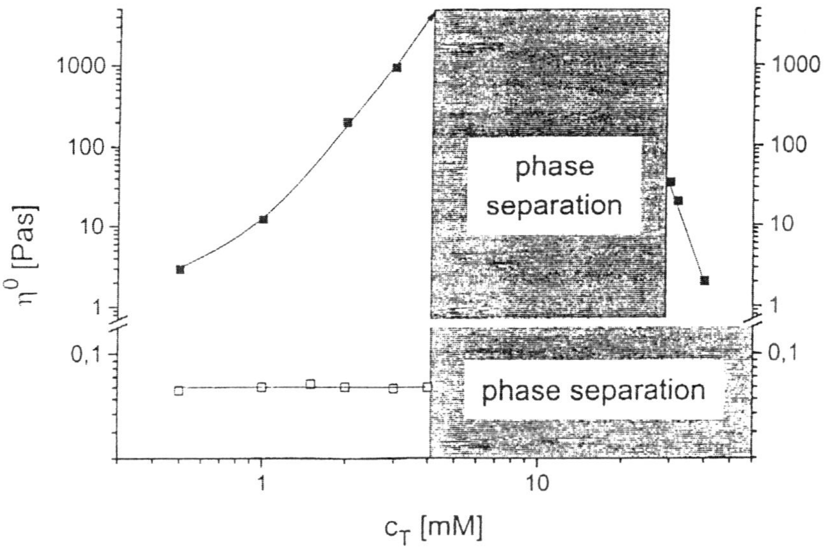

Figure 22 Comparison of the zero-shear viscosities of two polyelectrolytes with the same molecular weight (150,000 g/mol), substitution degree (DS = 0.1), and solution concentration (1 wt%) as a function of the concentration of oppositely charged surfactants: (■) cat-HEC+SDS and (□) Na-CMC, VI+DTAB (pH 4). (Reprinted from Ref. 90 with kind permission of Elsevier Science-NL, Sara Burgerhartstraat 25, 1055 KV Amsterdam, The Netherlands.)

and lobster). Chitin is comprised of one repeating monosaccharide, *N*-acetyl-β-D-(1,4)-glucosamine (**19**), that, like cellulose, can be randomly derivatized by adding sodium chloroacetate at the two available hydroxyl groups. It is important, during swelling and subsequent reaction of the chitin, to minimize alkaline hydrolysis of the acetamide. Such hydrolysis affords a free primary-amine-containing polysaccharide known as chitosan discussed in more detail in Section III.B.1.

Chitin's β-(1,4)-linked *N*-acetylated glucosamines mimic the glycosidic bonding seen in cellulose, and, indeed, these two polysaccharides share many common traits. Chitin is water-insoluble. Because of the extensive intermolecular hydrogen bonding, especially through the acetamide groups, it swells only sparingly and this retards its reactivity. Freezing temperatures are required to minimize the hydrolysis and to rupture the interpolysaccharide bonding, and concentrated caustic is used to swell the chitin fibers prior to derivatization sodium chloroacetate. Carboxymethylchitin, once formed, is quite water-soluble.

The presence of carboxymethyl groups on chitin confers solution behavior similar to that of CMC. The carboxymethyl groups are prone to complex with polyvalent cations, which can cause precipitation of the polysaccharide. Carboxymethylchitin builds viscosity through chain entanglement. Increasing the chain length of its solvated rigid helices increases its aqueous solution viscosities.

3. *Additional Formulating Concerns*

The anionic polysaccharides, though structurally diverse, share some common characteristics. Most of those described above interact strongly with multivalent cations; calcium ion (Ca^{2+}), in particular, binds tightly. This binding can be beneficial, e.g., the gel formation of

19

20

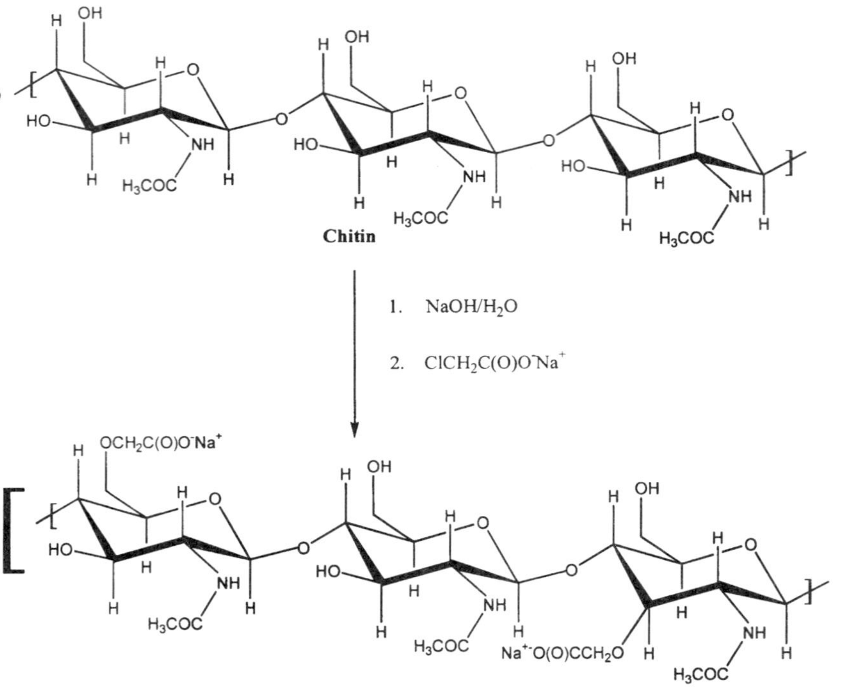

Figure 23 Partial structure and synthesis of carboxymethylchitin, **20**, showing repeating *N*-acetyl-β-D-(1,4)-glucosamine repeating monosaccharides, **19**.

alginic acid and kappa-carrageenan, or deterimental, e.g., the precipitation of carboxymethylcellulose even at low concentrations. Regardless of its effect at low concentrations, the addition of more polyvalent cation will finally precipitate most of these anionic materials. It is common to add sequestrants, like EDTA, to help mitigate the impact of these cations.

Anionic polysaccharides respond in similar fashion to surfactants. They are relatively unaffected by anionic surfactants like sodium or ammonium lauryl sulfate. On the other hand, they form strong ionic complexes with cationic surfactants like dodecyltrimethylammonium chloride, even at cationic surfactant concentrations below the critical micelle concentration (cmc), or concentration at which the surfactant molecules form micelles in solution (92,93). The behavior of polyelectrolytes in the presence of surfactants is summarized in Chapter 5 and has been reviewed (94).

The addition of cationic surfactant to an anionic polysaccharide solution shows its greatest effect near the surfactant cmc. As the surfactant concentration increases beyond the cmc, the polysaccharide may go back into solution or it may form an insoluble complex, flocculate, and settle out of solution. In general, as the polysaccharide's anionic charge increases, so does its interaction with cationic surfactants. As an example, alginic acid binds more strongly to cationic surfactants than carboxymethylcellulose.

The behavior of anionic polysaccharides with nonionic and amphoteric surfactants (betaines) is more complex. For example, nonionic surfactants can form charge transfer complexes with highly charged polysaccharides. Amphoteric surfactants can have various charges and various degrees of interaction with anionic polysaccharides depending on the pH of the solution. These surfactants can be anionic, cationic, or charge neutral (a behavior characteristic also of amphoteric polysaccharides discussed later) depending on the formulation pH. Each species interacts differently with the anionic polysaccharide whose own charge is affected by pH. Unfortunately, there is no rule of thumb to guide the formulator in the use of nonionic and amphoteric surfactants together with anionic polysaccharides; trial and error is often the only recourse.

B. Cationic Polysaccharides

The cationic polysaccharides of cosmetic interest consist primarily of a group of synthetically altered polyglycans. The reason is relatively straightforward: Nature does not stock a variety of polysaccharides containing nitrogen capable of carrying cationic charge. For a polysaccharide to have a cationic charge usually requires synthetic intervention. Chitosan, the one naturally occurring cationic polyglycan, is cationically charged only at pH values below 7.0.

Cationic polysaccharides, however, have a unique advantage: they bind tightly to anionic surfaces. The isoelectric point of the proteins of human skin and hair are near 5.0 and 3.2, respectively. This causes amino acids comprising the proteins of the skin and hair to be negatively charged over the cosmetically useful pH range of 5–8 (71,72,95–99). This is especially true after the skin or hair has been treated by a surfactant, and dyeing and perming further increase the anionic charge of these surfaces. Because of their opposite charge, cationic polysaccharides have been found to be useful as damage control agents, i.e., conditioners. Some cationic polysaccharides, because of their film-forming characteristics, are also finding applications in hair fixative formulations.

Almost any polysaccharide can be made cationic through synthetic manipulation. Only three cationic polyglycans, however, have achieved commercial significance in cosmetics: cationic hydroxyethylcellulose, cationic guar, and cationic hydroxypropylguar. While some cationic polysaccharides have found widespread use in other industries, like cationic starch in paper making, the aesthetic properties of cellulose and guar have given them a role in personal care.

1. Naturally Occurring Cationic Polysaccharides

a. Chitosan. Chitosan is distinct among the cationic polysaccharides: it is the only naturally occurring, commercially available polyglycan that can carry a cationic charge. Chitosan (Fig. 24) (**21**), naturally available in noncommercial quantities from insect exoskeletons and various bacterial parasites, is more practically isolated by alkaline hydrolysis of the acetamide of crustacean chitin (**19**) (Section II.A.2.b) (100). Chitosan is a random copolymer comprised of two monosaccharides, *N*-acetyl-β-D-(1,4)-glucosamine and β-D-(1,4)-glucosamine generally in a 1:4 ratio in commercial materials.

Chitosan is not cationic or water-soluble unless the pH is below 7.0. It is neutralized at these low pH values to the water-soluble chitosonium salt (**22**). Because every free β-D-glucosamine is neutralized to the positively charged ammonium salt at these low pH values, it is strongly cationic. Commercially, the polysaccharide is often found neutralized with a cosmetically functional carboxylic acid such as lactic acid or glycolic acid, both α-hydroxy acids, or 2-pyrrolidone-5-carboxylic acid, a component of the natural moisturizing factor found in skin.

Chitosan, employed as its salt, has strong substantivity to anionic surfaces like skin and hair (101–106). It is also a film-forming polysaccharide that has been used in fixative

19

21

22

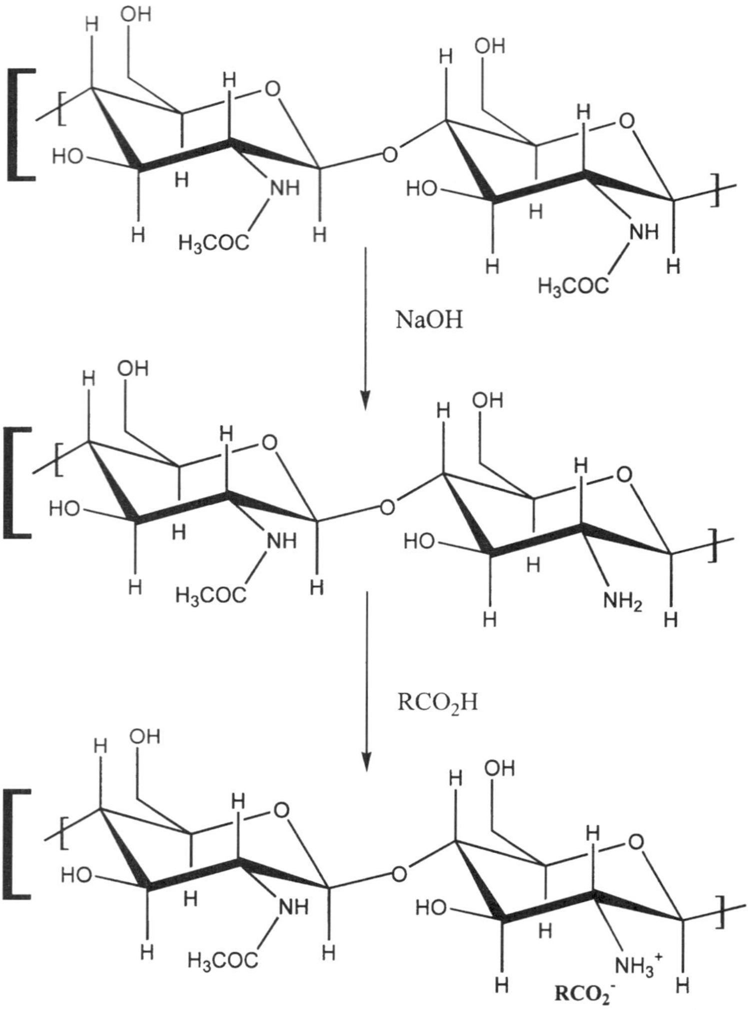

Figure 24 Formation of chitosan, **21**, and chitosan salts, **22**, from native chitin, **19**.

formulations and 2-in-1 shampoos. But because of the extraordinary level of cationic charge on the chitosan backbone, it forms strong water-insoluble associative complexes with most anionic surfactants. It can also complex some polyvalent metal cations, like Cu^{2+}, which are less common in cosmetic formulations. Evidence suggests that chitosan aids in the healing of wounds and damaged skin; this aspect is discussed further in Section III.F.2.

Because chitosan is one of the few naturally occurring cationic polysaccharides, and because of its biocompatibility with the human body, it has been employed extensively in the development of anionic/cationic polysaccharide matrices for drug delivery (107). Such matrices include, for example, combinations of chitosan with xanthan or alginate, which form strong polyelectrolyte ionic gels capable of trapping active materials. Additionally, the strongly cationic polysaccharide has been shown to be mucoadhesive (108).

That is, it will bind to the glycoproteins of moist body tissue such as those lining the eyes and throat.

2. Seminatural Cationic Polysaccharides

a. Cationic Hydroxyethylcellulose. The product that has found its most successful niche as a conditioning polysaccharide is cationic hydroxyethylcellulose (HEC) (109). The structure of cellulose was above in the discussion of cellulose gum (Fig. 20, in Section III.A.2.a), and will be seen again in the discussion of nonionic polysaccharides (Section III.C.2.a). Cellulose is comprised of β-D-(1,4)-glucose monosaccharides and, in its native form, is water-insoluble. Treating cellulose with the reactive alkylating reagent ethylene oxide (**23**) under alkaline conditions produces a water-soluble cellulose derivative known as hydroxyethylcellulose (**24**) (Fig. 25).

Hydroxyethylcellulose is employed extensively in industrial and personal care applications as an aqueous viscosifier. (The personal care applications will be discussed in greater detail in Section III.C.2.a.i.) It is possible to further derivatize HEC with various cationic reagents, for example, **25** or **26** (Fig. 25), which add quaternary charges randomly along the HEC backbone (110). These reactions are usually run in aqueous organic diluents that suspend and swell both the HEC and the cationic HEC products (**27** and **28**) without dissolving either. Although manufacture of **27** is typically conducted using caustic, **28** is made by free-radical polymerization using techniques of emulsion polymerization. Here, the HEC and resulting product are suspended as tiny beads in an organic medium during the grafting reaction. Isolation of the final cationic HEC derivatives is often achieved by centrifugation. Both of these cationic HEC derivatives can be characterized by their cat-

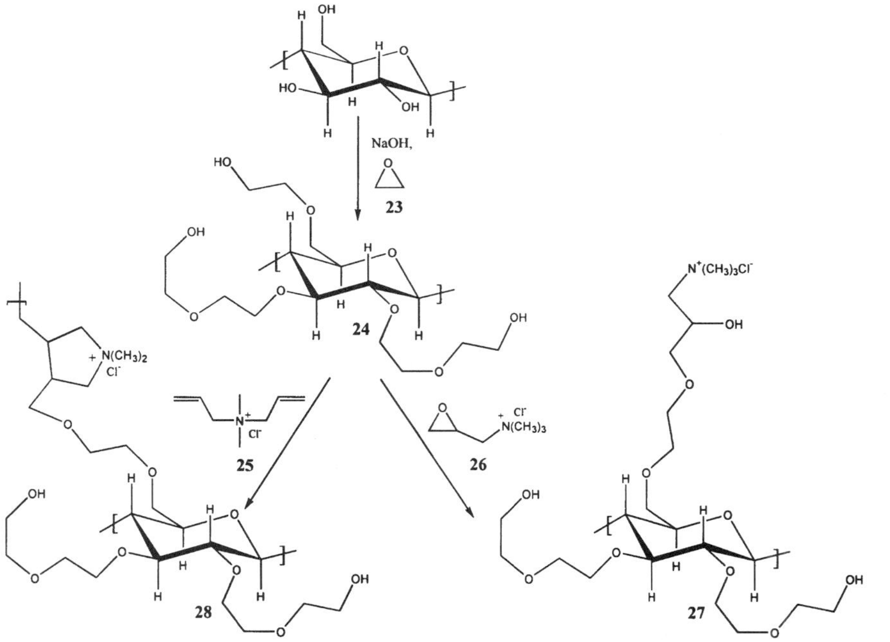

Figure 25 Synthesis of polyquaternium-10, **27**, and polyquaternium-4, **28**, from hydroxyethylcellulose (HEC), **24**.

ionic substitution (CS) level, the molar amount of quaternary nitrogen grafted onto the backbone.

Although both commercially successful cationic HEC derivatives (**27** and **28**) are based on the hydroxyethylcellulose backbone, because of their unique quaternary nitrogen structures, they have found different niches in the personal care industry. Cationic HEC, **27**, more commonly known by its International Nomenclature Cosmetic Ingredient (INCI) name, polyquaternium-10, is used as a conditioner delivered from shampoo and conditioner formulations. The cationic HEC, **28**, known by its INCI name, polyquaternium-4, is found as a conditioning and fixative adjuvant in hair fixative formulations such as mousses.

Most of the scientific investigation into the interaction of cationic HEC with anionic surfaces and surfactants has been carried out and recently reviewed by Goddard (92,101,111,112). It is generally accepted that cationic cellulose-based polysaccharides interact weakly with cationic surfaces and surfactants. However, in the presence of an anionic surface, like hair or skin, or in the presence of an anionic surfactant, the cationic polysaccharides respond vigorously. It has been suggested that the delivery of polyquaternium-10 to bleached, i.e., heavily damaged, hair can be further moderated and its beneficial effects improved when it is combined with high-molecular-weight nonionic cellulose ethers (113).

It was seen that anionic surfactants interact with the positive charge of cationic polysaccharides even at concentrations well below the surfactant's cmc. There is a rapid increase in the viscosity of 1.0 wt% polyquaternium-10 solutions as the anionic surfactant begins to neutralize the charge on the cationic polymer (Fig. 26). As shown earlier (Fig. 22), this solution viscosity response is characteristic of the cationic HEC/anionic surfactant combination and does not appear to occur in the juxtaposed anionic cellulose/cationic surfactant combination.

The viscosifying effect clearly depends on the molecular weight of the cationic HEC, increasing molecular weight affording increased solution viscosity (112). But the viscosifying effect of the polysaccharide/surfactant complex is also concentration dependent; e.g., 0.1 wt% solutions of polyquaternium-10 (in the dilute regime) in the presence of sodium dodecyl sulfate cause viscosity suppression at the point of charge neutralization (Fig. 27) (114). However, regardless of the polymer concentration, the charge-neutralized polymer-surfactant complex is forced to phase-separate (115). Depending on surfactant type, the cationic polysaccharide then either redissolves or precipitates from solution as a complex as the surfactant concentration continues to increase. Independent of polymer concentration, Figures 26 and 27 both indicate that further surfactant addition lowers the viscosity. At high concentration of anionic surfactants, the rheological effects of the cationic polymer are shadowed by the greater viscosity contributions of the surfactant alone.

Polyquaternium-10 has also been shown to be mucoadhesive, implying that it adheres to the proteoglycans of the mouth, eyes, vagina, or nasal cavity. This expands its potential use in formulations such as ocular delivery vehicles or oral therapeutics (116,117).

b. Cationic Guar/Cationic Hydroxypropylguar. Guar gum is a naturally occurring polysaccharide (Fig. 28) that is commercially isolated from the seeds of several leguminous plants (118–120). It is comprised of linear chains of β-D-(1,4)-mannose (**29**), with alternating mannose sugars having branching α-D-(1,6)-galactose units (**30**). Guar is often referred to as a galactomannan because of its constituent monosaccharides. The branching galactose sidechains give the polymer a comb-like structure along the random coils of the

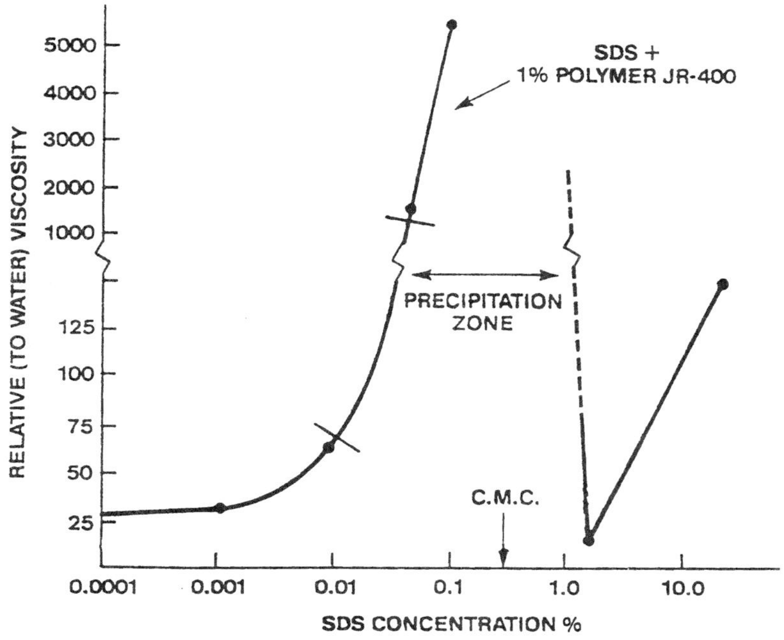

Figure 26 Relative viscosity verses surfactant (SDS) concentration for 1.0 wt% polyquaternium-10. (Reprinted from Leung PS, Goddard ED, Han C, Glinka CJ. A study of polycation-anionic surfactant systems. Colloids Surfaces 1985; 13:47–62, with kind permission of Elsevier Science-NL, Sara Burgerhartstraat 25, 1055 KV Amsterdam, The Netherlands.)

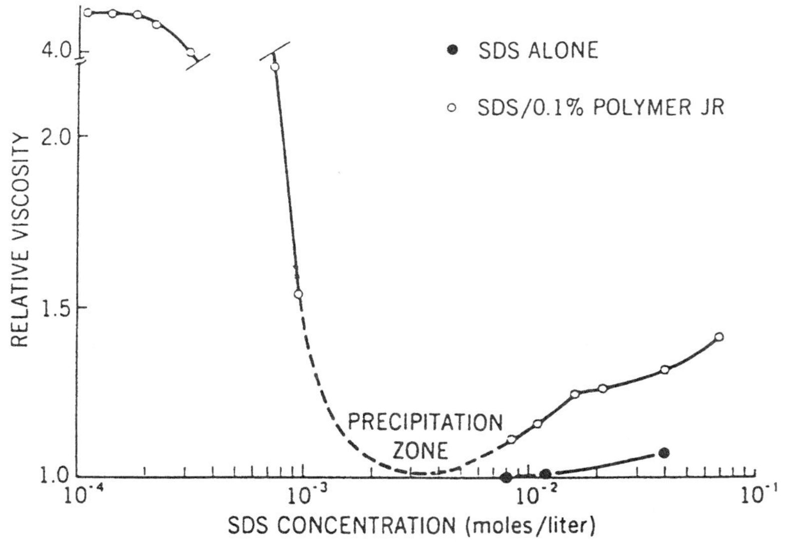

Figure 27 Relative viscosity versus surfactant (SDS) concentration for 0.1 wt% polyquaternium-10. (Reprinted with permission from Ref. 114.)

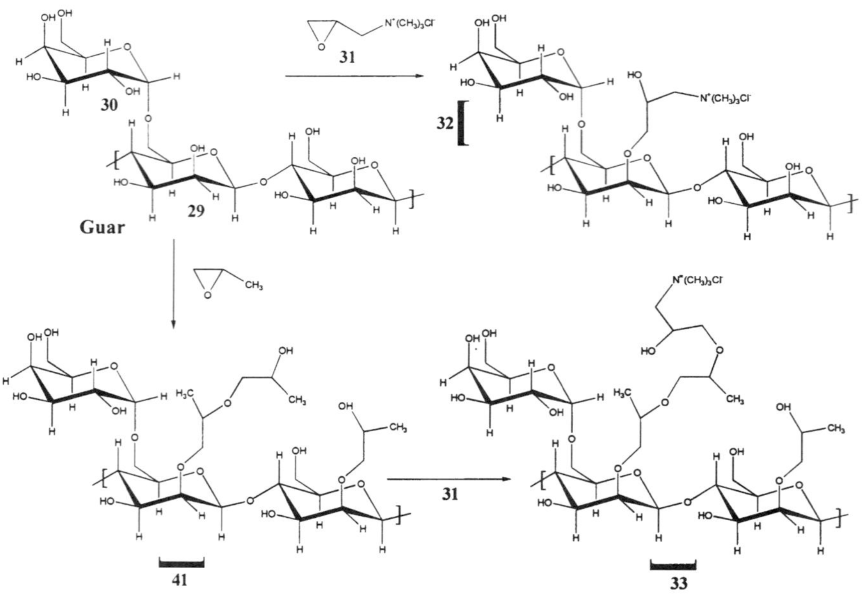

Figure 28 Structure of native guar comprising repeating β-D-(1,4)-mannose, **29**, with alternating α-D-(1,6)-galactose, **30**, sugars and its derivative products, cationic guar, **32**, hydroxypropylguar, **41**, and cationic hydroxypropylguar, **33**.

mannose main chains and are partly responsible for the water solubility of unmodified, native guar. Guar gum is employed extensively in a variety of industrial applications; its use in personal care will be addressed in Section III.C.1.c.

Guar, like HEC, can be cationically modified by alkoxylation with a quaternary epoxide (**31**) to improve its cosmetic characteristics (121). Cationic derivatization of native guar affords an inexpensive, cationic polysaccharide (**32**). One disadvantage is that solutions of cationic guar are normally hazy due to residual lipids and proteins left over from isolation of the gum. Guar manufacturers have found it advantageous, prior to derivatization with the quaternizing reagent, to treat the guar with propylene oxide to give nonionic hydroxypropyl guar (**41**) (Section III.2.C). Such treatments diminish the haziness of quar solutions (122). The resulting cationic hydroxypropylguar, which carries the INCI designation guar hydroxypropyltrimonium chloride (**33**), produces much clearer cosmetic formulations.

Cationic guar and cationic hydroxypropylguar behave comparably to cationic HEC in the presence of other charged materials. Cationic surfactants and surfaces do not interact strongly with cationic guar or cationic HP-guar, but anionic ones interact strongly with both. The behavior of cationic guar mimics to some extent that of cationic HEC in the presence of anionic surfactants: a viscosity maximum occurs near the point of charge neutralization followed by possible precipitation of a coacervate complex at higher surfactant concentrations. Still further increasing surfactant concentrations generally resolubilize the cationic polyglycan. Cationic guar as well as cationic HP-guar are both substantive to anionic surfaces like skin and hair (123–125). Thus, both are well suited as conditioning polysaccharides and widely used in shampoos and conditioners. One of guar's distinctive features is the lubricious feel it lends to cosmetic formulations, particularly in its fully hydrated state.

The *cis*-relationship of the C2 and C3 carbon hydroxyl groups on the mannose rings of guar imparts to the polysaccharide an ability to bind certain metal ions, particularly borate ions. Borate will bind to the mannose hydroxyls to create junction zones similar to those observed when calcium ion is added to a solution of alginic acid (Section III.A.1.a). The resulting aqueous solution experiences pronounced viscosity increases and subsequent gelation. The binding effect is pH-induced, occurs on the alkaline side, and is disrupted on the acid side owing to protonation of the borate salt. If the hydroxyl groups at C2 or C3 are screened, as occurs, for example, from hydroxypropylation and cationization of guar, the gelling effect of boric acid is diminished or eliminated. The gelling action of borate with unmodified guar is discussed further in Section III.C.1.c.

C. Nonionic Polysaccharides

Nonionic polysaccharides, as the name implies, are those polyglycans that do not carry a formal charge. This is not to say, however, that nonionic polysaccharides are not significantly affected by nearby species that can impact their charge characteristics. Thus, changes in solvent polarity, brought about by the addition of salts, surfactants, polymers, and other components, can affect the solution behavior of the nonionic polysaccharides.

Nonionic polysaccharides have found their usefulness in cosmetics as rheology modifiers and thickeners. The seminatural, nonionic polysaccharides, in particular, which include the family of ether-modified cellulose and guar-based materials, are used extensively in personal care. The natural, nonionic polysaccharides, although not as commonly used in personal care, are some of the least expensive thickeners.

1. *Naturally Occurring, Nonionic Polysaccharides*

a. Starch. Next to cellulose, starch is one of the most abundant polysaccharides available for commercial exploitation (126–129). It is an energy-storage polyglycan found in all green plants and is isolated commercially from a variety of crop plants including corn, potato, rice, wheat, and tapioca (other sources being less commercially viable). Production typically involves isolation of a starch ''granule'' from the food plant by some type of milling process. The starch granule must be separated from a host of other plant components, which might include lipids, proteins, and hemicellulose. The isolated granule, which can be thought of as a packet of tightly bound starch molecules, is composed of two basic polysaccharides, amylopectin (**34**) and amylose (**35**) (Fig. 29). Native starches are characterized primarily by the ratio of amylopectin to amylose contained within the starch granule.

Amylopectin is comprised of a central chain of repeating α-D-(1,4)-glucose monosaccharides to which, in a random fashion, α-D-(1,4)-glucose chains are attached through a α-D-(1,6)-glucose linkage. This branching allows amylopectin to grow to enormous molecular weights within the granule, typically greater than 500,000,000 g/mole. Amylose is comprised of repeating α-D-(1,4)-glucose monosaccharides and is, in fact, a diastereomeric allotrope of cellulose. Amylose is much lower in molecular weight than amylopectin, typically on the order of 1,000,000 g/mole. It is a linear polysaccharide that can assume tight helices in solution.

Starch is an inexpensive, nontoxic polyglycan used primarily as a rheology modifier. The thickening effects of starch range from water-thin viscosity to that of a gummy gel. The viscosity is related to the ratio of amylose to amylopectin found in the particular starch used. The higher the ratio of amylose to amylopectin, the greater the thickening

34
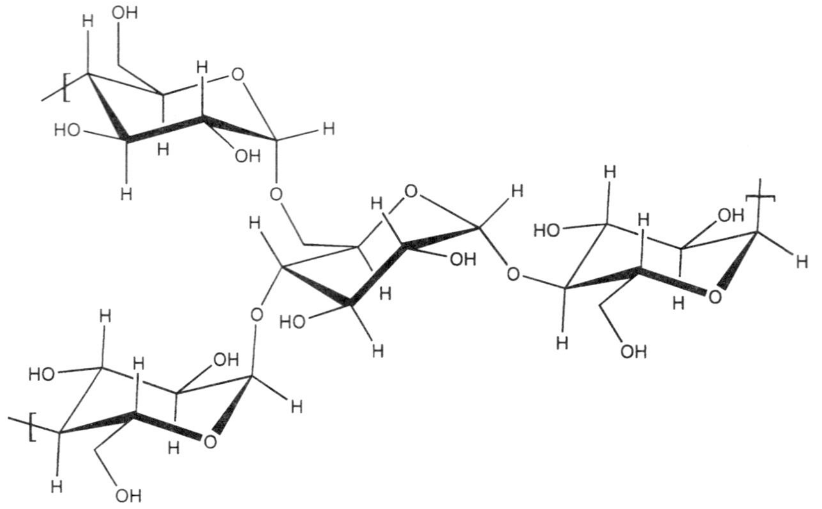

35
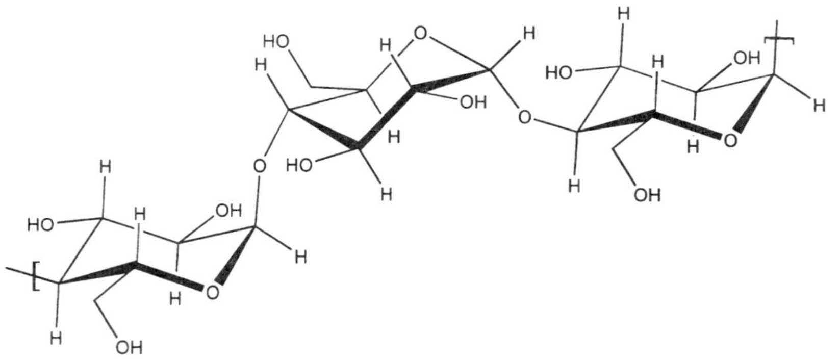

Figure 29 Structure of amylopectin, **34**, and amylose, **35**.

effect from the polysaccharide. This is contrary to the expectation that the amylopectin should have higher solution viscosity because of its enormous molecular weight. But in solution, amylose, which disperses readily in very hot water, unlike its diastereomeric cousin, cellulose, which remains water insoluble, intermolecularly intertwines with itself upon cooling through a process known as ''retrogradation.'' Retrogradation of low-molecular-weight amylose produces very firm gels, and such gels have found applications as noncaloric fat substitutes because of their fat-like properties. The intertwining occurs primarily through hydrogen bonding and can be interrupted by salts and surfactants.

Unfortunately, the same strong hydrogen bonding that causes retrogradation also makes dissolution of amylose into water more difficult. Usually, some type of steam or pressure cooking is required to dissolve it, and manufacturers will frequently supply high-amylose starch as a precooked powder to alleviate some of these difficulties. Its thickening effects can be improved when the starch is combined with inorganic thickeners such as bentonite (130). Solutions of starch tend to be hazy, which limits their effectiveness in clear formulations. This is the result of residual lipids and proteins, which are difficult to remove without unusual and expensive procedures that significantly increase the cost of the starch.

It is well known in the food industry that surfactants inhibit the retrogradation process. The reason for this lies in a well-known property of starch to combine with fatty acid and other materials through complexation of the fatty group inside the helix (131). Whether amylopectin forms complexes in a similar fashion is still being discussed although, generally, it is felt to be true. Formulators using fatty components such as surfactants and emulsifiers must remember this proclivity to complex, which can effectively reduce the concentrations of these surface-active materials. The starch may also complex more critically important components, such as perfumes and actives, if these components are present in the formulation when the starch is uncoiled, i.e., when the formulation is hot.

b. Maltodextrins/Cyclodextrins. Maltodextrins are hydrolysis products isolated by enzymatic or chemical degradation of native starch. Converting starch to a maltodextrin is a simple and inexpensive method to reduce its thickening and speed its hydration characteristics. Solutions containing maltodextrins are clear but have much lower viscosity than that of the parent starch. Maltodextrins have found limited use in personal care.

Cyclodextrins, on the other hand, are used extensively in cosmetic and drug delivery applications (132–136). Cyclodextrins, as the name implies, are cyclic amyloses comprised of 6 (α-), 7 (β-), and 8 (γ-), α-D-(1,4)-glucose monosaccharides (Fig. 30). Their small size classifies them as oligo- instead of polysaccharides, which places them somewhat outside the scope of this chapter. Nevertheless, cyclodextrins are important components in many cosmetic formulations where they function as hosts and solubilizing agents for water-sensitive or water-insoluble materials.

The ring-closed structure of cyclodextrins creates a molecule that looks something like a donut. The interior portion of the cyclodextrin is a lipophilic ("oil-loving") environ-

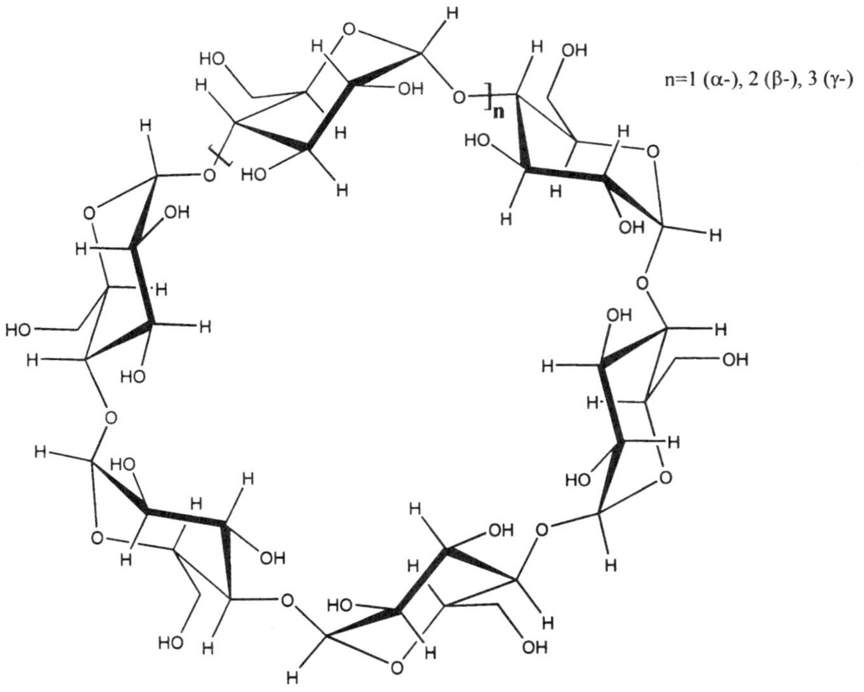

Figure 30 Structure of cyclodextrins: n = 1 (α); n = 2 (β); n = 3.

ment that binds lipophilic materials. If the lipophilic materials are water-insoluble, their complex with a cyclodextrin may render them more water-soluble. The size of the lipophilic moiety must fit the interior diameter of the cyclodextrin, such interior measurements being well established. Because of the preponderance of hydroxyl groups, the exterior of the cyclodextrin is hydrophilic, which makes the cyclodextrins, as a class, water-soluble. Although this is a general rule, some cyclodextrins, such as β-cyclodextin, are only moderately water-soluble and must be chemically modified to improve their solubility.

c. Guar/Locust Bean Gum. Guar, or guaran gum as it is sometimes called, and locust bean gum are energy-storage polysaccharides isolated from the seeds of various bean-growing plants (118–120). These gums, like starch, are isolated by milling processes. Both guar and locust bean gum are composed of β-D-(1,4)-mannose, (**29**) as the backbone monosaccharides from which branching α-D-(1,6)-galactose monosaccharides (**30**) appear intermittently (Fig. 28) (Section III.B.2.b). The ratio of mannose to galactose repeat units varies from approximately 1:2 for guar to 1:3 for locust bean gum depending on the source. The synergistic viscosity enhancement of locust bean gum with xanthan gum was noted earlier (Section III.A.1.d). Commercially, locust bean gum has received limited use in the personal care industry.

Guar has found broader appeal as a natural thickening agent for aqueous compositions (122). Solutions of guar are quite viscous at low solid levels owing to its high molecular weight. A disadvantage is that such solutions tend to be hazy, a result of residual oils and proteins left in the commercially available products. Removal of these residuals requires unusual or extended washing of the raw gums and this increases the cost of the product. One unique and attractive feature of guar solutions is their lubriciousness, or silky feel they bring to formulations.

Guar gum's utility as a rheology control additive is enhanced by its ability to complex multivalent metal ions, particularly borate ions (118). Addition of borate to a solution of guar at alkaline pH forms junction zones between the borate ion and the *cis*-hydroxyl groups at carbons C2 and C3 on the mannose backbone (Fig. 31). The gelation phenomenon is strictly pH dependent and disappears at acidic pH where the borate ion and the mannose hydroxyl groups become protonated.

d. Sclerotium Gum. Sclerotium gum, or scleroglycan, is isolated commercially as an exocellular fermentation product (137). It is comprised of a main chain of β-D-(1,3)-glucose residues to which, on approximately every third glucose, a branching β-D-(1,6)-glucose is attached (Fig. 32). The glucose combinations are like those in cellulose, except the main chain of sclerotium gum is linked β-(1,3), not β-(1,4). The combination of (1,3)-linkages and the branching glucose moieties reduce its crystallinity and increase its solubility compared to cellulose.

Scleroglycan, like xanthan gum (Section III.A.1.d), is capable of stabilizing oil-in-water emulsions even at low gum concentrations. The shear stress versus shear rate relationship of sclerotium gum seen in Figure 33 is similar to that seen in Figure 15 for xanthan gum. Low levels of sclerotium gum generate significant viscosity and the solutions have a yield value. Unlike xanthan, however, scleroglucan does not synergistically thicken in the presence of gluco- or galactomannans. Sclerotium gum solutions are relatively insensitive to heat, pH, and salts, although a combination of low pH and heat will hydrolyze the anhydroglycosidic linkages of the gum. Hydrolysis reduces its suspending ability and solution viscosity. Sclerotium gum, like guaran gum (above), forms gels in the presence

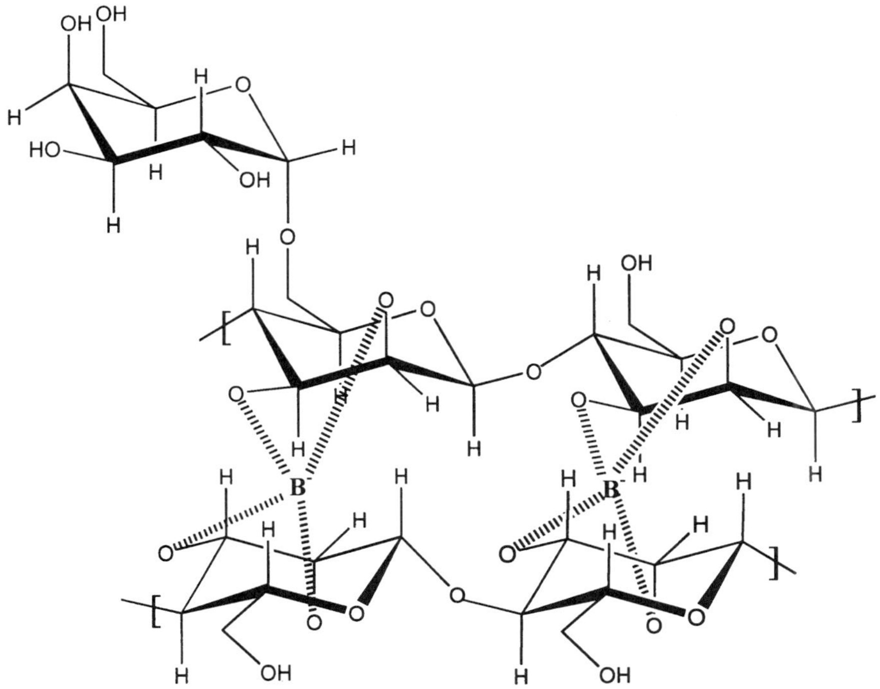

Figure 31 Junction zones occurring between guar and borate ion, B^-.

of borate ions under alkaline conditions. Despite its many benefits, sclerotium gum enjoys only modest use in personal care.

2. *Seminatural, Nonionic Polysaccharides*

a. The Cellulose Ethers. The nonionic cellulose ethers are, perhaps, the most popular and useful rheology control materials employed in the personal care industry (138,139). The reasons for this are many, not the least of which is their history of safe

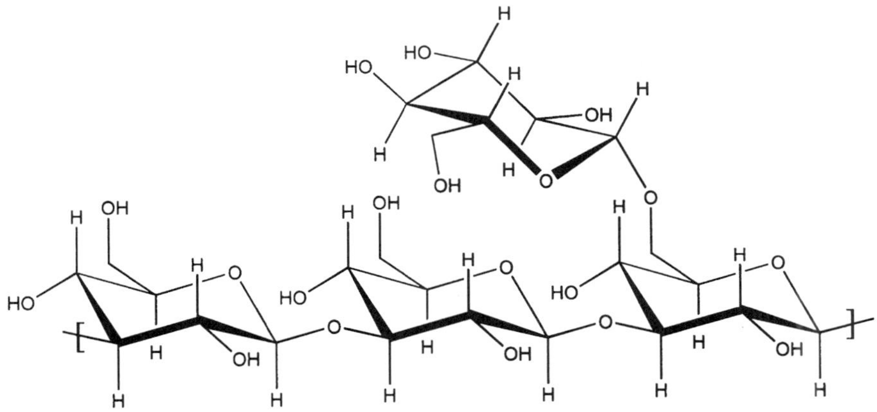

Figure 32 Partial structure of sclerotium gum.

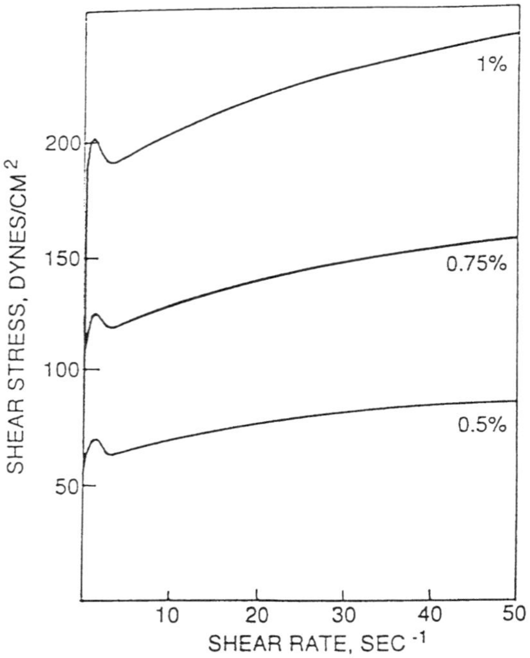

Figure 33 Shear stress versus shear rate for various concentrations of sclerotium gum. (Reprinted with permission from Ref. 137.)

and effective use (140). Personal care is a small segment of the enormous industrial applications in which these ethers are found. Most of the cellulose ethers covered in this section are GRAS for use in cosmetics and several have Food and Drug Administration approval for use in foods and pharmaceuticals. Modification of cellulose through etherification affords a variety of products having diverse and effective solution properties including associative thickening, a topic covered in Section III.E.

It was previously mentioned in the discussion of cellulose gum (Section III.A.2.a) that unmodified cellulose is water-insoluble. While native cellulose can be made to dissolve in cosmetically useless solvents such as dimethyl formamide and strong alkali solutions (where it carries the industrial name ''viscose''), it is necessary to disrupt the highly crystalline packing of the cellulose fibers to make the polysaccharide water-soluble. This can be done by reacting cellulose with various alkylating reagents under alkaline conditions (141). Each repeating β-D-(1,4)-glucose moiety comprising cellulose has three unreacted hydroxyl groups appended to it. Alkylation of these groups weakens the interchain hydrogen bonds within the cellulose. When enough reagent has been attached to the cellulose backbone, the polysaccharide will disperse into water.

The available cellulose ethers are generated from basic cellulose pulp and can be grouped, loosely, into a family tree (Fig. 34). Starting from cellulose, the polysaccharide can be treated with ethylene oxide to give hydroxyethylcellulose (HEC) (**36**), with propylene oxide to give hydroxypropylcellulose (HPC) (**37**), or with methyl chloride to give methylcellulose (MC) (**38**). These cellulose ethers can then be further treated to create new cellulose ethers. Thus, HEC can be treated with an activated ethylating agent to make ethylhydroxyethylcellulose (EHEC) (**39**), and hydroxypropylcellulose can be further

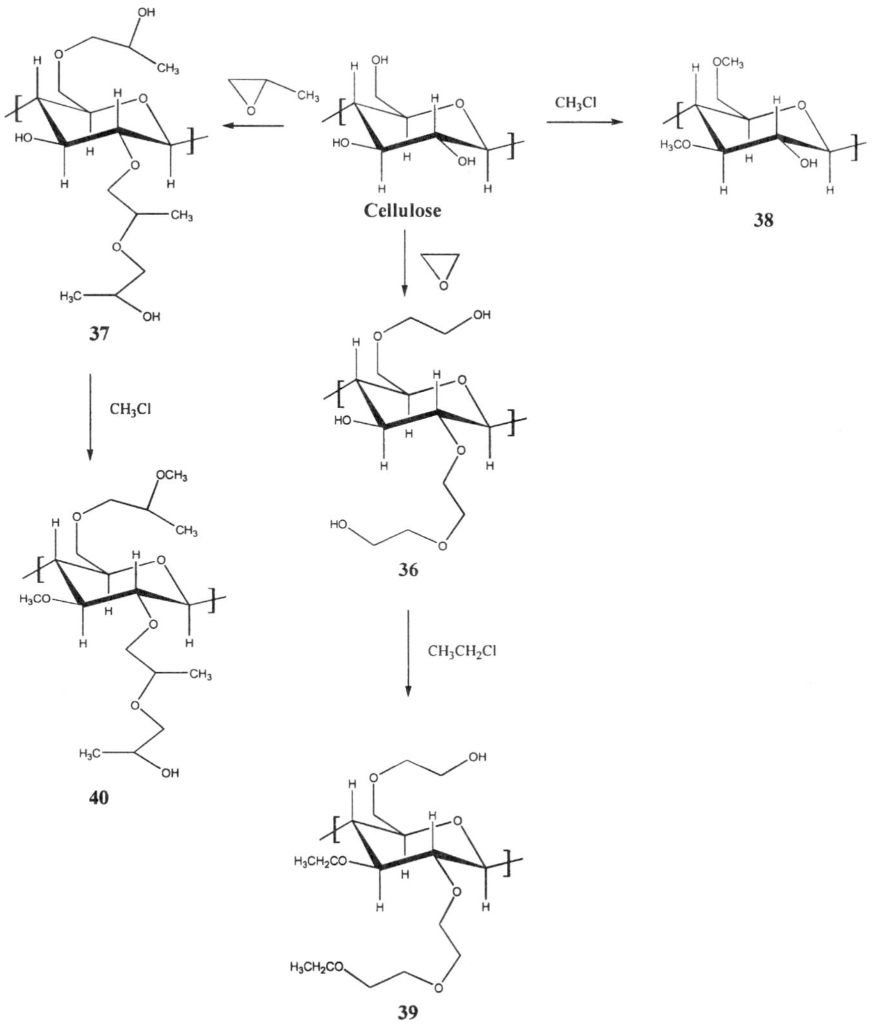

Figure 34 The cellulose ethers: hydroxyethylcellulose, **36**; hydroxypropylcellulose, **37**; methylcellulose, **38**; ethylhydroxyethylcellulose, **39**; and hydroxypropylmethylcellulose, **40**.

treated with methyl chloride to afford hydroxypropylmethylcellulose (HPMC) (**40**). The reaction of cellulose with ethylene or propylene oxide creates an ether group that itself has an additional terminal hydroxyl. Consequently, the term "degree of substitution (DS)" is insufficient to describe the chemistry because the epoxides can react with the terminal ether hydroxyls to form polyether chains. To address this, manufacturers use the term "molar substitution (MS)," the moles of alkylating agent added per mole of anhydroglucose available, to characterize the cellulose ethers.

The cellulose ethers are usually manufactured in batch reactors where a nonsolvent, such as aqueous 2-propanol, acetone, or butanol, swells the cellulose without allowing the resultant cellulose ether to dissolve. The alkylating agents are added and react with hydroxyls on the polysaccharide backbone. The products are then filtered in conventional equipment, washed, and dried.

The cellulose ethers share some common aqueous solution characteristics. Each particular cellulose ether, however, has unique characteristics owing to its unique chemistry. Generally all of the cellulose ethers dissolve in water at room temperature and ambient pressure. They dissolve in aqueous medium by hydration of the high-molecular-weight cellulose backbone, hydration made possible because the ether appendages interrupt interpolysaccharide hydrogen bonding. Essentially, each polysaccharide chain develops a sheath of tightly bound water molecules. This allows the chains to expand, uncoil, and dissolve, and then create the entangled network that builds viscosity (Fig. 35). Influences that change the nature of the hydration sheath, such as solvent polarity or the presence of other polymers or surfactants, affect the solution behavior of these polysaccharides. Salts, for example, increase the solvent polarity, which reduces the solubility of more lipophilic cellulose ethers such as HPC and HPMC. Contrariwise, surfactants can increase the solubility or viscosity of slightly surface-active cellulose ethers, such as HPC and HPMC. The effects, difficult to predict, are best evaluated experimentally.

The solubility of most cellulose ethers decreases as their solution temperature increases. This occurs as increasing thermal energy is imparted to the watery sheath surrounding each chain and increasing numbers of hydrogen bonds between these water molecules and the cellulose chain are broken. As the temperature continues to increase, finally the polysaccharide collapses upon itself and precipitates from solution. The temperature at which a cellulose ether falls out of solution is characteristic of that ether and is known as the cloud point (cp).

The cellulose ethers build significant viscosity at low concentrations, primarily the result of entanglement of the high-molecular-weight, rigid cellulose molecules. Control

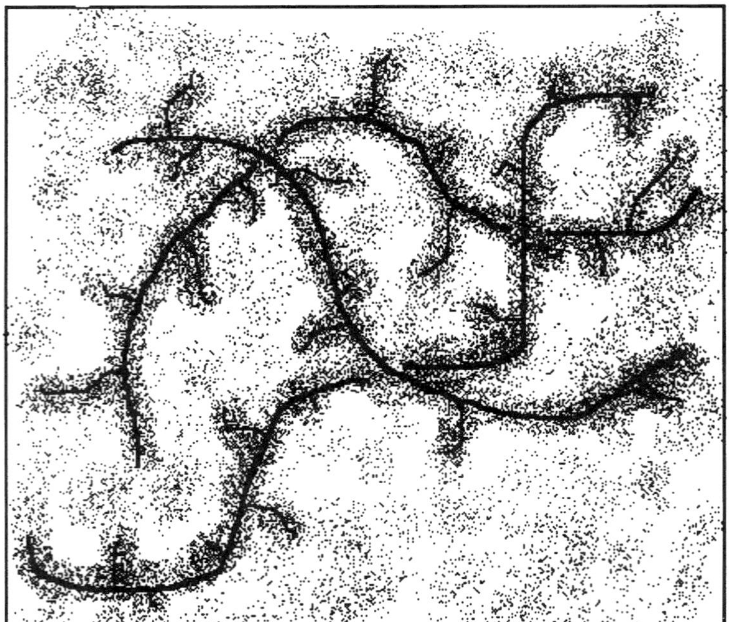

Figure 35 Cellulose ether hydration sheath.

of the viscosity is achieved through selection of the molecular-weight range of the parent cellulose. None of the cellulose ethers can, by itself, act as a suspending agent for water-insoluble materials. The cellulose ethers do not possess yield values. This characteristic is achieved only by blending with other yield stress-imparting materials such as xanthan gum, in the case of polysaccharides.

i. Hydroxyethylcellulose. Hydroxyethylcellulose (**36**) is unique among the cellulose ethers in this section for its lack of a cp, which, at ambient pressure, would be above 100°C (87,142–145). Hydroxyethylcellulose is the most hydrophilic and most widely used cellulose ether. It is not soluble in many cosmetically practical organic solvents including the hydroalcoholic solvents.

The polyethylene oxide chains attached to the cellulose backbone in HEC lack the hydrophobic influences of the pendent methyl groups (—CH_3) present in the methyl (MC, HPMC) ethers, or from the methyl groups of propylene oxide (HPC, HPMC) found in the other cellulose ethers mentioned. As a result, HEC is more tolerant to extremes of pH, salts, and surfactants than the other cellulose ethers. Hydration of HEC can be troublesome because the polysaccharide lacks a cp; this inverse solubility allows the other cellulose ethers to disperse at high temperatures and then rapidly hydrate as the temperature is lowered through the cp. Care must be taken to assure that small, only partially hydrated spheres, or ''fisheyes,'' do not form while HEC solutions are dissolving.

Recently, particularly in Europe, concerns have arisen over the use of ethoxylated products like HEC in personal care formulations (146). The concern is residual ethylene oxide. A recent study, however, suggests that such concerns are unfounded and that exthoxylated products should not cause adverse health effects.

ii. Hydroxypropylcellulose. Hydroxypropylcellulose (**37**) has its cp at about 45°C (87,147–150). Above this temperature, it will not hydrate when added to water; if already dissolved, it will fall out of solution upon heating to 45°C. Hydration of the polysaccharide is best done by adding it to hot water, where it fully disperses, and upon cooling completely dissolves without clumping.

Because of the pendent methyl groups on the propylene oxide side chains, hydroxypropylcellulose is much more lipophilic than HEC. This allows HPC to dissolve in and thicken many organic systems such as ethyl alcohol, aqueous ethyl alcohol, and propylene glycol. Hydroxypropylcellulose is also thermoplastic: it can be melt-processed as films, fibers, and structural components. The methyl groups on HPC can create hydrophobic domains, which help explain why highly concentrated solutions of HPC exhibit liquid crystalline morphology (151).

Certain HPC melts have been found to form thermotropic liquid crystal mesophases. The ordering of this category of liquid crystals is a function of temperature. In lyotropic liquid crystals, the ordering depends on concentration (152,153). Both structural and chemical features drive the organization of lyotropic liquid crystals (154). In aqueous solutions, hydrophilic and lipophilic character in the same molecule can generate such phases. Although this description fits low-molecular-weight surfactants, which, indeed, form lytropic liquid crystals, it also applies to polymers, including polysaccharides like xanthan gum and HPC (52,151,155–157).

As a polysaccharide dissolves into water at the proper concentrations, lipophilic and hydrophilic regions associate with one another into ordered structures. This association can assume a number of ''orientations'' depending on such factors as temperature, polysaccharide concentration, and ionic content of the water (Fig. 36). For HPC, the most preferred is the cholesteric. The onset of liquid crystalline morphology can usually be

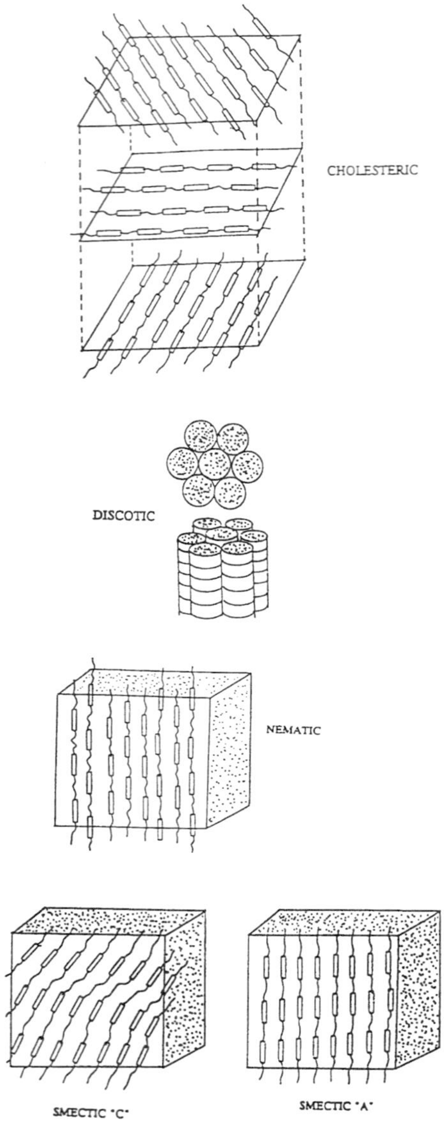

Figure 36 Liquid crystal phase morphologies. □ represents the lipophilic portions of the polysaccharide chain. (Reprinted with permission from Ref. 152.)

observed microscopically; under cross-polarized light the liquid crystalline domains appear as colorful diffraction patterns. Also, the onset of liquid crystallinity may be accompanied by reduced viscosity, which allows the normally viscous polysaccharide solutions to flow.

Surfactants and salts have an influence on aqueous solutions of HPC (158). In solutions of sodium dodecylsulfate and hydroxypropylcellulose, self-association of the surfactant is nucleated by lipophilic domains on the polysaccharide ether, at concentrations well below the critical micelle concentration (Fig. 37), a behavior even more highly pronounced

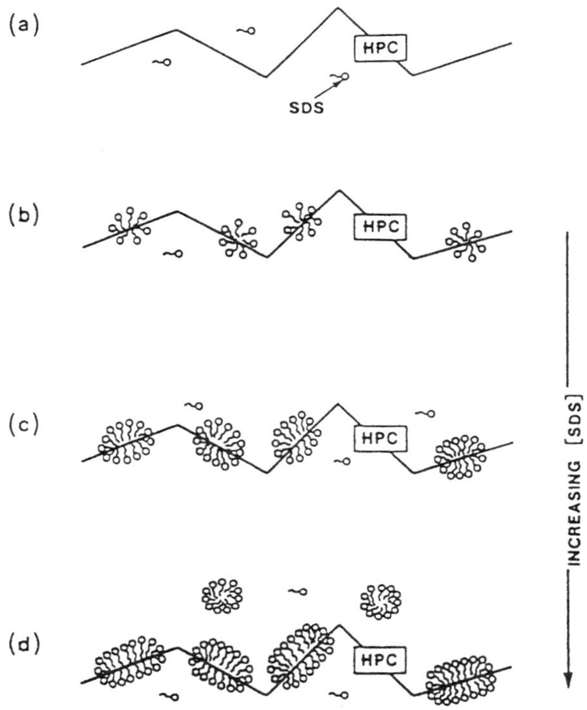

Figure 37 Proposed model of interaction of HPC with increasing concentrations of sodium dodecylsulfate. (Reprinted with permission from Ref. 158.)

in hydrophobically modified cellulose ethers (Section III.E). Increasing salt concentrations cause the polysaccharide hydrophobes to bind to one another, resulting initially in a viscosity increase through interpolysaccharide cross-linking and followed eventually by a viscosity reduction caused by salting out of the cellulose ether. Hydroxypropylcellulose, being nonionic like HEC, is relatively insensitive to pH fluctuations.

iii. Methylcellulose. Methylcellulose (**38**) has a gel point near 45°C and can be hydrated as described above for HPC (159–161). Above 56°C the polysaccharide precipitates from solution as a hazy cloud. Methylcellulose (MC) shares many of the same solution attributes of HPC's chemistry, but because it lacks the hydrophilic polyoxide chains, it tends to be more lipophilic. This enables it to dissolve and thicken a broader range of nonaqueous solvents including ethylene and propylene glycol, glycerin, and some oils.

Methylcellulose is compatible with most surfactant systems; it has been suggested that it enhances surfactant foam strength through a mechanism known as "interfacial gelation" (162). In the warmth of a shower, for example, the MC approaches its gel point and increases the viscosity of the films surrounding bubbles. This slows liquid drainage from bubble walls, making the bubbles and foam more durable. Regardless of the mechanism, MC improves foam generation and strength.

iv. Hydroxypropylmethylcellulose. Hydroxypropylmethylcellulose (**40**) shares most of the characteristics of methylcellulose (159,160,162,163). But the presence of the hydroxypropyl groups affords hydrophilic domains lacking in MC. This allows the HPMC to function better in some systems in which MC shows only marginal success.

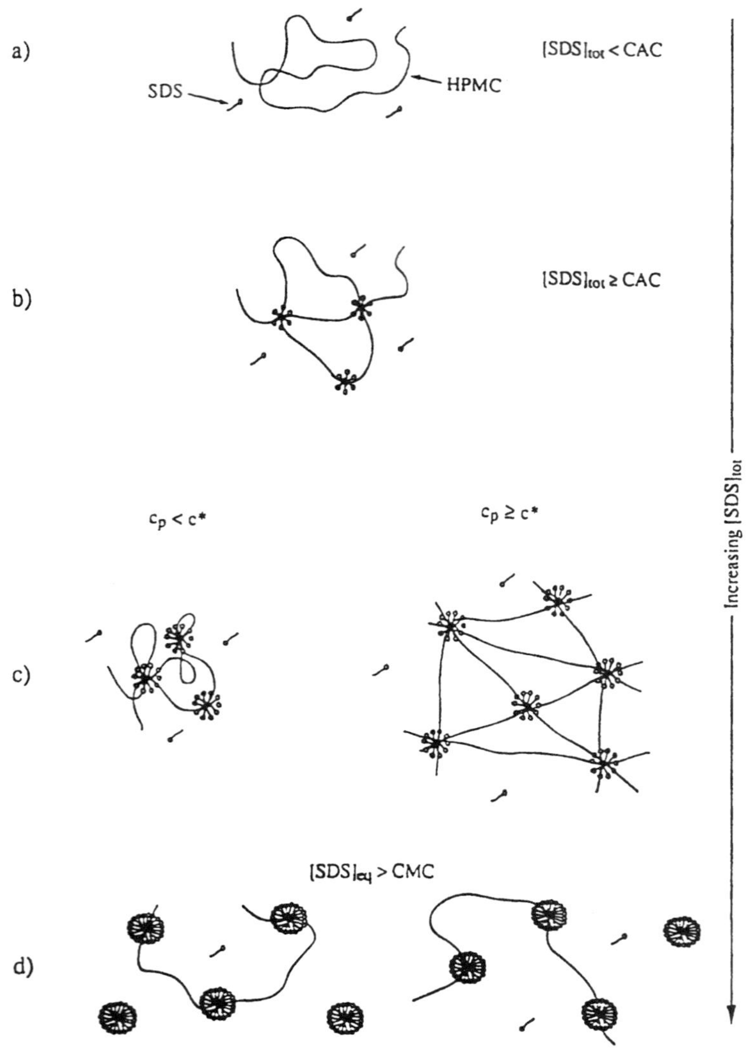

Figure 38 Proposed interaction of HPMC with increasing concentrations of SDS in water where CAC is the critical aggregation concentration, c_p is the concentration of the polysaccharide, c* is the critical overlap concentration for the polysaccharide, and CMC is the critical micelle concentration. (Reprinted with permission from Ref. 163. Copyright 1995 American Chemical Society.)

For combinations of surfactants and HPMC, Figure 38 shows that surfactant micelles create more intermolecular chain entanglement as the concentration of SDS increases than was seen in Figure 37 for SDS and HPC. In Figure 38, entanglement requires the polymer concentration, c_p, to exceed a critical overlap concentration, c* (i.e., the polymer must be in the concentrated regime), or the polysaccharide tends to collapse and the viscosity drops. It is currently felt that at sufficiently high surfactant concentrations, both HPC and HPMC become fully extended and the lipophilic domains become enshrouded in surfactant micelles.

Hydroxypropylmethylcellulose shares characteristic solution properties of both HPC and MC. It has been suggested that HPMC, like MC, enhances surfactant foaming through interfacial gelation (164). Because of its inherent lipophilicity and surface activity HPMC maintains stable oil-in-water emulsions even after heat sterilization (165,166). This provides unique opportunities to prepare sterile creams and lotions for pharmaceutical and dermatological applications.

v. Ethylhydroxyethylcellulose. EHEC (**39**) is included here even though it has limited applications in personal care. The interest in EHEC stems from its ability to gel at temperatures only slightly above 30°C, particularly in the presence of anionic and cationic surfactants (167–169). The hydrophobic domains on EHEC build strong interpolysaccharide cross-links as the polysaccharide solution is warmed. This thermal gelation effect is sensitive to the concentrations of the EHEC and surfactant employed (169). The lipophilic nature of the ether substituents on EHEC all but qualify it as a hydrophobically modified HEC (Section III.E.).

In one application, EHEC plays a role in the delivery of therapeutics to the eye (167). When an EHEC solution with a particular active is administered to the ocular surface, the salts and warmth of the eye cause the polysaccharide solution to thicken or gel. This reduces the cleansing effect of natural tearing and enhances the drug's residence time on the ocular surface.

b. Nitrocellulose. Nitrocellulose is one of the oldest-known modified cellulose derivatives (170). It is manufactured by treating cellulose pulp with a combination of nitric and sulfuric acids. Treatment with this acid combination creates nitrate esters on the cellulose hydroxyl groups (Fig. 39). Levels of commercial nitration are extremely critical because cellulose, nitrated to levels greater than 12% nitrogen, is commercially used as an explosive. Between 11 and 12% nitrogen, cellulose is soluble in various organics including many alcohols, ketones, and aromatic solvents.

Nitrocellulose is an excellent film-forming polymer cast from an organic medium. Rapid drying of the solvent leaves tough, shell-like films that still allow oxygen permeation. This combination of characteristics has made nitrocellulose the premier polymer for use in nail enamels and polishes (171–173).

c. Hydroxypropylguar. Hydroxypropylguar (HP-guar) is a chemically modified derivative of guaran gum, which has already been discussed in detail in Section III.C.1.c. The structure of HP-guar (**41**) is shown in Figure 28 (122). Guar is water-soluble in its native underivatized form. Nevertheless, solutions of guar are typically hazy and pituitous. Guar's exclusive solubility in water constricts its use in cosmetics. Derivatizing guar with propylene oxide yields hydroxypropylguar, which gives much clearer aqueous solutions

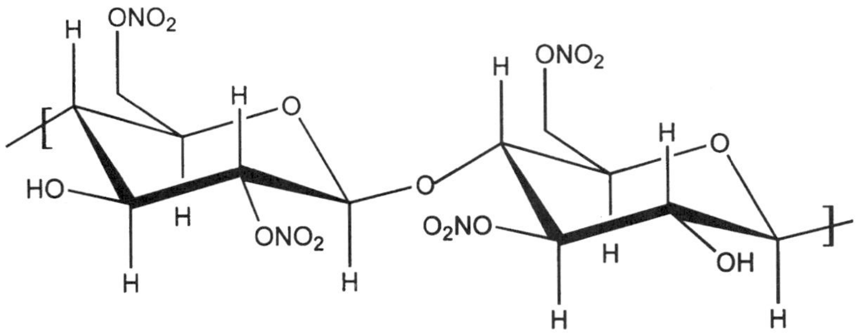

Figure 39 Structure of nitrocellulose.

and allows solubility in a wider range of cosmetic solvents such as aqueous alcoholic solutions.

Guar is hydroxypropylated much like cellulose. The native guar gum is swollen in an aqueous nonsolvent, like aqueous 2-propanol and, under the influence of caustic, is derivatized with propylene oxide. The product is filtered, washed, and dried. Viscosity ranges for the HP-guar are controlled principally by the molecular weight of the native guar.

HP-guar shares many of the solution characteristics of hydroxypropylcellulose. It is readily soluble in water and builds high viscosities at low solids through the mechanism of chain entanglement. HP-guar, like HPC, has a cp near 40°C, which allows easy dispersion in hot water and dissolution in cold. The guar ether is sensitive to salts and surfactants as is HPC. In the presence of either component, the hydrophobic domains of HP-guar associate and build viscosity; more extensive association, if too much salt or surfactant is added, results in precipitation of the HP-guar. Hydroxypropylation of guar minimizes its ability to complex borate ions, making solutions of HP-guar more tolerant to these types of multivalent ions.

D. Amphoteric Polysaccharides

Amphoteric polysaccharides are those polyglycans capable of carrying both cationic and anionic charges on the same chain. The term ''amphoteric'' derives from the Greek *amphoteros*, which means ''both.'' There are very few naturally occurring amphoteric polysaccharides; most of those used cosmetically are seminatural derivatives. Amphoteric polysaccharides are relatively unknown and underutilized in cosmetics although the use of amphoteric surfactants in personal care is quite common.

Amphoteric polysaccharides are, perhaps, the most chemically sophisticated polysaccharides, which may explain the reluctance of formulators to explore them. Depending on the pH of a cosmetic formulation, the amphoteric polysaccharide can be cationic, anionic, or both; i.e., it can be a quasi-nonionic species or zwitterionic (Fig. 40). A zwitterion is a molecular species wherein a proton from the acidic portion of the amphoteric resides on the basic. The resulting molecule has positive and negative charges in close proximity, effectively canceling one another and leaving the polysaccharide nonionic overall.

Amphoteric polysaccharides are challenging to formulate: they can be soluble when cationic or anionic, but insoluble in their zwitterionic form. These polyglycans can also have complex chemistries in the presence of salts and surfactants. Salts can modify the pH at which amphoteric polymers become zwitterionic. Surfactant behavior is more complex. When the amphoteric polymer is cationic, it is incompatible with anionic surfactants

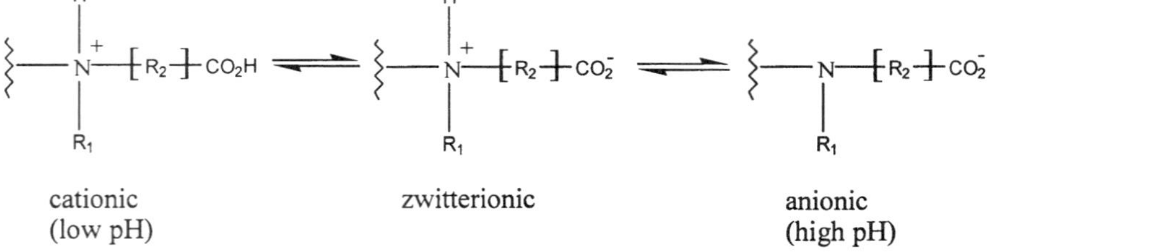

Figure 40 Effect of pH on an amphoteric species.

and polymers; when it is anionic, the opposite is true. The overall pH of the system drives these changes. Unfortunately, there are no rules of thumb for predicting a formula's stability in the presence of an amphoteric polysaccharide. Trial and error typically lights the way to a good formulation.

1. *Carboxymethylchitosan*

The most well-known amphoteric polysaccharide is carboxymethylchitosan (Table 4). The three varieties of carboxymethylated chitosan are *N*-(**42**)-, *O*-(**43**)-, and *N,O*-(**44**)-carboxymethylchitosan. The *N,O*-carboxymethylchitosan is the easiest to manufacture as it is made by the carboxymethylation of chitosan (Section III.B.1.a) using chloroacetic acid, the same reagent used to make cellulose gum (Section III.A.2.a). Under typical reaction conditions, the carboxymethyl group indiscriminately attaches itself either to the chitosan hydroxyls or to the primary amines. The other two derivatives, *N*-carboxymethylchitosan and *O*-carboxymethylchitosan, are more difficult to make, requiring several synthetic and separation steps.

The primary advantage for making chitosan amphoteric is to improve its water solubility. Chitosan is water-soluble only in acidic solutions; forming the amphoteric version allows this unique polysaccharide to dissolve under more alkaline conditions as well. Furthermore, placing anionic charge onto the glucosamine backbone begins to give this relatively inexpensive polysaccharide characteristics of more expensive, cosmetically interesting glycosaminoglycans like hyaluronic acid (Sections III.A.1.e. and III.F.1). Carboxymethylchitosan becomes zwitterionic and water-insoluble at a pH near 4.0. Low pH values, e.g., 1.0, are cosmetically unacceptable, but at these levels the amphoteric polysaccharide becomes cationic and redissolves. The presence or absence of cationic charge is also influenced by the amount of free, unreacted primary amines that remains on the polymer.

2. N-*[(2′-Hydroxy-2′,3′-dicarboxy)ethyl]chitosan*

Chitosan has recently been reported to undergo reaction with anionic epoxides like *cis*-epoxysuccinic acid (**45**) (Fig. 41) (176,177). The resulting amphoteric derivative, *N*-[(2′-hydroxy-2′,3′-dicarboxy)ethyl]chitosan (**46**), can have almost every single free primary amine group covered by a dicarboxylic acid, lower levels of substitution providing greater amounts of free primary amine groups. This places a concentrated level of anionic charge

Table 4 *N*-(**42**), *O*-(**43**), and *N,O*-Carboxymethylchitosan (**44**)

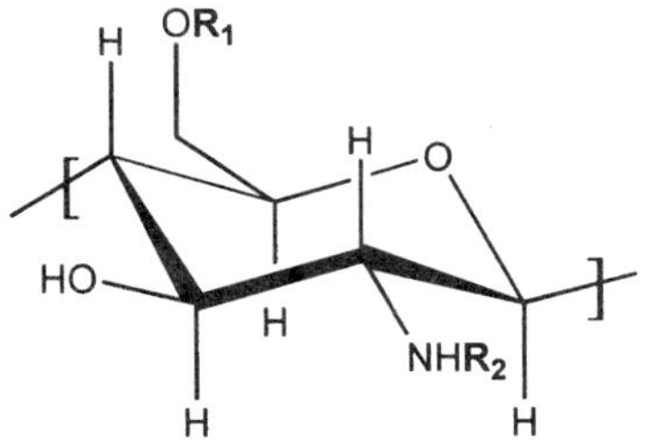

Name	#	R_1	R_2	Ref.
N-Carboxymethylchitosan	**42**	H	CH_2CO_2H	174
O-Carboxymethylchitosan	**43**	CH_2CO_2H	H	91
N,O-Carboxymethylchitosan	**44**	CH_2CO_2H	CH_2CO_2H	175

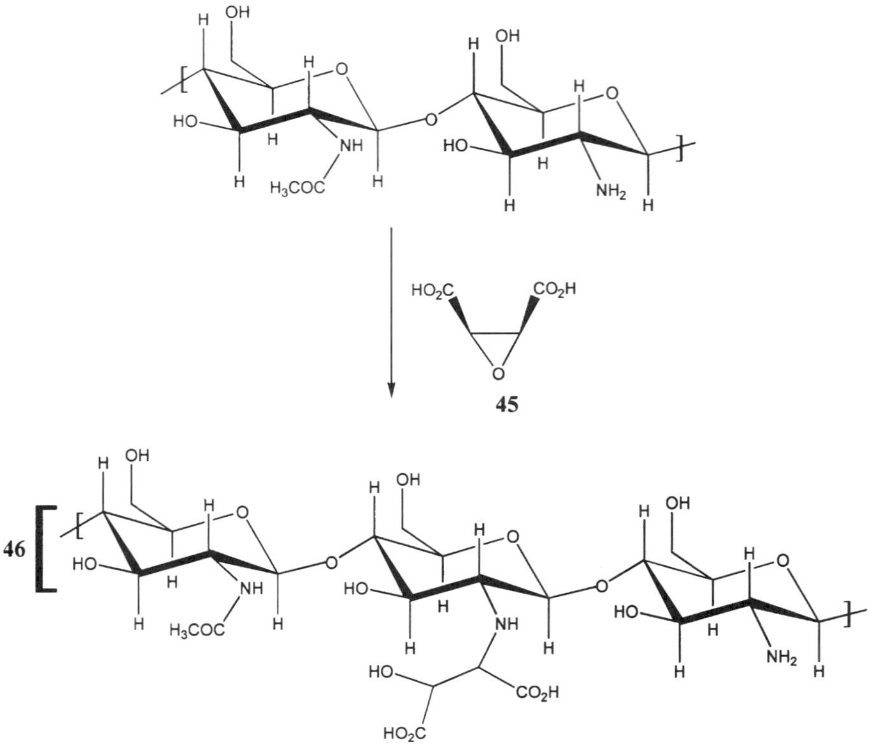

Figure 41 Synthesis of *N*-[(2′-hydroxy-2′,3′-dicarboxy)ethyl]chitosan from chitosan.

onto each glucosamine sugar. The new derivative shares many of the features of carboxymethylchitosan mentioned above. It is water-soluble, particularly at alkaline pH, but precipitates from solution near pH 4.0. The high concentration of anionic charge allows it to behave much like an anionic polysaccharide; like chitosan it gels in the presence of various multivalent cations and cationic polymers. It also shows good stability in the presence of anionic surfactants and anionic polymers, in sharp contrast with underivatized chitosan.

3. Potato Starch, Modified

Recently, an amphoteric polysaccharide derivative of potato starch was introduced (Fig. 42) (178,179). This material is derived from native potato starch (Section III.C.1.a) that has been derivatized with an amphoteric substituent. The starch ether has a high concentration of anionic charge surrounding the tertiary nitrogen, although it is only lightly modified with the amphoteric derivative. Because the level of amphoteric substitution is low, the starch has good solubility over the entire pH range. The amphoteric nature of the starch helps it to stabilize and thicken emulsions where ordinary starch fails. Also, the amphoteric substituent protects the starch backbone when it is exposed to more acidic conditions, circumstances that result in the hydrolysis of unprotected anhydroglucosidic linkages. Most likely the amphoteric ether acts to buffer the starch at these low pH levels.

E. Hydrophobically Modified Polysaccharides

The use of hydrophobically modified polysaccharides is an area of expanding interest in personal care. The term implies that a water-soluble polysaccharide is made less ''water-

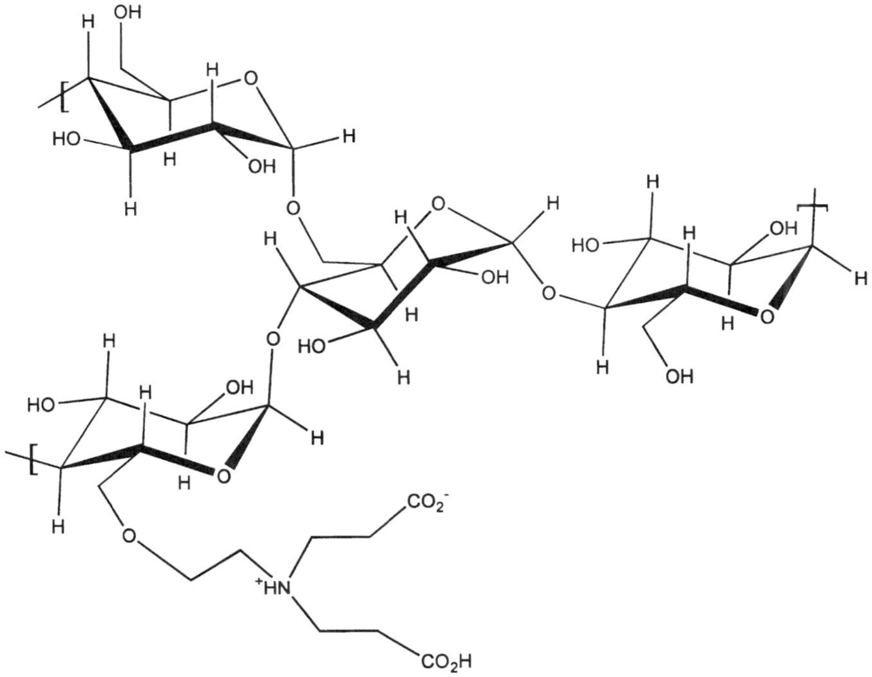

Figure 42 Amphoteric starch.

loving'' by lipophilic modification of the polysaccharide. The attachment of a lipophilic group typically occurs via etherification and causes the polysaccharide to assume new, often unusual solution characteristics.

When a water-soluble polysaccharide, like hydroxyethylcellulose (Section III.C.2.a.i), is dissolved in water, water molecules surround the polysaccharide chains and hydrate them; the water molecules create, in effect, a sheath around them (Fig. 35). This allows the chains to uncoil and expand in solution. The viscosity increases with concentration as chains begin to entangle. At a given concentration (in the absence of additional formulation influences, e.g., surfactants), solution viscosity is controlled primarily by the molecular weight of the polysaccharide. However, when the polysaccharide contains hydrophobic groups, for example, ethylhydroxyethylcellulose (Section III.C.2.a.v), its lipophilic moieties are thermodynamically uncomfortable in the aqueous medium. The affect of the water structure on these lipophilic species is entropy-driven and is termed the ''hydrophobe effect'' (180). Changes in the molecular structure of the water molecules near the hydrophobes and the development of molecular cavities in the water structure force the hydrophobic groups to congregate and form labile, noncovalent cross-links between the polyglycan chains. These cross-links have a profound influence on the solution behavior, particularly the viscosity.

Recent developments have led to improved types of hydrophobically modified polysaccharide ethers. In general, these are water-soluble polysaccharides modified with a long-chain, fatty alkyl group. The fatty group is introduced either through an alkyl epoxide, which generates a nonionic hydrophobe, or through a hydrophobically modified, cationic epoxide, which produces a cationic hydrophobe. Both are described below. Although each of these modifications confers unique properties, the principal effects of the hydrophobe are the same for both.

1. Cetyl and Nonoxyphenyl Hydroxyethylcellulose

Hydroxyethylcellulose (**36**) can be graft-modified with long-chain fatty alkyl epoxides, for example 1,2-cetyleneoxide (**47**), or with nonylphenol (**48**), to produce the corresponding HM-HECs (**49** and **50**), respectively, in Figure 43 (181–183). Like most etherification reactions that occur on HEC, the chemistry is usually carried out under alkaline conditions

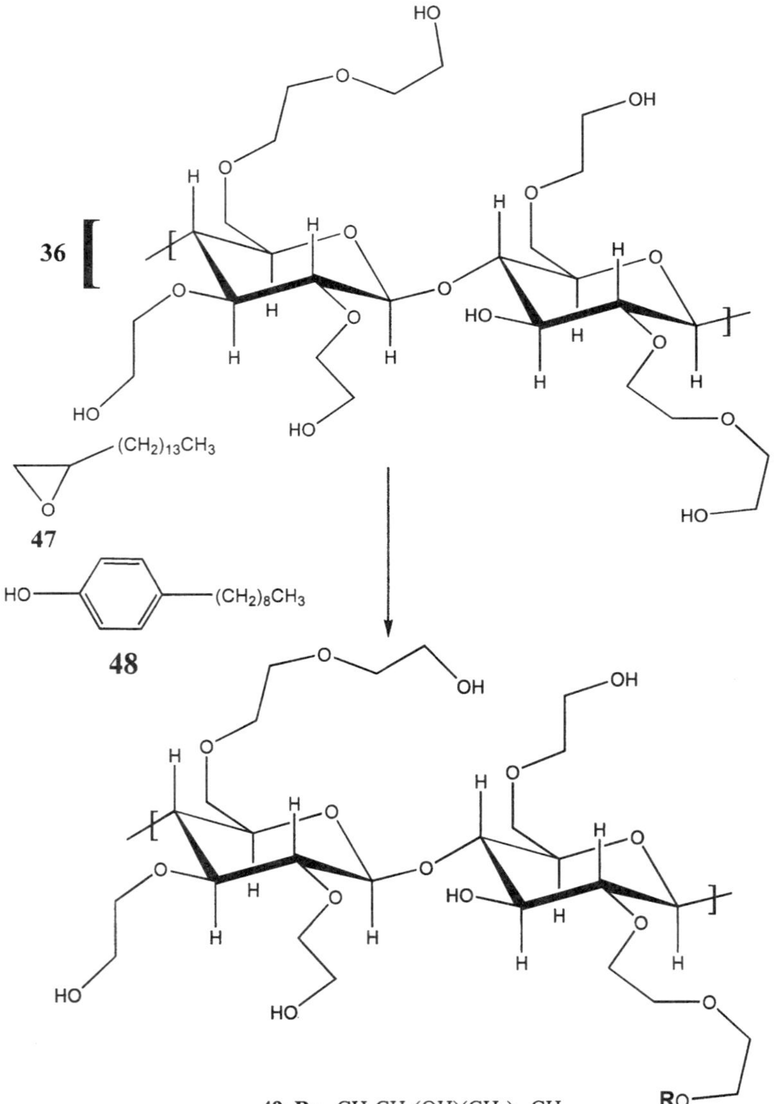

49, R= $-CH_2CH_2(OH)(CH_2)_{13}CH_3$

50, R= $-C_6H_4(CH_2)_8CH_3$

Figure 43 Synthesis of various hydrophobically modified hydroxyethylcelluloses (HM-HECs).

using a solvent that swells the HEC but does not dissolve either the HEC or the resulting HM-HEC. Aqueous alcohols or aqueous ketones are often employed in the manufacture of these HEC ethers. The percentage of hydrophobic substitution is relatively low because only small amounts of hydrophobe render HM-HEC water-insoluble. Recent concerns have occurred regarding the use of nonylphenols in personal care owing to their potential to mimic human estrogen. Because of this, the use of HM-HECs like **50** is suffering and will probably soon be discontinued.

The dissolution of HM-HEC in water is coordinate with hydration and expansion of the cellulose backbone as described above. The ''hydrophobic effect'' results in the formation of ''pseudo-micelles'' along the polysaccharide chain. These pockets of concentrated hydrophobe diminish the internal energy of the polysaccharide, stabilizing the presence of the hydrophobes in the water. These transient cross-links build viscosity and impart a yield value to the solution; whereas normal HEC solutions cannot suspend water-insoluble oils, HM-HEC solutions can.

It has been demonstrated that surfactants are attracted to the hydrophobic sites of HM-HEC at levels well below the surfactants' cmc (183). The concentration of surfactant at which these molecules begin to associate at HEC hydrophobes is the critical aggregation concentration (cac). When the surfactant concentration is low, it is content to reside near the hydrophobic sites of the polysaccharide. Increasing the surfactant concentration toward the cmc is accompanied by increasing viscosity, the result of stronger interpolysaccharide cross-linking stabilized by the surfactant (184,185). When the cmc is reached, polysaccharide hydrophobes intimately incorporate into surfactant micelles to produce a highly cross-linked network (Fig. 44). The viscosity normally peaks at the surfactant cmc. Increased viscosity results from phase separation of the polymer/surfactant complex, and usually manifests itself by increased haziness of the solution. As more surfactant is added and the micelle density increases, each hydrophobe eventually acquires its own micelle, cross-linking diminishes, and the viscosity drops. Frequently, the HM-HEC/surfactant complex disrupts, and the solution becomes homogeneous again. At even higher surfactant levels, the effects of the surfactant overshadow the polysaccharide contribution and viscosity is determined by the surfactant's micellar morphology.

2. *Polyquaternium-24*

Hydroxyethylcellulose (**36**), made both cationic and hydrophobic, is called polyquaternium-24 (PQ-24) (**52**) (Fig. 45) (101,110,186). Reaction of HEC with a dodecyl-modified quaternary epoxide (**51**) produces a hydrophobically modified material in which the hydrophobic group binds directly to the cationic site.

The cationic charge on PQ-24 makes the polysaccharide substantive to anionic surfaces (101,187). In addition, the hydrophobic chains give PQ-24 some of the characteristics of HM-HEC. In the presence of strongly anionic surfactants, PQ-24 builds viscosity through interpolymeric cross-linking via surfactant micelles. Eventually, as the surfactant begins to neutralize the polysaccharide's cationic charge, an insoluble polysaccharide/surfactant coacervate precipitates. In the presence of anionic surfactants, the rheology behavior is clearly reminiscent of that described above for the HM-HECs (Fig. 44). Considerable effort has been expended trying to understand the effect that both cationic charge and hydrophobic modification have on the behavior of PQ-24 in the presence of both cationic and anionic surfactants (185,188–190).

As mentioned above, the cationic charge of PQ-24 causes it to behave like a standard polyelectrolytic in solution; therefore, the addition of anionic polymers to PQ-24 solutions

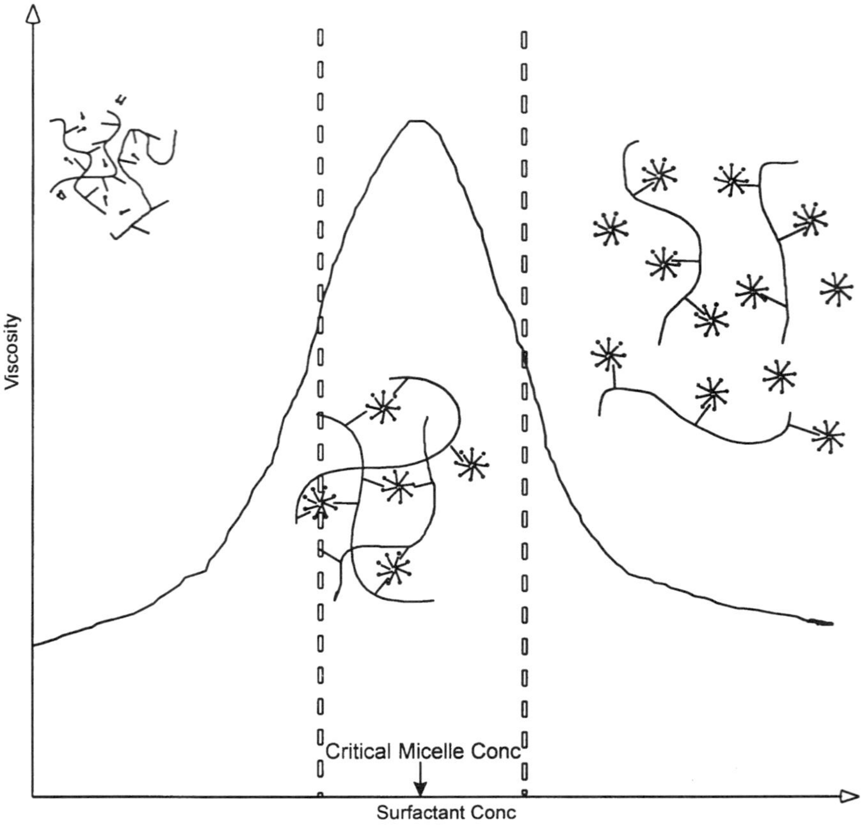

Figure 44 Effect of increasing surfactant concentration on HMHEC solution viscosity.

produces a water-insoluble polyelectrolyte complex. It has been suggested, however, that if the anionic polyelectrolyte is also hydrophobically modified, the tendency toward formation of this precipitate can be moderated (191). It is proposed that interaction of the hydrophobes creates enough separation of the charges to prevent precipitation of the complex. This may be useful in the development of conditioning/fixative gels and sprays.

A unique and useful complex of PQ-24 and hyaluronic acid (Sections III.A.1.e and III.F.1) has been described (74,192). The strong ionic interaction of anionic hyaluronic acid and cationic PQ-24 is tempered by the hydrophobic groups allowing stable solutions containing both components. The PQ-24 aids in delivering the hyaluronic acid, anchors the expensive anionic polysaccharide to the skin, and takes greater advantage of its beneficial effects before the polysaccharide is washed off the skin.

It has also been demonstrated that the presence of the cationic hydrophobe may afford a unique blending synergy with amylose, the linear component of ordinary starch (Section III.C.1.a) (193). The combination of these two natural polymers imparts improved yield stress to solutions of PQ-24, which allows them to better suspend water-insoluble oils. It has been proposed that the polymer blend is a mixture in which the amylose, because of its ability to encase fatty alkyl groups, forms a three-dimensional network by tying hydrophobic groups of the PQ-24 together (Fig. 46). The ability of solutions of the blend

36

52

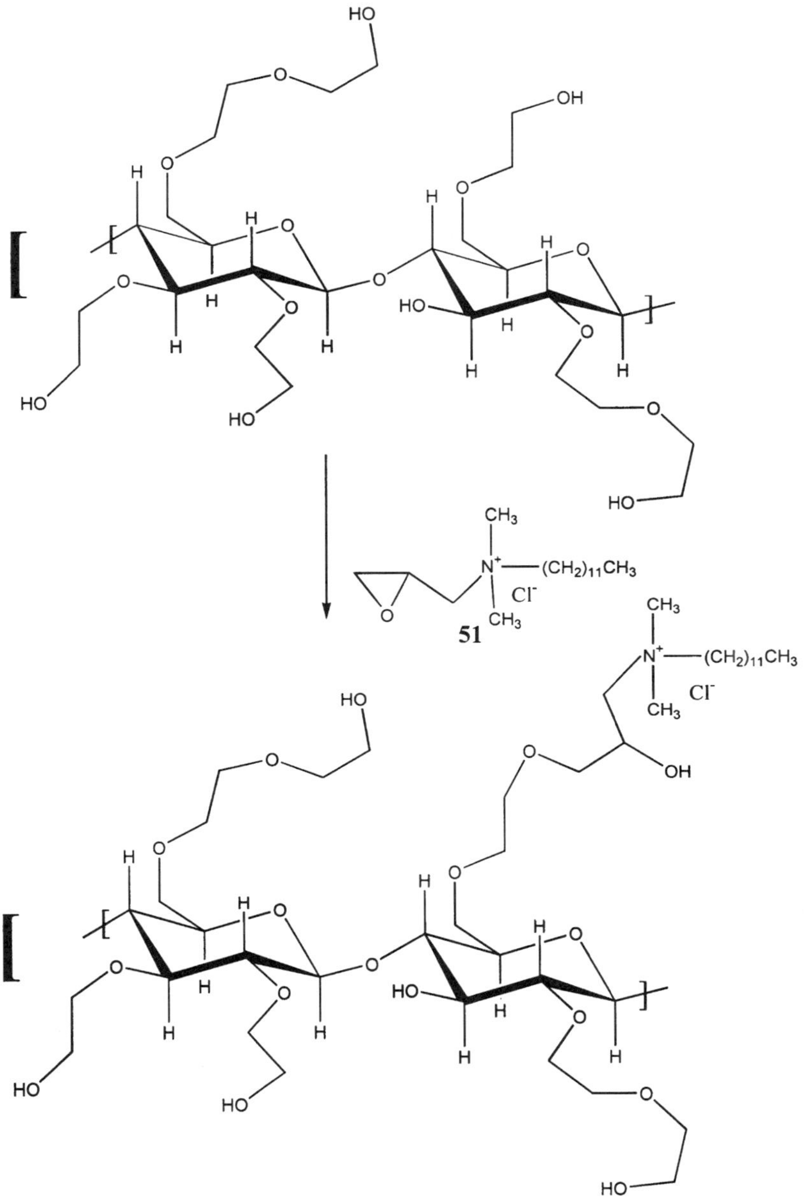

Figure 45 Synthesis of polyquaternium-24.

to stabilize emulsions may allow emulsifier-free formulations in which the conditioning polymer also serves as the primary viscosifier.

F. Polysaccharides with Topical Physiological Effects

The human body is composed of many polymeric components including, for example, polypeptides, proteoglycans, and polysaccharides. Many polysaccharides, when ingested

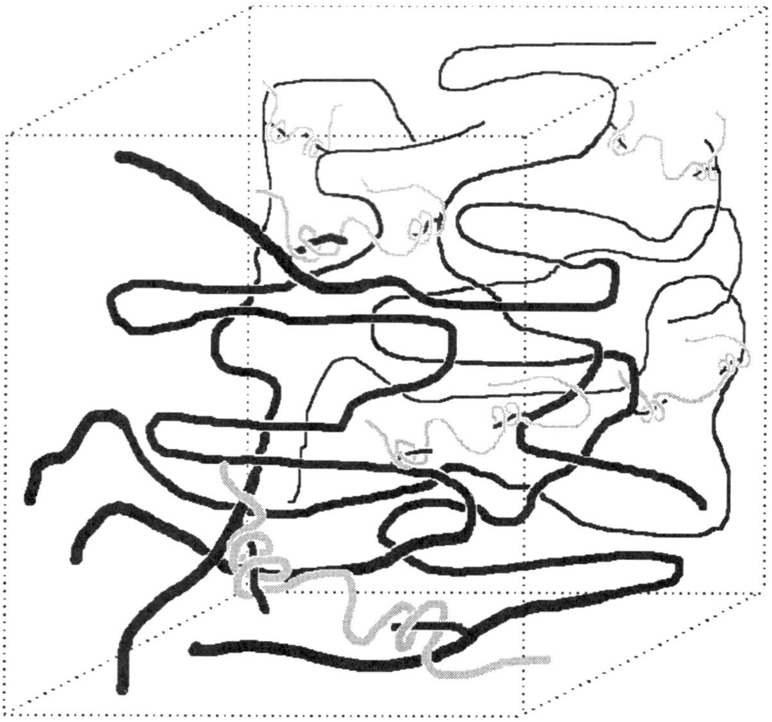

Figure 46 Three-dimensional polysaccharide network formed between polyquaternium-24 and amylose.

into the body, have a physiological effect. Ingested starch (Section III.C.1.a), for instance, is converted to glucose, which the body then uses for energy. Conversely, starch applied topically to the skin remains there and provides no benefit. The skin and, to a much lesser extent, hair cannot digest topically applied starch.

Nevertheless, the skin is a biochemically active organ. Old cells on the surface epidermis continually slough off and are replaced by new cells rising from the dermis below (194). When the skin is assaulted, as occurs from injury or irritation, the body responds rapidly through the process of healing, which is only partially understood (195). During healing, the presence of several polysaccharides applied to the wound can have a beneficial effect by reducing the time and nature of the healing process. Some of these polysaccharides are discussed below.

The use of these physiologically active materials borders on therapeutic or medicinal practice. In this capacity, their usage may or may not attract the attention of regulatory agencies such as the Food and Drug Administration. Regardless of these eventualities, the materials discussed below are considered safe for topical use.

1. Hyaluronic Acid

Hyaluronic acid (HA), discussed in detail in Section III.A.1.e, is a component of human skin that occurs in the interstitial fluids of the epidermis and, because of its water-absorbing capacity, lends turgidity, viscolasticity, and firmness to the skin. Changes in HA concentrations have been noted in skin as the body ages (196). In aging skin free of chronic sun

53

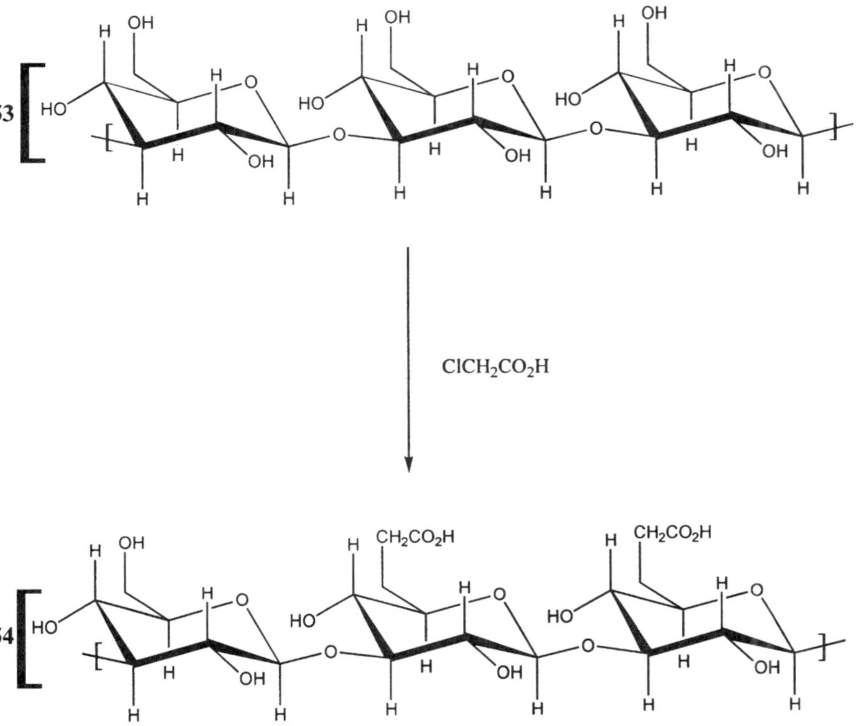

54

Figure 47 Structure of β-(1,3)-glucan, **53**, and carboxymethyl β-(1,3)-glucan, **54**.

damages or photodamage, the concentration of HA gradually diminishes. In contrast, heavily photodamaged skin maintains relatively high concentrations of HA as the skin ages. This may be the body's attempt to respond to the photo-induced loss of collagen and elastin, proteins that give skin its structure and that are not readily replaced in aging, damaged skin.

When the skin is wounded, the body counters with a cascade of biological responses. It has been demonstrated, for example, that when fetal tissue is injured, the wound is rich in hyaluronic acid and tends to heal without scarring (197). On the other hand, wounds in adult skin have lower levels of HA and scarring is more pronounced. Topical application of HA to wounded skin minimizes scarring and improves the healing process, although some controversy exists (65,198). The ability of HA to enhance wound repair must arise from its interaction with the biochemical healing cascade. Exactly how HA fits into this process is still being discussed, but the preponderance of evidence verifies its effectiveness.

2. Chitin and Chitosan

Chitin (Section III.A.2.b) and chitosan (Section III.B.1.a) are not naturally found in human skin. Their presence on the skin during wound healing, however, speeds healing and minimizes scarring (189). Both chitin and chitosan are slowly digested by lipases, enzymes present in the body used to digest triacylglycerols. It is not surprising that chitin and chitosan are immunopotentiating considering their similarities with hyaluronic acid through the common *N*-acetylglucosamine sugar. This sugar is common in the body's chemistry, especially in the many glycosaminoglycans and proteoglycans in body cells and fluids.

3. Beta(β)-(1,3)-Glucan

Beta(β)-(1,3)-glucan (**53**) is a natural polysaccharide comprised of β-(1,3)-glucose-repeating monosaccharides (Fig. 47) (200,201). It is obtained from yeast fermentation extracts that have been used topically for years to improve the skin's health. Beta-glucan stimulates the immune system and helps to heal wounded or irritated skin (202).

Beta-glucan is not water-soluble, and although it stimulates significant immunological response when applied as a solid, this form of delivery is not attractive from a cosmetic perspective. To improve it, the water solubility characteristics have been enhanced by carboxymethylating native β-glucan (**54**) (1,203–205). This modification does not appear to hamper the immune response and definitely improves the polysaccharide's personal care utility.

ACKNOWLEDGMENTS

The author is indebted to Mike Philbin, David Donabedian, Ray Rigoletto, Carmella Barbeito, and Jim Hatfield for their careful review of the manuscript and to Cathy Misner and her group for their help in locating literature references. In addition, the author would especially like to thank Freida Debaro for her help in preparing the manuscript.

REFERENCES

1. Zulli F, Suter F, Biltz H, Nissen HP, Birman M. Carboxymethylated β-(1,3)-glucan. Cosmet Toilet 1996; 111:91–96.
2. Guillot JP, Giauffret JY, Martini MC, Gonnet JF, Soule G. Safety evaluation of gums and thickeners used in cosmetic formulations. Int J Cosmet Sci 1982; 4:53–66.
3. Nicolaou KC, Winssinger N, Pastor J, DeRoose F. A general and highly efficient solid phase synthesis of oligosaccharides. Total synthesis of a heptasaccharide phytoalexin elicitor (HPE). J Am Chem Soc 1997; 119:449–450.
4. Rees DA, Morris ER, Thom D. Madden JK. Shapes and interactions of carbohydrate chains. In: Aspinall GO, ed. The Polysaccharides, Vol 1. New York: Academic Press, 1982:195–290.
5. Hoffman D. A new turn for Archimedes. Nature 1996; 384:28–29.
6. Mimura M, Urakawa H, Kajiwara K. Gelation and its relevance to the function of polysaccharides. Macromol Symp 1995; 99:43–55.
7. Watson JD, Crick FH. Molecular structure of nucleic acids. Nature 1953; 171:737–738.
8. Morris ER, Cutler AN, Ross-Murphy SB, Rees DA. Concentration and shear rate dependence of viscosity in random coil polysaccharide solutions. Carbohyd Polym 1981; 1:5–21.
9. Meadows J, Williams PA, Kennedy JC. Comparison of the extensional and shear viscosity characteristics of aqueous hydroxyethylcellulose solutions. Maromolecules 1995; 28:2683–2692.
10. Meer G. Natural gum polymers as ingredients in cosmetics. Cosmet Toilet 1984; 99:61–64.
11. Cottrell IW, Kovacs P. Alginates. In: Davidson RL, ed. Handbook of Water-Soluble Gums and Resins. New York: McGraw-Hill, 1980:Chapter 2, 1–43.
12. Clare K. Algin. In: Whistler RL, BeMiller JN, eds. Industrial Gums, Polysaccharides and Their Drivatives, 3rd ed. San Diego: Academic Press, 1993:105–143.
13. Yalpani M. Properties: alginates: In: Yalpani M, ed. Polysaccharides Synthesis, Modifications and Structure/Property Relations. Amsterdam: Elsevier, 1988:10–11, 108–109.

14. BeMiller JN. Carbohydrates. In: Kroschwitz JI, Howe-Grant M, eds. Kirk-Othmer Encyclopedia of Chemical Technology, 4th ed, Volume 4. New York: Wiley, 1992:941–942.
15. Clark M. Rheological additives. In: Laba D, ed. Rheological Properties of Cosmetics and Toiletries. New York: Marcel Dekker, 1993:69–73.
16. Draget KI, Skjak-Braek G, Smidsrod O. Alginate based new materials. Int J Biol Macromol 1997; 21:47–55.
17. Lee JW, Ashby RD, Day DF. Role of acetylation on metal induced precipitation of alginates. Carbohyd Polym 1996; 29:337–345.
18. Stokke BT, Smidsrod O, Bruheim P, Skjak-Braek G. Distribution of uronate residues in alginate chains in relation to alginate gelling properties. Macromolecules 1991; 24:4637–4645.
19. Djabourov M. Gelation—a review. Polym Int 1991; 25:135–143.
20. Clark, AH, Ross-Murphy SB. Structural and mechanical properties of biopolymer gels. In: Clark AH, Kamide K, Ross-Murphy S, Saito M, eds. Advances in Polymer Science. Berlin: Springer-Verlag, 1987:83:125–129.
21. Thom D, Grant GT, Morris ER, Rees DA. Characterization of cation binding and gelation of poly-uronates by circular dichroism. Carbohyd Res 1982; 100:29–42.
22. Pedersen JK. Pectins. In: Davidson RL, ed. Handbook of Water-Soluble Gums and Resins. New York: McGraw-Hill, 1980:Chapter 15, 1–21.
23. Rolin C. Pectin. In: Whistler RL, BeMiller JN, eds. Industrial Gums Polysaccharides and Their Derivatives, 3rd ed. San Diego: Academic Press, 1993:257–293.
24. Yalpani M. Properties: pectins. In: Yalpani M. ed. Polysaccharides Synthesis, Modifications and Structure/Property Relations. Amsterdam: Elsevier, 1988:110.
25. BeMiller JN. Carbohydrates. In: Kroschwitz JI, Howe-Grant M, eds. Kirk-Othmer Encyclopedia of Chemical Technology, 4th ed, Vol 4. New York: Wiley, 1992:943–944.
26. Clark AH, Ross-Murphy SB. Structural and mechanical properties of biopolymer gels. In: Clark AH, Kamide K, Ross-Murphy S, Saito M, eds. Advances in Polymer Science. Berlin: Springer-Verlag, 1987:83:130–132.
27. Guiseley KB, Stanley NF, Whitehouse PA. Carrageenan. In: Davidson RL, ed. Hardbook of Water-Soluble Gums and Resins. New York: McGraw-Hill, 1980: Chapter 5, 1–30.
28. Therkelsen GH. Carrageenan. In: Whistler RL, BeMiller JN, eds. Industrial Gums Polysaccharide and Their Derivatives, 3rd ed. San Diego: Academic Press, 1993:145–180.
29. Yalpani M. Properties: Carrageenans. In: Yalpani M. ed. Polysaccharide Synthesis, Modifications and Structure/Property Relations. Amsterdam: Elsevier, 1988:111–112, 457–461.
30. BeMiller JN. Carbohydrates. In: Kroschwitz JI, Howe-Grant M, eds. Kirk-Othmer Encyclopedia of Chemical Technology, 4th ed, Vol. 4. New York: Wiley, 1992:942.
31. Clark M. Rheological additives. In: Laba D, ed. Rheological Properties of Cosmetics and Toiletries. New York: Marcel Dekker, 1993:73–78.
32. Tye RJ. Carrageenan as a product ingredient. Drug Cosmet Ind 1991; November: 28, 30–32, 34.
33. Rochas C, Rinaudo M, Landry S. Role of molecular weight on the mechanical properties of kappa carrageenan gels. Carbohyd Polym 1990; 12:255–266.
34. Richardson RK, Goycoolea FM. Rheological measurement of κ-carrageenan during gelation. Carbohyd Polym 1994; 24:223–225.
35. Hermansson AM, Eriksson E, Jordansson E. Effects of potassium, sodium and calcium on the microstructure and rheological behavior of kappa-carrageenan gels. Carbohyd Polym 1991; 16:297–320.
36. Morris ER, Rees DA, Robinson G. Cation-specific aggregation of carrageenan helices: domain model of polymer gel structure. J Mol Biol 1980; 138:349–362.
37. Clark AH, Ross-Murphy SB. Structural and mechanical properties of biopolymer gels. In: Allan CH, Kamide K, Ross-Murphy S, Saito M, eds. Advances in Polymer Science. Berlin: Springer-Verlag, 1987:83:115–122.

38. Piculell L, Borgstrom J, Chronakis IS, Quist PO, Viebke C. Organization and association of κ-carrageenan helices under different salt conditions. Int J Biol Macromol 1997; 21:141–153.
39. Michel AS, Mestdagh MM, Axelos MAV. Physio-chemical properties of carrageenan gels in presence of various cations. Int J Biol Macromol 1997; 21:195–200.
40. Rochas C, Taravel FR. Polysaccharide-polysaccharide interactions. In: Salamone JC, ed. Polymeric Materials Encyclopedia. Boca Raton: CRC Press, 1996; 9:6704–6712.
41. Lundin L, Hermansson AM. Influence of locust bean gum on the rheological behavior and microstructure of K-κ-carrageenan. Carbohyd Polym 1995; 29:91–99.
42. Piculell L, Zhang W, Turquois T, Rochas C, Taravel FR, Williams PA. Effects of added galacto- and gluco-mannans on the NMR spectra of ^{133}Cs ions in kappa-carrageenan gels. Carbohyd Res 1994; 265:281–290.
43. Turquois T, Rochas C, Taravel FR. Rheological studies of synergistic kappa-carrageenan-carob galactomannan gels. Carbohyd Polym 1992; 17:263–268.
44. Williams PA, Clegg SM, Langdon MJ, Nishinari K, Piculell L. Investigation of the gelation mechanism in κ-carrageenan/konjac mannan mixtures using differential scanning calorimetry and electron spin resonance spectroscopy. Macromolecules 1993; 26:5441–5446.
45. Kang KS, Pettitt DJ. Xanthan, gellan, welan, and rhamsan. In: Whistler RL, BeMiller JN, eds. Industrial Gums Polysaccharides and Their Derivatives, 3rd ed. San Diego: Academic Press, 1993:341–371.
46. Cottrell IW, Kang KS, Kovacs P. Xanthan gum. In: Davidson RL, ed. Handbook of Water-Soluble Gums and Resins. New York: McGraw-Hill, 1980:Chapter 24, 1–31.
47. Christensen BE, Stokke BT, Smidsrod O. Xanthan—the natural water soluble cellulose derivative. In: Kennedy JF, Phillips, GO, Williams PO, eds. Cellulose and Cellulose Derivatives: Physico-chemical Aspects and Industrial Applications. Cambridge, England: Woodhead Publishing, 1995:265–278.
48. Quinn FX. Xanthan gum (overview). In: Salamore JC, ed. Polymeric Materials Encyclopedia. Boca Raton: CRC Press, 1996:11:8788–8801.
49. BeMiller JN. Carbohydrates. In Kroschwitz JI, Howe-Grant M, eds. Kirk-Othmer Encyclopedia of Chemical Technology, 4th ed, Vol 4. New York: Wiley, 1992:944–945.
50. Clark M. Rheological additives. In: Laba D, ed. Rheological Properties of Cosmetics and Toiletries. New York: Marcel Dekker, 1993:78–81.
51. Clark AH, Ross-Murphy SB. Structural and mechanical properties of biopolymer gels. In: Clark AH, Kamide K, Ross-Murphy S, Saito M, eds. Advances in Polymer Science. Berlin: Springer-Verlag, 1987:83:142–143.
52. Rees DA, Morris ER, Thom D, Madden JK. Shapes and interactions of carbohydrate chains. In: Aspinall GO, ed. The Polysaccharides, Vol 1. New York: Academic Press, 1982:245–248.
53. Sato T, Kakihara T, Teramoto A. Isotropic-liquid crystal phase equilibrium in semiflexible polymer solutions: xanthan, a rigid polyelectrolyte. Polymer 1990; 31:824–827.
54. Zatz JL, Knapp S. Viscosity of xanthan gum solutions at low shear rates. J Pharm Sci 1984; 73:468–471.
55. Zatz JL, Bernard KIP. Stabilization of oil-in-water emulsions by gums. J Soc Cosmet Chem 1986; 37:329–350.
56. Zatz JL. Physical stability of suspensions. J Soc Cosmet Chem 1985; 36:393–411.
57. Idson B. Polymers in skin care. Cosmet Toilet 1988; 103:64–65.
58. Xanthan gum—the natural water-soluble polymer for cosmetic and personal care products. In-Cosmetics Preprints, Vol II. Verlag fur Chem. Industrie H. Ziolkowsky GmbH, Augsburg: 1993:37–40.
59. Goycoolea FM, Richardson RK, Morris ER, Gidley MJ. Stoichiometry and conformation of xanthan in synergistic gelation with locust bean gum or konjac glucomannan: evidence for heterotypic binding. Macromolecules 1995; 28:8308–8320.

60. Chandrasekaren R, Radha A. Molecular modeling of xanthan: galactomannan interactions. Carbohyd Polym 1997; 32:201–208.
61. Nasr-El-Din HA, Noy JL. Flow behavior of alkali, surfactant, and xanthan solutions used for enhanced oil recovery. Rev Inst Fr Pet 1992; 47:771–791.
62. Chen CR, Zatz JL. Dynamic rheologic measurement of the interaction between xanthan gum and colloidal magnesium aluminum silicate. J Soc Cosmet Chem 1992; 43:1–12.
63. Volpi N. Glycosaminoglycans (overview). In: Salamore JC, ed. Polymeric Materials Encyclopedia, Vol 4. Boca Raton: CRC Press, 1996:2840–2849.
64. Schwartz NB. Carbohydrate metabolism. II. Special pathways. In: Delvin TM, ed. Textbook of Biochemistry with Clinical Correlations, 3rd ed. New York: Wiley-Liss, 1992:378–384.
65. Rieger MM. Hyaluronic acid in cosmetics. Cosmet Toilet 1998; 113:35–42.
66. Diaz VB, Fuentes EP, Martinez OE, Kraglievich AR. Chondroitin sulfate (overview). In: Salamone JC, ed. Polymeric Materials Encyclopedia, Vol 2. Boca Raton, FL: CRC Press, 1996:1262–1274.
67. Takahashi A, Kaburaki M, Oka Y. Hyaluronic acid (macroionic, rheological, and lubricity properties). In: Salamone JC, ed. Polymeric Materials Encyclopedia, Vol 5. Boca Raton, FL: CRC Press, 1996:3078–3082.
68. Milas M, Roure I, Berry GC. Crossover behavior in the viscosity of semiflexible polymers: solutions of sodium hyaluronate as a function of concentration, molecular weight and temperature. J Rheol 1996; 40:1155–1166.
69. Fiorentini G, Becheroni L, DiIorio G. Hyaluronic acid: analytical procedures for purity determination, polymerization degrees and comparative instrumental test ''in vivo.'' 15th IFSCC International Congress, Preprints, Vol A, 1988:139–151.
70. Hoshizaki S, Nakabata H. Application of water-holding polymers as a skin moisturizer. 12th IFSCC International Congress, Preprints, Vol 2, 1982:337–353.
71. Sarpotdar PP. Iontophoresis. In: Zatz JL, ed. Skin Permeation Fundamentals and Application. Carol Stream, IL: Allured Publishing, 1993:239–250.
72. Robbins CR. Chemical and Physical Behavior of Human Hair, 3rd ed. New York: Springer-Verlag, 1994; 204–207.
73. Idson B. Polymers in skin care. Cosmet Toilet 1988; 103:65.
74. Band PA, Brode GL, Goddard ED, Barone AG, Leshchiner E, Harris WC, Pavlichko JR, Partain EM, Leung PS. Interpolymer complexes between hyaluronan and cationic cellulose polymers. In: Gebelein CG, Cheng TC, Yang VC, eds. Cosmetic and Pharmaceutical Applications of Polymers. New York: Plenum Press, 1991:129–135.
75. Pavlichko JP. Polymer interactions to enhance the function of hyaluronic acid. Drug Cosmet Ind 1990; 147:21–24.
76. Whistler RL. Exudate gums. In: Whistler RL, BeMiller JN, eds. Industrial Gums Polysaccharides and Their Derivatives, 3rd ed. San Diego: Academic Press, 1993:309–339.
77. Meer W. Gum arabic. In: Davidson RL, ed. Handbook of Water-Soluble Gums and Resins. New York: McGraw-Hill, 1980:Chapter 8, 1–24.
78. Meer W. Gum karaya. In: Davidson RL, ed. Handbook of Water-Soluble Gums and Resins. New York: McGraw-Hill, 1980:Chapter 10, 1–14.
79. Clark M. Rheological additives. In: Laba D. ed. Rheological Properties of Cosmetics and Toiletries. New York: Marcel Dekker, 1993:61–62.
80. Stauffer KR. Gum tragacanth. In: Davidson RL, ed. Handbook of Water-Soluble Gums and Resins. New York: McGraw-Hill, 1980:Chapter 11, 1–31.
81. Clark M. Rheological additives. In: Laba D, ed. Rheological Properties of Cosmetics and Toiletries. New York: Marcel Dekker, 1993:63–64.
82. Feddersen RL, Thorp SN. Sodium carboxymethylcellulose. In: Whistler RL, BeMiller JN, eds. Industrial Gums Polysaccharides and Their Derivatives, 3rd ed. San Diego: Academic Press, 1993:537–578.

83. BeMiller JN. Carbohydrates. In: Kroschwitz JI, Howe-Grant M, eds. Kirk-Othmer Encyclopedia of Chemical Technology, 4th ed, Vol 4. New York: Wiley, 1992:945–946.
84. Majewicz TG, Podlas TJ. Cellulose ethers. In: Kroschwitz JI, Howe-Grant M, eds. Kirk-Othmer Encyclopedia of Chemical Technology, 4th ed, Vol 5. New York: Wiley, 1993:545–548.
85. Stelzer GI, Klug, ED. Carboxymethylcellulose. In: Davidson RL, ed. Handbook of Water-Soluble Gums and Resins. New York: McGraw-Hill, 1980:Chapter 4, 1–28.
86. Clark M. Rheological additives. In: Laba D, ed. Rheological Properties of Cosmetics and Toiletries, New York: Marcel Dekker, 1993:83–85.
87. Idson B. Polymers in skin care. Cosmet Toilet 1988; 103:64.
88. BeMiller JN. Carbohydrates. In: Kroschwitz JI, Howe-Grant M. eds. Kirk-Othmer Encyclopedia of Chemical Technology, 4th ed, Vol 4. New York: Wiley, 1992:932–933.
89. Ghannam MT, Esmail MN. Rheological properties of carboxymethyl cellulose. J Appl Polym Sci 1997; 64:289–301.
90. Kastner U, Hoffman H, Donges R, Hilbig J. Structure and solution properties of sodium carboxymethyl cellulose. Colloid Surf A 1997; 123/124:307–328.
91. Hirano S, Hirochi K, Hayashi K, Mikami T, Tachibana H. Cosmetic and pharmaceutical uses of chitin and chitosan. In: Gebelein CG, Cheng TC, Yang VC, eds. Cosmetic and Pharmaceutical Applications of Polymers. New York: Plenum Press, 1991:95–104.
92. Ananthapadmanabhan KP. Surfactant solutions: adsorption and aggregation properties. In: Goddard ED, Ananthapadmanabhan KP, eds. Interactions of Surfactants with Polymers and Proteins. Boca Rat. FL: CRC Press, 1993:5–58.
93. Jones MN, Chapman D. Micelles, Monolayers, and Biomembranes. New York: Wiley-Liss, 1995:Chapter 3.
94. Goddard ED. Polymer surfactant interaction. Part II. Polymer and surfactant of opposite charge. In: Goddard ED, Ananthapadmanabhan KP, eds. Interactions of Surfactants with Polymers and Proteins. Boca Raton, FL: CRC Press, 1993:171–202.
95. Goodard ED, Schmitt RL. Adsorption of cationic polymers. In: Cosmetic Toiletries Applied Research Series: Hair Care. Carol Stream, IL: Allured Publishing Corp, 1996:21–25.
96. Schmitt RL, Goddard ED. Adsorption of cationic polymers—Part 2. In: Cosmetic Toiletries Applied Research Series: Hair Care. Carol Stream, IL: Allured Publishing Corp, 1996:26–30.
97. Goddard ED, Faucher JA, Scott RJ, Turney ME. Adsorption of polymer JR on keratinous surfaces—Part II. J Soc Cosmet Chem 1975; 26:539–550.
98. Goddard ED. Substantivity through cationic substitution. Cosmet Toilet 1987; 102:71–80.
99. Hutter JM, Clarke MT, Just EK, Lichtin JL, Sakr A. Colloid titration: a method to quantify the adsorption of cationic polymer by bleached hair. J Soc Cosmet Chem 1991; 42:87–96.
100. Aruchami M, Gowri N, Sundara-Rajulu G. Chitin deacetylases in invertebrates. In: Muzarelli R, Jeuniaux C, Gooday GW, eds. Chitin in Nature and Technology. New York: Plenum Press, 1986:263–268.
101. Brode GL, Goddard ED, Harris WC, Salensky GA. Cationic polysaccharides for cosmetics and therapeutics. In: Gebelein CG, Cheng TC, Yang VC, eds. Cosmetic and Pharmaceutical Applications of Polymers. New York: Plenum Press, 1991:117–128.
102. Wachter R, Stenberg E. Hydagen® CMF in cosmetic applications: efficacy in different in-vitro and in-vivo measurements. In: Domand A, Jeuniaux C, Muzzarelli R, Roberts G, eds. Advances in Chitin Science. Lyons: Jacques Andre, 1996:381–388.
103. Wachter R, Hofmann M, Panzer C, Stenberg E. Hydagen® CMF: multifunctional agents of biomarine origin. Cosmet Toilet Manuf World 1997; 35–40.
104. Julia MR, Munoz I, Ayats A, Cot M. Sorption-desorption behavior of anionic surfactant on wool fibres treated with biopolymer. Agro Food Ind Hi-Tech 1996; March:13–16.
105. Onsoyen E, Dybdahl MK. The application and benefits of chitosan in cosmetics. Cosmet Toilet Manuf World 1991; 32, 34–35.
106. Lochead RY. The history of polymers in hair care. Cosmet Toilet 1988; 103:23–61.

107. Onishi H, Nagai T, Machida Y. Applications of chitin, chitosan and their derivatives to drug carriers for microparticulated or conjugated drug delivery systems. In: Goosen MFA, ed. Applications of Chitin and Chitosan. Lancaster: Technomic, 1997:205–231.
108. Ferrari F, Rossi S, Cristina B, Carmella C. Characterization of rheological and mucoadhesive properties of three grades of chitosan hydrochloride. Farmco 1997; 52:493–497.
109. Lochead RY. The history of polymers in hair care. Cosmet Toilet 1988; 103:39–40.
110. Gruber JV, Kreeger RL. Cellulose ethers, cationic. In: Salamone JC, ed. Polymeric Materials Encyclopedia, Vol 2. Boca Raton, FL: CRC Press, 1996:1113–1118.
111. Goddard ED. Cationic cellulosic derivatives. In: Kennedy JF, Phillips GO, Williams PA, eds. Cellulose: Chemistry, Biochemistry and Material Aspects. London: Horwood, 1993: 331–336.
112. Goddard ED, Leung PS. Anathapadmanabhan KP. Novel gelling structures based on polymer/surfactant systems. 16th IFSCC International Congress, Preprints, Vol 3. New York: Society of Cosmetic Chemists, 1990:193–209.
113. Hutter JM, Clarke MT, Just EK, Lichtin JL, Sakr A. The influence of nonionic cellulosic polymers on uptake of polyquaternium-10 by bleached hair. J Soc Cosmet Chem 1992; 43: 229–235.
114. Goddard ED, Hannan RB, Anionic surfactant complexes with charged and uncharged cellulose ethers. In: Mittal KL, ed. Micellization, Solubilization and Microemulsions, Vol 2. New York: Plenum Press, 1977:835–845.
115. Goldraich M, Schwartz JR, Burns JL, Talmon Y. Microstructures formed in a mixed system of a cationic polymer and an anionic surfactant. Colloid Surf A Physiochem Eng Asp 1997; 125:231–244.
116. Malmsten M, Ljusegren I, Carlstedt I. Ellipsometry studies of the mucoadhesion of cellulose derivatives. Coll Surf B Bioint 1994; 2:463–470.
117. Westwood A, Leder D, Donabedian D. Evaluation of an ophthalmic drug delivery system: Occumer Polymer™ and anionic therapeutics by ESCA and AFM. Polym Prep (Am Chem Soc Polym Mat Sci Eng) 1997; 76:130.
118. Maier H, Anderson M, Karl C, Magnuson K, Whistler RL. Guar, locust bean, tara and fenugreek gums. In: Whistler RL, BeMiller IN, eds. Industrial Gums Polysaccharides and Their Derivatives, 3rd ed. San Diego: Academic Press, 1993:181–226.
119. Seaman JK. Guar gum. In: Davison RL, ed. Handbook of Water-Soluble Gums and Resins. New York: McGraw-Hill, 1980:Chapter 6, 1–19.
120. BeMiller JN. Carbohydrates. In: Kroschwitz JI, Howe-Grant M, eds. Kirk-Othmer Encyclopedia of Chemical Technology, 4th ed, Vol 4. New York: Wiley, 1992:943.
121. Freeland MS, Holder I, Tucker J. Cationic guar gum. Cosmet Toilet 1984; 99:83–87.
122. Ricca JM. Guar gum: a versatile platform for transparent cosmetic products. Cosmet Toilet Manuf World 1996; 78, 80–84.
123. Pugliese P, Hines G, Wielinga W. Skin protective properties of a cationic guar derivative. Cosmet Toilet 1990; 105:105–106, 108, 110–111.
124. Lochead RY. The history of polymers in hair care. Cosmet Toilet 1988; 103:41.
125. Leporatti R, Pagnutti G, Rigano L, Trenti R. Le gomme cationiche condizaionanti: proprietcie applicazioni (conditioning cationic polymers: properties and applications). Cosmet News XVIII 1995; 102:199–210.
126. Zobel HF, Stephen AM. Starch: structure, analysis, and applications. Food Sci Technol 1995; 67:19–66.
127. BeMiller JN. Starch-based gums. In: Whistler RL, BeMiller IN, eds. Industrial Gums Polysaccharides and Their Derivatives, 3rd ed. San Diego: Academic Press, 1993:579–600.
128. Rutenberg MW. Starch and its modifications. In: Davidson RL, ed. Handbook of Water-Soluble Gums and Resins. New York: McGraw-Hill, 1980:Chapter 22, 1–83.
129. Clark AH, Ross-Murphy SB. Structural and mechanical properties of biopolymer gels. In:

Clark AH, Kamide K, Ross-Murphy S, Saito M. eds. Advances in Polymer Science 83. Berlin: Springer-Verlag, 1987; 83:133–135.
130. Besun N, Peker S, Kokturk U, Yilmaz H. Structure of starch-bentonite gels. Coll Polym Sci 1997; 275:378–389.
131. Mikus FF, Hixon RM, Rundle RE. The complexes of fatty acids with amylose. J Am Chem Soc 1946; 68:1115–1123.
132. Amann M, Dressnandt G. Cyclodextrins in cosmetics. Cosmet Toilet 1993; 108:90–95.
133. Szejtli J. Industrial applications of cyclodextrins. In: Atwood JL, Davies JE, MacNicol DD, eds. Inclusion Compounds. Vol 3: Physical Properties and Applications. London: Academic Press, 1984:331–390.
134. Citernesi U, Sciacchitano M. Cyclodextrins in functional dermocosmetics. Cosmet Toilet 1995; 110:53–58, 60–61.
135. Romberger ML. Cyclodextrins: altered states. Soap Perf Cosmet 1998; August:44–46.
136. Motwani M, Zatz JL. Applications of cyclodextrins in skin products. Cosmet Toilet 1997; 112:39–42, 44–47.
137. Brigand G. Scleroglucan. In: Whistler RL, BeMiller JN, eds. Industrial Gums, Polysaccharides and Their Derivatives. San Diego: Academic Press, 1993:461–474.
138. Lochead RY. The history of polymers in hair care. Cosmet Toilet 1988; 103:38–39.
139. Clarke MT. Water-soluble cellulose ethers for hair care products. Drug Cosmet Ind 1992; May:26, 28, 30, 95.
140. Musman DW. Properties of polymeric cellulose ethers, mainly sodium-carboxy methyl cellulose and its applicational effects in personal care. Gums, Polymers, Thickeners and Resins Symp. New York: Society of Cosmetic Scientists, 1986:1–17.
141. Doelker E. Cellulose derivatives. In: Pappas NA, Langer RS. Advances in Polymer Science, Vol 107. Berlin: Springer-Verlag, 1993:200–264.
142. Powell GM. Hydroxyethylcellulose. In: Davidson RL, ed. Handbook of Water-Soluble Gums and Resins. New York: McGraw-Hill, 1980:Chapter 12, 1–22.
143. Majewicz TG, Podlas TJ. Cellulose ethers. In: Kroschwitz JI, Howe-Grant M, eds. Kirk-Othmer Encyclopedia of Chemical Technology, 4th ed, Vol 5. New York: Wiley, 1993:548–553.
144. Clark MT. Rheological additives. In: Laba D, ed. Rheological Properties of Cosmetics and Toiletries. New York: Marcel Dekker, 1993:85–88.
145. Desmarais AJ, Wint RF. Hydroxyalkyl and ethyl ethers of cellulose. In: Whistler RL, BeMiller JN, eds. Industrial Gums Polysaccharides and Their Derivatives. San Diego: Academic Press, 1993:505–535.
146. Filser JG, Kreuzer PE, Greim H, Bolt HM. New scientific arguments for regulation of ethylene oxide residues in skin-care products. Arch Toxicol 1994; 68:401–405.
147. Butler RW, Klug ED. Hydroxypropylcellulose. In: Davidson RL, ed. Handbook of Water-Soluble Gums and Resins. New York: McGraw-Hill, 1980:Chapter 13, 1–7.
148. Desmarais AJ, Wint RF. Hydroxyalkyl and ethyl ethers of cellulose. In: Whistler RL, BeMiller JN, eds. Industrial Gums Polysaccharides and Their Derivatives. San Diego: Academic Press, 1993:516–522.
149. Majewicz TG, Podlas TJ. Cellulose ethers. In: Kroschwitz JI, Howe-Grant M, eds. Kirk-Othmer Encyclopedia of Chemical Technology, 4th ed, Vol 5. New York: Wiley, 1993:558–560.
150. Clarke MT. Rheological additives. In: Laba D, ed. Rheological Properties of Cosmetics and Toiletries. New York: Marcel Dekker, 1993:95–97.
151. Suto S. Hydroxypropyl cellulose (crosslinked, cholesteric liquid crystal). In: Salamone JC, ed. Polymeric Materials Encyclopedia, Vol 5. Boca Raton, FL: CRC Press, 1996:3167–3171.
152. Carraher CE. General topics: liquid crystals. Polym News 1996:21:306–309.
153. Cioca G, Calvo L. Liquid crystals and cosmetic applications. Cosmet Toilet 1990; 105:57–62.

154. Loll P. Liquid crystals in cosmetic emulsions. In-Cosmetics, Preprints, Vol. I. Verlag fur Chem. Industrie H. Ziolkowski GmbH, Augsburg: 1993:64–85.
155. Loll P. Liquid emulsions in cosmetic emulsions. Cosmet Toilet Manuf World 1994; 108–120.
156. Weigel P, Hirte R, Zenke D, Hartmann J. Flussig-Kristalline Zustande in Cellulose- und Cellulosederivatlosungen (liquid-crystalline state in cellulose and cellulose derivative). Acta Polymer 1984; 35:83–88.
157. Guido S. Phase behavior of aqueous solutions of hydroxypropyl cellulose. Macromolecules 1995; 28:4530–4539.
158. Winnik FM, Winnik MA. The interaction of sodium dodecylsulfate with (hydroxypropyl) cellulose. Polym J 1990; 22:482–488.
159. Grover JA. Methycellulose and its derivatives. In: Whistler RL, BeMiller JN, eds. Industrial Gums Polysaccharides and Their Derivatives. San Diego: Academic Press, 1993:475–504.
160. Greminger GK, Krumel KL. Alkyl and hydroxyalkylcellulose. In: Davidson RL, ed. Handbook of Water-Soluble Gums and Resins. New York: McGraw-Hill, 1980:Chapter 3, 1–25.
161. Majewicz TG, Podlas TJ. Cellulose ethers. In: Kroschwitz JI, Howe-Grant M, eds. Kirk-Othmer Encyclopedia of Chemical Technology, 4th ed, Vol 5. New York: Wiley, 1993:553–556.
162. Clarke MT. Rheological additives. In: Laba D, ed. Rheological Properties of Cosmetics and Toiletries. New York: Marcel Dekker, 1993:91–95.
163. Nilsson S. Interaction between water-soluble cellulose derivatives and surfactants. 1. The HPMC/SDS/water system. Macromolecules 1995; 28:7837–7844.
164. Conklin JR. The form and function of lather enhancer cellulosics in personal care products. In: Gebelein CG, Cheng TC, Yang VC, eds. Cosmetic and Pharmaceutical Applications of Polymers. New York: Plenum Press, 1991:15–24.
165. Daniels R, Rimpler S. Effect of heat sterilization on the stability of o/w emulsions containing hydroxypropylmethyl cellulose as emulsifier. Pharm Pharmacol Lett 1993; 3:80–83.
166. Hayakawa K, Kawaguchi M, Kato T. Protective colloidal effects of hydroxypropyl methyl cellulose on the stability of silicone oil emulsions. Langmuir 1997; 13:6069–6073.
167. Carlsson A, Karlstrom G, Lindman B. Thermal gelation of nonionic cellulose ethers and ionic surfactants in water. Colloids Surfaces 1990; 47:147–165.
168. Nystrom B, Lindman B. Dynamic and viscoelastic properties during the thermal gelation process of a nonionic cellulose ether dissolved in water in the presence of ionic surfactants. Macromolecules 1995; 28:967–974.
169. Nystrom B, Kjoniksen A, Lindman B. Effects of temperature, surfactant, and salt on the rheological behavior in semidilute aqueous systems of a nonionic cellulose ether, Langmuir 1996; 12:3233–3240.
170. Kimura J. Nitrocellulose. In: Salamone JC, ed. Polymeric Materials Encyclopedia, Vol 6. Boca Raton, FL: CRC Press, 1996:4582–4587.
171. Remz HM. Nail product rheology. In: Laba D, ed. Rheological Properties of Cosmetic and Toiletries. New York: Marcel Dekker, 1993:176–183.
172. Wimmer EP, Schlossman ML. The history of nail polish. Cosmet Toilet 1992; 107:115–120.
173. Remz HM. Polymers and thickeners in nail-care products. Cosmet Toilet 1988; 103:70–82.
174. Muzzarelli RAA. Amphoteric derivatives of chitosan and their biological significance. In: Skjak-Braek G, Anthonsen T, Sandford P, eds. Chitin and Chitosan Sources, Chemistry, Biochemistry, Physical Properties and Applications. London: Elsevier Applied Science, 1989:87–99.
175. Davies DH, Elson CM, Hayes ER. *N,O*-Carboxymethyl chitosan, a new water soluble chitin derivative. In: Skjak-Braek G, Anthonsen T, Sandford P, eds. Chitin and Chitosan Sources, Chemistry, Biochemistry, Physical Properties and Applications. London: Elsevier Applied Science, 1989:467–472.

176. Gruber JV, Rutar V, Bandekar J, Konish PN. Synthesis of *N*-[(3′-Hydroxy-2′,3-dicarboxy)-ethyl] chitosan: a new, water-soluble chitosan derivative. Macromolecules 1995; 28:8865–8867.
177. Gruber JV. Synthesis of *N*-[(3′-Hydroxy-2′,3′-dicarboxy)ethyl] chitosan: a new water-soluble, amphoteric chitosan derivative. In: Domard A, Jeuniaux C, Muzzarelli R, Roberts G, eds. Advances in Chitin Science, Vol 1. Lyon: Jacques Andre, 1996: 230–235.
178. Pasapane J, Ronco D. Novel amphoteric starch: a naturally derived rheology modifer for skin care. Cosmet Toilet Manuf World 1996; 175–179.
179. Cardinali S, Pasapane J, Greenburg J. Novel thickeners for hard-to-thicken personal care products. Drug Cosmet Ind 1997; May:42, 44–46, 48.
180. Silverstein TP. The real reason why oil and water don't mix. J Chem Educ 1998; 75:116–118.
181. Clarke, MT. Rheological additives. In: Laba D, ed. Rheological Properties of Cosmetics and Toiletries. New York: Marcel Dekker, 1993:88–91.
182. Thuresson K, Nilsson S, Lindman B. Influence of cosolutes on phase behavior and viscosity of a nonionic cellulose ether. The effect of hydrophobic modification. Langmuir 1996; 12: 2412–2417.
183. DeBruin JJ. Hydrophobically modified cellulose ether for personal care. SOFW-J 1994; 120: 944–948.
184. Tanaka R, Meadows J, Williams PA, Phillips GO. Interaction of hydrophobically modified (hydroxyethyl) cellulose with various added surfactants. Macromolecules 1992; 25:1304–1310.
185. Kastner U, Hoffmann H, Donges R, Ehrler R. A comparison of several samples of modified hydroxethyl cellulose and their interactions with surfactants. Prog Colloid Polym Sci 1995; 98:57–62.
186. Jones RT, Brown CA. The behavior of cationic cellulose derivatives containing fatty quat groups. Int J Cosmet Sci 1988; 10:219–229.
187. Shubin V. Adsorption of cationic polymer onto negatively charged surfaces in the presence of anionic surfactant. Langmuir 1994; 10:1093–1100.
188. Guillemet F, Piculell L, Nilsson S, Djabourov M, Lindman B. Interactions between hydrophobically modified polyelectrolyte and oppositely charged surfactant. Mixed micelle formation. Prog Colloid Polym Sci 1995; 98:47–50.
189. Winnik FM, Regismond STA, Goddard ED. Interactions of cationic surfactants with a hydrophobically modified cationic cellulose polymer: a study by fluorescence spectroscopy. Colloids Surfaces A Phys Eng Aspects 1996;106:243–247.
190. Winnik FM, Regismond STA, Goddard ED. Interactions of an anionic surfactant with a fluorescent-dye-labeled hydrophically-modified cationic cellulose ether. Langmuir 1997; 13: 111–114.
191. Thuresson K, Nilsson S, Lindman B. Effect of hydrophobic modification on phase behavior and rheology in mixtures of oppositely charged polyelectrolytes. Langmuir 1996; 12:530–537.
192. Band PA, Leshchiner A, Pavlichko JP. Expanding the topical applications of hyaluronan through complexation and derivatization. Cosmet Toilet Manuf World 1994; 243–246.
193. Konish PN, Gruber JV. Surfactant-free formulations employing a synergistic complex between a hydrophobically modified, cationic cellulose ether and amylose. J Cosmet Sci 1998; 49:335–342.
194. Glick AB, Yuspa SH. Regulating skin structure and function. In: Cosmetic Toiletries Applied Research Series: Skin Care. Carol Stream, IL: Allured Publishing Corp, 1995:9–14.
195. Martin P. Wound healing—aiming for perfect skin regeneration. Science 1997: 276:75–81.
196. Manuskiatti W, Maibach HI. Hyaluronic acid and skin: wound healing and aging. Int J Dermatol 1996; 35:539–544.
197. Moriarty KP, Crombleholme TM, Gallivan EK, O'Donnel C. Hyaluronic acid–dependent

pericellular matrices in fetal fibroblasts: implication for scar-free wound repair. Wound Repair Regen 1996; 4:346–352.
198. Stern R, Frost GI, Shuster S, Shuster V, Hall J, Wong T, Gakunga P, Csoka TB. Hyaluronic acid and skin. Cosmet Toilet 1998; 113:43–46, 48.
199. Horiuchi Y, Otoyama K, Kifune K, Nishioka K. Increase in epidermal ATPase-positive Langerhans cells following topical application of 70% deacetylated chitin (DAC-70) in DNCB-sensitized contact dermatitis in guinea pigs—preliminary report. J Dermatol Treat 1996; 7: 101–103.
200. Mansell PWA. Polysaccharides in skin care. Cosmet Toilet 1994; 109:67–72.
201. Wolk M, Danon D. Promotion of wound healing by yeast glucan evaluated on single animals. Med Biol 1985; 63:73–80.
202. Pauly M, Pauly G. New polysaccharides interest in care cosmetology. In-Cosmetics, Preprints, 1997. Dusseldorf: Verlag für Chemische Industrie H. Ziolkowsky GmbH, 1997:417–444.
203. Leibovich SJ, Danon D. Promotion of wound repair in mice by application of glucan. J Reticuloendothelial Soc 1980; 27:1–11.
204. Zulli F, Saecker C. CM-Glucan a new yeast polysaccharide for cosmetic use. Cosmet Toilet Manuf World 1994; 131–136.
205. Zulli F, Suter F, Blitz H, Nissen HP. CM-Glucan. A biological response modifier from baker's yeast for skin care. SOFW-J 1997; 123:535–538, 540–541.

9

Proteins in Cosmetics

Alessandro Teglia and Gianfranco Secchi
Kelisema Italy, Tavernerio, Italy

I. INTRODUCTION

A. Historical Use of Proteins in Cosmetics

Direct information on the ancient use of protein materials (cereal flours, animal blood, milk, and egg whites) for cosmetic purposes has come to us from all great ancient civilizations: Babylon, Egypt, Greece, Rome, China, and India (1), but the use of proteins for skin and hair care probably antedates recorded history. Traces of the remote self-beautification practices are still found from the residual primitive societies surviving on our planet. They tell us about the instinctive and empirical use of those protein substances which, after all with no capital modifications, are currently used and appreciated in modern cosmetology. For example, the migrant Eritrean shepherds of the Habab tribe still use, almost as unique cosmetic material, camel milk to clean the skin and hair, the Ainu fishers on the island of Hokkaido prepare facial masks with soy flour, the Badui tribe of Java treat hair with packs of rice flour and milk (2).

Actually, proteins should have been a marginal, though constant, presence in the inventory of cosmetic ingredients of prehistoric communities and early civilized societies: animal fats, plant oils and extracts, and mineral pigments were definitely far more attractive and pleasing. Moreover only few materials containing a high level of proteins were available (egg, milk) and extraction technologies were limited to milk curdling and mechanical separation of egg white. The use of whole or curdled milk, egg whites, cereal flours, and few other raw protein materials was handed down through centuries with no significant changes until the beginning of the 20th century and the first rational uses of proteins in cosmetics dates to the 1950s.

A great deal of the early published information on the subject is of European origin but scientific and practical interest in this topic soon spread to the United States. The beneficial effects obtainable from the topical application of protein-rich substances were recognized, and proteins were soon considered useful ingredients for the establishment of a suitable environment for healthy skin and hair as the result of their ability to retain water. Further scientific investigations were carried out in the following years, and at the beginning of the 1960s the binding properties of proteins and peptides to skin and hair were explored and their potential role as hair-conditioning agents was suggested. For their substantivity, proteins were considered useful to impart gloss, softness, and manageability to the hair, and because of their amphoteric and buffering properties, the use of protein hydrolysates was proposed for permanent-waving treatments to prevent damage to hair fibers (3). The mechanisms of substantivity of protein hydrolysates and their protective effects in skin and hair detergency were then investigated and first attempts were made to elucidate the relationship between their molecular characteristics and cosmetic properties (4–10). Since those early pioneer works the role of protein ingredients in cosmetics was gradually consolidated, an assortment of modified proteins was developed to enhance their functionalities, and deeper understanding of their activities was attained. In the last years, the environmental/ecological concern and the growing public sentiment against the use of animal ingredients in cosmetics have been new driving forces in the research and development efforts on protein derivatives.

II. SOURCES AND MANUFACTURING

A. Animal, Vegetable, and Other Sources

The term ''protein'' includes a wide range of polymeric compounds varying from low to very high molecular weights, made up of one or more polypeptide chains, which in turn are composed of many amino acid residues linked together by a peptide bond. More complex proteins, conjugated proteins, are made of amino acids and other groups forming part of the molecule. Most of the amino acids found in nature are α-amino acids having an asymmetric carbon atom and the general formula R—CH(NH_2)COOH. Some 20 different amino acids, all having an L-configuration, have been isolated from proteins (Table 1).

Proteins (from the Greek word *proteios* = of primary importance) play dominant roles in almost all biological processes in living beings. Principal functions are: enzyme catalysis, transfer and accumulation of small molecules and ions, coordinated movement, mechanical support, immunity protection, production and transmission of nervous impulses, and control of growth and differentiation (11). A general classification of proteins based on their chemical composition is provided in Table 2.

Most protein derivatives for cosmetic purposes are obtained from simple proteins (fibrous and globular), while conjugated proteins (proteoglycans and nucleoprotein derivatives) are far less frequently used, mainly as low-purity extracts from animal and plant tissues.

With regard to the origin, both animals (mammals, fish) and plants (angiosperms) give suitable proteinaceous materials for the preparation of cosmetic ingredients; proteins obtained from inferior organisms (algae, fungi) have only recently gained some success.

Availability and low cost have so far been the principal criteria for the selection of the sources; to these factors, the increasing public aversion for animal-derived ingredients and ecological concerns have been added since the early 1980s.

1. *Animal Sources*

Collagen and other scleroproteins of animal tissues were the first and most successfully used in the modern cosmetics industry, and, in spite of the decreasing popularity of animal ingredients in the last decade, they continue to represent the major sources of protein derivatives in cosmetics.

Collagen is present in all multicellular organisms; it is the principal protein constituent of the connective tissues, skin, tendon, and bone. In the skin it represents 70% of the weight of the dermis.

The basic structural unit of collagen (tropocollagen) has a molecular mass of about 285 kDa and consists of three polypeptide chains of the same length (about 300 nm) having a regular helical shape (α-helix), wound round each other to form a triple helical coil. The amino acid composition of this protein is unique: one amino acid residue in every three is glycine and two hydroxylated amino acids, hydroxyproline and hydroxylysine, rarely found in other proteins, are present in a considerable amount. The sequence glycine-proline-hydroxyproline is frequently repeated over the polypeptide chains. The α-helical structure of each single chain is stabilized by regularly occurring hydrogen bonds between the CO group of the residue n and the NH group of the residue $(n + 4)$. The small dimension of glycine allows the narrow coiling of the helical turns and the three chains to come in close contact. The three helices are linked together by numerous cooperative hydrogen bonds between the NH peptide groups of glycine and CO groups of other residues. The hydroxyl groups of hydroxyproline residues are also involved in the formation of interchain hydrogen bonds and must play an important role in the stabilization of the triple helix, since its thermal stability is directly related to the hydroxyproline content (11).

Collagen is synthesized in the cytoplasm of fibroblasts as larger precursor molecules (procollagen) where the triple helix is linked at the N-terminal part with peptides poor in glycine and hydroxyproline and at the C-terminal part with cystine-containing peptides (Fig. 1). The role of these propeptides is to prevent premature formation of collagen fibers in the fibroblasts.

Procollagen monomers are then secreted in the extracellular matrix and the terminal peptides liberated by the action of specific proteases. In the intercellular fluid, tropocollagen molecules cross-link by formation of intermolecular covalent bonds between hydroxylysine residues, to form fibrils and larger fibers. The molecules of tropocollagen in the fibers are arranged in parallel and overlapped for about one-fourth of their length. By this reticulation process, insoluble fibers highly resistant to traction are formed, which are responsible for the mechanical properties of the connective tissues (11,13). Thus, three types of native collagen are present in the connective tissues: (1) neutrosoluble, nonreticulated tropocollagen, in very small amount, (2) acid-soluble collagen at the reticulating stage, comprising 10–15% of total collagen, and (3) mature polymerized collagen. Soluble collagen retaining the triple-helix structure can be extracted from the first two types. By denaturation or hydrolysis procedures larger quantities of collagenic substances can be obtained. Common sources for collagen extraction are bovine hides and bones, pigskin, and fish skin.

Elastin is a highly cross-linked, insoluble scleroprotein rich in nonpolar amino acids. Two types are known: type 1 from bovine neck ligaments (ligamentum nuchae), aorta, skin, and type 2 from cartilage. Elastin fibers are located in the connective tissues of those structures of the body that are subject to periodic and repeated stress, such as the walls of the major arteries (aorta), lungs, skin, and neck ligaments. After collagen, elastin is the most abundant constituent of the connective tissues; bovine neck ligaments contain about 70% of their protein as elastin. In the dermis its fibers form an elastic network of strongly hydrophobic polypeptide chains, cross-linked with one another by means of covalent bridges.

The amino acid composition of elastin is similar to that of collagen with regard to glycine and hydroxyproline content, but hydroxylysine is absent. Repeating sequences of

Table 1 Physiological Amino Acids Classified by Side-Chain Type

Side chain type	Side chain structure	Amino acid	Abbr.	MW	pK_{a1} α-COOH	pK_{a2} $\alpha\text{-}NH_3^+$	pK_{a3} side chain	Isoelectric point
Acid	$—CH_2—COOH$	Aspartic acid	Asp	113.10	2.10	9.82	3.86	2.98
	$—CH_2—CONH_2$	Asparagine	Asn	132.12	2.02	8.80		
	$—CH_2—CH_2—COOH$	Glutamic acid	Glu	147.13	2.10	9.47	4.07	3.08
	$—CH_2—CH_2—CONH_2$	Glutamine	Gln	146.15	2.17	9.13		
Hydrophobic	$—CH(CH_3)_2$	Valine	Val	117.15	2.29	9.72		6.00
	$—CH_2—CH(CH_3)_2$	Leucine	Leu	131.17	2.33	9.74		6.04
	$—CH(CH_3)—CH_2—CH_3$	Isoleucine	Ile	131.17	2.32	9.76		6.04
	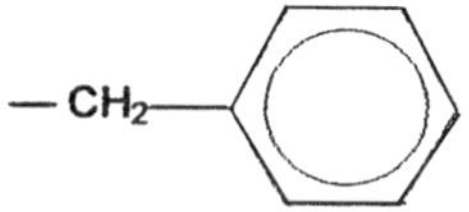	Phenylalanine	Phe	165.19	2.58	9.24		5.91
	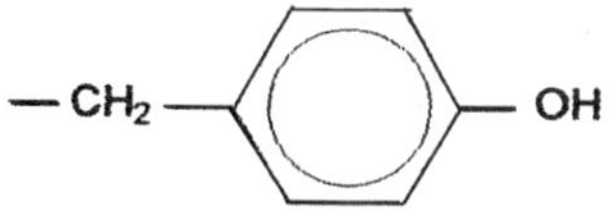	Tyrosine	Tyr	181.19	2.20	9.11	10.07	5.63
	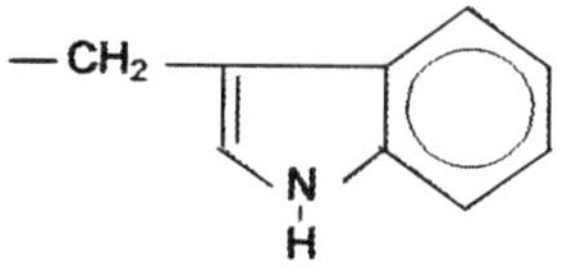	Tryptophan	Trp	204.22	2.38	9.39		5.88

	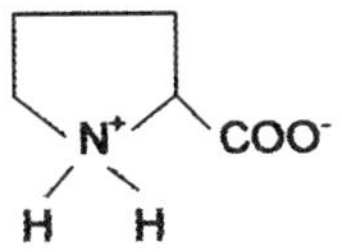	Proline	Pro	115.13	2.00	10.60		6.30
	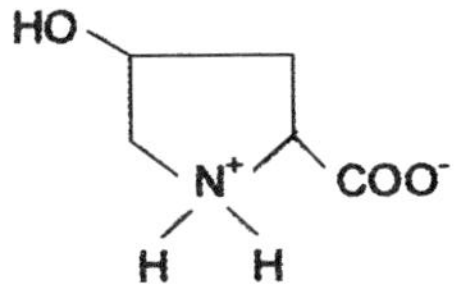	Hydroxyproline	OH-Pro	131.13	1.92	9.73		5.82
S-containing	—CH_2—CH_2—S—CH_3	Metionine	Met	149.21	2.28	9.21		5.74
	—CH_2—SH	Cysteine	Cys	121.16	1.80	10.80	8.33	
Basic	—CH_2—CH_2—CH_2—CH_2—NH_3^+	Lysine	Lys	146.19	2.18	8.95	10.53	9.74
	—CH_2—CH_2—CH(OH)—CH_2—NH_3^+	Hydroxylysine	OH-Lys	162.18				
	—CH_2—CH_2—CH2—NH—C(—NH_2)=NH_2^+	Arginine	Arg	174.20	2.01	9.04	12.48	10.76
	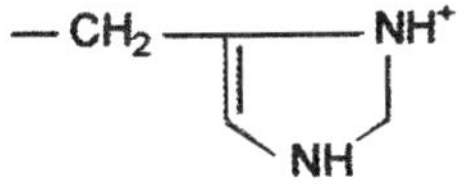	Histidine	His	155.16	1.77	9.18	6.10	7.64
Small netral	—H	Glycine	Gly	75.07	2.35	9.78		6.06
	—CH_3	Alanine	Ala	89.09	2.34	9.86		6.10
	—CH_2—OH	Serine	Ser	105.09	2.21	9.15		5.68
	—CH(OH)—CH_3	Threonine	Thr	119.12	2.15	9.12		5.64

Acidic ionization constants (water, 25°C) and pH values at the isoelectric points are reported.
Source: Refs. 11, 12.

Table 2 Classification of Major Protein Families on the Basis of Their Chemical Composition

Simple proteins (made only of amino acids)		Conjugated proteins (made of amino acids and other grouping substances)			
Fibrous (structural functions)	Globular (biological functions)	Nucleoproteins	Chromoproteins, metalloproteins	Glycoproteins	Lipoproteins
Collagen	Globulins	Deoxyribonucleins	Hemoglobins	Proteoglycans	Membrane proteins
Elastin	Albumins	Ribonucleins	Myoglobin	Fibroin	Blood lipoproteins
Keratins	Protamines		Cytochromes	Sericin	
Myosin	Istones		Enzymes	Extensin	
	Prolamines			Immunoglobulins	
	Enzymes				

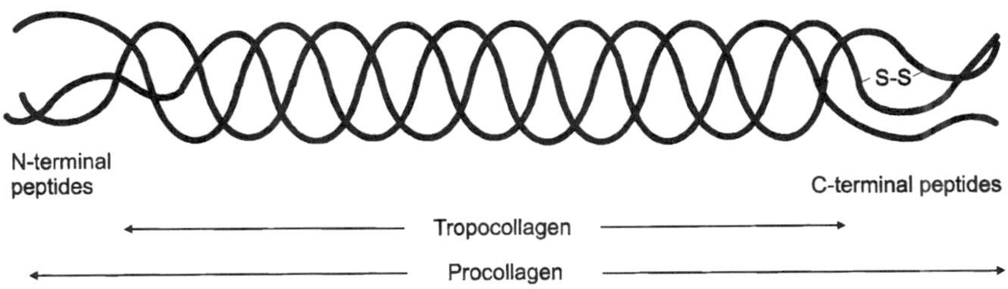

Figure 1 Schematic representation of the triple-helix structure of tropocollagen with the amorphous terminal peptides (telopeptides) of its precursor (procollagen).

valine-proline-glycine-valine are present in this protein, and thought to give a helical β-folded structure to the molecule, which would account for its elastic deformability. Elastin forms highly reticulated fibers by intermolecular condensation of two lysine residues (lysinonorleucine) or three (isodesmosine) or four (desmosine). Mature elastin contains many of these cross-linkages, which makes it insoluble and nonextractable in the native form (11,14). Soluble elastin, suitable for cosmetic use, is obtainable only as partial hydrolysate and is normally extracted from bovine nuchal ligaments. Powdered insoluble elastin, obtained by fine-grinding defatted and dried ligaments, is also of use in decorative cosmetics.

In spite of its animal origin, the use of keratin derivatives in cosmetics is generally well accepted by the supporters of animal rights as the protein can be obtained without cruelty from wool and hairs.

Mammalian keratins consist of filaments about 7 mm in diameter, embedded in a nonfilamentous matrix. The filaments are composed of helical structures of relatively low sulfur content (α-keratins); the matrix consists of two groups of nonhelical proteins, one cystine rich (18–45%, β-keratins), the second rich in glycine and tyrosine (γ-keratins). The high content of cystine residues is considered to be the special characteristic of keratins. While the individual peptide chains have molecular weights of the order of 50,000 Daltons, cross-linking of peptide chains by disulfide bridges results in huge aggregates having molecular weights of many millions, highly insoluble and resistant to the action of chemicals and enzymes (15). Major sources for keratin extraction include poultry feathers, animal hoofs and horns, wool, and human hair.

Milk was probably the first proteinaceous cosmetic ingredient used. Milk proteins are composed of about 80% casein, an acidic phosphoprotein present as colloidal dispersion, and a soluble protein fraction composed of lactalbumine and lactoglubulins, which are found in milk serum after acid precipitation of casein. These three protein substances are useful as cosmetic ingredients as partial hydrolysates (casein, lactalbumin) or in native form (lactoglobulin).

Silk is a continuous protein filament secreted by special glands located in the head of the silkworm (larva of the *Bombix mori*). The special structure of the silk fiber is made of two distinct strands of fibroin, coated and connected by a second protein (sericin) exuding from other glands together with fibroin. When emerging into air, this secretion is rapidly coagulated, forming a continuous, insoluble film. Silk powder, whole silk protein hydrolysates, and sericin hydrolysates are the most common silk derivatives used in cosmetics. Fibroin is a glycoprotein formed of two subunits of 370 and 25 kDa connected by disulfide bonds. It is mainly composed of three amino acids, glycine, alanine, and serine, in the ratio 3:2:1, forming repeating sequences of six residues (Gly-Ser-Gly-Ala-

Gly-Ala) over the polypeptide chain. This particular sequence allows the protein to resume a β-antiparallel, pleated-sheet structure, which is responsible for the flexibility and mechanical resistance of the silk fiber (11,13). As silk is composed of about 70–80% fibroin, products obtained by hydrolysis of whole silk are mainly fragments of fibroin. The second protein of silk, sericin, is a group of glycoproteins with a small carbohydrate content of about 3% and composed of five to six principal species having molecular masses between 65 and 400 kDa. It is particularly rich in hydroxylated amino acids and serine alone represents about 33% of total residues. The carbohydrate moiety and the hydroxylated amino acids are considered to be responsible for the binding and coating of fibroin fibrils by sericin. Because of the binding properties of sericin and in analogy with its function of coating polymer in the silk fiber, sericin derivatives have been proposed as protective film formers and conditioning agents in hair care cosmetics (16,17). In the first step of silk fabric processing, sericin is removed from the raw fiber by washing with tenside or enzyme solutions, or using hot water under pressure (degumming). Large amounts of sericin-containing wastes (0.5–2% sericin) are therefore available for sericin recovery and processing to cosmetic raw materials.

Besides collagen, elastin, keratin, milk, and silk protein derivatives, originating from low-cost and largely available materials, a variety of more specific animal proteins have been used in cosmetic products, including reticulin and fibronectin (two of the specialized proteins linking the cells of the connective tissues to the collagen fibers of the extracellular matrix), used as partial hydrolysates, and proteoglycan extracts. Proteoglycans are complex glycoproteins of the connective tissues made of long, complex polysaccharides (glycosaminoglycans) held together by a small part of protein, which possess extraordinary water-binding capacity and are responsible for the viscoelastic properties of anatomical joints and other tissues subject to mechanical stress. Any solid scientific evidence supporting a cosmetic effect of these particular ingredients, related to their biological functions in the living tissues, is missing.

Raw extracts from animal tissues and organs like thymus, placenta, heart, and bone marrow have also been of use in cosmetics; part of their cosmetic functions are attributed to their protein content.

A recent and promising chapter on the use of proteins in cosmetics is related to enzymes. Two distinct categories of application can be considered: the use of proteases as cleansing and skin-purifying agents based on the proteolytic action on skin keratins and sweat proteins, and the use of specific enzymes like superoxide dismutase to promote a biological effect in the skin, provided they can reach the site of action by topical delivery. To these, recent use of enzymes (glucose oxidase and lactoperoxidase) as bacteriostatic agents must be mentioned.

2. Vegetable Sources

Animal protein materials are widely available at low cost and high purity as by-products and solid wastes from slaughterhouses and tanneries, which, unless used in cosmetics, would contribute to the environmental problem. This has been one of the reasons for their success as cosmetic ingredients, but perhaps more important factors are the presence of the same proteins in human skin and connective tissues and their vital role in skin and hair physiology, which seemed to rationalize their use in topical products. Nevertheless, since all proteins, whatever their source, are polymers of the same 20 natural amino acids, there should not be big differences between animal and vegetable proteins for use as cosmetic ingredients. Though this is entirely true only for proteins that have lost their spatial architecture, such as hydrolyzed, low-molecular-weight peptides, the overall low specificity of the cosmetic activity of proteins contributed to the addition of vegetable and plant proteins to skin and hair care preparations. In the last decade vegetable proteins have become very popular as sources of cosmetic ingredients, a trend strongly supported by consumers' increasing repudiation of animal-derived ingredients and the desire to use renewable and environmentally friendly resources. Furthermore, increasing quantities of vegetable proteins from cereal grains and oilseeds have become available on the world market of food ingredients as high-purity isolates and concentrates, with a low content of carbohydrates and other extraneous substances, perfectly suitable for processing to cosmetic raw materials.

In higher vegetable organisms large amounts of proteins are concentrated in seeds as reserve materials to be used by the young plant in the first stages of growth. These are mainly insoluble proteins (globulins, prolamines), water insolubility being necessary to prevent their depletion when in the ground. Flours from cereal grains (wheat, oat, rice, corn) and defatted oilseeds (soy, peanut, sunflower, almond, sesame) are cheap and widely available sources of vegetable proteins. Oilseed globulins are usually rich in lysine and low in methionine and cysteine, whereas cereal proteins are generally low in lysine while containing a considerable amount of sulfur amino acids. High-protein vegetable materials most commonly used as starting substances for the manufacture of cosmetic ingredients are wheat and corn gluten (protein content 60–80%), soy, rice, and oat protein concentrate (70% protein) and isolate (90% protein), defatted oilseeds (35–50% protein), and a variety of other protein-containing materials from lupine, fava bean, grape seeds, sesame, and so forth.

Leaves and subterranean plant organs are additional sources of protein materials. Potato proteins are largely available as a by-product of the starch extraction. A promising source of soluble proteins is represented by the leaves of many species: leaves contain about 80–90% water and 10–20% organic material, a small part of this (10–30%) is made of proteins. About 50% of the proteins are water soluble and can be extracted and purified as a crystalline protein fraction with a molecular weight in the range 10–60 kDa, suitable for food and cosmetic purposes (leaf protein concentrate) (18).

Of the variety of vegetable proteins from which cosmetic ingredients are obtained, wheat gluten and soy proteins are of the widest use and interest.

Wheat gluten is a unique cereal protein owing to its property of high elasticity when hydrated. This elasticity allows the formation of gas cells in flour dough and is the main factor responsible for the texture of bread. Wheat gluten is a protein-lipid-carbohydrate complex, formed when flour is hydrated; when the starch is washed away with more water, the gluten coheres as an elastic, insoluble, rubber-like mass, which can be dried to give a cream-colored powder (19). The major proteins responsible for the properties of gluten may be fractionated into two components: gliadin, which is soluble in neutral 70% ethanol, and glutenin, the alcohol-insoluble component. Gliadin consists mainly of many different single-chain proteins of relatively low molecular weight (25–150 kDa) whose conformations are stabilized by intramolecular disulfide bonds. Glutenin is made of subunits of many sizes, joined through disulfide bonds into proteins with molecular weights ranging into the millions (20). Similarities between glutenin's subunits and gliadin molecules have led to the theory that glutenin consists, at least in part, of gliadin-like subunits joined by intermolecular disulfide bonds (21,22) (Fig. 2).

The low solubility of gluten proteins has been attributed to their high molecular weight, the presence of interpolypeptide —SS— bonds, and the cooperative hydrophobic

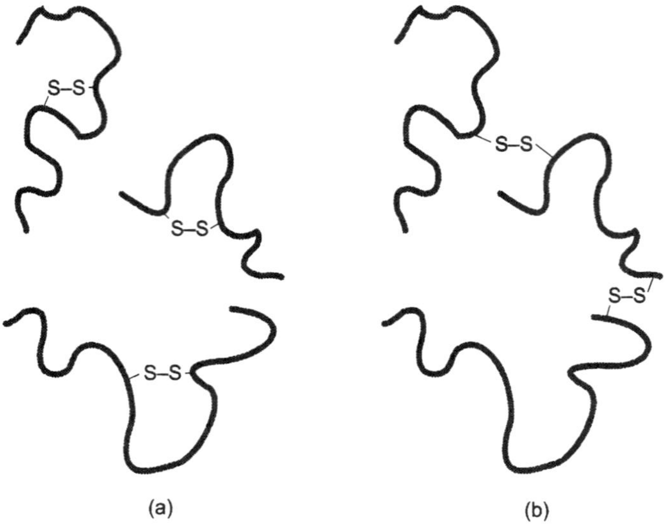

Figure 2 Location of stabilizing disulfide bonds (schematic) in the two main fractions of wheat gluten proteins: (a) gliadin and (b) glutenin.

interactions that cause the protein chains to resume a folded shape. The amino acid profile of wheat gluten fractions includes as major components glutamic acid (33–40% on a molar basis) and hydroxyproline (13–15%); cysteine residues are reported to be 2% in gliadin and 1.5% in glutenin. Sulfide-disulfide interchange reactions occurring in hydrated gluten are reported to be responsible for the rheological behavior of dough (23) and are one of the mechanisms of the cosmetic activity of its derivatives.

Soy isolate (90% protein) is the main industrial source for soy protein transformation into cosmetic ingredients. It is obtained from undenatured, defatted soy flour by dissolving the flour in dilute alkali (pH 8), removing the insoluble materials by centrifugation or filtration, and final precipitation of the proteins at their isoelectric point (pH 4.5). The major components of soy proteins are classified according to their sedimentation properties. Approximately 90% of them are storage globulins (glycinine, the 11S globulin, and conglycinin, the 7S globulin), with molecular weights ranging from 20 to 400 kDa. Constituent polypeptides form α-helix, β-structure, and random coils; subunits are aggregates by —SS—, hydrogen, and hydrophobic bonds. Undenatured soy proteins are widely used as food ingredients and for their gelling, whipping, emulsificating, and lipid-absorbing properties (24).

Several different protein derivatives from oilseeds (peanuts, almond, sunflower), cereals (corn, rice, oat), and a miscellany of other vegetable sources (potato, lupine, cottonseed, fava bean) have also been proposed for use in cosmetics. Nearly all these derivatives are hydrolysates, and as their amino acid composition is similar, they should not have any advantage over traditional wheat and soy protein derivatives. Corn proteins, rich in sulfur amino acids (Met+½Cys > 5%), oat proteins, and almond proteins are the most useful in this group.

Source vegetable proteins used for the preparation of cosmetic ingredients are usually complex mixtures of several different molecular species with variable size and conformation. An exception to the rule is a group of vegetable proteins containing a high percentage of hydroxyproline residues, which has recently raised the interest of cosmetic chemists for its affinity to animal collagen. They are glycoproteins composed of 40% carbohydrate and with about 10% hydroxyproline in the protein moiety. The carbohydrate part is mainly composed of arabinose and galactose. Early work on these plant proteins dates to 1960 (25). It was found that a protein with high hydroxyproline content was located in the cell wall of different plant species, and the first hypotheses on its physiological role were presented. Because of its similarities with collagen and elastin it was thought to be a tissue growth factor and given the name "extensin." Several different theories were later advanced: it has been proposed to have a role in the process stopping cell growth (supported by observations that accumulation of extensin occurs when the elongation process of the stem in different plants ceases), and a role in the response of plants to physical injuries and microbial contamination. Histochemical studies have confirmed that extensin is a component of the cell wall, whose rigidity and resistance to physical stress are due to the tight network of insoluble polysaccharide fibers linked in a protein matrix. Extensin seems to be the principal linking cement protein in this structure, and it shows functional analogies with the interconnective proteins of animal organisms (fibronectin, reticulin), rather than with collagen.

The molecule of extensin has a molecular weight of about 200 kDa (including the carbohydrate fraction) and it is likely to form a helical structure as the result of the numerous hydroxyproline and glycine residues, similarly to collagen. Major constituent amino acids are serine (18%), glycine (12%), lysine (12%), and hydroxyproline (10%). Extraction of native extensin from the cell wall of higher plants presents great difficulties because of probable formation of covalent attachments with other macromolecules, and only small glycopeptide fragments can be obtained, whereas larger polypeptides are extractable from Cyanophyceae and other species of algae. As a cosmetic ingredient it is available as partial hydrolysate with molecular weights in the range 1,000–50,000 Daltons with a significant content of carbohydrates. It is offered as an alternative to animal collagen for its film-forming and moisturizing effects. A positive smoothing effect on the skin has also been reported (26).

The amino acid composition of the principal source proteins of cosmetic interest is shown in Table 3.

B. Extraction, Hydrolysis, Derivatization

More than a hundred different proteins and protein derivatives are listed in the *International Cosmetic Ingredient Dictionary*, 6th edition, 1995 (29) (Table 4).

Unmodified proteins are a small minority; most of them are partial hydrolysates and condensation derivatives. Full naturalness is maintained only for a few pure molecules (soluble collagen, serum albumin) and probably for proteins contained in organ and tissue total extracts (not included in the table). The majority of protein ingredients for cosmetics can only be said to be natural-derived materials, having undergone a more or less extended degree of chemical manipulation. Protein hydrolysates are prepared to gain protein solubility and retain part of the natural character of the original substances, being composed only of amino acids; alkylated and acylated proteins are semisynthetic derivatives designed to enhance cosmetic performance and benefit and conserving little of the naturalness of the parent protein.

The principal procedures adopted to obtain useful protein materials, suitable for cosmetic use, and the features of the resulting products are reviewed in the following sections.

Table 3 Amino Acid Composition of the Principal Source Proteins of Cosmetic Interest

		Collagen (gelatin)	Elastin (bovine nuchal ligaments)	Keratin (human hair)	Silk (fibroin)	Silk (sericin)	Wheat gluten	Soy (flour protein)	Corn (protein isolate)	Casein	Yeast protein
Nitrogen-to-protein factor, f_N		5.55	5.55	6.25	5.8	6.65	5.7	6.25	6.25	6.38	6.5
Amino acid composition in g free acid per 100g ($N \times f_N$)											
Acid side chains	Asp	6.6	0.9	4.9	1.5	14.5	3.3	12.3	6.4	7.1	9.7
	Glu	11.4	2.4	11.4	1.5	6.0	40.2	19.7	25.6	22.0	14.3
Hydrophobic side chains	Val	2.6	15.7	5.8	3.0	3.8	4.6	5.0	5.0	6.7	7.4
	Leu	3.4	8.3	5.8	1.0	2.9	7.4	8.0	18.9	9.5	8.4
	Ile	1.7	3.3	2.6	1.0	1.6	4.4	5.1	4.6	5.4	5.3
	Phe	2.3	4.8	1.6	1.0	1.0	5.6	5.0	6.9	5.2	4.2
	Tyr	0.2	1.1	2.0	5.0	1.5	3.9	3.6	5.4	5.8	3.8
	Trp	0.0	0.0	0.0	0.0	0.0	1.1	1.3	0.5	1.7	1.3
	Pro	16.5	14.5	8.4	1.0	1.0	14.2	5.3	10.6	11.6	5.7
	OH-Pro	14.4	3.0	0.0	0.0	0.0	0.0	0.0	0.0	0.0	0.0
S-containing side chains	Met	0.8	traces	0.6	1.0	1.0	1.7	1.2	2.8	2.8	2.9
	Cys	traces	traces	17.8	1.0	1.0	2.3	1.2	2.0	0.4	1.4

Basic side chains	Lys	4.7	0.6	2.7	1.0	3.0	1.5	6.2	1.5	8.1	7.6
	OH-Lys	1.0	0.0	0.0	0.0	0.0	0.0	0.0	0.0	0.0	0.0
	Arg	8.9	1.0	5.8	1.0	3.7	3.2	7.2	2.7	3.8	6.3
	His	0.8	0.0	0.9	1.0	1.0	2.3	2.5	1.9	2.9	2.3
Small neutral side chains	Gly	27.6	25.6	6.4	44.0	16.5	3.4	4.2	2.8	2.0	4.8
	Ala	11.3	20.3	4.6	30.0	7.1	2.7	4.4	9.9	3.1	7.6
	Ser	4.2	0.8	11.7	12.0	28.4	5.3	5.1	5.6	6.0	5.1
	Thr	2.3	0.8	6.8	1.0	6.4	2.7	4.0	3.6	4.7	4.6
Weight fractions											
% acid		14.9	3.2	16.3	2.8	20.4	39.6	31.6	27.4	26.8	23.4
% hydrophobic		34.1	49.1	26.3	11.2	11.8	37.5	32.8	44.5	42.2	35.1
% S-containing		0.7	0.0	18.4	1.9	2.0	3.6	2.4	4.1	2.9	4.1
% basic		12.8	1.6	9.4	2.8	7.7	6.4	15.6	5.2	13.6	15.7
% small		37.6	46.1	29.6	81.3	58.2	12.9	17.5	18.8	14.4	21.5
MW of amino acids		109	106	118	90	107	132	131	128	132	1125
Theoretical hydrophobicity $H\Phi_{ave}$ (cal/mole)		798	1008	741	293	245	945	890	1064	1135	953

Percent weight fractions of amino acids with different chain type and average molecular weight of amino acids are also reported. Theoretical hydrophobicity values are calculated by the authors following Δf_t values given in Ref. 65 (see Section III.A.4).

Source: Refs. 15, 17, 27, 28.

Table 4 Tentative List of Protein Ingredients for Cosmetics

Nonhydrolyzed proteins
Albumen; atelocollagen; calcium caseinate; casein; collagen; corn gluten proteins; cytochrome C; desamido collagen; elastin; keratin; lactoglobulin; milk protein; oat protein; reticulin; sericin; serum albumin; serum protein; silk; sodium caseinate; soluble collagen; sweet almond protein; wheat germ protein; wheat germ gluten; wheat protein; whey protein; zein
Hydrolyzed proteins
Ammonium hydrolyzed collagen; gelatin; hydrolyzed (actin, albumen, casein, collagen, conchiorin, corn protein, elastin, fibronectin, gadidae protein, hair keratin, hemoglobin, human placental protein, keratin, lactalbumin, lupine protein, milk protein, oat protein, pea protein, placental protein, potato protein, reticulin, rice bran protein, serum protein, silk, soy protein, spinal protein, sweet almond protein, vegetable protein, wheat gluten, wheat protein, yeast protein, zein); MEA-hydrolyzed (collagen, silk); zinc hydrolyzed collagen
Quaternized proteins
Cocamidopropyl dimethylaminohydroxypropyl hydrolyzed collagen; cocamidopropyl dimethylammonium C_8–C_{16} isoalkylsuccinyl lactoglobulin sulfonate; cocamidopropyldimonium hydroxypropyl hydrolyzed collagen; cocodimonium hydroxypropyl hydrolyzed casein; cocodimonium hydroxypropyl hydrolyzed (collagen, hair keratin, keratin, rice protein, silk, soy protein, wheat protein); hydroxypropyltrimonium (gelatin, hydrolyzed casein, hydrolyzed collagen, hydrolyzed keratin, hydrolyzed rice bran protein, hydrolyzed silk, hydrolyzed soy protein, hydrolyzed wheat protein); lauryldimonium hydroxypropyl hydrolyzed (wheat protein, casein, collagen, keratin, silk, soy protein); oleamidopropyldimonium hydroxypropyl hydrolyzed collagen; quaternium-79 hydrolyzed (collagen, keratin, milk protein, silk, soy protein, wheat protein); steardimonium hydroxypropyl hydrolyzed (casein, collagen, keratin, rice protein, silk, vegetable protein, wheat protein); steartrimonium hydroxyethyl hydrolyzed collagen; triethonium hydrolyzed collagen ethosulfate; wheat germamidopropyldimonium hydroxypropyl hydrolyzed wheat protein
Condensates
AMP-isostearoyl hydrolyzed collagen; AMP-isostearoyl hydrolyzed soy protein; AMP-isostearoyl hydrolyzed wheat protein; capryloyl hydrolyzed collagen; capryloyl hydrolyzed keratin; cocoyl hydrolyzed (collagen, keratin, soy protein); ethyl ester of hydrolyzed (animal protein, keratin, silk); hydrolyzed wheat protein/dimetichone copolyol phosphate); hydrolyzed wheat protein hydroxypropyl polysiloxane; iodized corn protein; iodized hydrolyzed zein; isostearoyl hydrolyzed collagen; myristoyl hydrolyzed collagen; oleoyl hydrolyzed collagen; palmitoyl hydrolyzed (collagen, milk protein, wheat protein); potassium abietoyl hydrolyzed collagen; Potassium cocoyl hydrolyzed (casein; collagen; keratin rice bran protein; silk; soy protein; wheat protein); potassium lauroyl hydrolyzed (collagen, soy protein); potassium mirystoyl hydrolyzed collagen; potassium oleoyl hydrolyzed collagen; potassium stearoyl hydrolyzed collagen; potassium undecylenoyl hydrolyzed collagen; Rosin hydrolyzed collagen; sodium soy hydrolyzed collagen; sodium cocoyl hydrolyzed (collagen, keratin, rice protein, soy protein, wheat protein); sodium lauroyl hydrolyzed (collagen, silk); sodium myristoyl hydrolyzed collagen; sodium oleoyl hydrolyzed collagen; sodium stearoyl hydrolyzed collagen; sodium succinoyl gelatin; sodium/TEA-lauroyl hydrolyzed (collagen, keratin); sodium/TEA-undecylenoyl hydrolyzed collagen; sulfurized hydrolyzed (corn protein, zein); TEA-cocoyl hydrolyzed (collagen, soy protein); TEA-isostearyl hydrolyzed collagen; TEA-lauroyl hydrolyzed collagen; TEA-myristoyl hydrolyzed collagen; TEA-oleoyl hydrolyzed collagen; TEA-undecylenoyl hydrolyzed collagen; undecylenoyl hydrolyzed collagen
Enzymes
Amylase; bromelain; catalase; glucose oxidase; lactoperoxidase; lipase; papain; pepsin; superoxide dismutase; urease

Ingredients are classified into five main categories. Protein-containing materials such as thymus extract and mixtures are not reported.

Source: Extracted from Ref. 29.

1. Extraction

Materials employed for the manufacture of protein cosmetic ingredients include a variety of raw animal and plant organs and tissues where protein substances are present together with many other ingredients. Extraction and fractionation procedures are requested to obtain high-purity proteins in the native form, directly suitable for use in cosmetics or for further derivatization.

Preliminary extraction and purification steps are in many cases performed in routine industrial processing for the preparation of food ingredients, giving high-protein-content materials (wheat gluten, soy isolate, gelatin, casein), which are used as starting substances by manufacturers of cosmetic ingredients. Other unrefined materials, like bovine hidesplits, bones, horns and hoofs, pigskin, poultry feathers, sericin wastes, cereal flours, and oil-extraction residues of oilseeds, may be specifically processed for the preparation of cosmetic-quality derivatives. Finally, raw total extracts in aqueous or hydroglycolic vehicles are obtained from animal and vegetable organs and tissues rich in proteins, with little or no further purification. Extraction of soluble protein material is often performed by denaturation and hydrolysis procedures discussed below.

Isolation and purification procedures greatly differ for the various proteins and are too heterogeneous to be exhaustively reviewed here; only extraction of native soluble collagen from bovine dermis is briefly described.

Major sources of collagen for cosmetic purposes are untanned hidesplits and skin trimmings largely available in tanneries and slaughterhouses. During the processing of hides and skins for conversion into various types of leather, huge quantities of solid wastes such as raw hide/skin trimmings, fleshing, leather shavings, and other wastes found at various stages of pretanning and posttanning operations are available. Collagen in these materials is in its native form without much decomposition or much change in the protein structure. Residual keratinous matter and fat must be removed to obtain high-quality, soluble collagen preparations (30).

As in the maturation process collagen changes progressively from a monomeric neutrosoluble form to less soluble polymerized fibers, only a small part of collagen is obtainable in the native and soluble form. The relative amount of soluble collagen extractable from bovine skin corium decreases with increasing biological age: the citrate-soluble collagen content of 18-month steer skin is 10 times lower than in corium fetal skin (31). Thus, hides of young cattle are preferred for the preparation of cosmetic collagen.

The general procedure consists of preliminary removal of the hair, pretreatment with diluted alkali solution, to remove fats and carbohydrates, and extraction with aqueous citrate buffer (pH 3–4) containing variable amounts of sodium chloride or other salts to give a medium of appropriate ionic strength. Alkaline pretreatment and acid extraction should be mild enough to prevent disruption of the triple-helix structure by breakage of the stabilizing hydrogen bonds. By the slightly acidic treatment partial hydrolysis of the linkages that interconnect the terminal regions of tropocollagen occurs and soluble collagen is obtained. Yields of soluble collagen can vary from less than 1% to about 10% for alkali and neutral salt extractable material and up to 20% for acid extraction. The solution obtained can be colorless or milky depending on the concentration of collagen and the extent of residue cross-linking of the collagen molecules. Dialysis is sometimes used to remove excess electrolytes from the extract, although moderate ionic strength must be maintained for best stability of the final solution. Partial deamidation of asparagine and glutamine residues is performed by proper adjustment of the alkaline treatment, resulting in a more hydrophilic and soluble derivative (desamido collagen) that still retains the triple-helical structure. Other extraction methods can be used to obtain the fibrous form of collagen: by lyophilization of fibrous collagen dispersion compresses and sheets of polymerized collagen are prepared, which can be directly applied to the skin to give moisturization and sheen.

Fishes are a profitable source of native collagen since, in contrast to mammalian collagens, the extractability of the fish skin collagen in acid is higher and does not change significantly with age in many species. Soluble collagen obtained from fish is cheaper than the bovine-originated product; it has, however, lower stability to thermal denaturation (see Section III.A.6).

2. *Hydrolysis*

Because of their poor water solubility (the main technical requisite for the use of proteins in cosmetic formulations) and the difficulty of extraction from the matrix, most proteins are unsuitable for use in the manufacture of cosmetic preparations in the form in which they occur in nature. Only a few native proteins, such as collagen, serum albumin, and enzymes, can be isolated as soluble native proteins. To make proteins suitable for use in water-based cosmetic products and in a wide range of applications, natural proteins need to be converted into a soluble form; this is usually attained by the hydrolysis procedure, i.e., cleavage of the protein macromolecule by disruption of some of the peptide bonds.

Hydrolysis of the peptide bond proceeds rapidly and efficiently only when activated by a chemical (acidic or alkaline) or biological (enzymatic) catalysis, or when a combination of temperature and pressure is applied (Fig. 3).

Besides obvious considerations about the cost of the process, the choice of the activation mechanism depends chiefly on the desired degree of hydrolysis and prevailing charge of the resulting peptide mixture. It is, however, remarkable that the quality and performance of the products obtained are strictly related to the type and characteristics of the hydrolytic process (32).

Chemical hydrolysis is carried out in presence of a given concentration of hydrogen ions (acidic hydrolysis) or hydroxyl ions (alkaline hydrolysis); in acidic catalysis a nucleophilic attack of the water molecules on the protonated amide occurs; in alkaline hydrolysis the highly nucleophilic hydroxyl ion OH^- is directly involved in the cleavage mechanism. The speed and yield of reaction can be improved by providing kinetic energy in form of heat. The number of peptide bonds cleaved per mole of protein, i.e., the average size of resulting peptides, can be controlled through three important variables: concentration of H^+/OH^-, temperature, duration of the process.

In spite of the advantage represented by its low cost, chemical hydrolysis has several negative aspects that impair the final quality of the product. A first drawback, common to acidic and alkaline hydrolysis, is the very low specificity of the cleavage: hydrogen and hydroxyl ions do not distinguish one peptide bond from another, or do so minimally,

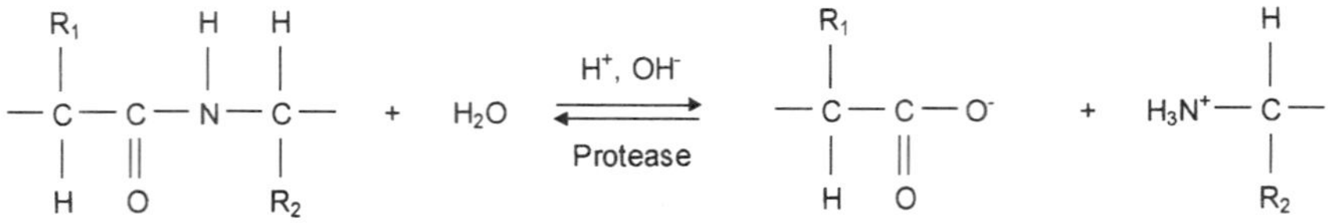

Figure 3 Cleavage of the peptide bond by acid, alkaline, or enzymatic hydrolysis.

and operate with almost equal probability along the protein chain, almost irrespective of the type of amino acids linked. Cleavage is only facilitated in the terminal positions of the chain because of the higher steric availability of the peptide bonds in this position, and the attack on the last peptide bond is slightly thermodynamically favored because of the liberation of a highly soluble free amino acid. The products of chemical hydrolysis always contain a variable amount of free amino acids and the molecular weight range of the resulting peptides is usually wider than for enzymatic hydrolysis.

A second negative consequence of chemical (acidic) hydrolysis is the occurrence of Maillard condensation between peptides and carbohydrates (often present in the starting protein materials), which gives dark-colored products, pungent in odor, hardly acceptable for cosmetic use. Moreover, protein derivatives obtained by chemical hydrolysis have a high content of inorganic salts, which generally have undesirable effects on the skin and make their powder preparations highly hygroscopic.

Strongly alkaline treatments can cause degradation of some amino acids and formation of nonphysiological, potentially toxic molecules. Some of these transformations occur through dehydroalanine, a reactive molecule that is formed via β-elimination of H_2S from cysteine or via dehydration of serine. Dehydroalanine can condense with the ε-amino group of lysine, whereby the unnatural amino acid lysinoalanine is formed, or react with a second molecule of cysteine to give lanthionine (Fig. 4) (33,34).

Apart from the unknown dermatological effects of these nonphysiological molecules, loss of cysteine and serine occurs, with alteration of the amino acid composition of the natural source protein. Other unnatural amino acids such as ornitinoalanine and β-aminoalanine can be formed when proteins are exposed to high pH values and/or high temperatures (35).

Finally, acidic and alkaline treatments cause deamidation of the amino acids asparagine and glutamine; the resulting amino acids are still natural (aspartic and glutamic acid), but formation of an additional negative charge for each $-NH_2$ group removed will occur, with consequent lowering of the average isoelectric point of the product, and free NH_3 is released in the product.

The problems occurring with the chemical hydrolysis of proteins can be reduced by appropriate process controlling, or partially corrected by posthydrolysis treatments (free NH_3 formed by deamidation can be removed by ultrafiltration). In spite of its limitations, chemical hydrolysis is the preferred method when a very high degree of hydrolysis is

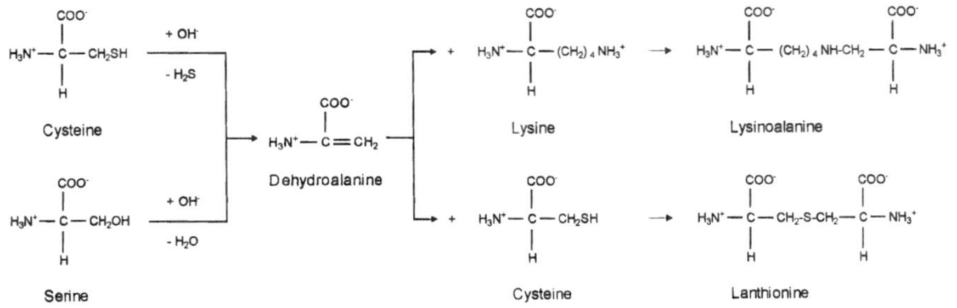

Figure 4 Chemical route of formation of nonphysiological amino acids by exposure of cysteine and serine to alkali. Lysinoalanine is formed by condensation of the reactive intermediate dehydroalanine with the ε-amino group in lysine; lanthionine results from the condensation of dehydroalanine with cysteine.

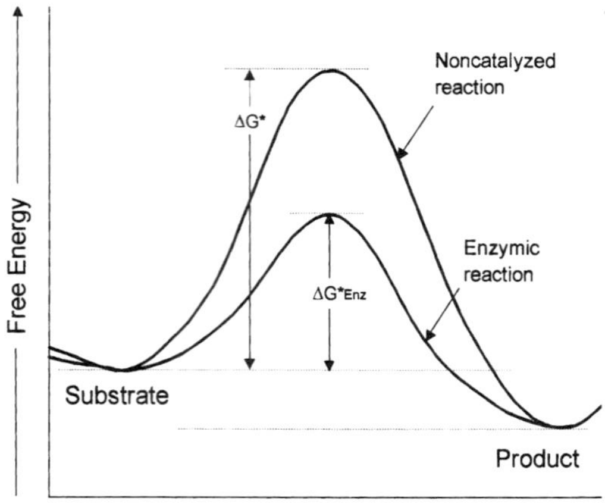

Figure 5 Schematic profiles of the Gibbs free energy of activation ΔG^* of a noncatalyzed and an enzyme-catalyzed reaction. Enzymes are able to lower the ΔG^* of a chemical reaction via an alternative, more favorable mechanism, based on the formation of a specific enzyme-substrate complex.

wanted (not attainable with enzymatic hydrolysis, which barely gives a final product with average molecular weight <500 Daltons), or when complete hydrolysis, with total liberation of free amino acids, is to be reached.*

When chemical hydrolysis is used for the preparation of soluble proteins for cosmetics, acidic treatment is preferred to alkaline for two main reasons: (1) the average isoelectric point of the peptides obtained is lower than after alkaline processing (36,37) (deamidation is favored in alkali), and (2) degradation of amino acids is easier to avoid.

Cleavage of the peptide bond can be obtained by biological catalysis (enzymatic hydrolysis), which allows operating at pH values close to neutrality and temperatures approaching those of living beings, with the important advantage of preventing possible degradation of amino acids and formation of hazardous by-products. The resulting products are light in odor and color and generally better accepted for use in cosmetic preparations than the relevant chemical derivatives.

Like all catalysts, proteolytic enzymes (specific proteins obtained from animals, vegetables, or, more extensively, from microbial cultures) do not shift the reaction equilibrium. Enzymes are able to open an alternative pathway, with a lower energy barrier, and accelerate the hydrolysis by lowering the free energy of the transition state (Fig. 5) (11).

The nucleophilic attack on the carbonilic carbon atom of the peptide bond is facilitated by a specific interaction of the enzyme with the side chains of adjacent amino acids and formation of an enzyme-substrate complex. This complex offer an exposed and activated peptide bond to water molecules or OH^- ions, and hydrolysis is facilitated. The result of the catalysis is an acceleration of the reaction by a factor of 10^5–10^{20}.

The mechanism of catalysis of most proteases can be summarized in three steps as follows (38).

* Preparation and cosmetic properties of free amino acids are not covered in this chapter.

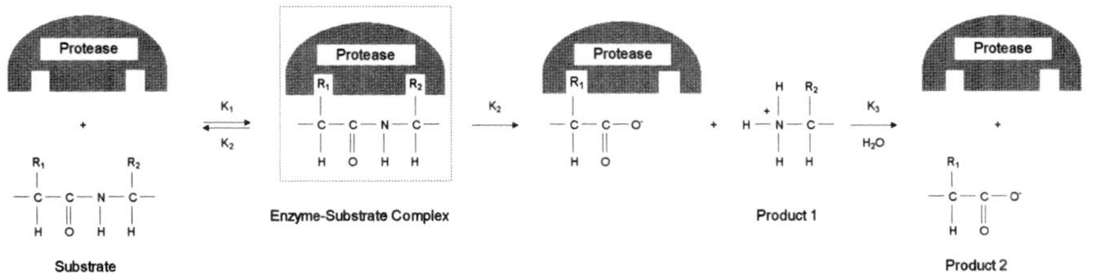

Figure 6 Enzymatic catalysis of proteolysis. The overall reaction rate is determined by K_2 and the Michaelis-Menten constant K_m is approximately equal to the dissociation constant K_2/K_1 of the enzyme-substrate complex (38).

1. Formation of the Michaelis complex between the original peptide chain (substrate) and the enzyme
2. Cleavage of the peptide bond to liberate one of the two resulting peptides
3. Nucleophilic attack on the remainder of the complex to split off the second peptide and to reconstitute the free enzyme (Fig. 6)

The deacylation step, i.e., the second of the three reactions, is the rate-determining step. Concerning the third and last step, it must be emphasized that free amino groups of peptides can act as nucleophiles and compete with H_2O to give the alternative reaction illustrated in Figure 7.

This competitive reaction (transpeptidation) determines a change in the amino acid sequence of the original protein. The transpeptidation scarcely occurs in acidic environment, because at low pH values the terminal amino groups are almost totally protonated and have no nucleophilic character; the same is true at high pH values, because in this case the strongest nucleophilic species present is the hydroxyl ion OH^-, much more reactive than amino groups. At pH values close to neutrality the enzyme can easily catalyze the transpeptidation, because although the hydrolysis is favored by the high concentration of H_2O, the nucleophilic attack by free amino groups proceeds many times faster (39). This can have the important practical consequence of the resynthesis of longer insoluble peptides, which can form haze and precipitate in the solutions of protein hydrolysates and their preparations, and is one of the main reasons that complete inactivation of the enzyme (or use of immobilized enzymes, easily removable and reusable) is required after completion of the process.

Enzymatic activity is pH and temperature dependent; activity curves are given for each particular enzyme preparation, which describe the initial reaction rate on a specific substrate as a function of pH and temperature. The optimum pH value can be very different for the different enzymes. It ranges from 1–2 (pepsin) to 10 and more for alkaline micro-

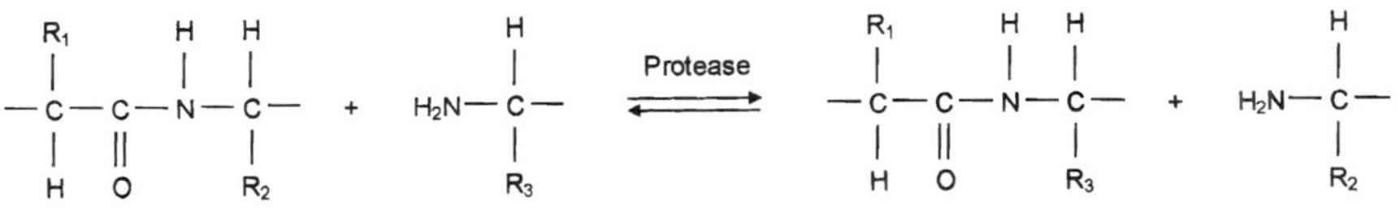

Figure 7 Free amino groups can react as nucleophiles and cleave the peptide bond when activated by the enzyme-substrate complex formation. This competitive reaction (transpeptidation) results in resynthesis of peptides with an amino acid sequence not present in the original substrate.

bial proteases. Protein hydrolysis performed with enzymatic catalysis at such extreme pH values is not totally free from unwanted chemical interference; e.g., deamidation easily occurs at alkaline pH, particularly if heat is provided. The optimum temperature value for most proteases is in the range 35–60°C, with a slow reduction of enzyme activity with temperature decrease and a steeper drop with temperature increase. The choice of the enzyme or enzyme mixture for a protein hydrolysis process is also guided by considerations about the need to preserve amino acids from degradation and the cost to provide adequate heating to the system. Other conditions being equal, enzymes with maximum activity at the lower temperature and at pH close to neutrality are preferred.

It is not always possible to apply enzymatic hydrolysis directly to proteins as they are in the native form. Native, globular proteins (e.g., from soy, corn, almond) or fibrous insoluble proteins (e.g., collagen, keratins, elastin) are generally resistant to proteolysis; this is generally explained by the compact tertiary structure of the protein that protects most of the peptide bonds. In the denatured, unfolded form the peptide bonds are exposed and available for enzymatic cleavage. As native proteins in aqueous solution are in dynamic equilibrium with a number of more or less distorted forms, part of which can be considered denatured and thereby accessible to enzyme attack, the initial break of a few peptide bonds can destabilize the protein molecule and cause irreversible unfolding: in some cases (e.g., hydrolysis of egg albumin by pepsin) this mechanism allows the protease to perform the hydrolysis to a remarkable extent. More frequently, especially when covalent bonds (disulfide bonds) stabilize the native form of the protein, a preliminary partial or extended denaturation is needed to make enzymatic hydrolysis possible; this is normally achieved by heating or chemical attack, or a combination of the two.

The capability of performing hydrolytic cleavage in mild, physiological conditions is not the unique advantage of enzymatic catalysis; in fact, it is also possible to cleave the polypeptide chain in correspondence of certain amino acids by using enzymes having specificity of action. Exopeptidases possess specific activity for the peptide bond that connects the terminal amino acids in the peptide chain (N-terminal or C-terminal or both); they liberate single free amino acids and are used (mainly in association with endopeptidases) when free amino acids are desired in the final product. A second, more numerous category of proteases are endopeptidases, enzymes that possess a specific hydrolytic activity for internal peptide bonds, adjacent to certain amino acids. This specificity is related to their ability to arrange a sort of molecular receptacle in their structure, which recognizes and houses amino acid side chains having precise electronic and steric characteristics. The protease-protein interaction can be more or less specific: specificity can be directed to basic positively charged side chains (trypsin), or to aromatic or large nonpolar aliphatic side chains (chymotrypsin), or to small uncharged residues (elastase). The use of a given protease, having precise specificity, makes it possible to plan the type of amino acids that will be preferentially located in the terminal position of the resulting peptides. The relative position of amino acids in the product of hydrolysis, together with its size, will influence its physicochemical characteristics and can be important for projecting the cosmetic properties of protein hydrolysates (see Section III.A.4).

The most critical quantitative aspect of protein hydrolysis (whether chemical or biological) is the extent of the cleavage, which determines the size of the resulting peptides. The average length and size distribution of protein hydrolysates will also affect the cosmetic behavior of these ingredients. The extent of cleavage is the most important parameter in protein hydrolysis and should be adequately measured and controlled to obtained peptides of the desired average size. It is expressed by the number of cleaved peptide bonds per amount of protein (mEq/g protein). The degree of hydrolysis is:

$$DH = \frac{h}{h_{\text{tot}}} \cdot 100\%$$

where

h = number of cleaved peptide bonds per amount of protein (mEq/g protein)
h_{tot} = total number of peptide bonds in a given protein (in mEq/g), determined from the amino acid composition of the protein, simply as the sum of mmoles of the individual amino acids per g protein (27)

Though solubility measurements (trichloroacetic acid solubility index) and molecular size evaluations (size exclusion chromatography) can be useful for estimating the extent of protein cleavage, the degree of hydrolysis is correctly assayed determining the increase of free amino groups, by formol titration (40), ninhydrin reaction (41), and trinitrobenzene sulfonic acid reaction (42). All parameters in a hydrolysis process are directed to attaining a certain degree of hydrolysis. The principal steps in a hydrolysis process for the manufacture of protein hydrolysates for cosmetics are schematically illustrated in Figure 8.

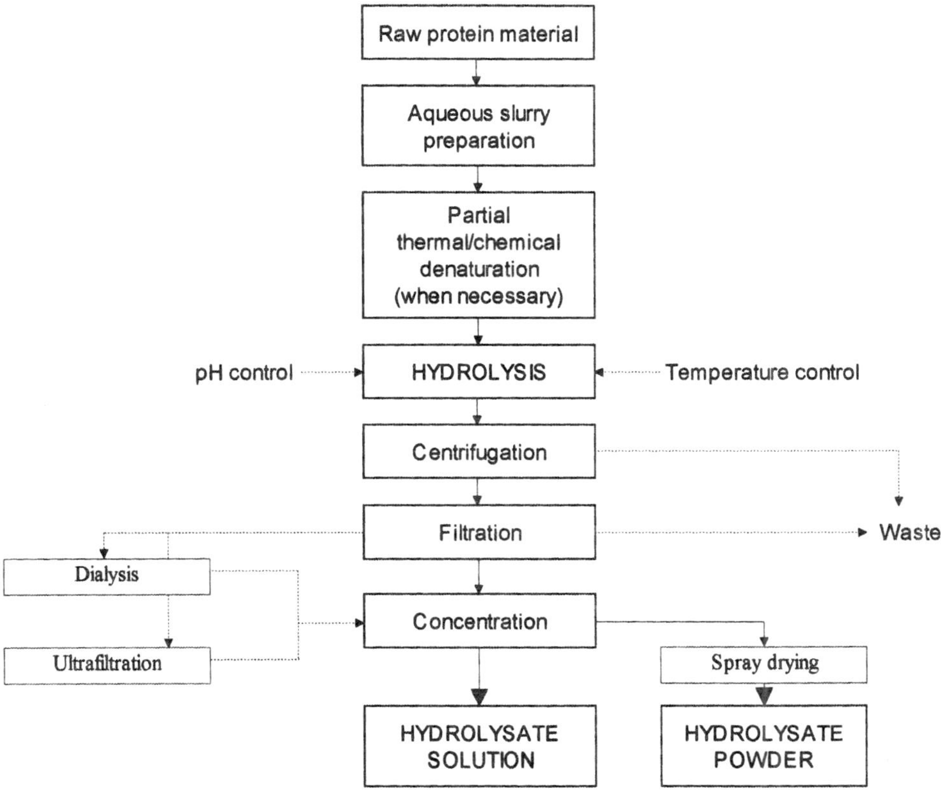

Figure 8 Process flow for protein hydrolysate manufacture.

3. Derivatization

Many different derivatizations have been tested on native proteins and protein hydrolysates in recent decades, to enhance and refine their functionality, impart new features and properties, or simply improve solubility and cosmetic acceptance. Some of the resulting products have been proved effective and commercially successful, others remain elegant laboratory curiosities, others may represent interesting prospects for future cosmetic applications. In the following survey, protein derivatives are classified according to the kind of reactive groups involved in the derivatization.

a. Amino Groups Derivatization. Most protein and peptide derivatizations are carried out with the reactive terminal amino groups and ε-amino groups of lysine as sites of chemical attachment and transformation. The pK value (25°C) of ^+H_3N— in polypeptides is estimated to be 7.5–7.8 (43). Free amino groups will therefore be fully protonated at pH < 6, partially protonated at pH 6–9.5, and unprotonated at pH > 9.5. It is easy to take advantage of the nucleophilic character of amino groups at neutral pH or slightly alkaline pH to condensate a carboxylic acid derivative by a simple acylation reaction that gives substituted amides as final products. N-alkylation is also possible, which adds a secondary group that may or may not bear an ionic charge. The characteristics and properties of the product of condensation depend on those of the added species as well as on the features of the starting substances.

N-acylation with a fatty acid radical was historically the first useful and successful protein derivatization for cosmetic purposes and still remains one of the most important. As a result of the reaction, each amino group with its potentially positive charge is masked by conversion into an amide, nonprotonable at neutral or lower pH value, while an additional lipophilic chain is added. The resulting molecule has an enhanced anionic character and gains amphiphilic properties when suitable-size hydrophilic and lipophilic moieties are involved (Fig. 9).

The reaction is generally carried out with a nature-originated fatty acid mixture derivative at pH 7–9. Neutralization during reaction is required and various alkalis (sodium and potassium hydroxides, triethanolamine) are used. Unwanted by-products are soaps, formed by hydrolysis of the acylchloride and acylamide, derived by condensation of the fatty acid

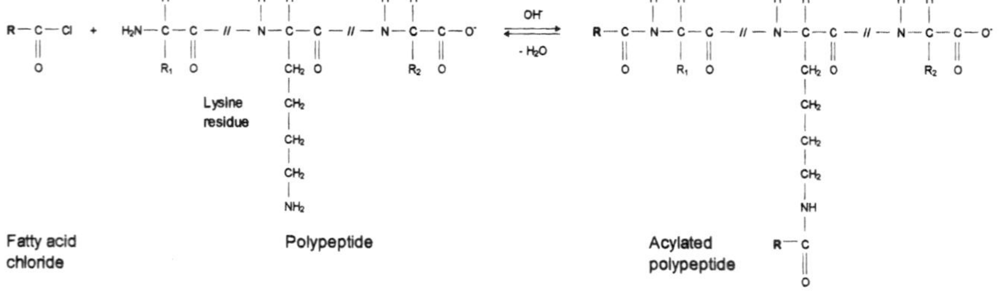

Figure 9 N-acylation of peptides with a fatty acid chloride. Condensation occurs at N-terminal amino acids and ε-amino group of lysine residues. The reaction mixture is maintained at pH 7–9, by continuous titration of the liberated carboxyl groups and in order to have a suitable concentration of unprotonated, nucleophilic —NH_2 groups. At higher pH values, side —$CONH_2$ groups of asparagine and glutamine are subject to hydrolysis giving free NH_3, which easily react with acylchlorides forming unwanted acylamides. Appropriate reaction parameters are chosen to prevent release of free fatty acids.

chloride with NH_3, when present in the starting protein substance. The substrate is usually a protein hydrolysate obtained by enzymatic hydrolysis; catalysis with endopeptidases is preferred when a low content of free amino acids and resulting acyl derivatives is desired. In commonly adopted reaction conditions, not only terminal amino groups and ε-amino groups of lysine side chain are acylated, but also other reactive side groups of amino acids (hydroxyl groups of serine, tyrosine, threonine, and hydroxyproline, free thiol group of cysteine); however, the condensation products of these reactive groups are generally less stable than N-acylated products and are easily subject to hydrolysis. The degree of cleavage and amino acid composition of the hydrolyzed starting protein must be known, to dose precisely the equivalent amount of acylchloride needed to react. Depending on the composition of the starting protein material, members of this group may contain acylation products derived from peptides as well as free amino acids. Protein–fatty acid condensates are mild cleansing and emulsifying agents, with a long history more than 30 years, of safe use. They have high skin and eye tolerability, good washing and foaming activity even in hard water, and considerable solubility in organic solvents, especially ethanol. Acyl peptides are widely used in association with anionic tenside in cleansing cosmetic formulations; their skin/eye compatibility and synergetic interactions with conventional anionics make it possible to achieve appreciable reduction in the irritation potential of less compatible tensides. The acyl peptides are amides and subject to hydrolysis; their formulations usually require a pH value > 5.

The anionic character of polypeptides can be increased at a higher extent by introducing ionizable carboxyl groups by amino group acylation with internal anhydrides of dicarboxylic acids, such as succinic anhydride or maleic anhydride (Fig. 10).

The increase in negative charge results in electrostatic repulsion, unfolding, and dissociation, which generally improve solubility, water absorption, emulsifying, and foaming properties (44–46). The resulting products have high water solubility and good stability in the pH range 5–8. At pH < 5 their solubility drops drastically and hydrolysis easily causes splitting of the polypeptide and dicarboxylic acid. These derivatives have extended application in the food industry as technical enhancers of emulsified preparations, but they have had poor success in cosmetic products. Only one of these derivatives (sodium succinoly gelatin) is listed in the *International Cosmetic Ingredient Dictionary*, 6th edition (29). They could be of use as rheological modifiers in emulsions and gels or as electrostatic coupling or bridging agents, which may help in the attachment of some other ionic or polar molecule to the skin or hair.

Much greater commercial success and experimentally substantiated effectiveness have been obtained with protein derivatives by implantation of positively charged radicals to amino groups. Increase of cationic character by covalent attachment of a quaternary group to protein hydrolysate is designed with the aim of facilitating and potentiating electrostatic binding to hair and skin keratins, which possess a net negative charge at physiological pH. In this way it is possible to combine the functional properties of polypeptides with the conditioning qualities of cationic substances, resulting in highly substantive products, especially useful and effective in rinse-off applications, imparting lubricity, flexibility, and combability to hair. "Quaternization" is based on the attachment of a quaternary ammonium radical to free amino groups of protein hydrolysates (Fig. 11, 12). Condensation with a trimethylammonium derivative results in quaternized polypeptides with enhanced hair/skin substantivity and increased resistance to rinse, but displaying overall conditioning properties not significantly different with respect to the original hydrolysate. Improvement of the conditioning, perceivable effects (mostly on hair) is obtained by at-

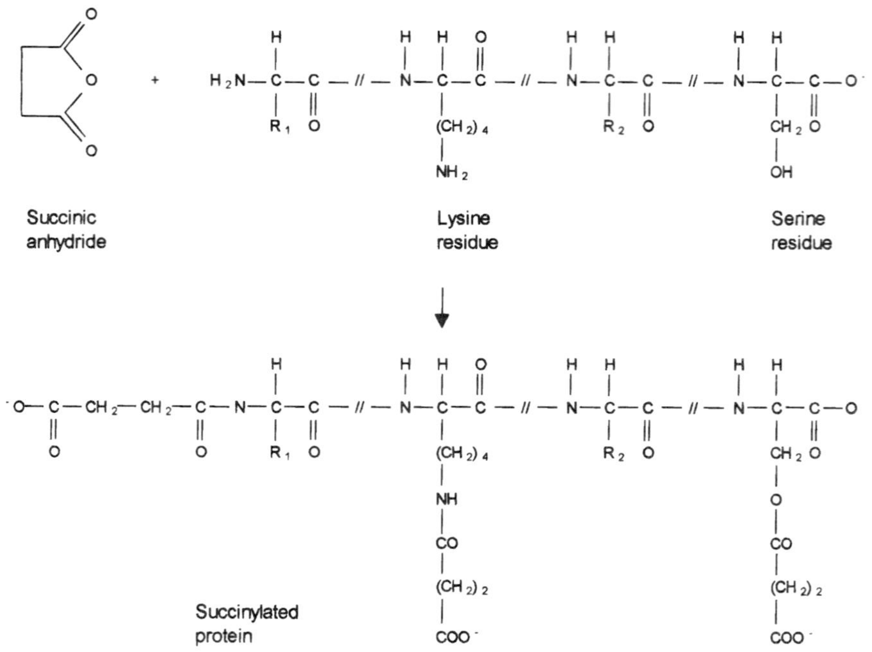

Figure 10 Schematic representation of acylation of peptides with succinic anhydride. N-succinylation of α- and ε-amino groups and O-succinylation of the serine side chain are shown. O-succinylation of tirosine and threonine and S-succinylation of cysteine are also reported to occur (44).

tachment of an alkyldimethylammonium derivative, where a lipophile linear alkyl chain (12 or more carbon atoms) provides ''fatty'' character to the product, a determining factor for conferring body, lubricity, and smoothness to the hair.

In contrast to the original amino group, which is protonated only at low pH values, the quaternized group is positively charged in a wide pH range and a distinct increase of

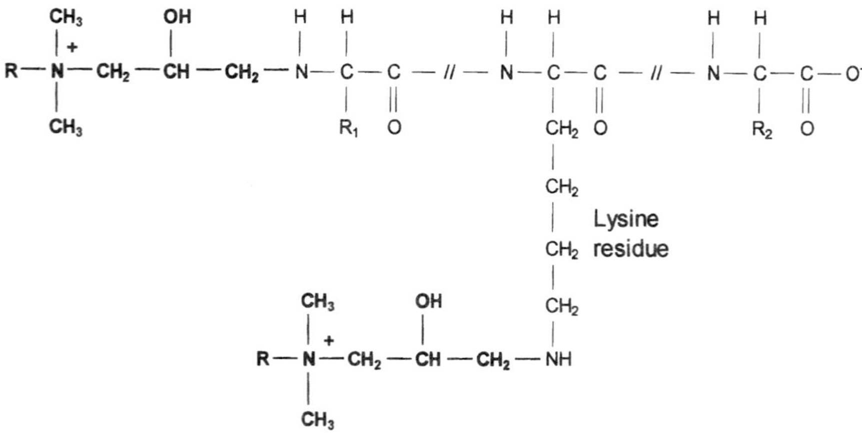

Figure 11 Chemical structure of an alkyldimonium hydroxypropyl polypeptide. R is usually an alkyl group derived from coconut or other oils and fats.

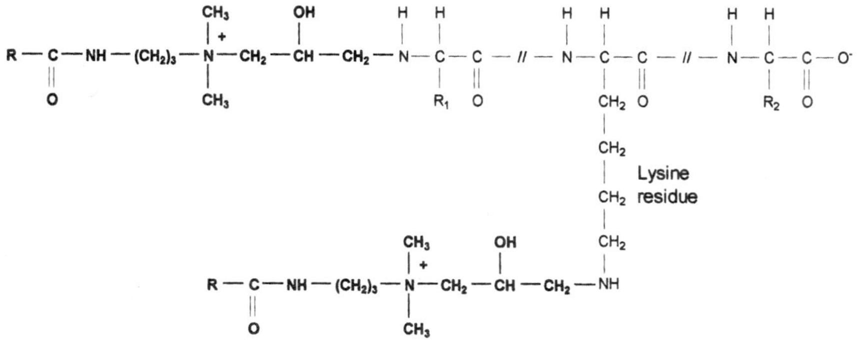

Figure 12 Chemical structure of an alkylamidopropyldimonium hydroxypropyl polypeptide. RCO-represents a cocoyl/oleyl/palmitoyl acid radical.

net charge of the polypeptide is obtained. The isoelectric point of protein hydrolysates, which ranges from 4 to 7 for most of them, can be raised to 9–12 by quaternization. As protein substances exhibit a positive net charge only below their isoelectric value, in the majority of cosmetic applications (with reference to pH), quaternized proteins have a prevailing positive charge. These derivatives have surface activity, moderate wetting and foaming properties, and water solubility; they are generally compatible with ionic and nonionic tensides and have skin/eye compatibility intermediate between that of the starting hydrolysate and the cationic group. They are widely used as conditioning and filming copolymers in hair cleansing and treatment preparations.

A more recent development in the derivatization of proteins for specific cosmetic purposes resorted to new protein-silicone copolymer derivatives, designed to combine the functional properties of protein derivatives with those of silicone oils. These ingredients have been proposed as hair conditioning agents and are reported to give glossiness, smoothness, and wet/dry combability to hair. Their general structure is shown in Figure 13.

The silanol derivative is covalently attached to terminal amino groups (and possibly ε-amino groups of lysine residues) of the hydrolyzed polypeptides. Terminal silanol groups are reactive and reported to give cross-linking bridges with a second silanol group from another molecule of the derivative, forming a siloxane bond (Si—O—Si) between protein chains. Formation of a protein-silicone network is said to occur in dehydrating conditions (as for hair blow-drying), after application of the product in solution form, creating a protective conditioning film on the hair surface. These protein-silicone copolymers are freely soluble in water at pH above 5.5 and display limited water tolerance at lower pH values (47).

b. Derivatization of Other Reactive Groups of Proteins. Reactions carried out on reactive sites of protein other than amino groups have not yet yielded products useful for cosmetic applications. It is, however, worthwhile briefly surveying some of these derivatizations for their potential usefulness in future preparation of cosmetic ingredients.

Phosphorylation of the serine hydroxyl group has been tested to improve the functional and technical properties of food proteins. Increase of water solubility, water-holding capacity, emulsifying, and foaming properties have been obtained by this derivatization (48). One possible chemical route for protein phosphorylation is based on the reaction with cyclic sodium trimetaphosphate (Fig. 14). Cyclic sodium trimetaphosphate is strongly

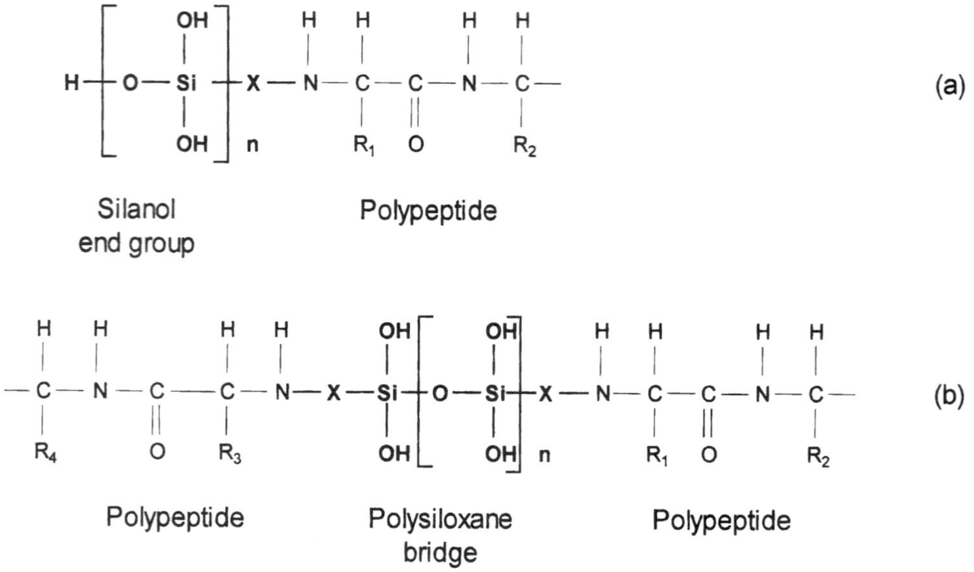

Figure 13 Structure of hydrolyzed protein polisiloxane copolymers with silanol-terminated chains (a) and siloxane cross-linked chains (b). X is a generic attachment group.

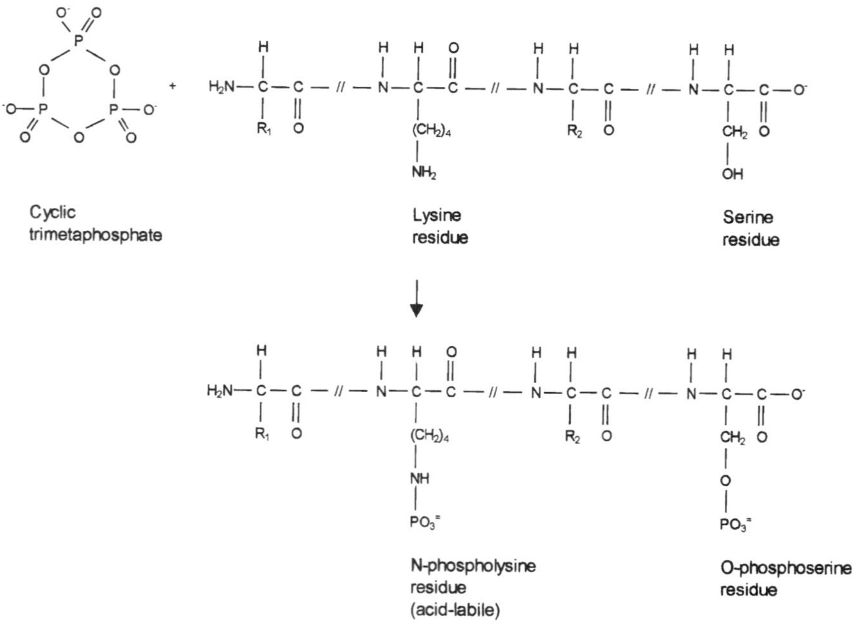

Figure 14 Polypeptide phosphorylation by reaction with cyclic sodium trimetaphosphate. O-phosphoesterification of serine and N-phosphoramidation of lysine easily occur at alkaline pH.

electrophilic in alkali and easily produces phosphoesterification of the primary hydroxyl groups of serine residues (preferred to the secondary hydroxyl groups of threonine) and phosphoramidation of the ε-amino group of lysine. The phosphoramidic bond created on lysine is acid-labile and can be cleaved by acidification to below pH 5, whereas O-phosphoserine residues remain unaffected. The covalent attachment of anionic phosphate groups to polypeptide chains causes an increase in net electronegativity and enhances solubility and surface activity, analogously to protein succinylation. The resulting products have structural affinities with two natural phosphoproteins present in the egg: ovalbumin and phosvitin. The cosmetic usefulness of this derivatization could conceivably be in enhancing solubility and extractability of high-serine proteins like silk sericin and fibroin and preparing high-molecular-weight proteins with useful rheological properties.

An interesting enzymatic-driven derivatization of proteins has been extensively studied and proposed for the preparation of new protein surfactants (49,50). These researches were originated by observations of the occurrence of plastein formation from proteolysates. Plasteins are gel-like substances that can be produced incubating a concentrated protein hydrolysate in the presence of a protease. The reaction was originally believed to be resynthesis of the protein, but this hypothesis was gradually abandoned and a transpeptidation mechanism was proposed and confirmed (51,52). Through the transpepdidation reaction, an enrichment of hydrophobic amino acids will occur for some of the peptides; these hydrophobic peptides, which have poor water solubility, condense to small particles and form the insoluble plastein. The plastein reaction was found to be suitable to incorporate amino acid esters in the peptide chain through a transpeptidation mechanism. Conditions necessary for the reaction are a very high concentration of the substrate (20–25%), alkaline pH (9–10), and the presence of a suitable protease as reaction catalyst. The reaction is stereospecific and occurs only with esters of L-amino acids. The scheme of the reaction is shown in Figure 15.

A lipophilic long-chain amino acid ester can be used to implant a high degree of lipophilicity to protein substances. Products obtained are amphoteric surfactants with a net prevailing charge either positive or negative depending on the pH of the medium and with a isoelectric point value similar to that of the source polypeptide. These amphiphilic protein derivatives differ substantially from acyl peptides, being C-esters and not acylamides. These products have proved to have gelling activity and excellent emulsifying properties, giving stable O/W systems with very fine oil dispersion (53).

c. Special Derivatives. In this section two additional modifications of proteins, not involving covalent attachment of additional substances, will be considered: disulfide bond recombination in sulfur-containing proteins and protein-surfactant complexation. The

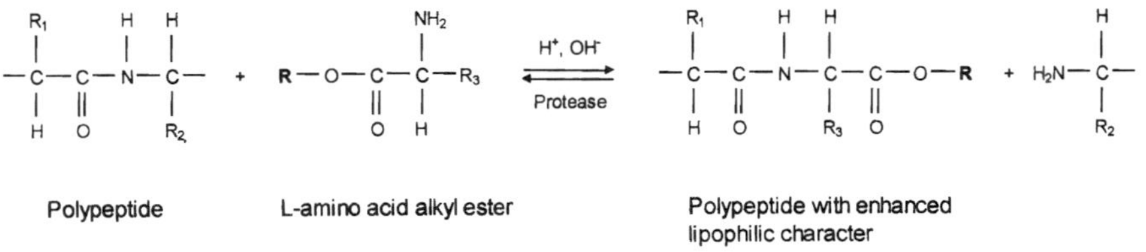

Figure 15 Covalent incorporation of amino acid esters into proteins by a transpeptidation reaction catalyzed by proteases. The reaction is based on the stereospecific nucleophilic attack of the —NH_2 group of L-amino acid alkyl ester on the carboamide bond of the polypeptide activated by the enzyme.

main purpose of both transformations is to achieve water solubility of high-molecular-weight, otherwise insoluble proteins and to make them suitable for use in cosmetic formulations.

The tertiary and quaternary structure of many proteins (keratins, soy globulins, wheat gluten proteins, corn zein) is stabilized by disulfide bridges between cysteine residues located in the same protein chain or in different chains. This —SS— cross-linking makes proteins insoluble and resistant to enzymatic hydrolysis. Cleaving of disulfide bonds with reducing agents is a practical tool for unfolding proteins, exposing peptide bonds to hydrolytic agents, and is the first step of a transformation procedure consisting in a controlled disulfide recombination, giving soluble, nonhydrolyzed, long-chain peptides. Reduction and opening of disulfide bridges (see Section III.A.2) is rapidly followed by reoxidation and reformation of —SS— linkages when reducing agents are removed. Random recombination causes both intra- and intermolecular cross-linking, with possible formation of large, insoluble aggregates. Two different procedures can be adopted to maintain protein solubility without cleavage of the peptide backbone: the first is based on irreversible inhibition of free —SH groups by oxidation to cysteic acid residues —SO_3H (which causes partial loss of the cosmetic potentialities of sulfur proteins); the second, more elegant, method consists in favoring intramolecular recombination with formation of smaller, more soluble polypeptides than those present in the starting material. Since, in diluted solutions, intramolecular recombination is predominant compared to interchain cross-linking (due to the lower probability of intermolecular interactions), this can be obtained by extensive dilution of the polypeptides after the reduction step and subsequent removal or neutralization of the reducing agent. By this procedure, water-soluble, high-molecular-weight, nonhydrolyzed polypeptides with undamaged reactive cystine residues can be obtained from high-sulfur proteins such as keratins and wheat gluten proteins; the resulting ingredients have specific use in hair permanent applications (54).

Complexation of proteins with surface-active substances in an aqueous environment is a second method by which solubilization of "reluctant" native proteins can be attained. Formation or recombination of covalent bonds is not involved in this procedure: only weak chemical interactions (ionic, hydrophobic, hydrogen bonds) act cooperatively in the formation and stabilization of a new entity, the protein-surfactant complex, whose physicochemical behavior and properties differ from those of the original species. Protein-surfactant interactions have been well explored by many authors and are discussed for their cosmetic implications in several sections of this chapter; they are of fundamental theoretical and practical concern for understanding the action of surfactants on skin/hair proteins and the role of exogenous proteins in detergency. In all cosmetic systems where surface-active agents and protein ingredients coexist, these interactions occur, more or less independently of the formulator's control. The two species give rise to a series of attraction-repulsion events that can affect the physicochemical and cosmetic properties of the product.

The binding of ionic surfactants to proteins is made possible by cooperative, nonspecific, noncovalent bonds, which can replace the intra- and intermolecular forces stabilizing the three-dimensional conformation of the protein. This results in unfolding of the protein coil (to a variable degree), while the surfactant molecules turn from a hydrated or micellar form into a bound species (Fig. 16).

Large amounts of tenside molecules are bound by proteins only after they have undergone a drastic unfolding that exposes many binding sites otherwise inaccessible to the ligand. A new species (complex) is formed: the water solubility of the protein is increased

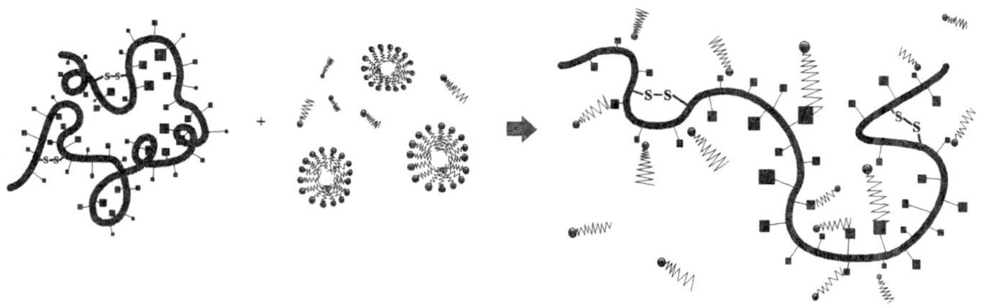

Figure 16 Protein-surfactant complexation produces unfolding of the polypeptide coil by ionic and hydrophobic interactions. The unfolding causes exposure of hydrophobic residues of amino acids and increases the surface hydrophobicity of the protein. (The black squares represent the lipophilic amino acid side chains; their size indicates the hydrophobicity degree.)

as well as its stability to thermal degradation. The unfolding leads to exposure of hydrophobic side chains of amino acids, increasing the surface hydrophobicity (see Section III.A.4) and the number of binding sites. The complexation is generally reversible and the protein can resume its native, folded conformation by removal of the ligand. For each ligand-protein pair a binding isotherm can be described, showing the molar or weight ratio between the two species in the complex at a given temperature. It has been demonstrated that the affinity of proteins to surfactants increases with their hydrophobicity. The hydrocarbon moiety of the ligand contributes the major share of the binding energy; for anionic tensides coulomb forces appear to make a subsidiary contribution. The binding of anionics is dependent on the pH (55–59).

By surfactant complexation it is possible to obtain relatively high-concentrated solutions of low-soluble proteins like reticulated collagen, wheat proteins, and keratins. Preformed protein-surfactant complexes have been proposed as cosmetic ingredients for detergency as a suitable vehicle for incorporating long-chain, otherwise insoluble proteins in skin/hair cleansing products and as mild cosurfactants with increased skin/eye tolerability compared to pure tenside (60).

As the last mention in this necessarily incomplete review on protein derivatives, it is worthwhile to cite the use of proteins and polypeptides as carriers of inorganic ions (Zn, Mg, Mn, Cu etc.), which are thought to be useful in hair and skin cosmetic treatments.

III. CHEMICAL AND PHYSICAL ASPECTS

A. Molecular Characteristics

1. Amino Acid Composition and Sequence

The structure of natural proteins is organized on four possible levels. The primary structure is given by the covalent bonds (mainly —CO—NH— and —SS—) linking different amino acids within the polypeptide chain; it is therefore determined by the amino acid sequence and the possible presence of cystine residues (cysteine—SS—cysteine). The secondary structure is characterized by the spatial location of adjacent amino acid side chains, which, by hydrogen bonds and other weak linkages, can give rise to formation of regular periodic structures like the α-helix of the collagen molecule or the β-pleated sheet of the silk fibroin. The tertiary structure is related to steric interaction and spatial location of nonadjacent amino acid side chains; this organization level allows the protein chain to resume a folded shape and locate the hydrophobic residues in the internal regions of the molecule, reducing the unfavorable interaction with water. The tertiary structure is characteristic of globular proteins. The quaternary organization is related to association and spatial arrangement of two or more polypeptide chains (subunits) cross-linked by hydrophobic and hydrogen bonds or disulfide bridges. Higher levels of structural organization (supersecondary structure, domains) have also been found and studied for their biological role and importance (11).

Most proteins and protein derivatives for cosmetic use (with the significant exception of soluble collagen and enzymes) maintain little of the spatial architecture of the source proteins, and generally, in the view of their cosmetic properties, the conformational aspects of these molecules have little practical relevance.

The proteins of all living organisms, from bacteria to humans, are built with the same 20 fundamental amino acids (Table 1). The amino acid composition characterizes the different proteins, but obviously the most important factor of specificity and identity is given by the amino acid sequence, genetically predetermined. The three-dimensional organization and biological activity of proteins is entirely designed by amino acid sequence and yet this factor, crucial in biology, has negligible importance for the cosmetic properties of most protein derivatives. Collagen, elastin, keratins, and other physiological scleroproteins play important roles in the human body, especially for structural and mechanical purposes in the connective tissues, and these functions result from their specific amino acid composition and, above all, amino acid sequence. The cosmetic effects of these proteins and their derivatives, as applied topically, are, however, only marginally linked to their spatial conformations, and the effect of most cosmetic proteins on the skin and hair should be regarded as nonspecifically or low-specifically related to the sequence of constituent amino acids.

Soluble native collagen could be considered a significant exception. It is well proved that the triple-helical structure of tropocollagen and its ability to reticulate by forming side interchain linkages are fundamental for the building of the fibrous hydrophilic skeleton in the connective tissues, and that this is the consequence of its characteristic amino acid pattern, with repeating sequences of glycine-proline-hydroxyproline and a glycine residue every three amino acids. These features are the basis of the biological properties of collagen in living tissues and possibly play important roles (together with molecular size and net charge) for the film-forming and moisturizing effects that exogenous native collagen exhibits on the skin surface. When collagen is denaturated or hydrolyzed, the spatial architecture of the original protein is likely to be entirely lost and relationships between cosmetic effects and three-dimensional structure can no longer be invoked.

2. *Thiol Groups and Disulfide Bridges*

Thiol groups of the cysteine side chain have great importance in protein chemistry and biochemistry and can play important roles in the cosmetic activity of protein ingredients. Cysteine is present in many proteins, usually at low percentages, with the striking exception of keratins (Table 3). The cysteine —SH group is ionizable (the typical pK is 8.5), but most prominent are the oxidation-reduction properties of —SH and —SS— groups. Cysteine is easily oxidized to cystine with formation of a disulfide bridge; in this stable form it is usually present in natural proteins. The formation of intra- and intermolecular disulfide bridges is a fundamental mechanism for the conformational arrangement of proteins, by which they resume the most stable and the biologically active form. By disulfide coupling, proteins restrict the accessibility of reactive sites (peptide bonds and functional groups of amino acid side chains), and this has consequences on protein solubility, resistance to denaturation, hydrolysis, and complexation with surfactants. Proteins not containing —SS— groups bind approximately 50% more sodium dodecyl sulfate than proteins with —SS— groups and in about half the time (59); because of their tight structure stabilized by numerous disulfide bonds, natural keratins are little affected by proteolytic attack unless pretreated with reducing agents or other chemicals capable of disrupting part of the —SS— bridges. The susceptibility of —SS— bonds to nucleophilic attack depends on their location in the polypeptide structure: when confined in hydrophobic and folded regions they are unlikely affected by reducing agents also at high concentrations. Total cleavage may sometimes be attained only by combined application of hydrogen bond disrupters (urea, guanidine) with a strong reducing agent (thioglycolate, dithiothreitol).

Reaction of —SS— groups with sulfite or thioglycolate ions causes cleavage and formation of highly reactive mercaptan ions susceptible of a variety of chemical derivatizations. The generally accepted mechanism for the reaction of thioglycolate (the reagent most frequently used for the reduction of hair in permanent waving treatments) proceeds through a two-step nucleophilic displacement (61):

$$\text{Protein—S—S—protein} + {}^{-}\text{S—CH}_2\text{—COO}^- \Leftrightarrow \text{protein—S}^- + \text{protein—S—S—CH}_2\text{—COO}^-$$

$$\text{Protein—S—S—CH}_2\text{—COO—} + {}^{-}\text{S—CH}_2\text{—COO}^- \Leftrightarrow \text{protein—S}^- + {}^{-}\text{OOC—CH}_2\text{—S—S—CH}_2\text{—COO}^-$$

To attain the maximum cleavage it is necessary either to use a large excess of thiol or to run the reaction under strongly alkaline conditions, indispensable for generation of the attacking nucleophile-mercaptide ion.

Another possible method for reduction of —SS— groups is based on reduction with sulfite ions. The mechanism proposed for sulfitolysis is based on the formation of the cysteine—S—sulfonate residue:

$$\text{Protein—S—S—protein} + \text{SO}_3^{=} \Leftrightarrow \text{protein—SSO}_3^- + \text{protein—S}^-$$

The mechanism of the nucleophilic attack in this reaction is not completely known; it is still not clear whether species responsible for cleavage of the cystine are the sulfite ($SO3^{=}$) or bisulfite ($HSO3^-$) or disulfite ($S_2O_5^{=}$) ions. Products of the reaction are a free thiol residue and a cysteine—S—sulfonate residue, also known as Bunte salt. Though totally ionized at pH values above 1, Bunte salts are capable of a number of reactions, including reformation of disulfide bonds.

Cystine reduction by sulfitolysis is generally preferred for processing and derivatization of cosmetic proteins, because it takes places at slightly acidic pH and room temperature, with no degradation of other amino acids.

Procedures involving cleavage and reformation of disulfide bridges are adopted in the manufacture of protein derivatives from cystine-containing source proteins. Partial disruption of —SS— linkages by sulfitolysis or alkaline treatments or (rarely) by use of mercaptide ions may be needed to expose a higher number of peptide bonds to proteases in the preparation of protein hydrolysates or to solubilize long polypeptides from wheat, soy, and keratinic proteins to make them suitable for cosmetic use. After cleavage it is necessary to neutralize the reactivity of thiol residues to prevent random recombination of —SS— bonds with possible formation of insoluble aggregates causing haze and precipitation in their solutions. The oxidant most commonly used for this purpose is hydrogen peroxide, although air oxidation in the presence of metal salts as catalysts is also effective. Little is known about the mechanism of these reactions: a free-radical mechanism is supposed to be the most probable leading to recombination of disulfide bonds (61):

$$\text{Protein—SH} + H_2O_2 \Leftrightarrow \text{protein—S}\cdot + \text{OH}\cdot + H_2O$$

$$\text{Protein—SH} + \text{OH}\cdot \Leftrightarrow \text{protein—S}\cdot + H_2O$$

$$\text{Protein—S}\cdot + \cdot\text{S—protein} \Leftrightarrow \text{protein—S—S—protein}$$

By this method 80–90% of the cysteine residues formed during the reduction step are converted back into cystine, while the remaining residues are probably oxidized to cisteic acid.

An alternative procedure to obtain cleavage of disulfide bonds and protein unfolding is direct oxidation of —SS— bonds to cisteic acid with hydrogen peroxide:

$$\text{Protein—S—S—protein} + H_2O_2 \Rightarrow 2\text{proteinSO}_3\text{H}$$

This reaction is carried out at alkaline pH, when the perhydroxyl anion HO_2^- is the predominant reactive species responsible for attacking the disulfide bond. Cisteic acid residues are stable and the resulting polypeptides will not recombine, but this method gives unwanted degradation of several amino acids (62) and produces additional negatively charged sites that cause deep changes in the protein structure. Only one protein derivative obtained by this method (Oxidized keratin) is reported in the *International Cosmetic Ingredients Dictionary 6th edition. (29).*

Severe alkaline treatment of cystine-containing proteins can also cause scission of disulfide bonds probably by a multiple mechanism not yet entirely understood. One proposed route is based on the already mentioned β-elimination from cysteine and formation of dehydroalanine (see Section II.B.2).

In addition to its usefulness in the manufacturing and processing of protein ingredients, reactivity of disulfide bonds is the basis of the specific action of some particular protein derivatives in permanent-waving treatments (see Section IV.C).

3. Molecular Size

Molecular size is one of the most important parameters affecting the physicochemical behavior and functional properties of peptides and proteins in cosmetic applications. The molecular mass of currently used cosmetic proteins can range from a few hundred to a million Daltons, corresponding to peptides made of few amino acids to huge polypeptide aggregates as in the case of nonhydrolyzed wheat gluten proteins and keratins. Numerous studies have tried to identify the optimum molecular size needed for a particular cosmetic effect. Though the results obtained are often contradictory, it has become clear that this parameter strongly influences the ability of proteins to link skin and hair keratin, their film-forming properties, and their interaction with other molecules.

The molecular size of a polypeptide is not directly related to its mass (given by the number and type of constituent amino acids), as its actual dimension in aqueous environment depends on the extent of the chain folding. When in aqueous environment, proteins tend to spontaneously resume the conformation corresponding to the lowest free-energy level, through suitable spatial arrangement of amino acid side groups. Nonpolar hydrophobic side chains point inward, forming tight aggregates by means of van der Waals interactions, while charged residues can point outward and establish stabilizing interaction with water by means of hydrogen bonds. Small side chains and polar neutral residues can be found in internal or exposed regions. By these arrangements the highest possible thermodynamic stabilization is reached for proteins in an aqueous environment (Fig. 17).

The actual dimensions of the molecule depend on the extent of chain folding and regulate many of its physicochemical properties. This, not the actual molecular mass, is the parameter commonly measured for cosmetic proteins and related to their properties and benefits.

Size exclusion chromatography (also referred to as gel filtration and gel permeation chromatography) is the most practical and frequently employed technique to fractionate polypeptides in function of their dimension and provides the basis to estimate the average molecular weight of protein blends. Exclusion columns contain porous particles of a hydrophilic polymer with different pore diameters. When a polypeptide mixture is forced to pass through the column, its components diffuse into those pores that have a diameter greater than their effective diameters (the effective diameter will include any molecules of solvation). If a solute is of such a diameter that it cannot diffuse into any of the pores, it will be unretained and elute in the void volume (V_0) of the column. Conversely, a polypeptide that is capable of diffusing completely into all of the pores will totally permeate the packing and require a much larger volume of solvent to achieve elution. The separation of molecules having different diameters is based on the extent of their diffusion through the pores and the different time needed to achieve their elution. An ideal size exclusion fractionation will occur when all solutes diffuse into part of the pores of the stationary phase. Size exclusion chromatography is a way of rapidly obtaining an estimate of the molecular weight of a sample, by comparison with authentic standards. To correlate the elution time of the polypeptides (which is a function of their size) with their molecular weight, the solutes and standards should have the same spatial conformation. For blends of molecules having homogeneous shape, over a considerable range, the elution volume is approximately a linear function of the logarithm of molecular weight. Practically, molecular masses of polypeptides are only approximately determinable as their hydrodynamic

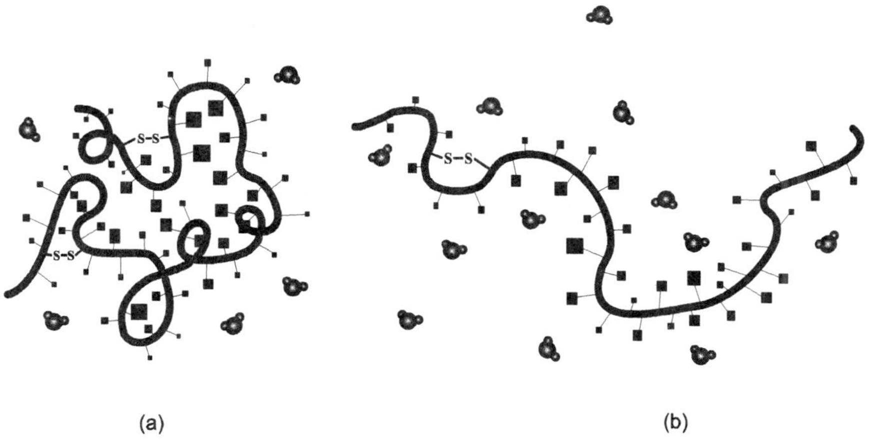

Figure 17 A hydrophobic polypeptide (a) resumes a folded shape in aqueous environment to minimize the unfavorable interactions of nonpolar side chains with water. A more hydrophilic polypeptide can be stabilized as a partially unfolded coil (b).

properties are rarely identical with those of the marker substances. For polypeptide mixtures as protein hydrolysates (the widely used protein ingredients in cosmetics), which are composed of hundreds or even thousands of different molecules, an average molecular weight or a molecular weight distribution can be estimated (Fig. 18).

Formol titration and other methods of determining terminal amino groups are also used to measure the average molecular weight of protein hydrolysates, but they are imprecise because —NH_2 groups of amino acid side chains also react and the molecular masses are usually underestimated.

Another method of determining molecular weight of macromolecules is by ultracentrifugation. The ultracentrifuge produces high centrifugal forces to measure the redistribution of sedimenting particles. The distribution of the particles is observed as an interference pattern from which a molecular weight can be calculated.

4. The Hydrophobicity of Proteins and Peptides

The importance of hydrophobic interactions in determining the spatial conformation of proteins and minimizing the free energy of their aqueous solutions has been stressed above. Formation and disruption of internal hydrophobic bonds is also essential for understanding denaturation phenomena of proteins and the mechanisms of their biological activity. The hydrophobicity of proteins and peptides affects their physicochemical behavior and may be of great value for their cosmetic effects and properties.

The hydrophobic character of proteins and peptides depends primarily on their amino acid composition, i.e., the relative amount and lipophilicity of nonpolar residues in the molecule. A measurement of protein hydrophobicity (average hydrophobicity $H\Phi_{ave}$) can be derived theoretically as the average of the individual Δf_t values based on the molar amino acid composition, where Δf_t is the change in free energy for the transfer of one mole of amino acid from ethanol to water (63–65). The average hydrophobicity values of the principal source proteins of cosmetic interest are listed in Table 3. A different way to express protein hydrophobicity is the so-called "surface hydrophobicity," an entity measured experimentally on proteins by the adsorption of a chemical compound (*cis-*

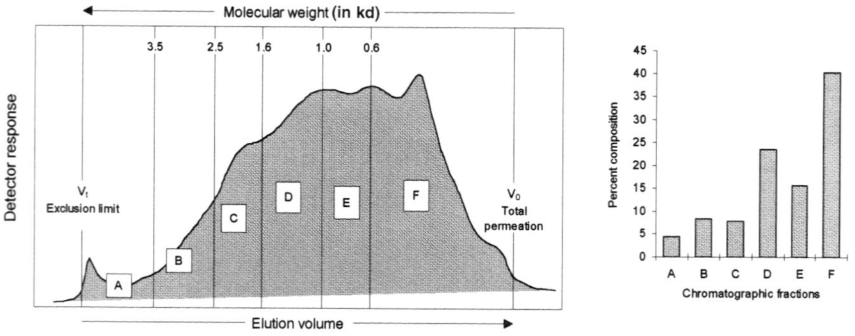

Figure 18 Size exclusion chromatography pattern of a wheat protein hydrolysate (left) and percent composition of the fractions having molecular mass within the known values of standard substances (right). Molecular weights of peptides are only approximately determinable, since their hydrodynamic properties are not necessarily identical with those of the marker substances. Chromatographic conditions: stationary phase TSKgel Toyopearl HW-40F (Tosoh Co., Japan) 10 × 500 mm; eluant 0.1 M NaCl in 0.1 M phosphate buffer pH 7.1; flow 0.4 ml/min; detection UV 220 nm. (Unpublished data.)

parinaric acid, an unsaturated fatty acid with conjugated double bonds) that fluoresces in a hydrophobic environment (66). Surface hydrophobicity has been found to influence protein solubility and stability, the rheological behavior of protein-containing systems, foaming and emulsifying properties, and interaction with surfactants and other molecules, and should be considered an important factor in determining the cosmetic properties of protein derivatives.

For protein hydrolysates, a qualitative theoretical relationship between molecular size, location of hydrophobic residues along the protein chain, and hydrophobicity has been proposed (27). For short peptides, if there is a relative excess of hydrophobic amino acids in the terminal positions of the chain, the actual hydrophobicity will be higher than if hydrophobic residues are preferentially located in the endo-positions. This is because folding of small peptides cannot prevent or significantly minimize the exposure of terminal hydrophobic groups to water. Conversely, longer peptides having the same amino acid composition will be less hydrophobic when lipophilicic residues are located in terminal positions, and the longer the peptide, the lower their actual hydrophobicity will be. Considering that proteolysis with enzymes having different specificity leads to peptides with a different location of hydrophobic/hydrophilic amino acids (see Section II.B.2), the hydrophobicity level of protein hydrolysates may, to a certain extent, be planned by selection of a particular enzyme and reaching a certain degree of hydrolysis. The relationships between enzyme specificity and molecular size and hydrophobicity of hydrolyzed peptides are illustrated in Figure 19.

Though some cosmetic features of protein hydrolysates can be improved with increasing hydrophobicity (foaming, surfactant binding capacity), highly hydrophobic peptides are generally less water soluble and easily form insoluble aggregates with formation of haze and precipitate in aqueous systems.

5. *Proteins as Ionic Substances*

The presence of terminal carboxylic and amino groups and other dissociable side chains in aspartic acid, glutamic acid, histidine, lysine, and arginine makes proteins ionizable substances, for which a dissociation equilibrium, pH dependent, is described (Fig. 20).

The pH value at which the number of protons combined with basic groups is equal

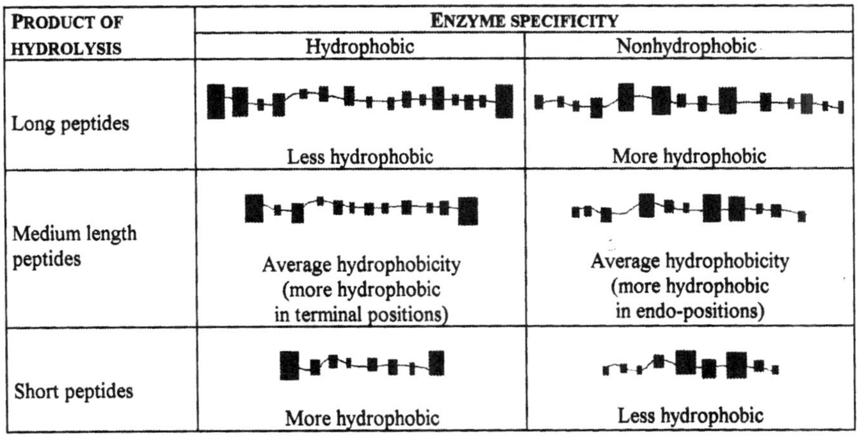

Figure 19 Schematic relationship between enzyme specificity, average hydrophobicity, and peptide chain length in enzymatic hydrolysis of proteins.

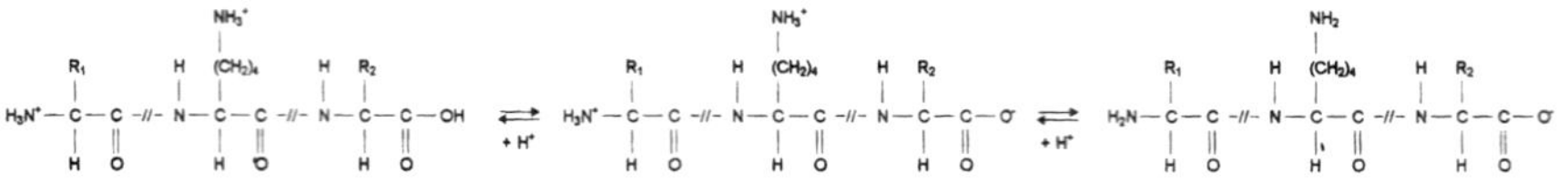

Figure 20 Ionization pattern of amino and carboxyl groups of peptides.

to the number of protons liberated from acid groups is the isoelectric point. This value depends on the values of the dissociation constants of acid groups and ionization constants of basic groups. Below their isoelectric point protonation prevails and proteins display a net positive charge; above the isoelectric point dissociation is preponderant and proteins possess a net negative charge. At their isoelectric point proteins have the lower solubility and stability in water, electric conductivity, osmotic pressure, viscosity, and surface tension.

Many of the interactions of protein substances with the skin and hair and other molecules present in cosmetic products are of ionic nature; hence the isoelectric point and pH of the medium play a basic role in their cosmetic effects. The isoelectric point value of a great number of pure natural proteins is known and principally determined by isoelectric focusing electrophoresis. All the transformations to which natural proteins are subject involving forming and disruption of covalent bonds (hydrolysis, alkylation and acylation, disulfide cleavage), and even conformational changes involving rearrangement of weak chemical bonds, may cause their isoelectric point value to change.

For polypeptide blends like protein hydrolysates an average isoelectric point value or range can be expressed. A simple method for evaluating this parameter is based on the ionic exchange chromatography technique (67). This is an approximate, though useful, indicator of the overall prevailing charge that these complex blends display at a given pH, as the result of the different isoelectric values of single constituent peptides. The average isoelectric point of most protein hydrolysates ranges from acidic to slight alkaline pH (4–8). Regardless of the amino acid composition of the source protein, the hydrolysis conditions and the molecular features of resulting peptides can determine a wide oscillation in the average isoelectric point of the product (2–3 pH units and more). This is because the dissociation pK values of —COOH and —NH_3^+ end-groups depend on the type of terminal amino acid and the peptide chain length (43). Moreover the extent of deamidation of asparagine and glutamine occurring during the hydrolysis causes a variable increase in the number of dissociable groups in the products.

Rather surprisingly, although peptide charge and size have been separately studied for their influence on skin/hair substantivity and surfactant complexation, the charge/mass ratio has never been investigated as a specific parameter affecting the cosmetic properties of protein derivatives.

6. *Protein Denaturation*

Few of the proteins of cosmetic interest retain their naturally occurring structure as supplied in raw materials, and not considering the special case of enzymes used as active ingredients in skin and hair care preparations, the maintenance of the undernatured form in finished formulations has relevance only for soluble collagen. Native (undenatured) tropocollagen is obtained by cold extraction with a slightly acidic medium from connective tissues of mammals and fishes. It consists of three α-helical polypeptide chains regularly twisted around each other to form a triple-helix structure. Cooperative intramolecular hydrogen bonds engaging all CO and NH groups stabilize the α-helical conformation and other interchain hydrogen bonds and water bridges keep the three chains tightly linked in the superhelix structure. In aqueous solution, soluble collagen forms a rigid rod with a diameter of about 1.4 nm and a length of 300 nm. The triple-helix structure is supposed to be responsible for the film-forming, moisturizing, and protective effects of soluble collagen, and denaturation to gelatin or partial disruption of the helical conformation would result in loss of its cosmetic properties. Collagen denaturation is caused by any chemical or physical agent capable of breaking the intra- and intermolecular hydrogen bonds stabilizing its conformation: heat, salts, surfactants, organic solvents, and substances containing hydroxyl or amino groups such as ethanol and urea. Exposure to high temperature is the most common cause of collagen denaturation in the preparation and life of cosmetic products.

When heat is provided to an aqueous solution of soluble collagen, many changes are observable in its physical behavior (drop of viscosity, changes in the optical-rotatory properties), which reveal that the helical structure has been lost. The cooperative hydrogen bonds are rapidly disrupted in a restricted temperature range with formation of a random structure (gelatin) that cannot be reformed into collagen. The denaturation of collagen is a two-step process, in the first of which the helical structure rapidly collapses as a consequence of the breaking of hydrogen cooperative bonds; the second step is much slower and results in strand separation. The temperature at which half of the helical structure is lost is the melting temperature T_m. Its value is different for collagen of different animal species and is correlated to the physiological body temperature. Chemically, a correlation has been demonstrated between the melting temperature and the content in the amino acids proline and hydroxyproline. The higher their content, the higher the T_m value. Soluble collagen obtained from codfish (body temperature 10–14°C) has a T_m of about 16°C (11). Evaluation of the melting temperature of collagen can be made by measuring the specific optical rotation. The value of $[\alpha_D^{20°C}]$ for native soluble bovine collagen is −400° and for the full denatured molecule is −120° (68).

The denaturation phenomenon is the basis for a simple test for the identification of native soluble collagen in cosmetic raw materials: from a homogeneous collagen solution, insoluble collagen fibrils can be obtained if sodium chloride is added to the solution to a final concentration of 5–7%. Fibrils from native collagen but not gelatinized or hydrolyzed collagen will be precipitated.

B. Physicochemical Properties

1. *Solubility and Stability*

Water solubility and stability in aqueous solutions and water-based cosmetic formulations is an indispensable requisite for protein derivatives, not only to obtain and maintain transparent preparations, but also because most of the expected cosmetic effects are possible only when the interacting species involved are solvated in an aqueous environment. The techniques and procedures adopted to obtain soluble derivatives (hydrolysis, complexation, etc.) have been described in the preceding sections.

Once solubility has been obtained it should be ensured its stability on time. The formation of less soluble protein species can occur in aqueous solution or finished cosmetic preparations, giving rise to haze, flocculation, or distinct precipitation of insoluble materials. (Destabilization phenomena related to interactions with other substances are described in Section V.E).

For protein hydrolysates the most frequent cause of loss of solubility is reaggregation of peptides by hydrophobic interactions. Hydrolysates obtained from hydrophobic proteins (casein, wheat, soy, corn) easily reform insoluble aggregates, but this effect is rarely observed for the highly hydrophilic peptides from collagen and silk proteins. Disulfide interchange reactions may also cause formation of larger interchained peptides with reduced solubility. Finally, elongation of the peptide chains can occur via a transpeptidation mechanism (see Section II.B.2) with formation of plastein aggregates when residual enzyme activity is present in the product.

A certain solubility in alcohol or other organic solvents is sometimes requested for use of proteins in hydroalcoholic lotions and nonaqueous cosmetic preparations. Hydrolysates with high surface hydrophobicity and derivatives obtained by the attachment of long lipophilic residues can partially comply with these requirements.

2. *Rheological Properties of Protein Derivatives*

The use of proteins as rheological modifiers and enhancers is highly important in food technology, where their physicochemical properties, rather than their nutritional value, will determine their acceptability as ingredients in prepared food. In cosmetic formulations, proteins are mainly considered (and expected) to be functional ingredients; thus poor emphasis has been given so far to their potential rheological activity. Yet high-molecular-weight natural proteins and a variety of modified proteins developed for food applications show interesting effects on aqueous and emulsified systems, and many protein derivatives suitable for cosmetic use are able to affect the physicochemical behavior of finished formulations.

Proteins having large molecular masses show water- and fat-binding capacity, air-trapping activity, gelling, thickening, and emulsifying properties. Gelation phenomena are often observed in protein solutions and dispersions; they are mainly due to the attraction-repulsion forces between charged groups in the protein, which leads to the formation of a three-dimensional network where water molecules are entrapped. This effect is generally amplified when an excess of ionized carboxylic groups is present, leading to prevailing repulsive forces with subsequent unfolding of polypeptide chains (69,70). This general behavior is supported by comparisons of the properties of native proteins with deamidated and succinylated derivatives, where additional carboxylic groups are introduced in the protein molecules. Protein gels are characterized by a relatively high viscosity, plasticity, and elasticity; they are used to provide a structural matrix for holding water, flavors, sugars, and other ingredients in food applications. Gelation has not been used so far in cosmetic systems, owing to the relatively high content of protein required and because the systems obtained are generally opaque, but development of enhanced modified protein will probably make this effect of some importance in cosmetic preparations.

The emulsifying properties of proteins can be explained by their amphiphilic character and surface activity. In oil-in-water systems, proteins tend to diffuse to the interface. The ionized environment at the interface shifts the conformational equilibrium, and unfolding of the protein occurs, with exposure of its hydrophobic segments to the oil interface and polar/ionic groups to the aqueous phase. This sequence, valid for high-molecular-weight proteins, involves protein denaturation, the extent of which depends on the flexibility of the molecule and conditions (temperature, pH, and ion effect) prevailing in the medium. Proteins with high molecular flexibility (flexibility is strongly reduced by disulfide bridges) show high surface activity, because unfolding is facilitated and exposition of hydrophobic residues enhances interfacial film formation (24). The emulsifying activity of proteins is well correlated with their surface hydrophobicity (71). Stabilization of O/W emulsions by proteins is the result of location of protein molecules at the interface, with formation of small oil droplets coated by a protein film, and, secondarily, of the increased viscosity of the aqueous phase. Chemical modifications like succinylation, leading to prevailing repulsive forces in the protein structure, facilitate unfolding of the polypeptide, exposure of more hydrophobic regions, and generally enhance their emulsifying properties. Hydrolysis generally results in a decrease of hydrophobicity, caused by increased charge density, and loss of emulsifying activity. Except for some protein–fatty acid condensates, which possess a distinct amphiphilic character and may be associated with primary emulsifiers in the preparation of O/W creams and lotions, the intentional use of proteins as emulsifiers in cosmetic formulations has not been reported. Nevertheless they can affect positively, but also negatively, the stability of cosmetic emulsions, by participation at the interface equilibrium.

Protein solutions are also known to foam easily. Protein foams consist of gas droplets encapsulated by a liquid cohesive film, containing unfolded surface-active proteins. Molecular flexibility and hydrophobicity are again important requirements for effective and stable foaming. Flexibility facilitates protein unfolding and subsequent increase of hydrophobicity; exposed hydrophobic regions cause association of polypeptides and increase of viscosity at the interface, resulting in more stable foaming (72,73). Though the foaming properties of protein derivatives are not comparable with those of most common surfactants, long-chain proteins and protein hydrolysates are sometimes associated with anionic and nonionic tensides to enhance foaming, foam stability, and foam feel of detergent formulations. In a limited number of cases, replacement of part of the basic tensides with an equal part of proteins will result in increased foam expansion and stability.

IV. ROLE AND FUNCTIONS OF PROTEINS IN COSMETICS

A. General Aspects

The efficacy of proteins as functional cosmetic ingredients has frequently been overstated. The use of collagen, elastin, and fibronectin in skin care products is often associated with the assertion that these substances can impart structure, firmness, and viscoelastic and elastic properties compensating for the loss and aging of these macromolecules in the human skin. Misleading conclusions about the ability of exogenous proteins and peptides to promote fibroblast activity, stimulate protein biosynthesis, restructure the endogenous protein network in the dermis, and neutralize free radicals in the deep layers of the skin are all based on the largely unfounded assumption that percutaneous transport of these molecules below the healthy horny layer occurs. For most protein derivatives, this hypothesis is strongly refuted by the fact that passive permeation of the stratum corneum barrier of substances with a molecular weight more than 3000 Daltons is not documented and only smaller molecules are thought to diffuse in the epidermis after topical application. The ionic and prevailing hydrophilic character of protein derivatives is another factor that restricts their possibility to permeate the stratum corneum barrier: they have generally low affinity for the lipids of the intercellular domains of stratum corneum, which is thought to be the major pathway of percutaneous absorption. Moreover, from a regulatory and ethical point of view, the penetration of cosmetic ingredients into the skin should be avoided or, at least, should not be emphasized and pursued. The local and systemic effects that chemical substances might have when the natural skin barrier would be crossed are almost totally out of the control of cosmetic chemists and dermatologists, and the role of cosmetic products and ingredients, as stated by most national and international regulations, ceases at the surface of the skin.

Only a few studies have been concerned with the percutaneous absorption of protein ingredients from cosmetic products and some controversial results have ensued. Most of these works dealt with the potential absorption of soluble collagen and were based on simple application models and selective detection of the exogenous protein radiolabeled with ^{14}C or ^{125}I (74,75).

^{14}C labeling was made by subcutaneous injection in rats of proline tagged with ^{14}C and subsequent extraction of the neosynthesized collagen where the radiolabeled amino acid was incorporated; ^{125}I labeling was made by electrophilic substitution with $^{125}I_2$ on the aromatic ring of tyrosine of the collagen molecule. Both labeling procedures were considered to not alter the general structural characteristics of collagen: the first because no changes in the side chains of amino acids were caused, the second because modifications involved the side chain of an amino acid present in small quantity in the collagen molecule. After application of a cream containing radiolabeled collagen to the skin of rats, the percutaneous absorption was evaluated by autoradiography and the molecular features of recovered collagen were investigated by gel electrophoresis and size exclusion chromatography. While ^{14}C-labeled collagen did not penetrate the stratum corneum, it was found that intact ^{125}I-labeled collagen was rapidly and efficiently absorbed in the dermis.

Other authors (76), also on the basis of experiments carried out in their laboratories, substantially rejected the conclusions of these studies and interpreted the results obtained as suggesting that excess radioactivity of free ^{125}I was entrapped in the hydrophilic moiety of unlabeled collagen during sectioning, autoradiography, or extraction procedures and that only endogenous collagen had been actually recovered.

Although the hypothesis that the large molecule of soluble native collagen, 1.5×300 nm in length, could penetrate the skin is generally refuted today, the discussion about the potential penetration of smaller peptides is still open. Absorption and accumulation of free amino acids is well documented to occur in the stratum corneum (77,78), yet this does not necessarily mean that larger polymers of these small molecules could penetrate.

Much more data support the view that cosmetic properties of protein ingredients are mainly related to their ability to be adsorbed onto the surface of the skin and hair, and unless direct evidence of permeation of the stratum corneum and cuticle cells of the hair fiber is shown, the cosmetic benefits obtainable should be regarded as final effects of a ''surface'' activity. ''Substantivity'' (which generally indicates the capacity of chemical substances to be sorbed to various surfaces) is the term adopted by cosmetic scientists to express the binding properties of proteins to the skin and hair and appears to be the key mechanism of many cosmetic actions of these ingredients. Well-documented improvements in the appearance and feel of skin and hair attained by the use of protein ingredients are the consequence of their substantivity. The most successful use of protein ingredients is in fact in hair treatment, where protein-substrate interactions are amplified for extension of the keratinic surface available. The consumption of protein materials in shampoos and hair conditioners can be estimated to match their use in all the other cosmetic categories.

A second crucial series of benefits is related to the interaction of proteins with other components of cosmetic formulations. Complexation of surfactants will reduce their potential irritancy and is at the basis of their protective effect in detergent formulations. Less emphasized and probably underestimated are their technical properties: proteins can be used as buffering agents, foaming enhancers, viscosity regulators, powder compactants, and for their water- and oil-binding properties and emulsifying capacity.

B. Protein-Skin Interactions

In numerous technical bulletins on protein derivatives, an exciting series of biological actions that these ingredients could perform on the skin biochemistry are claimed. These include stimulation of fibroblast respiration and regeneration, increase of protein synthesis in the epidermal cells, antielastasic activity, anti-free-radical scavenging, and a variety of others that are plausible only if a direct intervention of these molecules in the deep layers of the skin were to occur. Such strong claims are often supported by tests performed in vitro on fibroblast cultures or even in pure chemical systems, and a series of potential cosmetic effects (prevention of skin aging, increase of skin elasticity and firmness) are speculatively extrapolated. As direct scientific evidence that topically delivered proteins are capable of interacting with fibroblasts and other biological structures in the epidermis and dermis is still missing, a more realistic view of their effects on the skin is based on their well-documented ability to be adsorbed on the skin surface by linking the keratin matrix of the stratum corneum. Subsequent effects, such as skin hydration and protection, pH buffering of the hydrolipidic layer, and a series of measurable changes in the microrelief and mechanical properties of the skin, appear to be the consequence of the interactions of proteins with the structure of the stratum corneum.

Protein substantivity on the skin has been investigated by in vivo and in vitro studies. The adsorption of collagen peptides on human callus, morphologically and chemically similar to the stratum corneum of normal skin, has been demonstrated to occur rapidly from aqueous solutions and detergent formulations, even at very low protein content, and is quantitatively comparable to the adsorption on hair (79).

The moisturizing effect of proteins on the skin is frequently affirmed. The water-binding properties of protein derivatives are mainly related to the formation of hydrogen bonds with the water molecules. The free hydrogen and oxygen atoms in the peptide bond and many groups of amino acid side chains are available to link water molecules by hydrogen bonds. The peptide bond, the repeating unit of a polypeptide chain, has a rigid geometry; as the N—C bond has the partial character of a double bond, the CO and NH groups lie on the same virtual plane and are fixed in a *trans* configuration. This makes them sterically available for the formation of hydrogen bonds and allows stabilization of regular periodic structures like the α-helix and β-pleated sheet by intra- and intermolecular linkages. The side chains of 11 of the 20 basic amino acids are also involved in the formation of hydrogen bonds: (1) the side chains of triptophan and arginine are hydrogen donors, (2) asparagine, glutamine, serine, and threonine can be hydrogen donors or acceptors, (3) the ionizable side chains of aspartic and glutamic acid, lysine, tyrosine, and histidine can be hydrogen donors or acceptors depending on the pH. The water-binding property of proteins is therefore inherent to the presence and steric availability of the peptide bonds and amino acid side groups (Fig. 21).

The data available in the scientific literature and technical information of the manufacturers on the moisturizing effects of protein derivative are incoherent, and neither the relationship of the molecular features of protein ingredients with their hydrating effects nor the time course pattern of skin moisturization is clarified. Many of the data suggesting a moisturizing effect on the skin are indirect: some are based on measurements of the

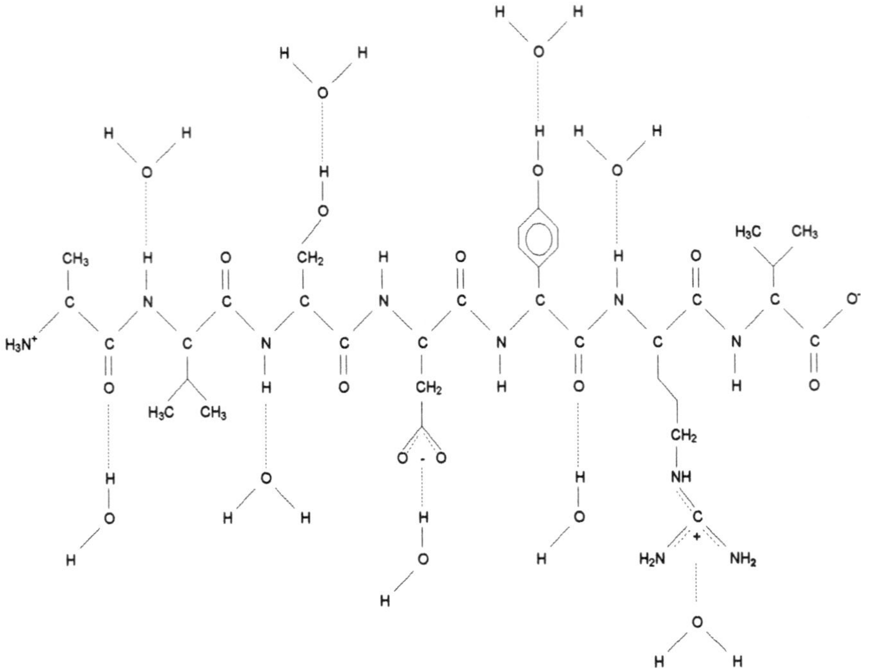

Figure 21 Binding of water molecules with =NH and —CO peptide groups and amino acid side chains by hydrogen bonds (schematic).

hygroscopic effects of protein derivatives; others relate the increase of the thickness of epidermis to hydration (76).

Direct testing of cutaneous hydration after application of protein substances showed a short-term increase of skin humidity after the use of soluble and reticulated collagen (80) and a sericin derivative (81). A test performed on O/W and W/O emulsions and aqueous lotions containing desamido collagen and hydrolyzed collagen showed that while desamido collagen caused skin moisturization comparable to that obtained with well-known humectants (urea, sodium pyrrolidone carboxylate), no significant increase of skin capacitance was revealed for the preparations containing hydrolyzed collagen, which was even found to cause dehydration (82).

In a more recent study, an increase of the skin microcirculatory patterns (skin temperature and blood flow/velocity in the skin capillaries) consequent to application of pure soluble collagen has been reported. These effects were related by the authors to a short-term inhibition of the transepidermal water loss, causing indirect uptake of excess water by the biopolymers in the dermis and consequent increase of elasticity and pulsation efficacy of the small blood vessels (83). These tests are largely heterogeneous and the results obtained not comparable, being based on different exposure and evaluation methodologies; however, all studies report only short-term moisturizing effects.

A smoothing effect on the skin microrelief consequent to the use of proteins in skin care products has also been documented (26,76,81). Mechanisms invoked are the formation of a smooth colloidal film on the skin surface, water uptake and moderate swelling of the stratum corneum caused by a direct water-binding action or partial blocking of transepidermal water flow, and a stretching effect on the micro furrows of the skin surface due to gradual loss of bound water from the polypeptides deposited on the skin. The skin-smoothing effect should, however, be regarded as a nonspecific result of all cosmetic maneuvers designed to increase the water content of the horny layer (84).

As mentioned above, collagen and other protein substances are also reported, in technical literature and product claims, to be useful to counteract the biological and actinic aging. As manifest cutaneous aging is the result of disorganization and depletion of collagen fibers in the dermis and direct intervention of exogenous proteins on these structures is still undemonstrated, only surface mechanisms giving a reduction of its effects are acceptable. Moisturization of the horny layer and film forming over the skin surface may have moderate effects on the skin microrelief, the component of the skin determined by the structure of its most superficial layer (85).

A generic skin protective effect is also claimed for protein ingredients. Their ability to reduce the adverse effects of surfactants on the skin is well documented, whereas a shielding action on other irritants or physical agents has been not convincingly demonstrated. An indirect protective property of protein derivative (mostly hydrolyzed proteins) is related to their buffering capacity. This can be advantageously used to favor maintenance or restoring of the physiological pH value on the skin, aiding prevention of pathogenic microflora colonization and impairment of the skin barrier function.

Particular uses of cosmetic proteins in the skin and scalp treatments that are worth mention are the use of collagen–fatty acid condensates in the treatment of acne and other skin impurities supported by abnormal microbial proliferation (86) and the use of an abietoyl protein condensate in the treatment of greasy scalp and hair (87).

C. Protein-Hair Interactions

In a greatly simplified description, which omits the fine details of hair architecture, human hair fiber is composed of two main structural components: the cuticle, composed of 5–10 layers of overlapping flat cells containing nonfibrous keratin with a high content of cystine residues (1 for 2.7 amino acids on average); and the cortex, the dominant structural element of the hair (60–90% of the fiber), which is responsible for its mechanical and elastic properties. The cortex is composed of long, spindle-like cells aligned with the fiber's axis, filled with microfibrils of low-sulfur α-keratin embedded in a high-sulfur β-keratin matrix (88). Whereas the interior of the hair fiber is widely believed to have little significance with respect to hair condition, the outside layer, the cuticle, is responsible for the tactile and optical perception of hair, governs the frictional properties of the fibers, and, by extensive disulfide cross-linking of its keratin, protects the inner cortex from fibrillation by mechanical or chemical aggression. Even though the cuticle is highly resistant to physical and chemical aggression, it is not immune to damages caused by a variety of mechanical stresses (friction, pulling, bending), exposure to environmental factors (ultraviolet radiation, wind, moisture) and chemical substances. Repeated and long-term exposure to these causes alteration of its surface geometry (roughness) and optical properties (opacity), breakdown and loss of cuticle cells, and exposure of the cortex, which can result in brittleness, splitting, complete fibrillation of the fiber, and finally breakage. Daily grooming procedures of combing, brushing, and towel drying progressively cause uplifting of the cuticles, resulting in an increase of the frictional forces between the hair fibers and the comb and triboelectric charging of the hair (flyaway effect) (89). Exposure of the fibers to high temperature during washing, blow drying, or by heat-styling procedures with hot rollers, curling, and straightening irons accelerates hair damage. Cosmetic treatments involving the use of alkali, reducing agents, and oxidizers cause cystine damage, with solubilization and loss of keratin peptides and amino acids. Shampooing alone can progressively abrade the cuticle and lead to keratin loss. Wet hair has a lower resistance to abrasion and chemical aggression than dry hair, because of its swelling and partial replacement of keratin-keratin cross-links by water bridges, with water-keratin bonds.

Sebum secretion and filming on the hair surface is an effective self-defense mechanism to counteract cuticle damage. Spreading of sebum along hairs occur via mechanical contacts with body movement and hair handling. The lipidic layer lubricates the fibers, reduces the frictional forces, and provides a chemical protective barrier. By this and other mechanisms hair is maintained in a proper healthy state, characterized by shine, softness, easiness to comb and style, mechanical resistance, and elasticity. In the absence of external influences hair tends to remain in this conditioned state. The role of cosmetic conditioners is to help counteract damaging effects and to restore the healthy state of the hair.

The conditioning mechanisms of cosmetic ingredients can be different, but requisite to all conditioners is the ability to bind hair keratin and moderately resist mechanical and rinse removal. As for the nature of the binding forces involved in conditioner-hair interaction, different chemical linkages are possible. Because of the chemical structure of the hair cuticle, the presence of many ionizable groups, and the negative net charge at physiological pH value [cuticle keratin has an isoelectric point of about 3.7 (90)], the electrostatic interactions are of great importance.

Proteins and protein derivatives have generally high chemical affinity with hair keratin and their high capacity to be adsorbed on the hair surface (substantivity) is given by the many binding sites and reactive groups present in their molecules. Weak but numerous cooperative ionic, hydrophobic, and hydrogen bonds can be established between exogenous proteins and hair keratin, resulting in an overall tight complex formation. Moreover, covalent substantivity can occur between hair keratin and cystine-containing protein derivatives when appropriate conditioning procedures are followed.

It is, however, important to point out that hair substantivity is a necessary, but not sufficient, requisite for the conditioning effects, which are related to the specific molecular characteristics and physicochemical properties of each conditioning agent.

The substantivity of protein derivatives (especially protein hydrolysates) has been subject to numerous researches, often resulting in controversial data and conclusions. Some of the experiments published in scientific literature or reported in the technical bulletins of protein manufacturers are reviewed and discussed here, with special concern for the studies on the relationship between molecular characteristics and substantivity, quantitative evaluations of protein-hair interactions, and application aspects.

Ranganayaki et al. (91,92) have studied the effect of different variables (type of hair, molecular weight, concentration, application time, pH) on the hair substantivity of enzyme-hydrolyzed collagen. They found that when virgin, bleached, and cold-waved hair were treated with hydrolyzed collagen, there was an increase in the sorption of peptide depending on the degree of damage to the hair. Less peptide was sorbed on the virgin hair (0.03 g/100 g of hair), comparatively more was sorbed on the bleached hair (0.2 g/100 g of hair), and a still larger amount was sorbed on cold-wave-treated hair (3 g/100 g of hair). The maximum sorption occurred with collagen hydrolysate of low-molecular-weight range (0.17 g/100 g of hair), and sorption decreased as the molecular-weight range increased (0.07 g/100 g of hair) on virgin hair. Sorption was enhanced on all types of hair up to a concentration application of 5%, and no significant increase occurred at higher concentrations. With regard to the effect of the time of exposure, these authors found that the sorption of collagen peptides was rapid during the initial 15 min of treatment, irrespective of the type of hair used (virgin, bleached, cold-wave-treated) and later the rate of sorption decreased. The sorption increase with pH and its rate followed the order cold-waved-hair > bleached > virgin. These results are in good agreement with conclusions of other works and provide valuable quantitative data, but information about the test methodology and chemical characterization of the test products is lacking.

The same authors studied the effects of application of collagen hydrolysates on the stress-strain characteristics of different hair: 5 cm of virgin, bleached, and cold-wave-treated hair were taken and stretched to 30% index in water at a rate extension of 0.25 cm/min. After stretching, the fibers were allowed to relax overnight in water and restretched. Comparison of the stress applied (in kg/mm^2) versus strain percent was made before and after treatments with collagen hydrolysate. It was found that when collagen hydrolysate is sorbed to the hair there is an increase in its tensile strength, markedly observable on cold-waved hair.

Stern and Johnsen (93) studied the relationship between hair substantivity and molecular size of collagen hydrolysates. They separated an enzyme-hydrolyzed collagen on dextran gel obtaining four peptide fractions with different molecular size range: (1) molecular weight > 30,000 Daltons, (2) 30,000–5000, (3) 5000–1000, (4) <1000. Five percent active protein solutions of the fractions obtained were applied under standardized methodology (10 min exposure at room temperature followed by rinsing for 30 sec in warm, running tap water) to bleached and bleached/waved hair swatches. Substantivity was evaluated by total hydrolysis of the hair with barium hydroxide and hydroxyproline determination. The fraction containing peptides with average molecular weight of 1000–5000 Daltons was found to give the highest substantivity on both bleached and bleached-waved hair. Pure hydroxyproline at the same concentration was less substantive than peptides of molecular weight of about 1000.

Turowski and Adelmann-Grill (79), extensively studied the influence of peptide molecular weight and hair/skin substantivity and found results that openly contrast with those reported by others (9,10,93). In this work substantivity of collagen hydrolysates was tested in water solutions and tenside preparations under conditions resembling actual cosmetic application. Hair substantivity was evaluated on virgin and bleached/dyed hair by labeling peptides with ^{125}iodine and measuring radioactivity of the substrate after suitable treatment. Great care was given to radiolabeling procedures of peptides in this work, and the authors excluded the possibility that higher- or lower-molecular-mass fractions had preferentially been taken up by the radioactive label. Collagen hydrolysates were characterized for average isoelectric point and molecular weight distribution. In addition to the chemical characteristics of the tested hydrolysates, other variables investigated were: hydrolysate concentration in the application medium, time of incubation, type of hair (untreated and bleached/dyed), type of the vehicle (water, shampoos with different tenside composition), washing conditions. The main findings were the following: (1) dependence of the substantivity on the peptide concentration in the medium was almost linear and saturation was not attained at a concentration below 5%; (2) the amount of protein sorbed to the hair varied significantly with the washing conditions (amount of water used and rinse duration), especially when applied in shampoos; (3) the characteristics of the shampoo formulations strongly influenced both substantivity and permanence of the peptides on the hair after washing; (4) absorption of peptides on damaged hair was higher than on untreated hair when at low concentration in the medium and for short incubation time; this difference was less apparent for longer exposure and generally considered to be small; (5) maximal substantivity to hair was found when the molecular masses of the hydrolysates were between 7500 and 15,000 Daltons; (6) the most substantive of the tested hydrolysates had the lowest average isoelectric point and was the only sample present as net anion at the pH of application. It is not easy to reconcile these results with most of the observations about the influence of molecular mass and prevailing charge of peptides on substantivity. Nevertheless this work is valuable for having studied substantivity in realistic application conditions and gives much interesting quantitative information on the resistance of attached peptides on rinse.

A different experimental approach of substantivity evaluation was followed in a more recent study carried out by Mintz et al. (94). These authors have investigated and compared the molecular size of collagen polypeptides as applied to hair and after desorption procedures and substantially confirm the results of the majority of previous researches about the relationship between molecular size and substantivity. Virgin and treated (bleached-waved) hair was treated in standardized conditions with simple water solutions of a hydrolyzed collagen sample, well characterized for molecular size distribution of constituent peptides. After removal of nonspecifically adsorbed peptides by rinsing with warm, running tap water, removal of bound collagen peptides was accomplished by two sequential steps in the following order: (1) hair samples were maintained in a 50°C water bath for 45 min with 10-fold amount of deionized water; (2) they were subsequently soaked overnight at 25 °C in 10-fold amount of 0.5 M NaCl solution to remove any remaining peptides. The molecular-weight distribution of peptides removed by the two sequential procedures was determined by size exclusion chromatography; individual column fractions were assayed for hydroxyproline and primary amino group content using fluorescamine reaction. No hydroxyproline residue was demonstrated to remain on hair samples after the two-step desorption procedure. It was found that: (1) in both the high-temperature and high-salt soakings almost a double amount of fluorescamine-reactive peptides was released from bleached-waved hair than from virgin hair and a similar ratio was found for the hydroxyproline content of the desorption fractions; (2) about twice as much hydroxyproline-containing peptides was released from virgin hair in the high-temperature soaking as from the high-salt soaking, whereas in the bleached/waved hair the ratio of hydroxyproline-containing peptides between high-temperature and high-salt fractions was approximately 4:1; (3) the molecular-weight-distribution profile of the desorption fractions showed a major presence of low-mass peptides in the high-temperature extract and a relatively higher content of larger peptides in the high-salt fraction, which also had a much broader molecular-weight distribution. The authors concluded that small peptides are selectively bound to hair keratin of treated and undamaged hair; the high temperature of the extraction medium caused the hair structure to swell, allowing exit of these peptides from the hair shaft, whereas larger peptides were predominantly bound (in minor amount) via ionic interactions to the hair and removed by high-salt solutions.

A similar experimental methodology, based on a simple adsorbing procedure from water solution at controlled pH and a two-step desorption extraction with 50°C distilled water and NaCl solution, was used by Teglia et al. to evaluate the relationship between molecular characteristics and substantivity of different protein hydrolysates (32). More than 20 protein hydrolysates were selected after preliminary screening of about 50 commercial products of animal and vegetable origin or especially prepared in the laboratory to provide a suitable range of products with different molecular characteristics with regard to molecular size, ionic charge, and amino acid composition.

Substantivity was tested on virgin Caucasian hair, and damaged hair obtained by a standardized procedure based on oxidation with hydrogen peroxide, reduction with alkaline thioglycolate, and treatment again with hydrogen peroxide. The adsorption procedure consisted of immersion of hair swatches in 10-fold 2.5% protein solution for 1 hr at 20°C at pH 6.0. Unbound peptides were removed by extensive rinsing with running tap water at room temperature. Desorption was made in two sequential steps as in the work of Mintz et al. (94). Desorbed peptides were quantitated in the extraction fractions by fluorescamine reaction and the molecular mass distribution of desorbed peptides was analyzed by size exclusion chromatography. Quantitative results of the substantivity test are reported in Figures 22 and 23.

Main findings and conclusions were as follows: (1) The keratin hydrolysates tested had higher substantivity compared to other animal and vegetable derivatives. They were more substantive than hydrolysates having a higher isoelectric point and smaller average size. This probably indicates that the amino acid composition can have an important influence on hair substantivity and that covalent cross-linking between hair keratin and cystine-containing hydrolysates may occur on partially reduced hair by sulfide-disulfide interchange. (2) Substantivity of hydrolysates of the same origin increased with decreasing molecular size and increasing isolectric point. (3) The actual hydrophobicity of peptides (see Section III.A.4) was supposed to affect their substantivity to hair: in fact two wheat protein hydrolysates (M and N in Figs. 22 and 23) having similar average molecular size and net charge, but obtained by the action of two different protease (M by an enzyme with specificity for hydrophilic side chain amino acids and N by an enzyme with specificity for hydrophobic side chain amino acid), showed different substantivity. (4) Analyses of the molecular weight distribution of desorbed peptide compared to original products showed a preferential adsorption of smaller peptides for all samples, on both virgin and damaged hair; the higher-molecular-weight fraction bound was almost completely removed by high-temperature extraction and hardly detectable in the high-salt extracts (Fig. 24).

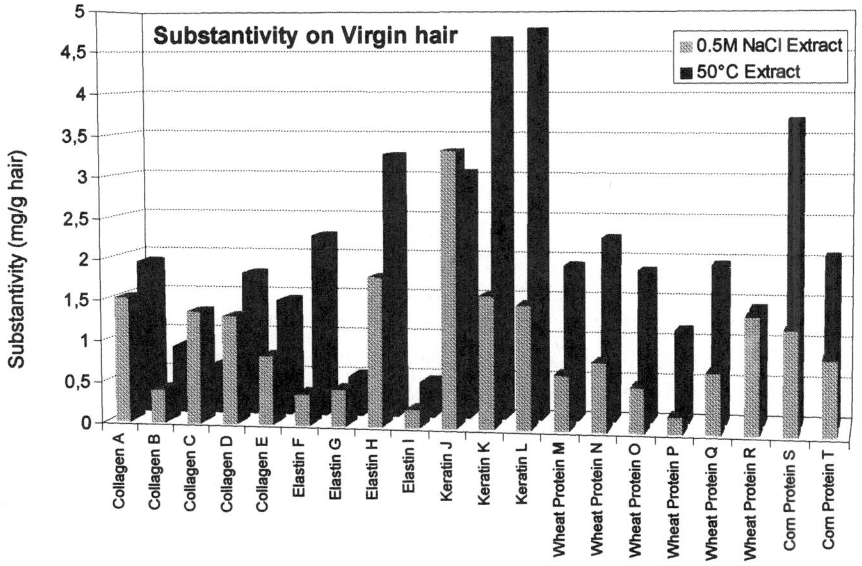

Figure 22 Substantivity on virgin hair of animal and vegetable protein hydrolysates (32).

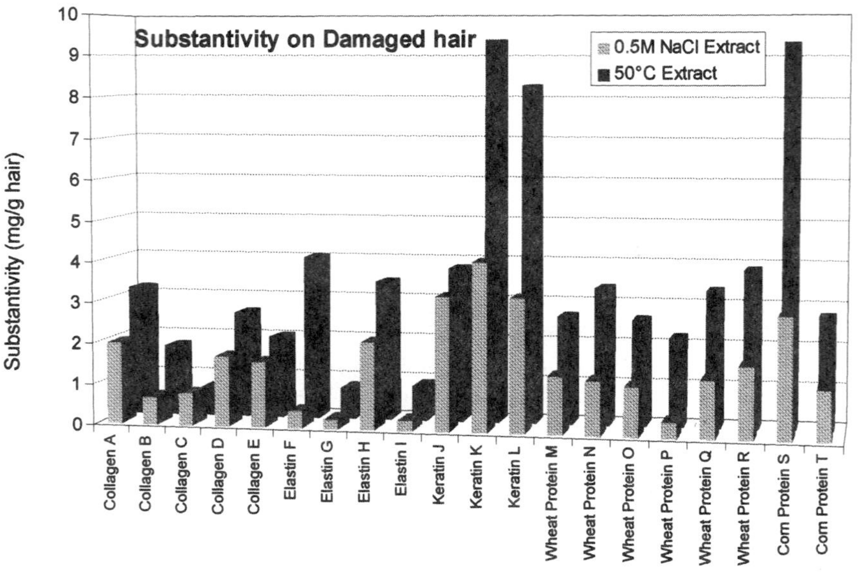

Figure 23 Substantivity on damaged hair of animal and vegetable protein hydrolysates (32).

The incompleteness and partial disagreement of the studies reviewed reflects the difficulties of an accurate experimental control on the many molecular variables of protein hydrolysates and is the consequence of the heterogeneous experimental models adopted for protein adsorption and substantivity evaluation. Some solid evidence can, however, be extracted from these researches and the multitude of technical data on protein substantivity reported in the technical bulletins of manufacturers: (1) Protein adsorption onto hair occurs; the binding is rapid and is proved to occur from water solutions and cosmetic actual formulations as well; (2) damage of the cuticle, chemical reduction, and swelling increase the capacity of hair to bind exogenous peptides, probably in relation to the formation of microcavities and fissures, which could physically locate large amounts of peptides and expose numerous binding sites; (3) small peptides exhibit generally higher substantivity than larger peptides; (4) peptide substantivity increases with isoelectric point.

Further aspects of protein substantivity to hair are of practical importance. The time course of binding and the relationship between substantivity, protein concentration, number of repeated applications, and characteristics of the vehicle are of great interest to cosmetic chemists to formulate properly with protein derivatives. Substantivity does not necessarily correlate directly with conditioning performance: for example, excessive accumulation of peptides on the hair surface can impart unwanted hair heaviness, rigidity, and triboelectric charging; therefore, detailed evaluation of the conditioning effects of protein derivatives should always be regarded as the key test for their utility in hair care applications.

Though accurate quantitative data on the kinetics of peptide adsorption onto hair are not available, many studies on substantivity suggest that the binding of hair keratin is rapid and efficient. This allows adsorption to take place in quick cosmetic procedures where the time of application and contact is restricted to a few minutes (shampooing, rinse conditioning). Karjala et al. (9,10) found that peptide binding to human hair is rapid

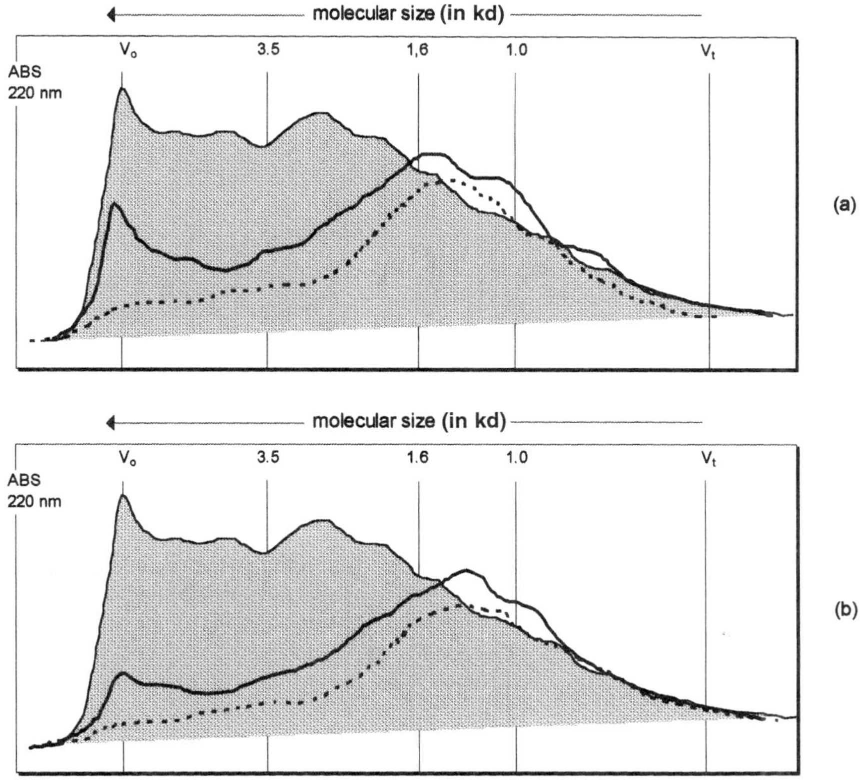

Figure 24 Size exclusion chromatography patterns of high-temperature (solid line) and high-salt (dotted line) fractions desorbed form damaged (a) and virgin hair (b) after application of a collagen hydrolysate. A higher amount of large peptides was adsorbed on bleached/waved hair than on virgin hair. Large peptides were found to be less effectively bound than smaller peptides, as they were selectively removed by hot water (32).

for the first 5–10 min of treatment of virgin or bleached hair and more rapid in damaged hair from aqueous solutions. Turowski and Adelmann-Grill, in the above-mentioned study (79), observed little dependence of hair substantivity of collagen hydrolysates within the interval 1–20 min, from both aqueous solutions and shampoo formulations: just 1-min incubation causes adsorption of 30–60% compared to a 20-min exposure.

As for the relationship between protein concentration and substantivity, the data reported show a similar pattern for most hydrolysates: substantivity increases almost linearly with concentration up to a certain concentration level, and then the slope of the adsorption curve decreases, reaching a plateau corresponding to saturation of the binding sites of hair keratin. A typical curve for this relationship is shown in Figure 25 (95).

As normal-use concentration of protein hydrolysates in hair care products seldom exceeds 1–2% as active substance, reaching keratin saturation is unlikely for single applications, whereas a buildup effect can realistically be expected after repeated use. An accumulation pattern derived experimentally for repeated applications of wheat peptides is shown in Figure 26.

Accumulation of peptides on the hair surface after repeated protein applications could

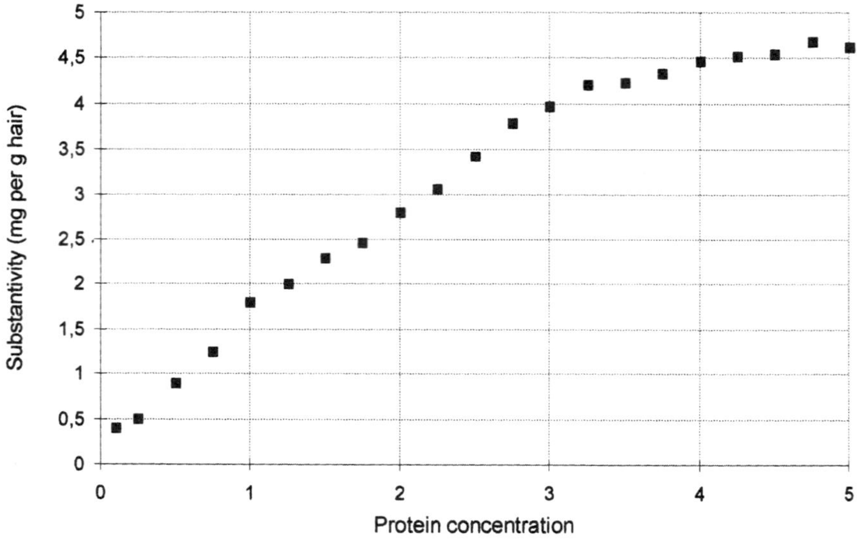

Figure 25 Relationship between substantivity and protein concentration in the medium. Applications were made by immersion of virgin hair tresses in water solutions of a wheat protein hydrolysate (hair/solution ratio 1:10 w/w) at 25°C for 2.5 hr, pH 5.5. Desorption consisted in extraction with 10-fold 50°C distilled water, after rinsing of the hair tresses. The amount of adsorbed peptides was determined by nitrogen determination on the extracts (95).

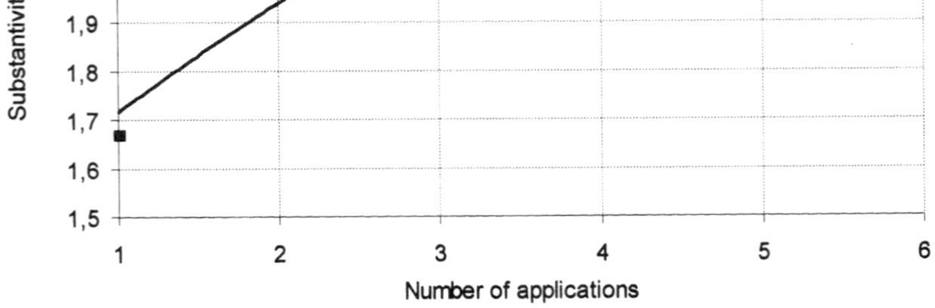

Figure 26 Substantivity test for repeated applications of a 1% wheat protein hydrolysate solution. Adsorption and desorption procedures as described in the legend of Figure 24. Each application was followed by thorough hair rinse with water at room temperature (95).

theoretically occur over the saturation level through the binding of newly supplied peptides to those previously attached to hair fibers. This normally has unwanted effects (hair heaviness, stiffness, and bad texture); it is therefore useful to know the adsorption pattern versus dose and number of applications of protein derivatives, to properly adjust the composition of relevant formulations. These data are sometimes provided by protein manufacturers, though mainly concerned with application of simple aqueous solutions of peptides; most helpful for formulators is direct testing of actual preparations with quantitation of substantivity or evaluation of the conditioning effect. An effective protein hydrolysate should attain saturation of keratin-binding sites at the lowest possible concentration with no excessive buildup on repeated use.

As the ionization pattern and net charge of amphoionic substances is pH-dependent, protein substantivity is significantly influenced by the pH of the medium. The dissociation of ionizable groups of hair keratin is also affected by pH, but since most hair care and hygiene products have a pH value in the range 5–7 and the isoelectric point of cuticle keratin is below 4, it exists as net anion in almost all cosmetic applications. For protein hydrolysates the pH of the formulation is more critical. Their isoelectric point may vary from about 4 to above 7, and since the strongest binding forces involved in protein attachment to the hair are thought to be ionic, the overall peptide substantivity is expected to increase with the increase of their cationic character. As a general rule, confirmed by experimental data, protein hydrolysates are more substantive at a pH value below their isoelectric point (96), yet when protein hydrolysates have a net negative charge, they are still substantive to the hair. This is because hydrophobic and hydrogen bonds also contribute to the binding with the substrate, and (perhaps most important) at a pH value up to 2–3 units above the overall isoelectric point, part of the peptides and ionizable groups still carry a positive charge. Moreover, in alkaline medium swelling of the hair may aid peptide penetration and moderately contribute to an increase of substantivity

Studies on the hair substantivity of protein derivatives other than pure hydrolysates are far less numerous and most available data are supplied in relevant technical bulletins.

Quaternized peptides show generally higher hair substantivity than underivatized hydrolysates. These molecules carry undissociable quaternary groups and display a net positive charge up to true alkaline pH values (9–12). These derivatives are reported to achieve maximum substantivity at far lower active concentration than the parent protein and to give negligible overaccumulation above saturation of the cuticle keratin (97,98). The adsorption ceases at a given concentration, possibly because repulsion between distinct positive molecules prevents further binding of newly supplied quaternized peptides.

The protein-hair interactions described so far involve coulomb attraction and other weak, noncovalent, cooperative chemical bonds (hydrophobic, hydrogen) that contribute to the overall binding force. As mentioned above, in special applications, protein derivatives containing a cystine residue may interact covalently with hair keratin, by means of a sulfide-disulfide interchange reaction. Keratin and wheat protein derivatives have been proposed as reactive ''covalent conditioners'' to be used in cosmetic treatments such as permanent waving and bleaching-dyeing where partial recombination or disruption of disulfide bridges of hair keratin is involved (99,100).

The proposed mechanism for the covalent attachment of cystine-containing peptides on reduced hair keratin is illustrated in Figure 27.

The reactive derivative can be used between the reduction and oxidation steps of waving or directly in the reducing solution (alkaline thioglycolate). In the first case, —SS— groups of the exogenous polypeptides undergo nucleophilic attack of mercaptide

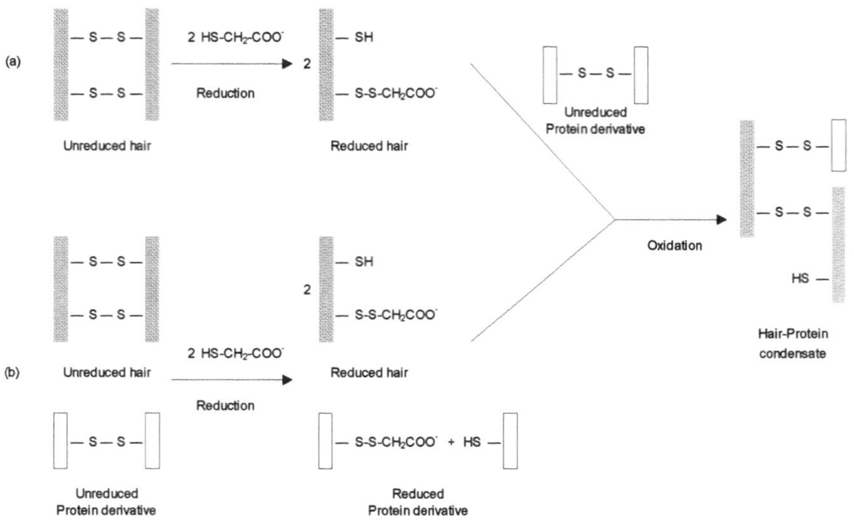

Figure 27 Proposed mechanism for covalent substantivity of exogenous protein to hair by sulfide-disulfide interchange in permanent waving treatment. The formation of new —SS— bonds between the two species can occur by nucleophilic attack of thiol groups of reduced hair on disulfide bonds of unreduced protein (a), or via contemporaneous reduction of hair and protein derivative (b). A third possible route (not shown) is based on a separate ''activation'' of the protein derivative by sulfitolysis with Na_2SO_3 at a concentration sufficient to reduce soluble peptides, but having negligible effects on the hair.

ions of reduced hair; the second route is based on separate reduction and activation of the polypeptides by the action of thioglycolate. By subsequent oxidation (with classical bromate or hydrogen peroxide preparations) cross-linking of hair keratin with external protein is obtained. The covalent attachment results in stable substantivity, highly resistant to repeated shampooing, as monitored by ^{125}I technique (96). Conditioning benefits reported consisted in improved dry combability, curl retention, and general feel. Best results were obtained with application of these ingredients on already reduced hair. When they are applied during or after the oxidation step, no immediate improvement in hair conditions results, but as relaxation of permed hair gradually occurs from partial cleavage of —SS— bridges, a use as postpermanent maintenance conditioners seems to be rational for these ingredients.

As it is not necessary for both hair keratin and external polypeptides to be in the reduced state for disulfide recombination to occur, a different way to obtain covalent substantivity from these derivatives has also been suggested. It is based on a separate ''activation'' of the protein derivative by sulfitolysis with Na_2SO_3 at a concentration (0.2%) sufficient to reduce soluble peptides, but having negligible effects on the hair. In this way covalent conditioning on nonreduced hair can be provided apart from permanent waving treatments (54).

Finally, the possibility that not only surface adsorption but also penetration of peptides into the hair fiber and deposition in the cortex could occur is supported by a study carried out by Cooperman and Johnsen (101). Low-molecular-weight collagen peptides were found to be absorbed on both virgin and damaged hair, but the low-specific-detection technique employed (ninhydrin staining of cross-sections of hairs) makes the results reported doubtful.

D. Proteins in Detergency

Surfactant interactions with proteins have been extensively studied by cosmetic scientists, with special interest in the effects of tensides on skin and hair keratin. Despite the increasing availability of highly skin-compatible surfactants that still retain excellent detergent properties, the adverse reactions potentially caused by these ingredients have never been underestimated by dermatologists and cosmetic chemists, and the subject persists as one of the key topics of cosmetology. The physicochemical aspects of protein-surfactant interactions have been investigated with a more theoretical approach in noncosmetic contexts by many scientists who exhaustively explored the behavior of binary systems of anionic tensides and native proteins (55–59).

The use of proteinaceous materials as protecting, anti-irritant agents in cleansing products for skin and hair owes its principles and success to both these research streams.

The mechanisms of the adverse effects produced by surfactants upon contact with skin and hair are not yet fully elucidated, but general agreement exists that the adsorption and interactions of their molecules to the keratin of the stratum corneum and hair cuticle are the initial determining step.

Observable toxic responses in the skin (irritation, allergic reaction) can be directly caused by the presence of surfactant molecules in the dermis, by inflammatory mediators (cytokines) liberated by keratinocytes, or by other substances penetrating the epidermis after the skin barrier function has been impaired by surfactants. The damage of hair fibers is closely related to the impairment of the cuticle layer, which can cause modifications in the mechanical and optical properties of the hair. Substantial differences exist between the mechanisms of skin damage and hair damage, but for the purposes of our discussion, only the common initial event of surfactant-keratin interaction will be considered.

One of the main characteristics of the behavior of surfactants in aqueous systems is their tendency to form larger aggregates (micelles) when a certain concentration is reached (critical micelle concentration, CMC). The CMC is specific for each given tenside at a given temperature, but the values given in the literature should be viewed with caution as it is also known that the size of the surfactant aggregates increases with concentration. When different species of surface-active substances are present in a solution, mixed micelles are formed and the CMC of the blend is different from that of each individual surfactant.

It is generally agreed that penetration of surfactants within the keratin matrix of the stratum corneum or cuticle cells of the hair fibers is the first step of skin/hair damage and that only monomeric surfactants can penetrate, while the hydrated micelles are too large to enter the tight network of keratin; thus, the concentration of tenside monomers (and hence the CMC) should be related to the skin and hair damage. This relationship has been actually demonstrated by tests in vivo and in vitro, and is strongly supported by the observation of the synergistic anti-irritant effect in tenside blends where the formation of large mixed micelles causes lowering of the CMC of the system and a reduction of its irritation potential (102). This theory has been a useful model to approach the relationship between the chemical characteristics of tensides and their adverse cosmetic effects, but it conflicts with the observation that in many test situations, toxic responses in the skin are correlated to the surfactant concentrations above the CMC (103,104). This discordance is only partly explainable by the fact that micelles are dynamic species, which form and reform readily, exchanging monomers with the solution, and that the binding of surfactant molecules to the skin and hair keratin causes the monomer-micelle equilibrium in the bulk solution to shift, reducing the concentration of the micellar species (105). (The possible penetration of micelles through glandular ducts and hair follicles in the skin adds another significant contribution to this model.) Pragmatically, it is important that by proper combination of surfactants with other molecules having amphiphilic properties, one can obtain a significant and measurable reduction of the damaging potential of the preparation.

The binding of surfactant molecules to skin and hair keratin occurs via ionic and nonionic interactions. The coulomb attraction of the ionic head of charged tensides to charged sites of keratin contributes a large share of the binding energy. This is indirectly supported by experimental data on the effect of pH on the swelling of epidermis caused by various tensides (106). Hydrophobic bonds are also involved; for anionic tensides, they produce new polar sites in the skin keratin and by this mechanism may play an important role in the swelling of the stratum corneum (107). A schematic representation of the ionic and hydrophobic bonds involved in protein-surfactant interaction is shown in Figure 28.

Once the initial attachment of surfactant monomers or small aggregates to the keratin surface has been satisfied, a series of other events and transformations may take place. When in the stratum corneum and hair cuticle, surfactants are supposed to cause denaturing effects on the keratin structure. This partial denaturation is supposed to be based on one or a combination of the following mechanisms: the hydrocarbon tail of surfactants penetrates into apolar regions of the keratin replacing the conformation-stabilizing hydrophobic interactions by ligand-segment interactions; the ionic head of surfactants produces attraction-repulsion forces on the charged groups of the keratin disordering its architecture; the formation of excess of positive or negative charges causes additional osmotic pressure,

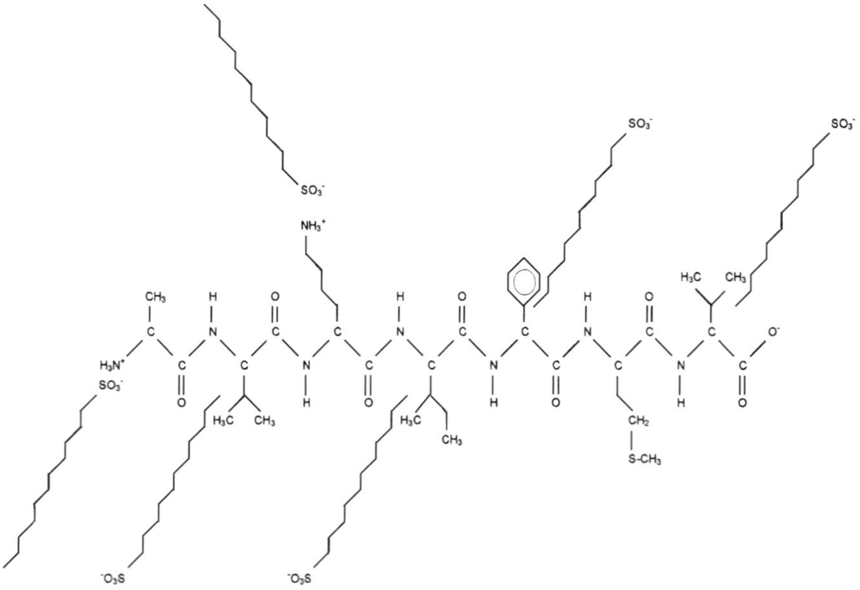

Figure 28 Sites of ionic and hydrophobic binding involved in protein-surfactant interaction.

leading to swelling of the matrix and increasing permeability (106). The degree of these alterations depends on the molecular characteristics of the surfactant (charge density and polarity of the nonionic heads, length of the hydrocarbon tail, type of the counterion) and on the physicochemical conditions of the medium (pH, ionic strength, CMC). Disordering of the keratin architecture causes swelling and increased permeability. By this mechanism the surfactant molecules or small aggregates find their way to deeper layers in the skin where, directly or perhaps as by-products resulting from enzymatic degradation, they cause the toxic effects. Disordering and swelling of the hair keratin in cuticle cells causes uplifting of cuticle scales and loss of peptides, up to exposure of the cortex and impairment of the mechanical properties of the hair fibers.

Numerous studies have found correlation between the protein denaturing and solubilization potential of tensides and their skin irritancy. The zein solubilization test (zein is a highly insoluble protein containing cystine residues) was proposed more than 30 years ago as an in vitro method to predict the irritancy of surfactant systems (108). Despite its strong theoretical limitations due to the structural differences of this protein and human keratins, a good correlation of the results obtainable by this test method with data obtained on wool keratin solubilization has been reported in more recent work (109). Another predictive test in vitro for detergent irritancy is based on the swelling response of a collagen membrane: the water uptake of an insoluble film of reticulated collagen immersed in a surfactant system is directly proportional to the ability of the tenside molecules to permeate, swell, and hydrate the collagen matrix and is well correlated to the in vivo irritancy of the system as determined by the classic soap chamber test procedure (110). Other methods that have been used to evaluate the degree of protein denaturation caused by surfactants and their blends were based on measurement of the denaturation of ovalbumin, human serum albumin, and other animal proteins by evaluation of their chromatographic behavior in a gel filtration system (111), and measurement of the change of specific rotation of their solution (112). Other authors have evaluated the amount of thiol groups (113,114) and amino acids (114,115) liberated from human skin and hair keratin after exposure to various tensides.

The mechanisms and effects of protein-surfactant interactions reviewed here are important for understanding the specific action of proteins in detergency.

The use of proteins in skin detergency dates to ancient times. The legendary habit of Cleopatra to bathe in milk, as well as modern use of luxurious native proteins in cleansers, reflects an intended use of proteins as skin care ingredients (aiding conditioning and moisturizing), to be distinguished from the rational association of protein derivatives with surfactants, designed to improve the tolerability and physicochemical properties of detergents. With regard to their interaction with tensides, protein derivatives may effectively display two type of advantages in detergency: modulating the adverse effects of detergents on skin and hair, and improving their technical properties.

The ability of exogenous proteins to reduce the skin and eye irritation potential of detergents was highlighted many decades ago in the cosmetic chemistry community. First extensive insights were probably those of Meinecke (4), who reported that addition of a protein hydrolysate or a protein–fatty acid condensate to a solution of a highly irritant surfactant (sodium alkylbenzene sulfonate) caused a remarkable increase in the skin tolerability of the product and postulated a protective effect based on the formation of a protein colloidal layer on the skin, which could prevent or minimize the direct interaction of tenside molecules with skin keratin. The same interpretation has been advanced more recently by other authors (116–118).

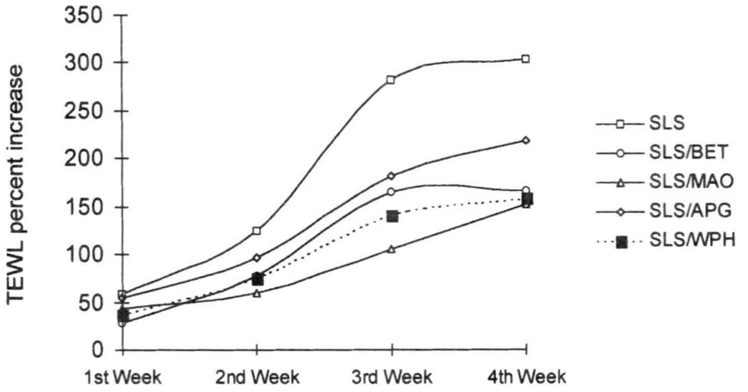

Figure 29 Time course of transepidermal water loss (volar side of forearm) as determined on repeated washing with sodium lauryl sulfate (SLS) plus anti-irritant substances: BET (cocamidopropylbetaine), MAO (cocamidopropylamine oxide), APG (alkyl C_{8-16} polyglucose), WPH (wheat protein hydrolysate MW 2200 Daltons) at the same concentration. WPH prevents the impairment of the skin barrier function caused by SLS as effectively as well-known mild tensides.

A different interpretation suggested an alternative mechanism based on the formation of complexes between proteins and surfactants within the detergent formulation, which produce larger mixed micelles and consequent lowering of the CMC of the system (119,120). This model was initially supported by the observation that some insoluble dyes, which were solubilized in tenside solutions above the CMC of the surfactant, could gain water solubility abundantly below the CMC when small amounts of protein substances were added to the system (121), and is therefore strictly linked to the hypothesis that only monomers of the surfactants can penetrate the skin keratin matrix and induce adverse effects on the skin. These two interpretations are not mutually exclusive and there could reasonably be contemporary cooperative occurrence of the two mechanisms.

The protective effect of protein derivatives in detergency has been tested in numerous studies and quantitative data are available in the technical literature. Native proteins, hydrolysates, and condensates are all reported to reduce the irritant effects of tenside on the skin. To compare the protective properties of protein substances with the well-known effect of amphoteric and nonionic tenside in detergent formulations based on anionic surfactants, a study was carried out based on intensive and repeated application on the skin of binary systems containing sodium lauryl sulfate and the anti-irritant test substance, and evaluation of some biophysical parameters for assessing skin damage (122). It was demonstrated that a hydrolyzed protein was as effective as some of the cosurfactants traditionally employed to inhibit the irritation potential of anionic tensides. Some of the results obtained are illustrated in Figure 29.

V. FORMULATING WITH PROTEINS

A. Proteins in Skin Care Products

Protein derivatives are used in a variety of skin care and makeup formulations. Soluble protein ingredients are suitable to be included in almost all common technical forms (emulsions, lotions, gels, powders). A few liposoluble protein derivatives, such as isostearoyl hydrolyzed collagen, are also available for inclusion in anhydrous lipidic systems. Insoluble proteins are also of use for some particular applications: insoluble elastin and keratin micronized powders are used in some cosmetic powders; compresses of fibrous insoluble collagen obtained by lyophilization of aqueous dispersions are moistened and applied on the skin, maintained for few minutes, and removed: transitory moisturization and increase of skin smoothness and shine are obtained (80). Silk powder produced by finely grinding pure degummed silk fibroin protein can be used in decorative cosmetics such as lipsticks, mascara, and anhydrous makeup preparations to give smoothness, lubricity, and luster to these preparations and to enhance their oil and water absorption properties.

Native proteins and hydrolysates with high average-molecular-weight masses are generally preferred in skin care applications for their film-forming properties. Soluble collagen and its partially deamidated derivative (desamido collagen) are traditional consolidated examples. Their long, rod-like molecules are able to form a continuous colloidal film on the skin surface, giving a smooth feel and softness. Since the filming properties of these substances are mainly due to the length of their molecules, and the hydrating effect is related to the large number of exposed hydrogen-binding sites available for linking water, and their conformation is stabilized by the triple-helix structure, it is important to avoid exposure to heat and denaturing agents in the preparation and life of relevant formulations. For this reason in the preparation of emulsions they are usually added after emulsification and cooling of the batch to a temperature at least 3–5 degrees below the melting temperature T_m.

With regard to the use of protein ingredients in emulsions, little is known about the location of their molecules in multiphase systems and the influence on their stability. As most protein ingredients have a distinct hydrophilic character, a preferred location in the aqueous phase is to be expected, and a participation in the interface structure and equilibrium may be hypothesized for derivatives that possess significant amphiphilicity and for high-molecular-weight proteins.

A wheat protein derivative with molecular weight of 250–500 kDa has been studied in aqueous solution and in an O/W emulsion for its effects on the viscoelastic properties of the skin. A slight increase in skin extensibility and elasticity was found and related to its moisturizing and film-forming effects. This derivative is proposed in skin care preparation for transient skin firming-tightening effects (54).

Protein hydrolysates are also employed in skin care products as conditioners, moisturizers, and film formers at active concentrations of 0.1–2%. Low-molecular-weight peptides are sometimes added to other humectants (glycerin, sodium lactate, sodium pyrrolidone carboxylate, free amino acids) in moisturizing products. In the preparation of emulsions, hydrolyzed proteins are generally incorporated into the aqueous phase prior to formation of the emulsion. At pH values around neutrality, they tolerate temperatures like those usually needed for emulsification (70–85°C), without any significant amino acid degradation or coagulation. The effects of protein hydrolysates on the stability of emulsions are not reported, but because of their ionic character and the presence of inorganic salts in their preparations, they are supposed to have a stabilizing effect on W/O emulsions and a negative effect on the stability of O/W emulsions. This trend is generally reported by formulators.

The pH of the formulation is an important factor for the skin substantivity of hydrolyzed peptides. Compatibly with the other needs of the formulation, it should be kept at a value below or close to their average isoelectric point, to have a considerable percentage of protonated amino groups, but not too low to cause the exposed carboxyl groups of skin keratin to be indissociated.

Fatty acid condensates are proposed as emulsifying agents in O/W preparations; they are reported to form homogeneous, highly dispersed creams (123).

The commonly used concentration levels of various protein derivatives in skin care formulations are listed in Table 5. The dose ranges reported are derived from the technical documentation of several suppliers and from the data of relevant scientific literature. They are given only as a general overview on the realistic and effective doses of these ingredients in actual cosmetic products and not intended to be a guide for formulators. As great differences may exist in the quality and cosmetic activity of derivatives of the same kind available on the market, users are strongly suggested to consider the specifications of each particular material and should be encouraged to perform their own tests to determine the convenient concentration for particular formulations.

B. Proteins in Hair Care Products

Hair hygiene and care formulations including shampoos, leave-on and rinse-off conditioners, dressing and coloring lotions, permanent waves, and hair straighteners are the cosmetic products for which the use of protein derivatives has been constantly most successful and frequent.

Proteins are claimed and proved to increase the tensile strength of hair, increase elasticity, impart body and softness, help repair split ends and cuticle damage, and protect from the adverse effect of detersion, chemical waving, and bleaching. Different protein derivatives are selected for specific hair treatments and products. Commonly used dose ranges in different hair care formulations are listed in Table 6.

Most of the conditioning effects of proteins are related to their ability to be adsorbed

Table 5 Suggested Use Concentration Ranges of Common Protein Derivatives in Skin Care Products

Protein derivative	Function in formula	Use concentration
Protein hydrolysates (almond, collagen, elastin, extensin, fibronectin, milk protein, oat protein, reticulin, silk proteins, soy protein, wheat protein, yeast protein)	Humectant, moisturizer, film former, skin conditioner, buffering agent	0.2–5% in creams and lotions, aftershave lotions
Soluble collagen, desamido collagen, serum albumin, sodium caseinate	Skin moisturizer, conditioner, protectant	0.01–0.1% in creams and lotions
Gelatin	Thickening agent, film former, humectant, emulsion stabilizer, skin protectant	1–2% in emulsions as stabilizer and thickener; 0.5–2% as skin moisturizer and protectant
Potassium and sodium cocoyl hydrolyzed (collagen, soy protein, wheat protein)	Coemulsifier	0.5–2% in O/W emulsions
Silk powder, insoluble elastin powder, insoluble keratin powder	Oil absorbent, cohesive agent, protectant	1–5% in powder makeup preparations

Data are drawn from relevant technical literature. Concentrations are given in active protein substance.

Table 6 Suggested Use Concentration Ranges of Common Protein Derivatives in Hair Care Products

Protein derivative	Function in formula	Use concentration
Protein hydrolysates (almond, collagen, keratin, milk protein, oat protein, silk proteins, soy protein, wheat protein, yeast protein, zein)	Hair conditioner, buffering agent	0.2–2% in shampoos, conditioners, cream rinses, lotions, waving preparations, styling products
Hydrolyzed wheat protein polysiloxane copolymer	Hair conditioner	0.5–3%
AMP-isostearoyl hydrolyzed protein	Hair conditioner	0.05–1% in alcoholic conditioner lotions
Alkyldimonium hydroxypropyl (or ethyl) hydrolyzed protein	Hair conditioner	0.5–2% in conditioners, cream rinses, conditioning perms, relaxers, lotions
Soluble (keratin, wheat protein)	Permanent conditioning protein	0.5–5% in conditioning perms
Potassium undecylenoyl hydrolyzed collagen	Antidandruff	0.5–2% in shampoos and conditioners
Potassium abietoyl hydrolyzed collagen	Scalp lipid regulator	1–2% in shampoos and conditioners

Data are drawn from relevant technical literature. Concentrations are given in active protein substance.

on the cuticle keratin or to react covalently with it. Substantivity to hair is easily obtained from simple aqueous solutions and many quantitative data are available for different derivatives. In the presence of surfactants, substantivity is considerably reduced, owing to competition between the protein and the tenside molecules and the washing effect, yet the attachment of proteins to hair keratin is also significant when they are included in shampoo formulations with high surfactant content and for the short time of contact of shampooing procedures. Thus, conditioning and protective effects can also be obtained in these unfavorable application conditions.

The use of protein hydrolysates and quaternized derivatives in shampoo formulations has been demonstrated to reduce the loss of tensile strength caused by anionic tensides on the hair fibers (124,125). This protective effect is higher for quaternized derivatives than for parent hydrolysates. A wheat protein hydrolysate was found to be more effective than a collagen hydrolysate. Since the two tested products had similar isoelectric point and average molecular size, the difference could be explained by the higher hydrophobicity of the vegetable derivative.

The effects of a shampoo containing sericin hydrolysate were extensively tested and compared to those obtained with placebo (16): it was found that sericin peptides caused increase of hair smoothness and combability and improvement of the skin/eye tolerability of the formulation.

Protection of the hair from the adverse effects of alkali treatment is also reported. Hair is treated with strong alkali solutions in the reducing step of the permanent-waving treatment and in bleaching/dyeing procedures. This exposure causes hair swelling and partial disruption of cystine bridges with solubilization and loss of keratin peptides and amino acids. Hair solubility in alkali is reduced by pretreatment with a shampoo containing hydrolyzed proteins (124). Hair swelling is also significantly prevented by pretreatment with a 5% protein solution. The scale of the protective effect for protein hydrolysates ranks in the order keratin > elastin > collagen (119).

By addition of 2% of lauryldimonium hydroxypropylamino hydrolyzed collagen in a sodium laureth sulfate–based shampoo improvement of wet combability and increase of tensile strength is obtained compared to placebo (125).

A wheat protein hydrolysate with a molecular weight range of 5000–10,000 Daltons used in 1% concentration in a shampoo formulation has been found to lower the average coefficient of friction of the hair, giving lubricity and enhanced wettability, improve hair smoothness, as evaluated by atomic force microscopy visualization, and increase foamability of the preparation more effectively than other vegetable and animal hydrolysates (126).

The foaming properties of protein derivatives are also important features for their use in shampoos. They enable formulators to reduce the level of active surfactants in shampoos without reducing overall foaming power. This becomes of great importance in the formulation of low-active, frequent-use type shampoos where overall foaming effects can still be maintained at low-active levels, minimizing skin and eye irritation.

C. Proteins in Cleansing Products

Addition of protein substances in cleansing formulations (mainly when based on anionic tensides) improves their skin and eye tolerability and reduces the potential adverse effects of intense and repeated detergency (skin dehydration, roughness, impairment of the barrier function of the horny layer). Quantitative data on this protective action are supplied in technical bulletins of protein derivatives and scientific literature, with particular reference to the use of soluble collagen, protein hydrolysates, and fatty acid condensates. Two studies carried out by the authors have compared the anti-irritant properties of wheat protein hydrolysates and mild cosurfactants in association with anionic tensides (122) and evaluated the protective effect of high-molecular-weight wheat protein in realistic cleansing preparations (60). In the first study it was demonstrated that a hydrolyzed protein was as effective as cocamidopropylbetaine and cocamidopropylamine oxide and superior to alkyl C8–16 polyglucose in preventing skin permeabilization, dehydration, and increased roughness caused by repeated washing with sodium lauryl sulfate and sodium laureth sulfate.

In the second study the dependence of protective effect and protein concentration in two bubble bath formulations (Table 7) was tested by the predictive test of skin irritancy based on the swelling response of a collagen film (see Section IV.D).

Some reduction of the swelling of collagen (predictive parameter of in vivo irritancy) was obtained at a surfactant-protein ratio of 10:1 and the protection was comparatively more effective for the formulation with a higher content of sodium laureth sulfate (Fig. 30).

High-molecular-weight protein–fatty acid condensates are reported to be more effective than acylated derivatives of smaller peptide in increasing the skin and eye tolerability of different anionic tenside, as evaluated by the red blood cell test (127) and quaternized derivatives also reported to possess anti-irritant properties when included in anionic-based formulations: the mucous membrane compatibility of sodium laureth sulfate, as determined by the Draize test, can be increased about fourfold, by replacing of one-third of the surfactant with a lauryldimonium hydroxypropyl hydrolyzed collagen (128).

Table 7 Basic Composition of the Detergent Formulations Tested for the Swelling Response of Collagen Membranes

Bubble bath formulations, ingredient	Weight percent	
	Formulation A	Formulation B
Sodium laureth sulfate	25.0	18.0
Cocamidopropylamine oxide	5.0	—
Disodium laureth sulfosuccinate	—	10.0
Disodium cocoamphodiacetate	3.0	6.0
Pearlescent 35% (Sodium laureth sulfate, glycol distearate)	5.0	3.0
Cocamide DEA	2.0	3.0
PEG-7 glyceryl cocoate	1.5	3.0
Glycerin	1.5	—
Citric acid	0.1	0.1
Preservatives, dyes, water	To 100 parts	To 100 parts

Common dose ranges of protein derivatives in different hair care formulations are listed in Table 8.

D. Technical Uses of Proteins in Cosmetic Formulations

Soluble native proteins, protein hydrolysates, and fatty acid condensates are sometimes used to improve and refine the physicochemical properties of cosmetic formulations. Many

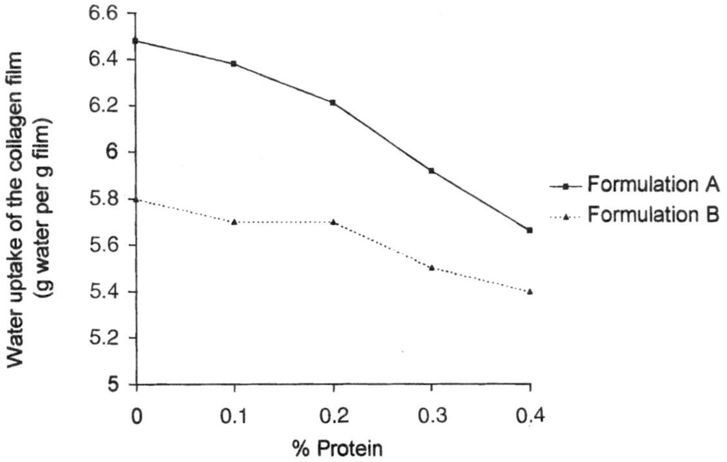

Figure 30 Swelling test of a collagen film. Water uptake for formulations A and B (see Table 7) at 1% active washing substance for both, in the presence of different amounts of nonhydrolyzed wheat proteins. Solutions were prepared in phosphate buffer 1 mM pH 6.0. Incubation was made at 50°C for 24 hr.

Table 8 Suggested Use Concentration Ranges of Common Protein Derivatives in Cleansing Products

Protein derivative	Function in formula	Use concentration
Protein hydrolysates (almond, collagen, elastin, extensin, fibronectin, milk protein, oat protein, reticulin, silk proteins, soy protein, wheat protein, yeast protein)	Anti-irritant, skin conditioner, moisturizer	0.2–5% in shampoos and skin cleansers
Soluble collagen, desamido collagen, serum albumin, sodium caseinate	Skin moisturizer, conditioner, protectant	0.01–0.5% in shampoos and skin cleansers
Gelatin	Thickening agent, film former, humectant, skin protectant	1–3% in shampoos and skin cleansers
Potassium and sodium cocoyl hydrolyzed (collagen, soy protein, wheat protein)	Detergent, foaming enhancer, anti-irritant	1–10% in shampoos and skin cleansers
Alkyldimonium hydroxypropyl hydrolyzed (collagen, wheat protein)	Anti-irritant, conditioner	1–5% in shampoos and skin cleansers

Data are drawn from relevant technical literature. Concentrations are given in active protein substance.

of these derivatives possess significant surface activity, which may help viscosization and gelification, foaming and emulsification.

Foam expansion and stability of detergent formulations can be increased by addition of small amounts of hydrophobic hydrolysates and long-chain polpeptides having a high surface value. Fatty acid condensates and also quaternized proteins are able to enhance foam stability and density of anionic detergents, though in most cases replacement of anionic surfactant with an equal amount of these derivatives will result in net decrease of the foam height.

The high buffering capacity of protein hydrolysates is used to stabilize the pH of cosmetic preparations; as a general rule, the lower the average peptide length (higher charge density), the higher the buffering power will be.

Insoluble gelatin is one of the components (together with vegetable gums) of the wall of microcapsules containing oils and mineral pigments used in detergents and makeup preparations and in soft gelatin capsules containing bath products (36).

E. Stability and Possible Interactions

Protein derivatives possess chemical reactivity, mainly due to the presence of free amino groups and cystine residues in their molecules, and may form noncovalent bonds with many other substances by the great number of functional groups of amino acid side chains, which can give rise to hydrogen, hydrophobic, and ionic interactions. Interactions of proteins with other common components of cosmetic formulations are therefore highly possible and some of these may result in unwanted changes in the physicochemical and functional properties of finished products.

Most of the proteins used in cosmetic systems are water-soluble and frequently supplied as aqueous solutions. Nevertheless, interaction with water itself may, paradoxically, be a cause of loss of stability, resulting in haze and formation of solid insoluble aggregates. Some hydrolysates and quaternized derivatives, supplied as clear and stable water solutions, may lose solubility by simple dilution with more water. The mechanism of this phenomenon is unclear, though for hydrolyzed polypeptides the ionic strength of the medium may be a factor (27). Protein hydrolysates normally contain a large amount of inorganic electrolytes (1–10% on protein substances) and these small ions should aid the conformational stabilization of the protein by linking water and subtracting part of its molecules into unfavorable interactions with the hydrophobic residues of polypeptides. When the hydrolysate is diluted with more water, the ionic strength of the medium is reduced and some of the polypeptides cannot remain in solution. This explanation is substantiated by the observation that in some cases, it is possible to remove haze or even redissolve precipitate by adding sodium chloride. Another possible interpretation, which would also explain the analogous behavior of some quaternized derivatives, is based on the hypothesis that only at high concentrations in water, i.e., at a high protein:water ratio, would the close proximity of polypeptides cause lipophilic groups to be effectively unexposed to the molecules of water, which are bound by the many hydrophilic amino acid chains. The formation of haze by these mechanisms of reaggregation/recombination may take time to occur and represent a subtle source of destabilization in water-based lotions of low ionic strength containing small amounts of hydrophobic peptides.

Inversely, the presence of ethanol and other alcohols in hydroalcoholic preparations may cause loss of solubility of hydrophilic peptides. In these products polypeptides with high hydrophobicity are preferred. The coefficient of ripartition 2-butanol/water (as nitrogen-partition coefficient) is used to estimate the lipophilic/hydrophilic balance of proteins: for hydrophobic hydrolysates the nitrogen-partition coefficient value is 0.1–0.15 and lower for more hydrophilic derivatives (129).

Inorganic salts can cause reversible or irreversible denaturation of native proteins by replacement and disruption of the hydrogen bonds stabilizing the structure: soluble collagen is totally precipitated from its solutions by addition of 5–6% NaCl. Long-chain, nonhydrolyzed proteins solubilized by complexation with surfactants can be precipitated by addition of a small amount of electrolytes, which break the ionic interactions between the ionic head of the tenside and charged groups in the protein. The solubility of peptides not exceeding 20 kDa is normally unaffected by addition of salts. The pH is obviously important in determining the solubility of proteins and their interactions with other molecules. These have been discussed in other sections of this chapter and are only mentioned here. Interactions of proteins with other ionic organic ingredients common in cosmetics are important when molecules with numerous charged sites are involved. Large polyanions like hyaluronic acid, cellulose gum, and mucopolysaccharides may form insoluble complexes with polypeptides containing numerous protonable groups, and polycations like quaternized guar gum may precipitate proteins with a net negative charge. Proteins with large molecular masses may be precipitated by tannins and other polyphenol derivatives contained in numerous vegetable extracts (rathany, tormentil, witch hazel). Other possible unwanted interactions involve the reaction of the free amino groups of proteins with aldehydic components of fragrances, giving changes reported by formulators.

Finally, proteins are reported to be potential inhibitors of numerous preservatives commonly used in cosmetics (130). The mechanisms involved are various and not fully understood: the reactivity of amino groups and electrostatic interactions are both possible.

Also, protein materials are generally good substrates for microbial growth and partial inactivation of the preservative system may be the result of the higher consumption of biocides needed to face an increased microbial proliferation. Formaldehyde intentionally used or liberated by relevant donor biocides is easily consumed by condensation with free amino groups of peptides. Protein hydrolysates, having a high percentage of reactive amines, are stronger inactivation agents than larger proteins, while large polypeptides may lose solubility by masking the few amino groups present into nonionizable derivatives. Quaternary preservatives such as benzalkonium chloride and cetrimonium bromide may be inactivated by electrostatic interaction with anionic peptides, and potential inhibition is also reported for phenols, phenoxyethanol, and isothiazolinones.

Loss of protein solubility with formation of haze and precipitate is also possible in finished formulations containing protein hydrolysates as a consequence of the transpeptidation mechanism (see Section II.B.2), provided residual enzyme activity is present and the chemical environment of the formulation allows the enzyme to work.

VI. SAFETY OF PROTEINS AND PROTEIN DERIVATIVES

A. Toxicological Aspects of Proteins in Cosmetic Applications

Thorough assessment of the risk associated with exposure to cosmetic ingredients has become a crucial strategy to guarantee that basic safety requirements of finished products are met. Toxicity data for cosmetic ingredients are, however, largely missing, and the share of raw materials still uncovered by reliable toxicity information mainly includes natural and natural-derived products, which often are nonhomogeneous mixtures of partly unknown substances.

Protein derivatives are generally composed of several different molecular species, as the result of the complex composition of source material and its processing to smaller peptides or condensates; moreover, many different additives, impurities, by-products, and contaminants may be present. A hydrolyzed protein preparation can be composed of thousands of different peptides, inorganic ions, sugars, lipids, ammonia, preservatives, antioxidants, and a variety of other possible impurities. Fatty acid condensates of hydrolyzed protein can contain, in addition, soaps and acylamides. Furthermore, products with the same INCI name, prepared by different manufacturing processes or from different source materials, will probably differ, also significantly, in their chemical composition.

From these considerations, two points become apparent: (1) the toxicological profile of these ingredients is the result of combined effects of their numerous components; (2) as the composition of protein materials having the same INCI name may vary depending on their manufacture, one can only generalize on the safety of each particular type of derivative.

Finally, the naturalness of proteins does not necessarily make them safe: some of the substances with the most powerful biological activity and potential toxicity are peptides and polypeptides (e.g., endorphins, tetanus toxin) and some proteins are known to cause allergic reaction after ingestion (e.g., milk casein, egg albumin, wheat gluten).

Collagen and its peptides are known to have a chemotactic effect, i.e., the ability to promote directional movement of inflammatory cells toward the site of administration (131–133), which induces a sequence of changes characteristic of inflammation. The use of collagen in wound-healing preparations is based on this mechanism, which is associated with an increase in formation and deposition of endogenous collagen. This effect, however, presumes the presence of collagen below the horny layer barrier, and the relevant risk of inflammation exists only when collagen is directly injected into the skin, whereas percutaneous transport after topical application on healthy skin is highly improbable.

The sensitizing potential of protein substances is generally considered to be low by topical administration and hydrolyzed proteins are thought to be less antigenic than native proteins. The acute toxicity of underivatized proteins, native or hydrolyzed, as reported by many suppliers, is also generally low: the LD_{50} determined by oral administration on rat/mouse ranges from 10 to 20 g/kg as pure protein substance. Hydrolyzed proteins are generally rated at the lowest values of eye and skin irritancy by in vivo and in vitro tests. Hydrolyzed collagen has been identified as a safe cosmetic ingredient in actual use and concentration from a wide range of tests: it is reported to be almost nontoxic when administered orally or dermally in acute and subchronic animal toxicity studies, and nonirritating or minimally irritating when tested full-strength in primary skin irritation assays and nonsensitizing (134).

Condensation of hydrolyzed proteins with fatty acid groups determines reduction of the skin and eye compatibility, resulting from the increase of their amphiphilic character; the skin/eye tolerability of acylated proteins is reported to increase with the average length of the peptide moiety (127). Quaternized derivatives are generally less compatible than fatty acid condensates (128). The irritation potential of protein-surfactant complexes is intermediate between those of the parent protein and the pure tenside.

B. The Risk of Chemical and Biological Contaminants in Protein Ingredients

Besides ubiquitous environmental pollutants, which can contaminate protein materials and their derivatives to a various extent (pesticides in cereals and oilseeds; heavy metals in fish and vegetables; polynuclear aromatics; polychlorobiphenols), few specific chemical and biological contaminants are of concern for cosmetic proteins, related to their source materials or their manufacturing procedures.

A specific heavy-metals contamination (chromium) was detected in collagen hydrolysates prepared from trimming/cuttings of chromium-tanned hides; up to 100 ppm of chromium was found in samples of powdered collagen hydrolysates on the market at the end of the 1970s (135). The oxidation state of chromium was not determined, but probably it was Cr^{III}, less toxic than Cr^{VI}, as in the tanning industry only basic salts of Cr^{III} are used.

A potential health hazard related to the use of vegetable derivatives in cosmetics is represented by a class of extremely toxic substances: mycotoxins. Cereals and protein-rich oilseeds may be contaminated with mycotoxins, toxins produced by several fungi, the most prominent of which, because of their carcinogenic activity, are aflatoxins (mainly produced by *Aspergillus flavus* and *Aspergillus parasiticus*) and trichothecenes (produced by fungi of the genus *Fusarium*). In contrast to aflatoxins, trichothecenes are able to affect human health not only by oral route, but also by dermal application (136). Even micrograms of type A trichothecenes cause skin irritation (137). Mycotoxins can contaminate cosmetic products via two pathways: either through contaminated raw materials or through biosynthesis by toxinogenic fungi in the finished products. Mycotoxins were found in unprocessed wheat bran for cosmetic use, but as they have low resistance to heat, the risk of their survival in heat-chemical processed materials as vegetable protein derivatives can be considered to be very low. Moreover, suitable preservation of finished cosmetic products has proved to be normally effective in suppressing the proliferation of the microbial species involved (136).

The recent quickly spreading epidemic of bovine spongiphorm encephalopathy (BSE) in Europe has caused a diffuse and mounting public alarm for possible transmission of the disease to humans via food, drugs, and cosmetics containing bovine derivatives. It is a paradox that greater concern has been raised by the media for the potential risk involved in the use of cosmetic products containing animal originated ingredients (collagen has been the preferred target) than for the far greater number and larger consumption of secondary foods (beverages, ice cream, sweets) and pharmaceuticals that contain bovine products (gelatin).

The European Community (EC) has recently banned the use of cosmetic ingredients derived from brain, spinal cord, and eye from cattle, sheep, and goats (138), whereas no restriction has been imposed on ingredients originating from connective and cartilaginous tissues, skin, and milk. Collagen, elastin, keratin, and other protein derivatives from these tissues are therefore permitted as cosmetic ingredients in Europe, provided source materials are not contaminated by the above-mentioned organs and do not come from countries where a high incidence of BSE is reported. In spite of this permission, the use of bovine collagen and elastin has dropped dramatically in the European cosmetic market and the manufacturing of protein derivatives has been more often addressed to vegetable materials. Further research and clarification on the matter are urgently required as the real hazard of BSE infectivity to humans via cosmetic applications is still uncertain.

BSE first came to the attention of the scientific community in November 1986 with the appearance in cattle of a newly recognized form of neurological disease in the United Kingdom. Between November 1986 and May 1995 approximately 150,000 cases of this new cattle disease were confirmed in the United Kingdom. Epidemiological studies at that time suggested that the source of disease was cattle feed prepared from carcasses of dead cattle. BSE is associated with a transmissible agent, the nature of which is not yet fully understood. The agent affects the brain and spinal cord of cattle and causes sponge-like changes visible with an ordinary microscope. It is a highly stable agent, resisting heating to normal cooking and industrial processing temperatures and even higher temperatures such as those used for sterilization, autoclaving, and drying. Although there is still no concrete proof that it is the actual cause of the BSE, or simply a by-product of the BSE disease, the transmissible agent associated with BSE is a protein (prion) always found in BSE-affected brain and absent in healthy organs. This protein contains no form of nucleic acid, yet its reproduction is clearly demonstrated. The disease is fatal for cattle within weeks to months of its onset.

BSE is one of several different forms of transmissible brain disease of animals. Others include scrapie, a disease common in sheep; diseases in humans with sponge-like findings in brain, and with severe and fatal neurological signs and symptoms, include kuru, which appears to be transmitted by human ritual handling of bodies and brains of the dead; and Creutzfeldt-Jakob disease (CJD). The World Health Organization (WHO) meeting held in 1995 compared the annual number of cases of CJD in France, Germany, Italy, Netherlands, and the United Kingdom, concluding that the epidemiological evidence in Europe did not indicate a change in the incidence of CJD that could be attributed to BSE and that if the measures taken in the United Kingdom regarding cattle feed and other precautionary measures at farm, slaughtering, and meat processing were being strictly implemented, the risk of BSE transmission, and therefore of possible transmission of BSE to humans, would be minimized. Nevertheless, in recent times, some cases in the United Kingdom have been identified with what appears to be a variant of CJD. Results of patient interviews and medical history, genetic analysis, and testing for other possible causes of this disease were reviewed by the United Kingdom Advisory Committee on Spongiphorm Encephalopathy, which concluded that although there is no direct evidence of a link on the basis of current data and in the absence of any credible alternative, the most likely explanation at present is that these cases are related to exposure to BSE before the introduction of the specified bovine offal ban in 1989.

At a consultation organized by WHO in Geneva on April 2–3, 1996 (139), a group of international experts reviewed the public health issues related to BSE and the emergence of the new variant of CJD (V-CJD). Based on analysis of clinical and pathological data of 10 recent cases of V-CJD, the group concluded that there is no definite link between BSE and V-CJD, but that circumstantial evidence suggests exposure to BSE may be the most likely hypothesis. This group also confirmed that BSE was greatly reduced by measures taken in the United Kingdom and made recommendations to further minimize transmission of BSE among animals and to reduce as completely as possible any exposure of humans to the BSE agent. With respect to specific products, the consultation reported that: tests on milk and milk products from BSE-infected animals have not shown any infectivity and are therefore considered safe; gelatin is considered safe for human consumption as its preparation involves a chemical extraction process that should destroy BSE infectivity; tallow is likewise considered safe if effective rendering procedures are in place. A previous WHO consultation in 1991 had issued guidelines for minimizing the risk of transmission of agents causing spongiphorm encephalopathy via medicinal products. These guidelines, together with a classification of animal tissues and body fluids on the basis of their potential infectivity, were officially adopted and published by the European Community in 1991 and still represent the official European guidance for the manufacture of medicinal and cosmetic derivatives from biological materials (140).

In this document, on the basis of experimental data on transmissible BSE, organs, tissues, and fluids are classified into four main groups bearing different potential risk (Table 9).

The majority of animal materials used for the extraction of cosmetic proteins are classified in the category of ''no detectable infectivity.'' Milk, connective tissues, skin, and hair are considered to be relatively safe and unlikely to present any risk of contamination. Organs like brain, spinal cord, and eye and others like placenta, bone marrow, and

Table 9 Relative Spongiphorm Encephalopathy Infectivity and Classification of Tissues and Body Fluids with Regard to Their Potential Risk.

Category I	
High infectivity	Brain, spinal cord, eye
Category II	
Medium infectivity	Ileum, lymph, nodes, proximal colon, spleen, tonsil, dura mater, pineal gland, placenta, cerebrospinal fluid, pituitary gland
Category III	
Low infectivity	Distal colon, nasal mucosa, sciatic nerve, bone marrow, liver, lung, pancreas, thymus
Cateogory IV	
No detectable infectivity	Heart, kidney, mammary gland, milk, ovary, serum, skeletal muscle, testes, fetal tissue, bone, cartilaginous tissue, connective tissue, hair, skin

Source: Ref. 140.

thymus, which have been used to obtain cosmetic ingredients, are strongly suggested or regulated to be avoided in the preparation of medicinal and cosmetic materials. The EC document indicates careful selection of source materials as the most important criterion for the safety of medicinal products. The use of source materials from countries where there is a high incidence of BSE is to be avoided. In addition, it should be ensured that there is no risk of BSE infection from the feeding to ruminants of animal protein derived from specified offal materials (brain, spinal cord, spleen, thymus, tonsil, intestine, placenta) and from the processes used in the rendering industry. The age of animals is also considered an important safety parameter: since natural scrapie or BSE has not been detected in animals under the age of 6 months, cattle yielding source materials should not be older than 6 months.

Suggested removal and inactivation procedures consist of: (1) autoclaving at appropriate conditions (recommended parameters are 134–138°C for 18 min for porous-load autoclaving and 132°C for 1 hr for gravity-displacement autoclaving); (2) treatment with sodium hydroxide (preferably 1 N solution for 1 hr at 20°C); (3) treatment with sodium hypochlorite (preferably solution containing at least 2% available chlorine for 1 hr at 20°C. Though none of these procedures guarantees complete inactivation of the infectious agents, combination of the technical measures specified, together with appropriate selection of source materials, is considered by the EC effective for the manufacture of safe animal derivatives for the pharmaceutical and cosmetic industry.

However, it would be prudent to consider that though hidesplits, connective tissues, and bones of BSE-infected animals are far less infectious than the central nervous system and other organs, as long as the agents are not definitely identified and not detectable by any sufficiently sensitive test, no tissue or body liquid can rigorously be declared free of infectivity. Skin and bones from infected animals could also be supposed to be infectious, because they are well supplied with blood and nerves. Furthermore, BSE prion is extremely resistant to acid-alkaline treatments and to heat, and although strong chemical or physical attack or a combination approach (141) may reduce the infectiousness of BSE-contaminated materials, there is no proof of a complete inactivation of the agent or any indication that a minimum dose is required for the transmission of BSE to other species. These considerations lead to the conclusion that animal derivatives without BSE infectivity and with no hazards to human health can be prepared only from healthy animals. The measures activated by the international community to eradicate the BSE epidemic and prevent contaminated materials from coming onto the market appear to be fundamental for the future fully safe use of these materials in cosmetics as well as in food and medicaments.

This brief overview of the specific potential health hazards from chemical and biological contaminants in protein derivatives and the emotional impact of the BSE affair should not cause exaggerated apprehension about the safety of these materials as applied topically. The overall risk does not appear to be greater than for the majority of current natural and synthetic cosmetic ingredients, provided suitable measures in the selection of source materials and manufacturing and quality surveillance are followed, and that humans will be able to discern what nature allows us to modify and what it does not.

REFERENCES

1. Rovesti P. Alla ricerca dei cosmetici perduti. Venice: Marsilio, 1975.
2. Rovesti P. Alla ricerca della cosmesi dei primitivi. Venice: Marsilio, 1977.
3. Burnett RS. Proteins in cosmetics. Am Perfum Cosmet 1963; 78:69–72.

4. Meinecke K. Über die reizwirkung oberflächenaktiver Stoffe auf die Haut. Arc Klin Exp Dermatol 1960; 211:370–378.
5. Riso RR. Protein derived detergents. Soap Cosmet Chem Spec 1963; 39:82–84.
6. Riso RR. Protein derived detergents. Soap Cosmet Chem Spec 1963; 39:151–160.
7. Bouthilet RJ, Karler A. Cosmetic effects of substantive proteins. Proc Sci Sect Toilet Goods Assoc 1965; 44:27–31.
8. Bouthilet RJ, Karler A. Cosmetic effects of substantive proteins. Part II. Proc Sci Sect Toilet Goods Assoc 1965; 45:27–29.
9. Karjala SA, Williamson JE, Karler A. Studies on the substantivity of collagen-derived polypeptides to human hair. J Soc Cosmet Chem 1966; 17:513–524.
10. Karjala SA, Karler A Williamson JE. The effect of pH on the absorption of collagen-derived peptides by hair. J Soc Cosmet Chem 1967; 18:599–608.
11. Stryer L. Biochemistry, 3rd ed. New York: WH Freeman, 1989.
12. Lide DR. CRC Handbook of Chemistry and Physics, 75th ed. Boca Raton, FL: CRC Press, 1994.
13. Dickerson RE, Geis I. The Structure and Action of Proteins. New York: Harper & Row, 1969.
14. Anwar RA. Comparison of elastins from various sources. Can J Biochem 1966; 44:725–734.
15. Gillespie JM, Marshall RC. The normal and aberrant hair keratins. In: Orfanos CE, Montagna W, Stüttgen G, eds. Hair Research. Berlin-Heidelberg: Springer-Verlag, 1981:76–83.
16. Engel W, Hoppe U, Pape W, Sauermann G. Eigenschaften eines sericinhaltigen puffernden Shampoos. Ärzt Kosmetol 1987; 17:91–110.
17. Hoppe U, Eichner W. Sericin. SÖFW-J 1992; 15:881–890.
18. Pasquon I, Zanderighi L. La chimica verde, 1st ed. Milan: Hoepli, 1987.
19. Wookey N. Wheat gluten as a protein ingredient. J Am Oil Chem Soc 1979; 56:306–309.
20. Crow MJA, Rothfus JA. Chromatography of proteins from wheat gluten on polyacrylamide gel. Cereal Chem 1968; 45:413–420.
21. Beckwith AC, Nielsen HC, Wall JS, Huebner FR. Isolation and characterization of a high-molecular-weight protein from wheat gliadin. Cereal Chem 1966; 43:15–28.
22. Bietz JA, Wall JS. Isolation and characterization of gliadin-like subunits from glutenin. Cereal Chem 1975; 50:537–547.
23. Nielsen HC, Beckwith AC, Wall JS. Effect of disulfide-bond cleavage on wheat gliadin fractions obtained by gel filtration. Cereal Chem 1968; 45:37–47.
24. Kinsella JE. Functional properties of soy proteins. J Am Oil Chem Soc 1979; 56:242–258.
25. Lamport D, Northcote D. Hydroxyproline in primary cell walls of higher plants. Nature 1960; 188–191.
26. Armengol R. A plant glycoprotein similar to collagen. SÖFW-J 1991; 117:717–721.
27. Adler-Nissen J. Enzymic Hydrolysis of Food Proteins. New York: Elsevier Science, 1986.
28. Sandberg LB, Soskel NT, Leslie JG. Elastin structure, biosynthesis and relation to disease state. N Engl J Med 1981; 304:556–579.
29. Wenninger JA, McEwen GN. CTFA International Cosmetic Ingredient Dictionary, 6th ed. Washington, DC:CTFA, 1995.
30. Ranganayaki MD, Ranganathan TS, Jayaraman KS. A novel technique for the preparation of collagen derivatives for cosmetics. Part 1. Preparation and characterisation of collagen product. Res Ind 1988; 33:205–210.
31. Miller AT, Karmas E, Fu Lu M. Age-related changes in the collagen of bovine corium: studies on extractability, solubility and molecular size distribution. J Food Sci 1983; 48:681–685.
32. Teglia A, Mazzola G, Secchi G. Relationship between chemical characteristics and cosmetic properties of protein hydrolysates. XVIIth IFSCC Congress, Yokohama, 1992, A207.

33. Groot de AP, Slump P. Effects of severe alkali treatment of proteins on aminoacid composition and nutritive value. J Nutr 1969; 98:45–56.
34. Nashef AS, Osuga DT, Lee HS, Ahmed AL, Withaker JR, Feeney RE. Effects of alkali on proteins. Disulfides and their products. J Agric Food Chem 1977; 25:245–248.
35. Finley JW, Friedman M. New aminoacid derivatives formed by alkaline treatment of proteins. Adv Exp Med Biol 1977; 86B:123–128.
36. Leopold T. Gelatine. Herstellung und Nutzung in der Pharmaindustrie. SÖFW-J 1990; 116: 639–645.
37. Steisslinger HW. Kollagen Hydrolysate. Parfüm Kosmet 1991; 72:556–566.
38. Svendsen I. Chemical modifications of the subtilisins with special reference to the binding of large substrates: a review. Carlsberg Res Commun 1976; 41:237–291.
39. Fastrez J, Fersht AR. Demonstration of the acyl-enzyme mechanism for the hydrolysis of peptides and anilides by chymotripsin. Biochemistry 1973; 12:2025–2034.
40. Taylor WH. Formol titration: an evaluation of its various modifications. Analyst 1957; 82: 488–498.
41. Moore S, Stein WH. Photometric ninhydrin method for use in the chromatography of amino acids. J Biol Chem 1948; 176:367–388.
42. Adler-Nissen J. Determination of the degree of hydrolysis of food protein hydrolysates by trinitrobenzenesulfonic acid. J Agric Food Chem 1979; 27:1256–1262.
43. Steinhardt J, Beychok S. Interaction of proteins with hydrogen ions and other small ions and molecules. In: Neurath H, ed. The Proteins, Vol 2. New York: Academic Press, 1964: 139–304.
44. Gounaris AD, Perlmann GE. Succynilation of pepsinogen. J Biol Chem 1967; 242:2739–2745.
45. Franzen KL, Kinsella JE. Functional properties of succinylated and acetylated soy protein. J Agric Food Chem 1976; 24:788–795.
46. Choi YR, Lusas EW, Rhee KC. Effects of acylation of defatted cottonseed flour with various acid anhydrides on protein extractability and functional properties of resulting protein isolates. J Food Sci 1982; 47:1713–1716.
47. Gallagher KF, Jones RT. Emerging technology in protein copolymerization. Cosmet Toilet 1993; 108(3):97–104.
48. Sung HY, Chen HJ, Liu TY, Su JC. Improvement of the functionalities of soy protein isolate through chemical phosphorylation. J Food Sci 1983; 48:716–721.
49. Yamashita M, Arai S, Amano Y, Fujimaki M. A novel one-step process for enzymatic incorporation of amino acids into proteins: application to soy protein and flour for enhancing their methionine levels. Agric Biol Chem 1979; 43:1065–1068.
50. Watanabe M, Toyokawa H, Shimada A, Arai S. Proteinaceous surfactants produced from gelatin by enzymatic modification: evaluation of their functionality. J Food Sci 1981; 46: 1467–1469.
51. Fujimaki M, Arai S, Yamashita M. Enzymatic protein degradation and resynthesis for protein improvement. Adv Chem Ser 1977; 160:156–184.
52. Monti JC, Jost R. Papain-catalyzed synthesys of methionine enriched soy plastein. Average chain length of the plastein peptides. J Agric Food Chem 1979; 27:1281–1285.
53. Shimada A, Yazawa E, Arai S. Preparation of proteinaceous surfactants by enzymatic modification and evaluation of their functional properties in a concentrated emulsion system. Agric Biol Chem 1982; 46:173–182.
54. Croda Ltd. Tritisol—high molecular weight wheat protein. Technical Bulletin, 1991.
55. Schwuger MJ. Über die Wechselwirkung zwischen Proteinen und Tensiden an der Modelsubstanz Zein. Kolloid-Z Z Polym 1969; 233:898–905.
56. Schwuger MJ. Komplexbildung zwischen Aniontensiden und Eialbumin in Wasser. Kolloid-Z Z Polym 1971; 246:626–635.

57. Ray A, Reynolds JA, Polet H, Steinhardt J. Binding of large organic anionis and neutral molecules by native bovine serum albumin. Biochemistry 1966; 5(8):2606–2616.
58. Reynolds JA, Herbert S, Polet H, Steinhardt J. The binding of divers detergent anions to bovine serum albumin. Biochemistry 1967; 6(3):937–947.
59. Pitt-Rivers R, Ambesi Impiombato FS. The binding of sodium dodecyl sulphate to various proteins. Biochem J 1968; 109:825–829.
60. Teglia A, Secchi G. New Protein ingredients for skin detergency: native wheat protein-surfactant complexes. Int J Cosmet Sci 1994; 16:235–246.
61. Wolfram LJ. The reactivity of human hair: a review. In: Orfanos CE, Montagna W, Stüttgen G. eds. Hair Research. Berlin-Heidelberg: Springer-Verlag 1981:479–500.
62. Gruber HA, Mellon EF. Oxidation products of amino acids and collagen. Anal Biochem 1975; 66:78–86.
63. Tanford C. Contribution of hydrophobic interactions to the stability of the globular conformation of proteins. J Am Chem Soc 1962; 84:4240–4247.
64. Bigelow CC. On the average hydrophobicity of proteins and the relation between it and protein structure. J Theoret Biol 1967; 16:187–211.
65. Bigelow CC, Channon M. Hydrophobicities of aminoacids and proteins. In: Handbook of Biochemistry and Molecular Biology, 3rd ed, Vol 1. Cleveland: CRC Press, 1976:209–243.
66. Sklar LA, Hudson BS, Simoni RD. Conjugated polyene fatty acids as fluorescent probes: synthetic phospholipid membrane studies. Biochemistry 1977; 16(5):819–828.
67. Lampson GP, Tytell AA. A simple method for estimating isoelectric points. Anal Biochem 1965; 11:374–377.
68. Lindner H, Lindner H. Möglichkeiten einer in vitro-Testung der Hautverträglichkeit von Tensiden am Kollagenmolekul. Parfüm Kosmet 1986; 67:372–378.
69. Ochiai-Yanagi S, Miyauchi H, Saio K, Watanabe T. Modified soybean protein with high water-holding capacity. Cereal Chem 1978; 55:157–167.
70. Cheftel JC, Cuq JL, Lorient D. Amino acids, peptides and proteins. In: Fennema OR, ed. Food Chemistry. New York: Marcel Dekker, 1985.
71. Voutsinas LP, Cheung E, Nakai S. Relationships of hydrophobicity to emulsifying properties of heat denatured proteins. J Food Sci 1983; 48:26–32.
72. Townsend AA, Nakai S. Relationships between hydrophobicity and foaming of food proteins. J Food Sci 1983; 48:588–594.
73. Kitabatake N, Doi E. Surface tension and foaming of protein solutions. J Food Sci 1982; 47:1218–1225.
74. Nagelschmidt M, Struck H. Kollagen als Cosmeticum? Arch Derm Forsch 1974; 250:237–243.
75. Huc A, Journot M, Hartmann D. Etude de la penetration in vivo dans la peau de rat du collagene acido-soluble en solution acide ou en melange dans une creme cosmetique. Int J Cosmet Sci 1981; 3:159–183.
76. Chvapil M, Eckmayer Z. Role of proteins in cosmetics. Int J Cosmet Sci 1985; 7:41–49.
77. Ruland A, Kreuter J. Transdermal permeability and skin accumulation of amino acids. Int J Pharm 1991; 72:149–155.
78. Sznitowska M. Percutaneous absorption of amino acids and their cosmetic efficacy. Cosmet Toilet 1993; 108(9):29–32.
79. Turowski A, Adelmann-Grill BC. Substantivity to hair and skin of ^{125}I-labelled collagen hydrolysates under application simulating conditions. Int J Cosmet Sci 1985; 7:71–84.
80. Morganti F, Randazzo SD, Cardillo A. Role of insoluble and soluble collagen as skin moisturizer. J Appl Cosmetol 1986; 4:141–152.
81. Voegeli R, Meier J, Blust R, Hofsteter R. Sericina: proteina naturale della seta. Cosmet News 1995; 103:236–242.

82. Schrader K. Studies on water-retaining cosmetics on the skin. Parfüm Kosmet 1981; 62:265–272.
83. Curri SB, Grifeo S, Ronchi C, Campagnoli G. Microcircolazione e idratazione cutanea: effetti dell' applicazione di collagene. Cosmesi Dermatol 1992; 41:51–72.
84. Hatzis J, Marks R. The relationship between conductance and capacitance measurements and skin surface contour during hydration of the stratum corneum. In: Marks R, Plewig G, eds. Stratum Corneum. Berlin-Heidelberg: Springer-Verlag, 1983:257–261.
85. Leveque JL, Corcuff P. The surface of the skin—the microrelief. In: Frosch PJ, Kligman AM, eds. Noninvasive methods for the quantification of skin functions. Berlin-Heidelberg: Springer-Verlag, 1993:3–24.
86. Nicolas JF, Mironneau I. Capryloyl-collagenic acid for acne vulgaris. Cosmet Toilet 1992; 107(11):57–59.
87. Busch P, Hensen H, Fischer D, Ruhnke A, Franklin J. An abietic acid protein condensate for treating greasy hair. Cosmet Toilet 1995; 110(2):59–68.
88. Robbins CR. Chemical and Physical Behaviour of Human Hair, 2nd ed. New York: Springer-Verlag, 1988:1–38.
89. Lunn AC, Evens RE. The electrostatic properties of human hair. J Soc Cosmet Chem 1977; 28:549–569.
90. Robbins CR. Chemical and Physical Behavior of Human Hair, 2nd ed. New York: Springer-Verlag, 1988:140–141.
91. Ranganayaki MD, Ranganathan TS, Jayaraman KS. A novel technique for the preparation of collagen derivatives for cosmetics. Part 2. preparation and characterisation of collagen derivative. Res Ind 1989; 34:183–189.
92. Ranganayaki MD, Ranganathan TS, Jayaraman KS. A novel technique for the preparation of collagen derivatives for cosmetics. Part 3. Functional properties of collagen derivatives. Res Ind 1990; 35:1–7.
93. Stern E, Johnsen V. Studies on the molecular weight distribution of cosmetic protein hydrolysates. J Soc Cosmet Chem 1977; 28:447–455.
94. Mintz GR, Reinhart GM, Lent B. Relationship between collagen hydrolysate molecular weight and peptide substantivity to hair. J Soc Cosmet Chem 1991; 42:35–44.
95. Kelisema Srl. Kelyamin. Technical Bulletin, 1996.
96. Jones RT. Substantivity and properties of wheat protein as applied to hair. XVIth IFSCC Congress, New York, 1990, A30.
97. Croda Ltd. Croquat. Technical Bulletin, 1991.
98. Croda Ltd. Hydrotriticum. Technical Bulletin, undated.
99. Naito S, Ooshima K. Sorption of keratin hydrolyzate to hair and the cosmetic effect. XIVth IFSCC Congress, Barcelona, 1986, S.5.15.
100. Croda Ltd. Kerasol. Technical Bulletin, 1990.
101. Cooperman ES, Johnsen VL. Penetration of protein hydrolysates into human hair strands. Cosmet Perfum 1973; 88:19–22.
102. Lang G, Spengler J. Surfactants in cosmetic formulations: skin irritancy and physical properties XIVth IFSCC Congress, Barcelona, 1986, L.1.3.
103. Fullerton A, Broby-Johanssen U, Agner T. Sodium lauryl sulphate penetration in an in vitro model using human skin. Cont Derm 1994; 30:222–225.
104. Van Neste D. In vivo evaluation of unbound water accumulation in stratum corneum. Dermatology 1990; 181:197–201.
105. Rieger M. Surfactant interactions with skin. Cosmet Toilet 1995; 110(4):31–50.
106. Zeidler U. Influence of surfactants on the swelling of epidermis. XVth IFSCC Congress, London, 1988, B.5.
107. Rhein L, Robbins C, Fernee K, Cantore R. Surfactant-structure effects on swelling of isolated human stratum corneum. J Soc Cosmet Chem 1986; 37:125–139.

108. Götte E. Chemistry, physics and application of surface active substances. Proc. IVth Int. Congr. on Surface Active Substances, Brussels, 1964, Vol III, 5.83.
109. Balaguer F, Garcia Domingues J, Parra JL, Pelejero CM. Comparative studies of the action of surfactants on some protein materials and their irritation potential on human skin. VIIIth IFSCC Congress, London, 1974, B7.
110. Blake-Haskins JC, Scala D, Rhein LD. Predicting surfactant irritation from the swelling response of a collagen film. J Soc Cosmet Chem 1986; 37:199–210.
111. Miyazawa K, Ogawa M, Mitsui T. The physico-chemical properties and protein denaturation potential of surfactant mixtures. Int J Cosmet Sci 1984; 6:33–46.
112. Imokawa G, Sumara K, Katumi M. Study on skin roughness caused by surfactants. J Am Oil Chem Soc 1975; 52:484–489.
113. Harrold SP. Denaturation of epidermal keratin by surface active agents. J Invest Dermatol 1959; 32:581–588.
114. Prottey C, Ferguson T. Factors which determine the skin irritation potential of soaps and detergents. VIIIth IFSCC Congress, London, 1974, B9.
115. Conrads A, Zahn H. A study of the interaction of sodium dodecyl sulphate with the proteins of human heel stratum corneum. Int J Cosmet Sci 1987; 9:29–46.
116. Johnsen VL. Proteins in cosmetics and toiletries. Drug Cosmet Ind 1980; 126:36–39.
117. Morganti P, Muscardin L, Fabrizi G. Protective effect of collagen upon irritation response of detergents. Int J Cosmet Sci 1983; 5:7–14.
118. Domsch A, Pospischil H, Schuster G, Tronnier H. Cosmetic dermatological effects of protein hydrolysates. Parfüm Kosmet 1980; 61:325–330.
119. Berg A, Lindner H. Schutz-Proteine in der Kosmetik. Parfüm Kosmet 1979; 60:74–88.
120. Schuster G, Domsch A. Proteinderivate in der Kosmetic: welche und warum. SÖFW-J 1982; 108(7):177–184.
121. Steinhardt J, Scott JR, Birdi KS. Differences in the solubilizing effectiveness of the sodium dodecyl sulfate complexes of various proteins. Biochemistry 1977; 16(4):718–725.
122. Teglia A, Secchi G. Evaluation of the protective efficacy of proteins and mild tensides against the adverse cutaneous effects of anionic detergents by means of tranepidermal water loss and profilometric measurements. XVIIIth IFSCC Congress, Venice, 1994, P073.
123. Frieß W, Nürnberg E. Kollagenhydrolysat-tensid 3000 als determinierender Bestandteil von hydrophilen Cremes. Pharm Ind 1994; 56:61–65.
124. Henkel KGaA. Gluadin. Technical Bulletin, 1995.
125. Busch P, Domsch A, Hensen H. Cationic protein derivatives for hair cosmetics. XVth IFSCC Congress, London, 1988, A23.
126. Kowata Y, Tamura H, Motoi H, Tabata Y. Performance of polypeptides from wheat protein as cosmetic material. XVIIth IFSCC Congress, Yokohama, 1992, A206.
127. Steisslinger HW. Improvement of the compatibility of binary systems containing a new high molecular weight protein surfactant. SÖFW-J 1992; 118:908–918.
128. Henkel KGaA. Cospha protein hydrolysates and protein derivatives. Technical Bulletin, 1992.
129. Adler-Nissen J. Peptide mixtures as emulsifiers. Novo Industri A/S Technical Bulletin A-05887, 1987.
130. CTFA Microbiology Committee. Interaction between cosmetic ingredients and preservatives. Cosmet Toilet 1995; 110(11):81–86.
131. Chang C, Houck J. Demonstration of the chemotactic properties of collagen. Proc Soc Exp Biol Med 1970; 134:22–24.
132. Houck J, Chang C. The chemotactic properties of the products of collagenolysis. Proc Soc Exp Biol Med 1971; 138:69.
133. Postlethwaite AE. Chemotactic attraction of human fibroblasts to type I, II and III collagens and collagen-derived peptides. Proc Natl Acad Sci USA 1978; 75:871–875.

134. Final report on the safety assessment of hydrolyzed collagen. J Am Coll Toxicol 1985; 4: 199–221.
135. Bader S, Gondoni A. Heavy metals content in protein derivatives for cosmetics (It). Diploma thesis, University of Ferrara (Italy), School of Cosmetic Science and Technology, 1982.
136. Meyer B, Gedek K, Heinzel M. Mycotoxins: relevance to cosmetics. Cosmet Toilet 1992; 107(5):75–79.
137. Chung CW, Trucksess MW, Giles AL, Friedman L. Rabbit skin test for estimation of T-2 toxin and other skin irritation toxins in contaminated corn. J AOAC 1974; 57(5):1121–1127.
138. EC Directive 97/1 1997.
139. World Health Organization. Press release WHO/28-3 April 1996. [http://www.who.ch/press/1996/pr96-28.html]
140. Guidelines for minimizing the risk of transmission of agents causing spongiform encephalopathies via medicinal products. Commission of the European Community III/3298/91-EN.
141. Schrieber R, Seybold U. Gelatine production, the six steps to maximum safety. Dev Biol Stand 1993; 80:195–198.

10

Measuring and Interpreting Polycation Adsorption

E. Desmond Goddard
Union Carbide Corporation, Tarrytown, New York

I. INTRODUCTION

Cationic materials (surfactants and, more recently, polymers) have been the traditional conditioners for keratinous substrates, especially hair. This is connected with the fact that these substrates are, normally, negatively charged because of their low isoelectric point (see below). Today polycations, employed either alone or together with a coconditioner, are by far the most predominant type. Accordingly, it is recognized that means of monitoring the adsorption and retention of polycations are central to the understanding of the mechanism of their action and effectiveness.

II. SURFACTANTS AS A MODEL

Because of their widespread use and well-recognized interfacial activity, we first consider the adsorption of ionic surfactants as a model for the adsorption of polyelectrolytes (polycations) and examine the dominant forces and factors governing the phenomenon:

a. The Charge of the (aqueous) Interface. Ordinary surfactants will be repelled from interfaces with charges of like sign to their own, and attracted to those of opposite sign. As pointed out in Chapters 2 and 4, such electrostatic forces are strong and of long range (except when the ionic strength of the contacting solution is high).
b. The Interfacial Free Energy (''tension'') of the Aqueous Interface. Media of low dielectric constant such as hydrophobic solids and fluids (e.g., air and oil) have a high interfacial energy against water. Such an unfavorable energy condition constitutes a potent factor promoting adsorption of a surfactant from a contacting aqueous solution to the interface.
c. The Length of the Alkyl Chain of the Surfactant. Traube's rule (1) states that, in a homologous surfactant series, the concentration (c) of surfactant required to lower the surface tension of water by a given amount decreases by a constant

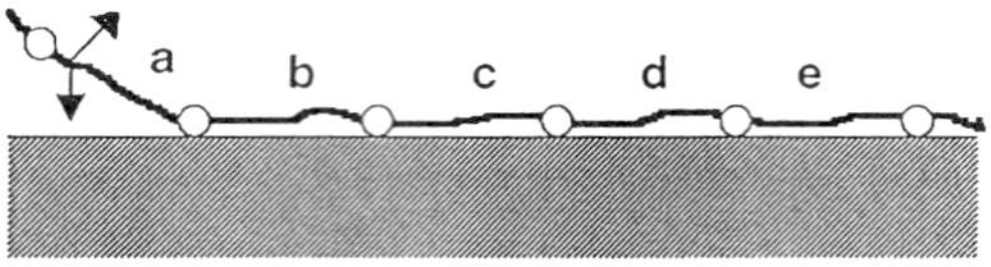

Figure 1 Simplistic depiction showing why polymer adsorption tends to be irreversible: segment ''a'' trying to ''escape'' is restrained by adsorbed segments b, c, d, and e (shown without ''loops''— see Final Comments).

factor for each unit increase of chain length, i.e., one CH_2 group. Thermodynamically, Traube's rule can be approximated by the expression, for chain lengths n and $(n + 1)$:

$$\Delta G_{\text{ads}} = -RT \ ln \ c_n/c_{n+1}$$

The derived value of ΔG_{ads}, ca. 1 kT/CH_2, means that the alkyl chain's contribution to the adsorption free energy in a typical surfactant will be in the range of 12–15 kT per molecule.

In the case of polymer adsorption, all three of the above items have potential relevance; items (b) and (c) would assume special importance in the case of hydrophobic or hydrophobically modified polymers. In addition, a factor of unique significance in the case of polymers is that even small energies of interfacial attraction, when expressed per monomer group, can become appreciable when summed up for the polymer molecule as a whole; smaller forces, such as dipole/dipole, which may be only of the order of 1 kT, become a substantial nkT when expressed for an n-mer. This is one of the reasons that the adsorption of polymer tends to be irreversible, as indicated in Chapter 2, and desorption is kinetically unfavorable. Also, put simplistically, a segment such as *a* endeavoring to desorb is restrained by segments *b*, *c*, *d*, etc., already adsorbed (Fig. 1).

III. SURFACE OF HAIR AND STRATUM CORNEUM (SC)

While the essentially keratinous bulk makeup of hair and skin (SC) is generally accepted, their surfaces are less well defined. It is obvious that the detailed properties of the latter will be pivotal in determining the adsorption behavior of added conditioning agents. Thus, it is recognized that a sebum layer is generally/frequently present on both of these substrates (see below). While such a layer can be regarded as a ''contaminant,'' a lipid layer can also be intrinsic to the surface. This aspect has been explored in some detail in the case of hair (2), the substrate of emphasis in this chapter. For details on the structure of hair the book by Robbins (2), and Chapter 12, may be consulted.

The presence of hydrophobic layers (either intrinsic or contaminant) on the substrate can obviously affect the deposition of additives from a solution contacting the substrate, through their influence on van der Waals forces, hydrophobic forces, and the like. It is thus essential to use standardized methods of cleaning and rinsing to prepare specimens for adsorption experiments. Long-range electrical forces, determined by the intrinsic surface charge of the keratin, while less likely to be affected, would be directly influenced if the contaminant were itself charged, for example an ionic surfactant. The history of hair, such as the extent of weathering, will also have an influence. Therefore, it is best, as far as possible, to use a standard source of hair and skin, for adsorption experiments.

The substantial uptake of water by hair and skin immersed in water is expected to have a major influence on their surface and bulk behavior toward solutes, including sorbing polycations.

For reasons that will become apparent it is convenient to divide discussion of the sorption of high-molecular-weight cationic conditioners into work done in two time periods, namely, the "early" period (pre-1980) and the "current" period (post-1980).

IV. MEASURING THE ADSORPTION OF CATIONIC POLYMERS

A. The Early Period: Radiotracers

The merits of the radiotracer method for studying physical interactions (including sorption) with hair were recognized quite early (3). In fact, up to 1980 it was the chief method that was used to study such interactions that involved hair-conditioning polycations. Some advantages of the method are:

a. The high sensitivity and accuracy of radioactive assay.
b. Tagging does not alter the interacting molecule chemically.
c. Assessments can be done in the presence of interfering or competing components, such as ionic surfactants.

A factor linked to advantage (a) concerns the limited surface area of natural keratins: even for hair, the nominal value (see below) is only ~0.1 m^2/g. For all of the above reasons, more (published) adsorption data in this field have been obtained by the radiotracer method than by any other—even though, for environmental reasons, use of the method has dwindled during the last decade.

1. *Polyethyleneimine*

Two early reports of the use of radiotagging (^{14}C) to study the uptake of a polymer by hair came from the Dow Chemical Company (4,5) and were concerned with the cationic polymer polyethyleneimine (PEI). Although this polymer was withdrawn from hair products in the 1970s it can be considered as an initial model for an adsorbing polycation. The first (4) of the two reports concerned a specimen of very low molecular weight (600), as much an oligomer as a polymer. (Its sorption properties were actually studied in connection with their bearing on a subsequent possible polymerization step for hair waving.) However, the results obtained merit mention because of several important findings. First, the uptake was found to be appreciable—of the order of several percent by weight of the hair. Second, once sorbed, the PEI was very difficult to remove by washing, even with a solution of untagged PEI. (See below for rationale.)

The study was expanded by Woodard (5) to include two other PEI-based polymers, a higher-molecular-weight homopolymer, PEI (60,000), and a similarly high-molecular-weight PEI/PEO copolymer. Further experimental details provided by Woodard were that the exposed hair samples were dissolved in hyamine prior to scintillation counting and that the "tagged ^{14}C PEI was prepared by reacting a small percentage of the amino groups with $^{14}CH_3I$" [so that it does not quite fully meet criterion (b) above].

Table 1 Sorption from 5% PEI on Hair

Time (min)	PEI 60,000 (%)	PEI 600 (%)
2	0.8	0.5
5	0.9	0.6
60	1.2	1.2

Considering only the results for the two homopolymers, MW 600 and 60,000, one can summarize the results of Woodard as follows:

1. Uptake of the polymer is substantial, exceeding 1% by weight in 60 min, as shown in Table 1.
2. Sorption is comparable for the 600 and 60,000 molecular weight materials.
3. Initial adsorption occurs almost immediately. (See Fig. 2.)
4. Bleaching of hair has a major effect on the uptake of PEI 60,000: after 1 hr a threefold increase from 1.2% to 3.4%. For PEI 600 the effect was much less: a 25% increase from 1.2 to 1.5%.
5. Reducing the concentration of PEI reduced the amount of sorption. An 80% reduction in concentration reduced the amount sorbed by 50%: thus, after 1 hr the uptake was 0.6% from a 1% solution of either PEI 600 or PEI 60,000.
6. As a function of pH (three values tested) sorption was highest at pH 7. The reduction observed at pH 10 probably reflects lower ionization of PEI; that at pH 2, reversal of the net sign of charge of hair (see below).

The results obtained by Woodard, namely high and fast uptake of PEI, led her to use

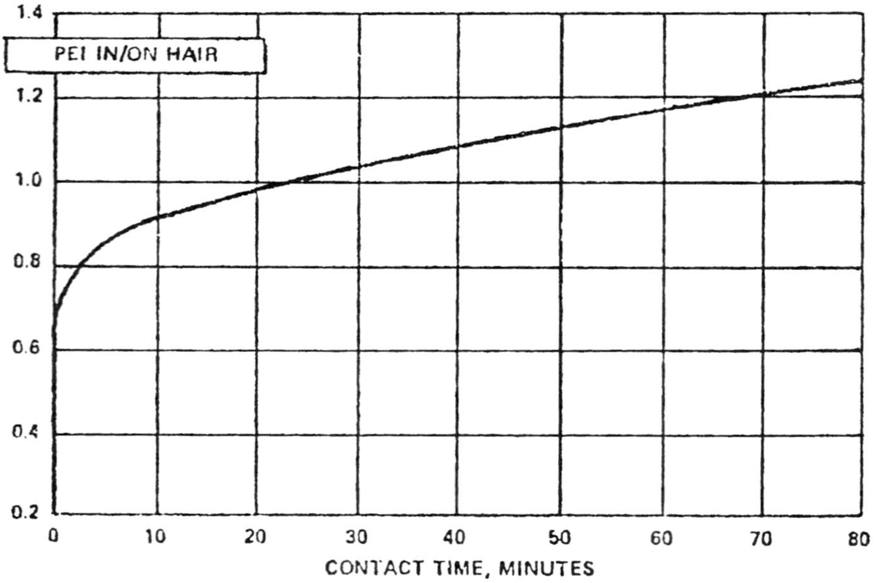

Figure 2 Sorption of ^{14}C-labeled polyethyleneimine (PEI 600) from a 5% aqueous solution by virgin hair; uptake is expressed in percent, based on weight of hair. (From Ref. 5.)

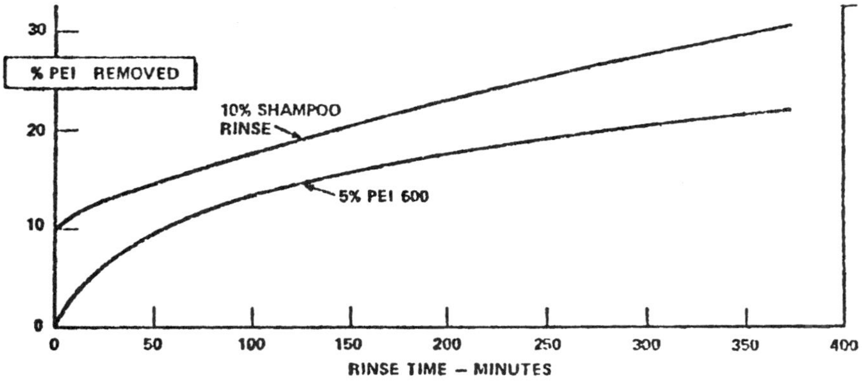

Figure 3 Desorption of PEI from pretreated hair: most of the presorbed PEI is retained. See text. (From Ref. 5.)

terms such as ''sorption'' and ''diffusion . . . into/onto the hair'' (5). Consequently, studying desorption became of interest. Two methods were explored: exposure to a solution of (untagged) polymer, and exposure to a shampoo solution. [The rationale for the former method is the recognition that adsorption of high-molecular-weight polymers tends to be ''irreversible.'' A simplistic picture of the removal mechanism is that, if a segment of an adsorbed (tagged) polymer desorbs momentarily, there is a statistical chance that its place can be taken by a segment of a (nontagged) polymer molecule in solution near the surface, which thus gains a ''foothold'' for adsorption of further segments.] The conditions chosen by Woodard were 24 hr exposure of hair to 5% *PEI-60,000 solution, four water washes, and then a time study of desorption into a 5% PEI 60,000 (untagged), or 10% shampoo ''rinse'' solution. The results in Figure 3 show the removal of presorbed PEI is very limited indeed, amounting to only 30% or less in 6 hr!

The results obtained by Woodard introduced a new concept of *penetration* of high-molecular-weight conditioning polycations in hair. This concept has still not been widely accepted in the industry. One possible interpretation of the observed results is that the polymer investigated, PEI, is a ''slender'' macromolecule whose narrow cross-sectional area might facilitate penetration into hair by a reptation process (Chapter 1) through its pores. The next section shows that this factor is not (solely) responsible for the observed behavior.

2. Cationic Cellulosic Polymers

The Polymer JR family of polymers from Amerchol Corporation is the most widely used and investigated among conditioning polymers. The generic formula is

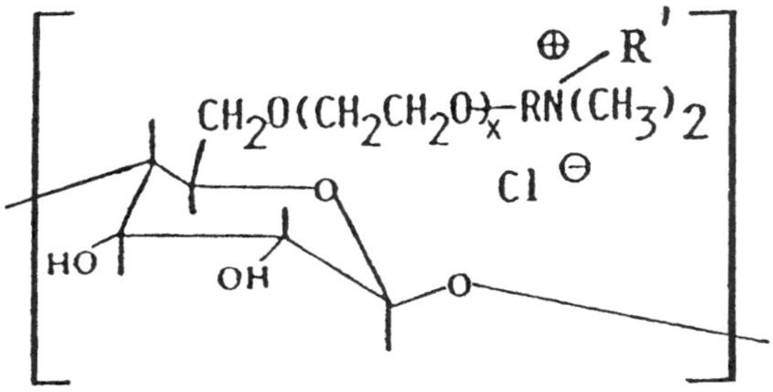

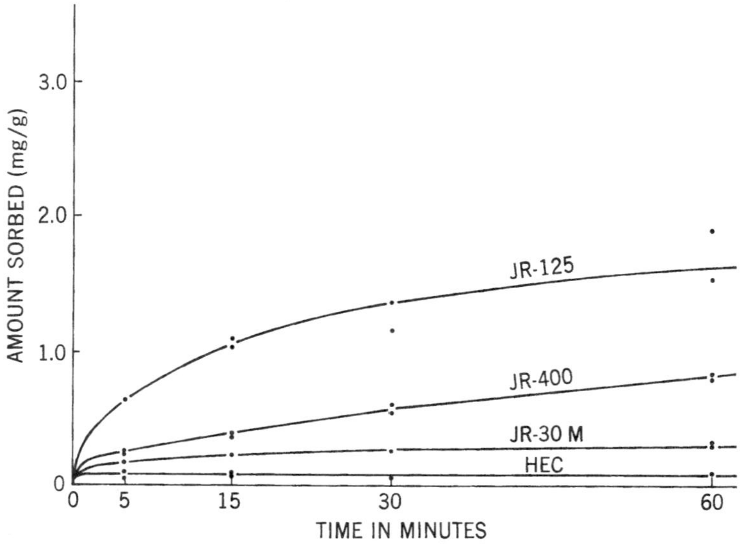

Figure 4 Sorption of ^{14}C-labeled polymers by virgin hair; 0.1% polymer solutions. Short exposure times. (From Ref. 8.)

The cross-sectional area of these macromolecules is clearly considerably larger than that of PEI.

As reported in a series of publications (6–10), studies of the sorption of three homologous members of this family were investigated over a wide range of conditions using the radiotagging technique. The methods used were essentially similar to those of Woodard except that a biological oxidizer (Packard) was used to dissolve the exposed hair samples rather than alkaline digestion employed in the early experiments. The three grades of polymer were JR125 (mol. wt. 250,000), JR 400 (mol. wt. 400,000), and JR 30M (mol. wt. 600,000). Radiotagged specimens were prepared by carrying out the polymer synthesis with ethylene oxide tagged with ^{14}C.*

The results of sorption experiments on virgin hair are presented in Figures 4 and 5. Though uptake rates and amounts sorbed are lower than those observed by Woodard for PEI 60,000, the pattern shown by these cationic cellulosic polymers is qualitatively similar. Some uptake occurs almost immediately, but it is again evident that sorption continues to increase over a period of minutes, hours, or even days. Within the cellulosic series there is a distinct trend of uptake decreasing as molecular weight increases.

The case of uncharged hydroxyethylcellulose (HEC), the ''parent'' molecule of JR polymers, deserves special mention. (The specimen chosen had a molecular weight of ~400,000, about the same as Polymer JR 400.) First, although the uptake is small, it is finite. Second, the isotherm is flat, typical of true adsorption but atypical of a process involving bulk diffusion. Using the BET surface area of hair, viz., 0.1 m^2/g (7), and con-

* As one of the papers (8), dealing with sorption studies on virgin hair in comparison with other substrates, appeared in a somewhat inaccessible assembly of conference papers it was decided to reproduce it as an auxiliary chapter to follow the present one. This decision has led to a minor amount of duplication of material between the two chapters.

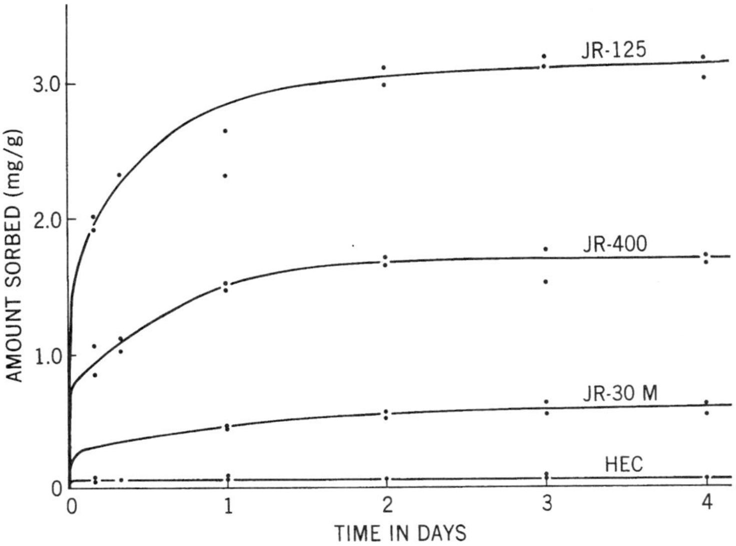

Figure 5 Sorption of ^{14}C-labeled polymers by virgin hair; 0.1% polymer solutions. Long exposure times. (From Ref. 8.)

verting the adsorption value of HEC, viz., 0.05 mg/g hair, to an area value per anhydroglucose residue (mol. wt. 250), one obtains a value of 85 A^2, consistent with a loosely packed monolayer of cellulose in flat orientation (8). According to this model the ''equilibrium'' (4 day) uptakes of Polymer JR30M, 400, and 125, correspond to 10, 30, and 50 monolayers—a completely unrealistic picture, especially the last-mentioned value (8).

A more realistic estimate of the area occupied per molecule can be made from adsorption studies of these positively charged polymers on glass (8), which, like hair, is negatively charged (see below). The estimate yields a value of ~30 A^2/anhydroglucose residue. On this basis the equivalent number of monolayers calculated for Polymer JR 30M, 400, and 125 on hair amounts to 4, 10, and 18, respectively: for bleached hair (7) the corresponding figures would be 15, 100, and 180 monolayers! These calculations show that the adsorption model is completely unrealistic. In a similar vein, calculations using Woodard's data for PEI (5) lead to multilayer adsorption values where the layers would be several hundred molecules thick. As suggested previously (5), the only feasible explanation is that these polymers are able to diffuse into the water-swollen hair fibers, with diffusion coefficients decreasing with increasing molecular weight. Estimates of the diffusion coefficients will be presented later.

Another result contraindicative of a monolayer adsorption process is that the molecular weight sequence of uptake given above is just the opposite of that anticipated for an adsorption process, in which the highest-molecular-weight homolog should display the highest adsorption affinity (Chapter 11). On the other hand, results obtained (8) with nylon fibers, for which no penetration is expected, did display this feature for the above set of polymers and, furthermore, demonstrated that equilibrium uptakes are achieved rather quickly—in minutes. In addition, being itself uncharged, nylon showed little difference in uptake between the charged Polymer JR 400 and its uncharged counterpart, HEC. This information supports a monolayer adsorption process in this case. Likewise, in the experiments with glass referred to above, equilibrium adsorption of Polymer JR 400 occurred rapidly and the uptake was consistent with an adsorbed monolayer of polymer in ostensibly flat configuration.

a. Bleached Hair. Though qualitatively similar, with trends following those of virgin hair, sorption studies with bleached hair, displayed much higher uptakes of polymer, indicative of the more damaged and porous nature of the fibers. [See Fig. 6 (7).] This trend was seen by Woodard for PEI 60,000. Furthermore, a substantial influence of polymer concentration on the course and amount of sorption was found. Thus the estimated number of adsorbed monolayers of Polymer JR 125 referred to above would double, from 180 to 360, if the polymer concentration were increased from 0.1% to 1%.

b. Influence of Salt. If postulated mechanisms involving an electrostatic driving force are valid, then a substantial influence of salt on the sorption of polycations on hair would be expected: through electrical shielding, the driving force, and hence the amount of sorption, should decrease. This has been confirmed for both bleached hair and brown hair (7,9,10). With simple salts, the amount of reduction increases with concentration of added salt (Fig. 7). For a given molarity of added salt the effect increases with the valence of the cation (Fig. 8). In other words, multiply charged cations are most effective at screening the negative charges of hair, following the well-known Schulze-Hardy rule (11) of colloids. (Little difference in adsorption accompanied changes in the anion of simple added salts.) Based on a series of experiments (9), the following sequence in the effect of added salt in reducing the adsorption of Polymer JR, from most effective to least effective, was $La^{3+} > Al^{3+} > Fe^{3+} > Ca^{2+} > Fe^{2+} > Cs^{+} > Na^{+} > Li^{+}$.

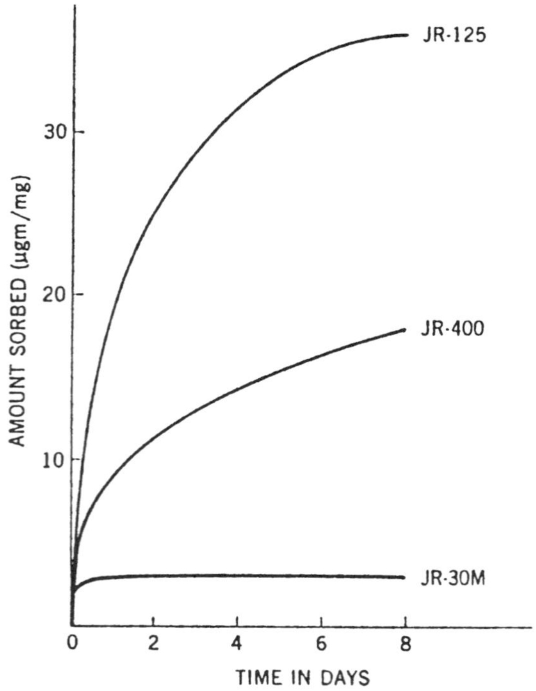

Figure 6 Sorption of different grades of Polymer JR by bleached hair; 0.1% polymer solutions. (From Ref. 7.)

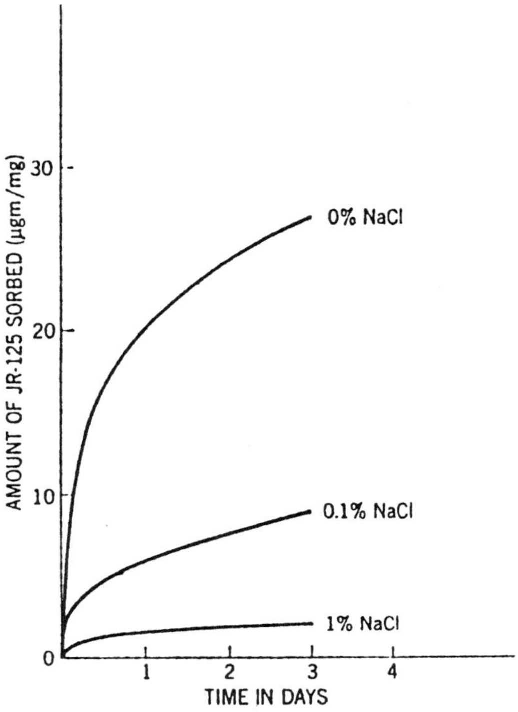

Figure 7 Effect of added salt on the sorption of Polymer JR 125 by bleached hair; 0.1% polymer solutions. (From Ref. 7.)

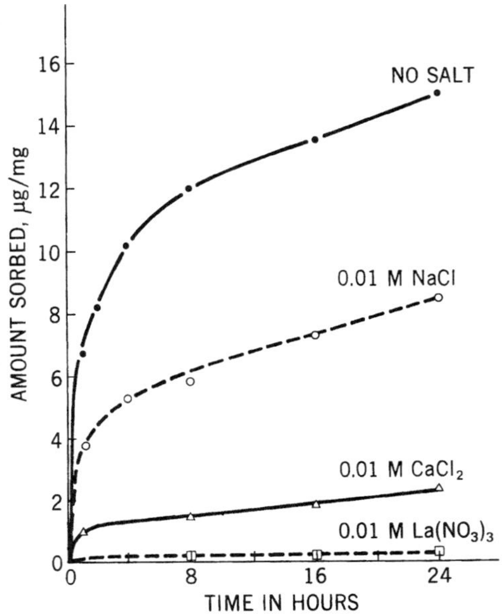

Figure 8 Effect of different salts on the sorption of Polymer JR 125 by bleached hair; 0.1% polymer solutions. (From Ref. 9.)

c. Effect of pH. If the above reasoning is valid, then pH should exert a substantial influence on polycation sorption, to the extent that pH can influence the net charge of the keratin substrate. This assumes, of course, that the polycation itself is a strong electrolyte, like Polymer JR, whose ionization is virtually unaffected by pH. Initial work (7) showed little variation of the sorption of Polymer JR 125 (on bleached hair) within the pH range 4–10. Later work (12), however, showed a catastrophic reduction in the sorption of this polymer on virgin hair when the pH was reduced below the isoelectric point (pH 3.7). (See Fig. 9.) Indeed, under these conditions the amount of uptake now approximated that displayed by the uncharged parent molecule, HEC. This result is testimony to the profound influence of electrostatic forces on polyelectrolyte adsorption.

d. Effect of Surfactants on Sorption. Early work (6) involving simulated shampooing had shown a major influence of the component surfactant on the uptake of Polymer JR on hair. In the extreme cases, with the nonionic Tergitol 15-S-9 as the "shampooing" surfactant, there was substantially "unimpeded" deposition, while anionic surfactants like lauryl sulfate (TEALS) and alkylbenzenesulfonate (LAS) led to considerable reduction. With Miranol CM-SF (an ampholytic based on imidazoline) as surfactant there was again substantial deposition of the polymer: this was also the case with a soap, perhaps through a coprecipitation effect involving water hardness.

In model experiments, employing 1% surfactant solutions in the presence of 0.1% Polymer JR 400, it was shown (8) that, in long-term (several days) exposure, SDS reduced the adsorption of polymer on virgin hair about 10-fold, while Tergitol 15-S-9 again had a comparatively minor effect. The effect of an amine oxide lay between the aforementioned. On the other hand, the cationic surfactant CTAB virtually eliminated the polymer's adsorption. The interpretation is that, being a much faster diffusing species, the cationic

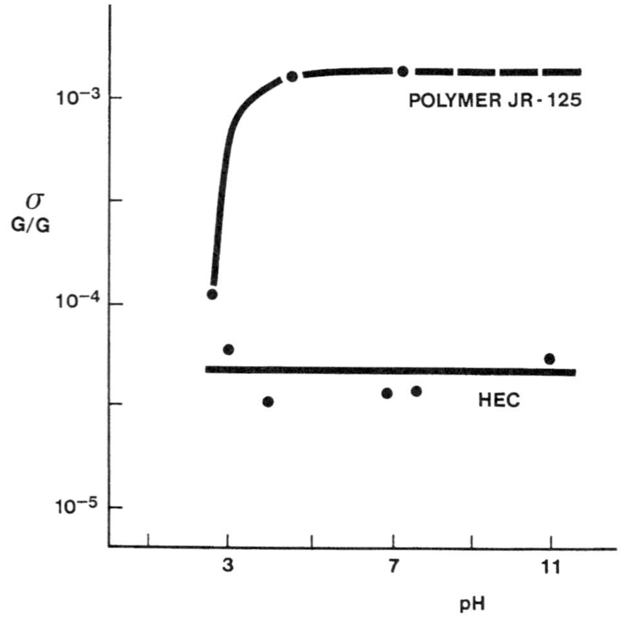

Figure 9 Sorption of Polymer JR 125 onto virgin hair as a function of solution pH; 0.1% polymer solutions. (From Ref. 12.)

surfactant is able to preempt the negatively charged adsorption sites on the hair. (See Chapter 5, Fig. 1; Chapter 11, Fig. 5.)

Experiments with bleached hair (7), in which the effect of ionic surfactants on deposition of the polycation was studied in more detail, yielded results that, in general, paralleled those obtained for virgin hair. One finding of obvious potential importance was that the sorption of polymer decreased approximately in proportion to the amount of anionic surfactant (SDS) present, presumably owing to progressive tie-up of the polycation in negatively charged complexes.

e. Sorption as a Diffusion Process. The results presented so far have given evidence that from aqueous solution cationic polymers are slowly sorbed into hair. Hence it is appropriate to consider the phenomenon as one involving a diffusion process. Such an analysis has been reported (7). As a first approximation the model chosen was one involving migration into a semi-infinite slab, with penetration limited to a region near the interface. Under these conditions, the equation governing diffusion is (13)

$$\frac{\partial c}{\partial t} = D \frac{\partial^2 c}{\partial x^2}$$

with the following boundary conditions:

$c = c_0$ at $x = 0$, for $t > 0$ (bulk concentration c_0 is constant)
$c = 0$ at $t = 0$, for $x > 0$ (x = distance parameter)

The solution of this equation is

$$Q(t) = 2c_0\,(Dt/\pi)^{1/2}$$

which is known as the Hill equation (13).

The experimental data were found to follow this equation reasonably well for at least the first few hours or so (7,8). Calculated values of D, the diffusion coefficient, in cm^2/sec, are given in Table 2.

While trends are generally consistent with expectations, the higher value of D for Polymer JR 400 in virgin hair than bleached hair is inconsistent. Furthermore, derived values of D for the diffusion of Polymer JR 125 into bleached hair showed a strong dependence on concentration (7). Some anomalies also exist in the desorption kinetics as discussed below. For these reasons the simple diffusion model can only be considered preliminary. Undoubtedly, effects associated with the structure of hair, as discussed in the conclusion of this chapter, are involved.

f. Desorption. Desorption studies carried out on hair previously exposed to Polymer JR solutions have been carried out (9,10). An interesting, if predictable, finding was that desorption tends to be rather slow and incomplete. A log-log plot showed that desorption (9) follows a 0.1–0.2 power of time law, as previously reported by Chow (4) for the

Table 2 Diffusion Coefficient (cm^2/sec)

	Virgin hair (8)	Bleached hair (7)	Stratum corneum (13,14)
Polymer JR 125	6.4×10^{-9}	1.3×10^{-8}	1.1×10^{-10}
Polymer JR 400	1.1×10^{-9}	7.1×10^{-10}	9.7×10^{-11}
Polymer JR30M	1×10^{-10}	3×10^{-10}	1.2×10^{-12}

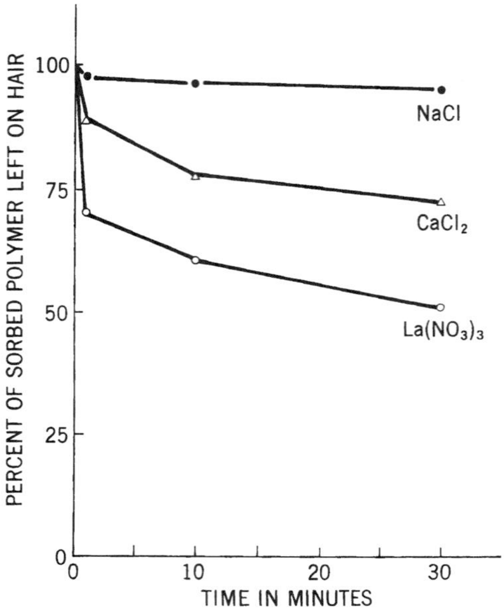

Figure 10 Desorption of preadsorbed Polymer JR 125 from bleached hair by 0.01 M salt solutions. (From Ref. 9.)

desorption of PEI: this behavior is quite different from simple diffusional release from a polymer matrix with its expected square root of time dependency. Experiments were carried out in the presence of added salts in the expectation that, through reduction of electrostatic binding forces, the salt would facilitate desorption. This was confirmed in the effects of cation valence, viz., $La^{3+} > Ca^{2+} > Na^{+}$, in removal efficiency (see Fig. 10). These results were obtained for bleached hair previously exposed for an hour to 0.1% Polymer JR 125 solution, rinsed, and then treated with 0.01 M "rinse" solutions (which were found the most discriminating as regards differentiation among the above cations). Results obtained for virgin hair (Table 3) showed that SDS was not much more efficient that $CaCl_2$ in removing presorbed Polymer JR 400; neither was a combination of NaCl and SDS (10).

The results shown in Table 3 reflect somewhat arbitrary laboratory conditions rather

Table 3 Desorption of Polymer JR 400 from Brown Hair

	Percent Amounts of Polymer JR Desorbed				
		0.1 M	0.1 M	0.1 M	0.05 M SDA/ 0.1 M
Time	H_2O	NaCl	$CaCl_2$	SDS	NaCl
1 min	8	41	49	53	48
5 min	9	45	56	61	41
10 min	10	47	59	66	48
30 min	14	58	60	69	56

Initial sorption: 1.63 mg polymer/g hair. Sorption conditions: 30 min exposure to 0.1% polymer.

than actual shampooing practice in which starting levels of polymer present in the hair are likely to be considerably lower than those employed here. This aspect is discussed further at the end of the chapter.

g. Experiments with Stratum Corneum Membranes. Results obtained with neonatal rat stratum corneum membranes (14–16) paralleled those obtained with hair fibers, with absolute uptakes of polymer being fairly close to those found for virgin hair. Thus the uptake values decreased in ascending order of molecular weight (Fig. 11), were time dependent, and decreased in the presence of added surfactant in the order cationic surfactant (biggest effect) >> anionic surfactant >> nonionic surfactant. (See Fig. 12.) When the sorbed amount of Polymer JR 400 was expressed per unit (apparent) area of the membrane and compared with a similarly expressed uptake value for glass [corresponding to "true" monolayer coverage, see above (8)], it vastly exceeded the latter. This again suggests a sorption process of the polymer into the water-swollen membrane. [See Fig. 13(8,15).] Experiments employing a diffusion cell showed, however, that even for the fastest-migrating homolog, viz. Polymer JR 125, a period of 2 weeks was required before any polymer penetrated all the way through a stratum corneum membrane (16).

Pretreating a stratum corneum membrane with Polymer JR 400 solution was observed to lead to a substantial reduction in the diffusion rate of SDS across the membrane, again

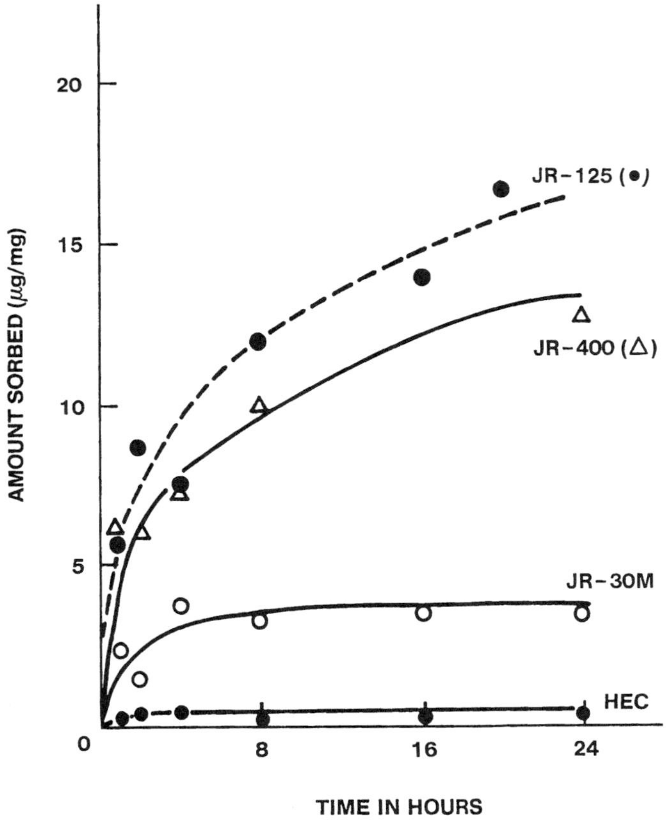

Figure 11 Sorption of various grades of Polymer JR and of hydroxyethylcellulose (HEC) by stratum corneum; 0.1% polymer solutions. (From Ref. 15.)

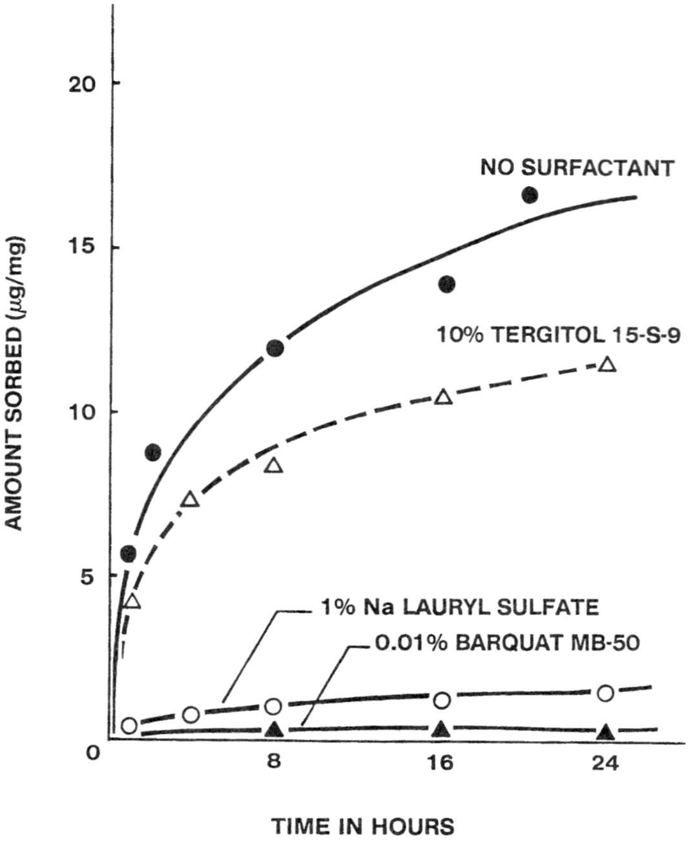

Figure 12 Effect of surfactants on the sorption of Polymer JR 125 by stratum corneum. (From Ref. 15.)

attesting to the presence of sorbed polymer in the treated membrane (14,16). Values of the diffusion coefficient, *D*, of the polymers into SC membranes were calculated by applying the Hill equation (13) to the radiouptake data (14,15). They are listed in Table 2. The values decrease with increasing molecular weight; also, they are generally lower than those observed for hair.

3. Polymers Based on Dimethyldiallylamine Chloride (DMDAAC)

The last of the radiotracer studies described here is concerned with the sorption of two polymers from Calgon Corporation, namely Merquat 100 and Merquat 550, on hair (17). Merquat 100 is a DMDAAC homopolymer (mol. wt. 100,000) and Merquat 550 is an acrylamide/DMDAAC copolymer (mol. wt. 500,000).

Methods were essentially similar to those used in the Polymer JR studies, viz., ^{14}C tagging, sample combustion, and scintillation counting, and the findings were similar in many respects. Thus, initial uptake was rapid and increased steadily with time, and uptake was substantial, reaching 1% in the case of Merquat 550 in 3 h on bleached hair (see Table 4). Other similar findings were that bleached hair sorbed substantially more polymer than did virgin hair (by three- to eightfold, depending on the cosolute present); salts de-

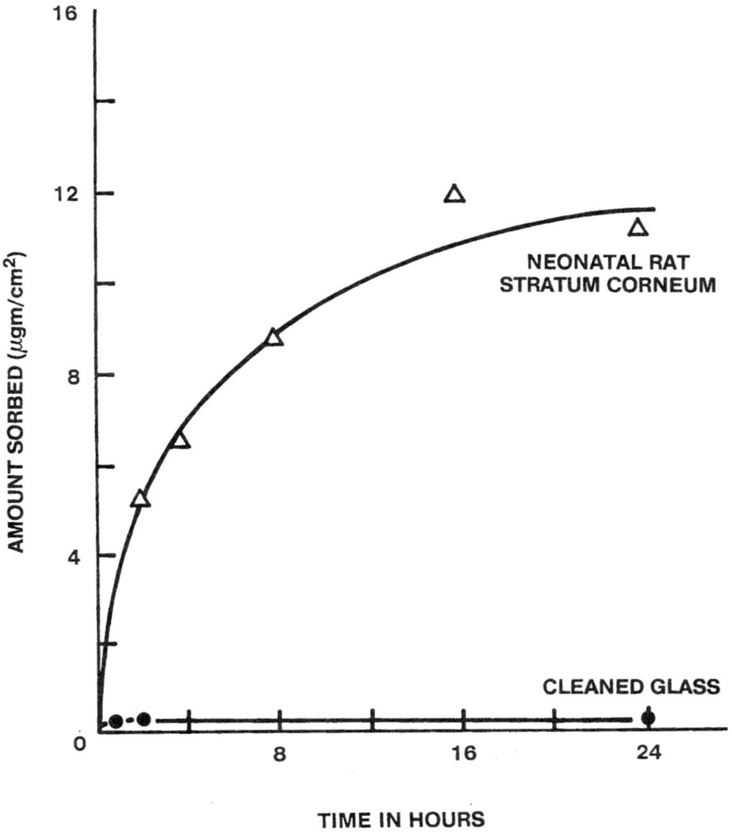

Figure 13 Sorption of Polymer JR by different surfaces; 0.1% polymer solutions. (From Ref. 15.)

Table 4 Effect of Temperature on the Sorption of 0.1% Merquat Polymers by Bleached Hair

	μg Polymer sorbed per mg hair			
	5 min	30 min	60 min[a]	180 min[a]
Merquat 100				
22°C	1.32	1.84	2.1	2.5
40°C	1.80	2.36		
Merquat 550				
22°C	5.44	7.28	7.5	10.0
40°C	7.40	9.25		

[a]Estimated.

creased sorption in order of the valence of the cation ($NaCl < CaCl_2 < AlCl_3$); and lowering pH led to lower uptake, especially as the isoelectric point of hair was approached. As shown in Table 4, increasing the temperature of exposure from 22°C to 40°C led to an increase (~30%) in uptake of both polymers, presumably due to further expansion of the water-swollen matrix. While anionic surfactants like SDS and TEALS sharply reduced polymer sorption, the effect of the ampholytic Miranol C2M was minor.

The substantially higher uptake observed for Merquat 550 was attributed (17) to its higher molecular weight. This is not consistent with the trends found in the Polymer JR family. An alternative explanation is that the Merquat 550 copolymer has more flexibility than the Merquat 100 homopolymer and, on the reptation model (Chapter 1), may be a more efficient diffusant into the hair.

B. The Current Period

1. *Surface Spectroscopic Techniques*

During the last few decades a number of sophisticated surface analytical techniques have been developed that involve irradiation and detection procedures. These include electron spectroscopy for chemical analysis (ESCA, sometimes referred to as X-ray photoelectron spectroscopy XPS), Fourier transform infrared-attenuated total reflectance (FTIR-ATR), electron probe microanalysis (EPMA), ion scattering spectroscopy (ISS), and secondary ion mass spectrometry (SIMS). Generally, it is a requirement that the adsorbate molecule possess an element or grouping sensitive to the measuring procedure and indicative of, and exclusive to, the said molecule. Until now, the limited reported use of these techniques for detection and quantification of polymers adsorbed on keratins probably reflects the generally high cost of the instrumentation (see Section VI). In this respect, published data appear to be largely limited to the first three techniques mentioned above, of which by far the most widely used has been ESCA.

a. ESCA. The basic process of ESCA involves irradiation of a surface with an X-ray beam, which causes emission of "core" electrons from surface atoms. The measured energy of these electrons characterizes the elements present, and the intensity allows estimates of the surface concentration of the elements. With regard to applicability to keratins, Robbins and Bahl demonstrated the utility of ESCA for studying the surface of hair and skin substrates themselves (18,19). For the present purpose the success of the method depends on the polymer's possessing, in sufficient atomic concentration, elements different from those of the substrate (keratin) or having elements in a different bonding (oxidation) state. With regard to cationic polymers, the quaternary nitrogen group itself is appropriate since natural keratins, though rich in nitrogen, possess few of these groups (unless through contamination). There are other possibilities: for example, if the polymer is rich in COH or COC groups (as in cellulosics) this carbon signal can be used as most of the carbon atoms in keratin are in the CH, CC, or C=O forms. For obvious reasons, ESCA would not be well suited to studying the adsorption of other proteins or protein hydrolysates, unless they were suitably "tagged." Another approach utilizing ESCA is to measure the *reduction* in signal from an identifiable element, such as sulfur, present in the keratin surface but not present in the adsorbing polymer. Though less sensitive and accurate, this approach is often useful qualitatively.

Hair. Investigation of the adsorption of several cationic polymers by the ESCA technique has been reported by Goddard and Harris (20,21). Typical results are illustrated in Figures 14 and 15 for Polymer JR 400 and in Figure 14 for Quatrisoft LM 200, a hydropho-

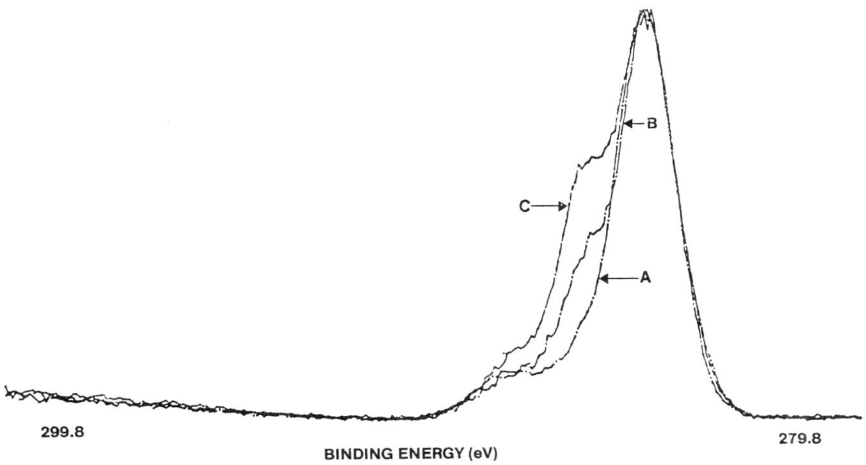

Figure 14 Carbon 1s high-resolution ESCA spectrum of control hair (A) and hair treated (30 min) with 0.1% Polymer JR 400 (B) and 0.1% Quatrisoft LM 200 (C) solutions. (From Ref. 20.)

bically substituted cationic cellulosic polymer. An interesting finding attesting to the importance of hydrophobic effects is the higher uptake of Quatrisoft (as is evident from the C—O shoulder in Fig. 14) despite its lower CS value. Quatrisoft also seemed to display more reproducible, as well as higher, deposition than Polymer JR, as shown in repeat experiments involving analytical scans along the length of separate hair fibers (20). Higher deposition at the tip (vs. the root) end of the fibers, seen with Polymer JR, was not seen with Quatrisoft treated hair. Higher deposition of the hydrophobically modified polymer was also evident on bleached hair. Equally interesting was the finding that deposition of Polymer JR 400 on bleached hair was about the same as that on virgin hair, in light of the much higher uptake by bleached hair that had been found in radiotracer studies (7).

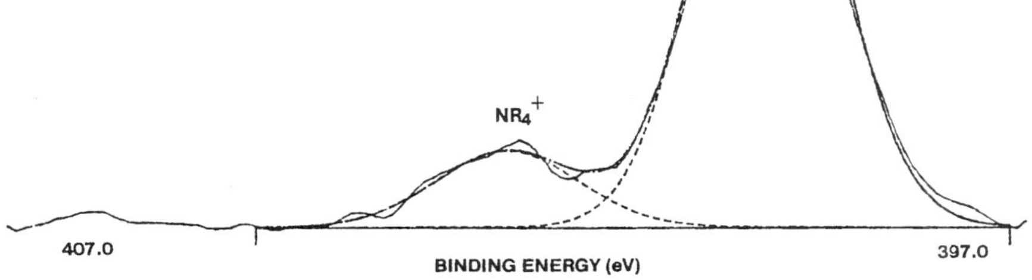

Figure 15 Nitrogen 1s high-resolution ESCA spectrum of hair treated with 0.1% Polymer JR 400 (30 min). (From Ref. 20.)

This equivalence of surface polymer content, as measured by ESCA, indicates that the elevated uptake observed radiometrically results from polymer migration into the damaged matrix of bleached hair. The high affinity of the surface reaction was demonstrated by the finding that reducing the concentration of both polymers 10-fold (from 0.1% to 0.01%) during deposition had little effect on the surface concentration observed by ESCA measurements (20).

Estimates of the surface coverage of hair can be made in several ways using the change in elemental makeup of the surface following adsorption. One approach is through the change in C/O ratio according to

$$\text{Measured (C/O)} = X(\text{C/O})_{\text{poly}} + (1 - X)\,(\text{C/O})_{\text{hair}}$$

where X is the fraction of surface covered. Estimates of surface coverage of hair treated with Polymer JR 400 and Quatrisoft thus obtained were 25% and 66%, respectively. Estimates based on N^+ content were somewhat higher (22). Two factors limiting the accuracy of such estimates are the unknown depth of the penetration profile of the polymers and the precise depth registered by ESCA measurements.

A point of interest is the removability of polycations, once adsorbed. Exposure of treated hair to 1% SDS solution for 5 min (a very gentle cleaning!) resulted (20) in substantial removal of polymer, but some ''contamination'' of the surface with sulfur atoms, suggesting coadsorption and retention of the surfactant under these conditions. This result emphasizes the fact that ESCA, like radiotracing, can be used to estimate adsorbed polymer in the presence of such ''contaminants.'' (Most of the studies reported, here, however, were ''model'' in the sense of not being done in the presence of surfactants or other additives.)

ESCA was also used (20) to demonstrate the deposition of three other conditioning polymers, namely Reten-220 (Hercules), Merquat 550, and Gafquat 755 (GAF). A point of interest was the finding that the ESCA data allow conclusions to be drawn regarding the stoichiometry of one of the adsorbed copolymers—illustrating its utility as a truly ''micro''-analytical technique.

The use of ESCA to study the adsorption on hair of amino functional silicones has been described by Wendel and DiSapio (23). These materials were shown to deposit more strongly than dimethiconols and to be quite resistant to removal by shampooing.

Stratum Corneum. Isolated membranes are readily examinable by ESCA, both per se (19) and for establishing the presence of deposited layers on them. For example, after exposure to solutions of several polycations (Polymer JR 400, Quatrisoft, and chitosan), clear peaks assignable to the C—O and N^+ groups were evident (21,22) in the spectra, similar to those shown in Figures 14 and 15. Table 5, however, reveals the extremely interesting fact that adsorption of Polymer JR and chitosan occurs only on the inner side of the membranes (which had previously been washed with water but not surfactant). By contrast, the hydrophobically substituted Quatrisoft showed, through both CO and N^+ peaks, evidence of substantial adsorption on both sides of the membranes. This difference was attributed to the presence of hydrophobic lipids on the original outer membrane surface. After membranes were washed (30-min exposure to 1% SDS solution to remove sebum suspected on the outer surface), all three polymers exhibited equivalent deposition on the inner and outer surfaces. Estimates (21) (according to the above equation) yielded values of approximately 50% coverage of the stratum corneum surfaces, but with Quatrisoft again showing the highest level.

Estimating the true *surface* coverage is hampered in the ESCA technique by the finite

Table 5 Substantivity on Unwashed Skin: High Resolution Results

	Atomic %					
	C				N	
Polymer	CH	C—O	C═O	COO	N	N^+
Polyquaternium-10						
Outer	68.5	9.6	3.6	2.6	2.7	ND
Inner	60.4	15.6	4.6	1.0	2.0	0.7
Polyquaternium-24						
Outer	53.1	17.8	3.7	1.5	0.7	0.4
Inner	53.4	23.4	3.7	0.3	1.0	0.4
Chitosan						
Outer	59.6	12.8	4.4	3.1	3.9	ND
Inner	56.4	16.4	4.7	1.8	2.0	0.8

All entries are average of two separate samples.
ND = not detected.

substrate penetration of the beam and then ejection of the characterizing electrons. One approach, though time consuming, to offset this effect is to carry out ''angle resolved'' ESCA in which irradiation is varied from high angle of incidence toward grazing incidence. For example, the measurements of Band et al. (24) shows a constant N/N^+ ratio to a depth of 56 A when angle-resolved ESCA was used to examine a skin sample treated with a mixture of Quatrisoft and hyaluronan. On the other hand, when the treatment was sequential (Quatrisoft, then hyaluronan), the measurements showed high hyaluronan content at the surface and, as before, elevated N^+ content, due to Quatrisoft, at 56 A depth. A recent illustration of the use of angle-resolved ESCA is provided in studies (25) on the adsorption of adhesive protein films.

b. Electron Probe Microanalysis (EPMA). An illustration of the use of this method is provided in the work of Yahagi (26) on the cationic polymer amodimethicone (ADMS) in which the *silicon* atoms constitute the identifying element in the EPMA procedure. The ADMS was applied to the hair as a 0.2% emulsion. Several interesting observations were made. For example, deposition and retention of ADMS was found to increase substantially (nearly fourfold) as one moves from the root to the tip of a hair. This was ascribed to mechanical weathering of the hair. Furthermore, the results indicate, in a scan along the length of a treated hair fiber, recurrent maxima in intensity of the silicon peak, at ca. 10 μ spacings, corresponding well to the separation of cuticle cell ''edges'' on the hair surface and suggesting accumulation of the treating agent in these areas. (See Fig. 16.) This seems to be a very significant finding. (See Section VI.)

c. Fourier Transform Infrared–Attenuated Total Reflection (FTIR-ATR Spectroscopy). Incorporating ATR capability (27) extends the utility of infrared (IR) spectroscopy to include surface analysis. For cosmetic science use, the substrates of interest (hair fibers, excised skin membranes, areas of live skin, etc.) would be pressed against a total internal reflectance prism, such as germanium, and a beam of IR rays passed through the prism, so experiencing multiple reflections at the prism surface. Each reflection involves a slight penetration (one to several microns) into the contacting medium, thus allowing development of an IR spectrum of the surface *region*. Until now, IR methods have not

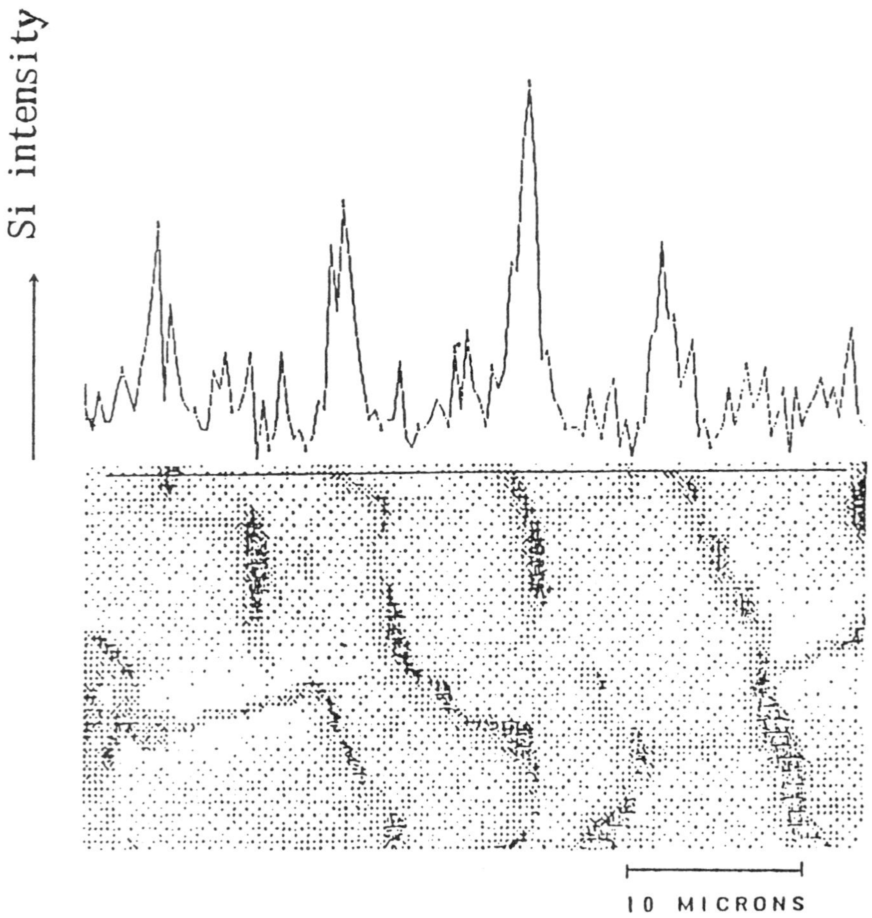

Figure 16 The distribution of Si atoms on the hair surface by EPMA (line analysis). The hair sample was treated with 0.2 wt% amodimethicone emulsion. (From Ref. 26.)

enjoyed wide use for determination of polymeric agents deposited on hair and skin, but they have been applied for assessment of moisturization of skin (28,29) and of damage to hair caused by weathering and bleaching (30). Although not connected with cationic agents, results of Klimisch and Chandra merit mention (31). They applied the FTIR method to the determination of silicones on skin, in vivo, using the Si—CH_3 band and, as reference, the amide II (protein NH) band of this substrate. Substantivity, assessed by removal during sequential soap washings, increased with the molecular weight of the silicone. Budrys indicated that the method can be applied to determine the presence and retention of conditioning polymers (Nalquat 2240 and Polymer JR) on hair (32).

2. *Measuring Changes of Intrinsic Surfaces Properties of Hair and Skin*

a. Surface Potential: Electrokinetic (Zeta) Potential.

Background. A charged surface in contact with an aqueous solution will create an electrical potential at that interface, which decays exponentially with distance into the solution and is accompanied by a similar distribution profile of counterions, near the sur-

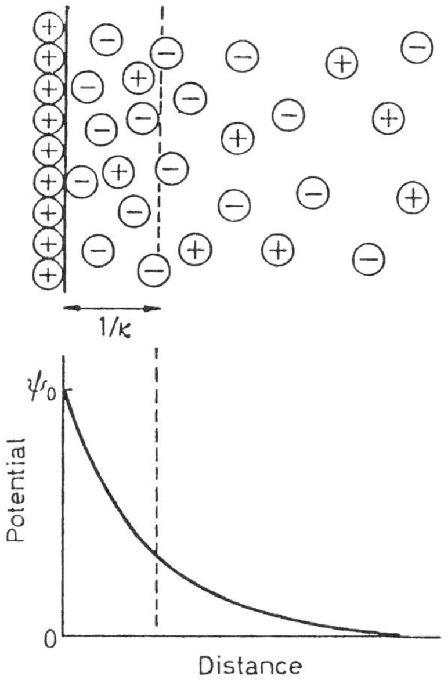

Figure 17 Schematic representation of a diffuse electrical double layer, of "thickness" $1/\kappa$, in contact with a positively charged surface. (From Ref. 33.)

face, the so-called electrical double layer. Its thickness is given by the parameter, $1/\kappa$. [See Fig. 17 (33).] Increasing ionic strength compresses the double layer (reduces $1/\kappa$) and reduces the electrical potential; hence, to maximize the latter, measurements are most often done under conditions of low ionic strength. One electrical double-layer model, due to Gouy and Chapman, which assumes point charges and a diffuse double layer, leads to the following expression for the surface potential, Ψ_0 (34):

$$\Psi_0 = \frac{2\ kT}{e} \sinh^{-1} \frac{134}{A\sqrt{c}}$$

Here e is the electronic charge, c is the ionic strength (assuming a 1-1 electrolyte in solution), and $^1/A$ is the charge density of the surface (per square angstrom).

The potential ζ, measured electrokinetically, corresponds to that in the "slip plane," which is just outside the plane of the surface where the potential is Ψ_0. To a first approximation ζ is often equated with Ψ_0. The charges of the keratin surface are evidently generated by the ionizable groups present in the side chains of the amino acids comprising this protein (35). The pH value at which the number of positive and negative charges are equal, viz., the isoelectric point (i.e.p.), is quite low: pH 3.8 for hair, and pH 5 for skin. For this reason, conditioning agents are generally positively charged to promote adsorption. Although the change in ζ potential they create is, in principle, linearly related to the amount of adsorption (36), the method has often been employed in a qualitative or semiqualitative way as a sensitive indicator of adsorption (or desorption) of the agent (37–39). The two main methods that have been employed for measuring zeta potential are electrophoresis and (to a lesser extent) streaming potential.

Electrophoresis. This technique involves measurement of the mobility of particles ("radius" a) of the substrate, suspended in various aqueous solutions, under an imposed electrical field. If the κa parameter is small (33), the equation of Hückel may be used to calculate the zeta potential, ζ.

$$\mu = \frac{\zeta D}{6\pi\eta}$$

where D is the dielectric constant of the aqueous medium, η is viscosity, and μ is the observed mobility. A severe limitation of this method in the present case is that the substrate must be in a finely ground state to yield a stable suspension. In generating this state, fresh surfaces of the hair or skin will result, which will be different from the original surface.

Some results (40), obtained using Laser Zee (Pen Kem) electrophoresis equipment, are presented in Fig. 18. Changes in the ζ potential/pH profile of skin particles in the presence of Polymer JR, cetyltrimethylammonium chloride (CTAC), and SDS give clear evidence of adsorption. The uncharged polymer, HEC, also does this; it diminishes the potential of skin on both the negative and positive sides of the isoelectric point, presumably by displacing the slip plane around the particle further into the electrical double layer. As

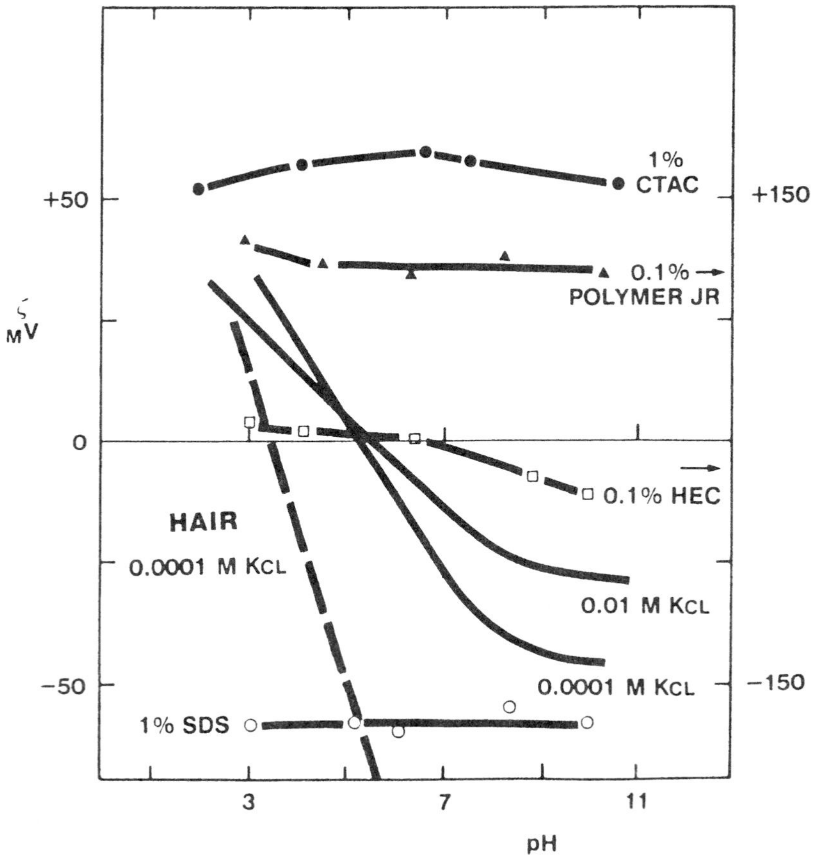

Figure 18 Zeta potential of skin, as a function of pH, in the presence of various additives. Profile for hair control is included. (From Refs. 12, 40.)

discussed earlier, this uncharged polymer must absorb by virtue of its possessing a large number of interacting polar groups.

Streaming Potential. Like electrophoresis, streaming potential is essentially a surface technique. It is, furthermore, the opposite of electrophoresis in which an electrical field is imposed across the finely divided substrate in suspension, and motion of the particles results. (See Fig. 19.) For streaming potential, relative motion is imposed by forcing liquid through a porous bed of the substrate: by Newton's law of action and reaction, an electrical potential will be generated across the bed.

Fibrous substrates, such as hair, lend themselves readily to this measurement. Results of studies (38,39) on the adsorption behavior of certain polycations are presented in Chap-

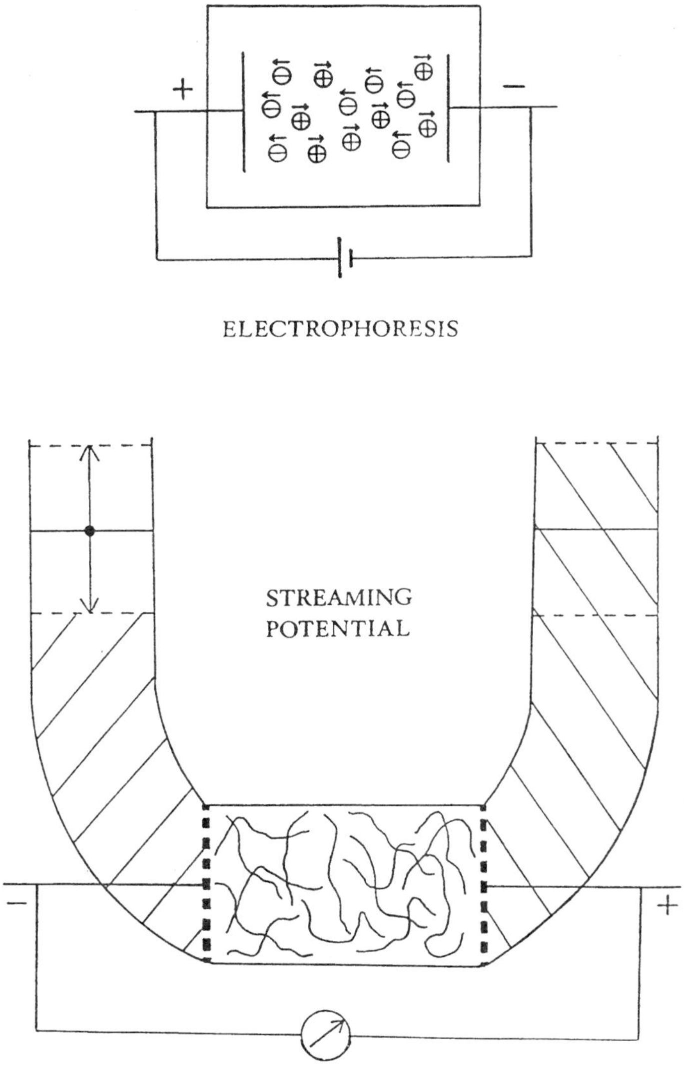

Figure 19 Schematic representation of electrophoresis (particles) and streaming potential (bed of fibers).

ter 12. These utilized a "pulsing" technique to generate the potential. Here we present some results (40,41) obtained by an "alternating direction of flow" technique (42).

The zeta potential is calculated from the measured potential, *E*.

$$\zeta = 9.690 \times 10^4 \lambda\eta E/P$$

where λ is the electrical conductance of the solution in mho/cm and *P* is the applied pressure in cm mercury. The ζ-pH profiles obtained for hair in the presence of CTAC, Polymer JR, and SDS are essentially similar to those displayed by skin (Fig. 18). An implication of the results is that both of the cationic species and, indeed, the anionic SDS appear to adsorb across the entire measured pH range.

The streaming potential method has a great advantage in that merely by replacing the contacting conditioning solution with water (or, strictly speaking, a weak electrolyte solution to control the electrical conductivity), one can study the *desorption* of the agent in situ. Typical desorption data are shown in Figure 20. Whereas the cationic polymers

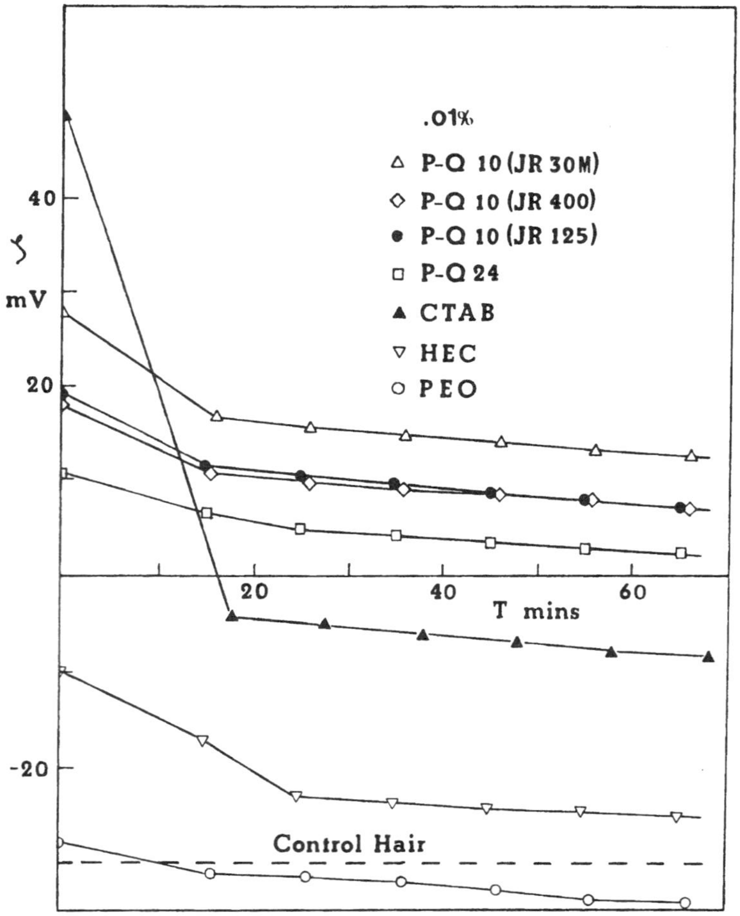

Figure 20 Decay of ζ-potential of hair during a 1-hr "rinse" (10^{-4} M KNO_3) after exposure to various treating solutions (0.01%). (From Refs. 12, 41).

Quatrisoft LM 200 and Polymer JR desorb to some extent (over a period of 1 hr), the positive potential of the keratin surface is maintained. This indicates strong retention.

In contrast it is seen that initial desorption of the cationic surfactant CTAC is rapid (if only partial), and the hair resumes a negative net charge. The uncharged polymer HEC is also seen to desorb over a 20-min period. Within the cationic cellulosic series, the strongest retention is that of the member with the highest molecular weight, Polymer JR 30M. There is little evidence of adsorption of polyethylene oxide.

b. Surface Energy: Contact Angle. Another intrinsic property of the keratin substrate is its surface energy. This is manifested in the contact angle (Θ) that a given liquid, such as water or aqueous solution, makes with the keratin surface. Of course, being an intrinsically surface technique, it will sensitively respond to any "contamination" such as sebum that may be present on the surface. For this reason the substrate, such as hair or skin, should be carefully cleaned and rinsed prior to measurement or, at least, reproducibly prepared.

The method has been used mainly for hair fibers; Chapter 12 describes two elegant procedures, viz., "immersion" and "liquid membrane," for the measurement. Among other findings it has been demonstrated that the method can clearly detect the presence of an adsorbing polycation and, indeed, its retention after rinsing. The method can also be used to study deposition from simulated shampoo systems, but in this case the effect of residual surfactant complicates interpretation of the results. Up to this point, this approach has been used largely in a qualitative sense; i.e., the measured contact angle has not been related quantitatively to the amount of deposition. Another approach, described briefly by Yahagi (26), is to measure the critical surface tension for wetting. This is determined by measurements of Θ for a series of liquids of diminishing surface tension and extrapolating to the value that would result in a zero angle, i.e., complete wetting. By this approach, as expected, a higher value of Θ for bleached hair (34°) was obtained over that for virgin hair (31°). Though not applied to a study of the adsorption of polycations, Yahagi's results show a clear reduction in wettability of hair treated with cationic surfactants and, especially, silicone—unlike the increase noted with a hydrophilic polycation found by Kamath et al. (43). This shows the importance of the nature of the adsorbing agent on the wetting property observed.

3. Scanning Electron Microscopy (SEM)

The electron microscope, which came into wide use shortly after World War II, extended the sensitivity of the microscope from the micron to the millimicron range. It has provided excellent images of the surface of hair. Although incapable of detecting a uniform monolayer deposited on this substrate (see below), it can be employed to demonstrate multilayer deposits, especially near the edges of surface cuticle cells, which may form during multiple cycling with some conditioning shampoos (44). While the precision and sensitivity of conventional SEM instrumentation continue to improve, an inherent limitation is the need for exposure of the sample to high vacuum and, furthermore, to a coating procedure to ensure its surface conductivity. These limitations are mitigated in the "environmental" SEM.

4. Atomic Force Microscopy (AFM)

The last two decades have witnessed the emergence of a new and powerful group of analytical methods for characterizing solid surfaces at the molecular level. The methods are referred to collectively as "scanning probe microscopy." By far the most widely used is "atomic force microscopy" (AFM), which, unlike the originally developed "scanning tunneling microscopy'' (STM), does not require that the sample be electrically conducting: not only can AFM be used under ambient atmospheric conditions, measurements can also be made on specimens immersed in water. In the AFM method a sharp tip (generally Si_3N_4) attached to a cantilever is used to measure the topography of the sample, which is scanned in the x, y plane (Fig. 21). The vertical displacement of the tip, detected by a reflected laser beam and photodiode, is used to adjust the sample position in the z direction to maintain constant force. The feedback voltage provides the topographical (z) data. In gross terms the method may be likened to the functioning of a phonograph stylus.

Although there were early reports of AFM's use for studying the adsorption of proteins (45), its first reported use for studying conditioning polycations seems to have been that by the author and R. L. Schmitt (46). A somewhat paradoxical problem was posed immediately: while the AFM technique clearly had the sensitivity to detect the presence of adsorbed polymer, the background topography (i.e., the surface of hair) was found to be grossly coarse at the discriminating magnifications required. For this reason, these authors used a model surface, namely mica, which, like keratin, is negatively charged at neutral pH, but unlike keratin is molecularly smooth. Indeed, at the magnifications employed for studying adsorption, the surface of mica was a featureless background (despite the fact that at higher magnification its molecular makeup could clearly be seen). Exposure of the mica to a solution of Polymer JR led to the appearance of a regular but ''loopy'' deposit in which the apparent height of the loops was 30–60 A. This phenomenon was shown to be partly an artifact that had to do with a mechanical ''sweeping'' effect caused by the stylus and previously seen with monolayers of proteins (47).

In the second set of experiments (48) a ''tapping'' mode AFM instrument was used (Digital Instruments Nanoscope III, Santa Barbara, CA). Here the contact force is reduced by 10–100-fold to ~0.1 μN and the probe lightly taps, rather than scrapes, the specimen, with a frequency of 330 kHz. The absence of specimen damage can easily be demonstrated by the reproducibility of the image in repeat scans (48). A typical scan, for an adsorbed layer of Polymer JR 400, is shown in Figure 22 where, again, a loopy but regular deposit is seen, reminiscent of the classical ''train and loop'' model of polymer adsorption. On the other

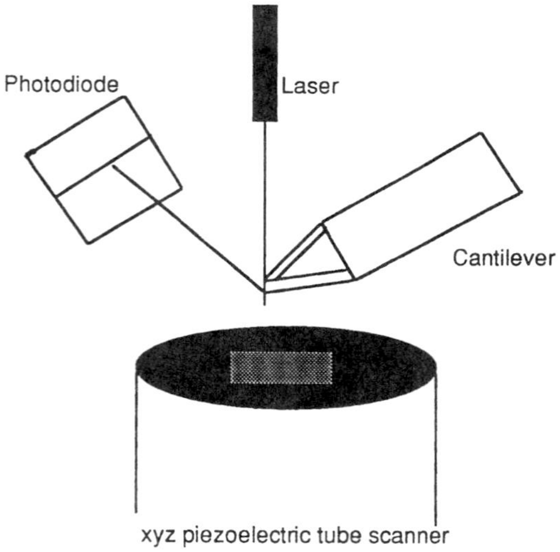

Figure 21 Schematic representation of atomic force microscope (AFM).

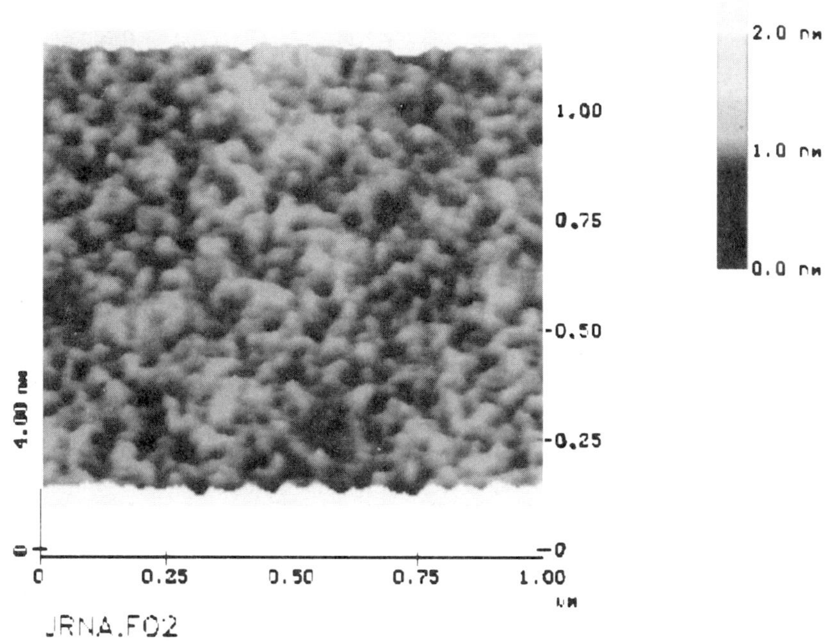

Figure 22 Tapping mode AFM image of mica exposed to 0.5% Polymer JR 400 solution for 15 min, then rinsed. Dimensions in nanometers. (From Ref. 48.)

hand, the deposit of this polymer from a mixed solution with SDS led to a much more textured image (48). An attempt to utilize a highly polished keratin as a replacement, and more realistic, substrate surface was judged unsuccessful because of residual roughness (46,48).

Because of the evident ease of the AFM method, more of its use in the personal care field can be anticipated. Thus, data on human hair have recently been presented by Hössel et al. (49). Despite the intrinsic roughness of the hair surface, these authors have published a series of micrographs that show definite topographical changes following exposure of the hair to conditioning polymers under a variety of conditions.

Current instrumentation allows AFM equipment to be used in a number of different ways, the choice made being dependent on the surface to be investigated, e.g., the elasticity mode, the adhesion (phase) mode, or the lateral (two-dimensional friction) mode. A recent example of the investigation of adsorbed protein films using the tapping mode can be found in Ref. 25.

5. *Surface Forces Balance (SFB)*

The SFB is a specialized apparatus, developed by Tabor and Winterton (50) and refined by Israelachvili and Adams (51), to study basic colloidal forces—specifically in this case to measure the interaction of orthogonally positioned hemicylinders (generally mica) as they are brought together (or separated) in aqueous solutions. Separations (D) can be measured with a precision of better than 5 A and forces (F) to a precision of 10^{-2} μN. Data are presented in plots of F/R versus D where R is the radius of curvature of the cylinders. Force/distance curves have been measured in the presence of electrolytes, adsorbing surfactants, and, as mentioned in Chapter 2, polymers. Here we will briefly discuss some of the results obtained in four studies (52–55) concerned with the adsorption of conditioning polymer-type polyelectrolytes.

Figure 23 (53) shows the force parameter/distance profiles observed in the presence of Polymer JR 400. While not recorded here, repulsive interaction between the adsorbed polymer layers was detected at a separation of ~1000 Å, and below 900 Å, it started to increase markedly. An interesting feature is the hysteresis evident after the first compression; thereafter, expansion and compression profiles coincided. These results again suggest a nonflat ("loopy") initial configuration and loops being compressed as the adsorbed polymer is forced into more intimate contact with the mica surface during the first compression. A schematic diagram of this sequence of events is presented in Figure 24 (52). Results (54,55) obtained with Quatrisoft LM 200 (the hydrophobically substituted cationic cellulosic of lower CS value) were interesting in the sense of revealing no difference between the first and second compression profiles and the *F*/*R* versus *D* characteristic very similar to that of Polymer JR compressions *after* the initial one. This suggests the formation of an initially more compact ("flatter") adsorbed layer in the case of Quatrisoft.

Interesting [and substantial (52)] effects were observed when the experiments were repeated with anionic surfactant, SDS, added to the polymer solution. Expansion of the force/distance profile suggested coadsorption of the polycation and the surfactant (55) in some cases; shrinkage of the profile, a displacement of the polycation (52) in others.

Finally, preadsorption of a cationic polymer (Quatrisoft) was shown to facilitate the adsorption of a negatively charged polymer (hyaluronic acid) onto the negatively charged

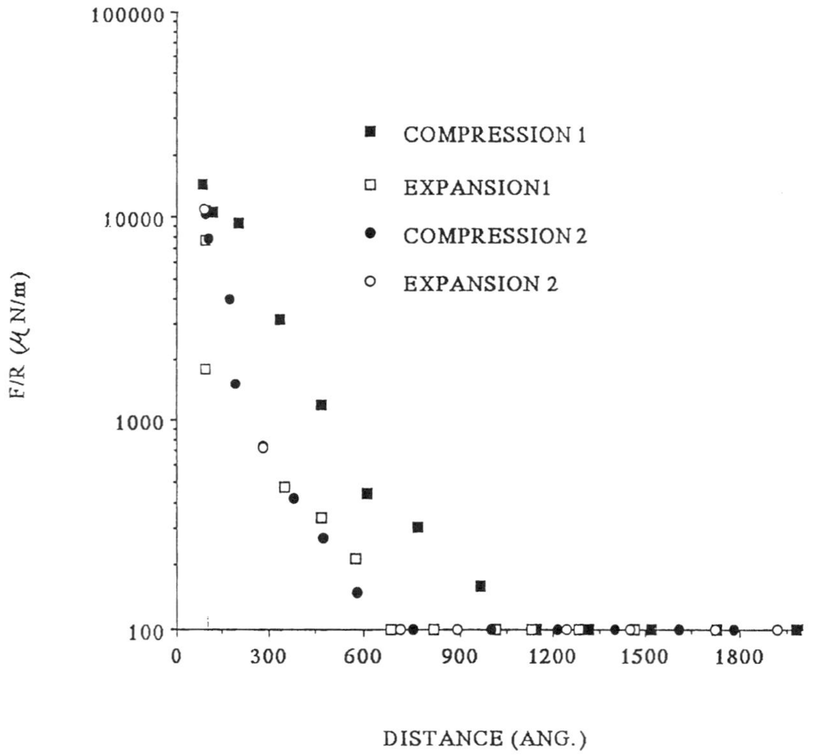

Figure 23 Force distance profiles for mica hemicylinders immersed in 0.1% Polymer JR 400 solution. (From Ref. 53.)

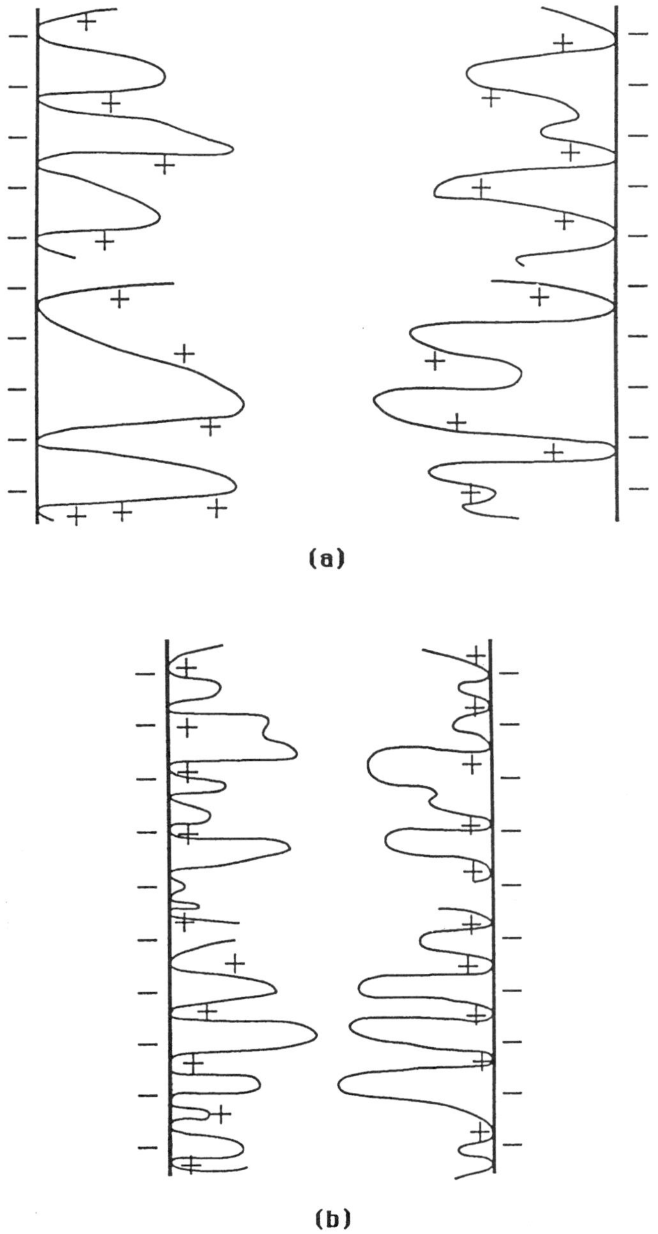

(a)

(b)

Figure 24 Schematic diagram of the configuration of the adsorbed layer of cationic polymer (a) before compression and (b) after first and subsequent compressions. (From Ref. 52.)

mica—a case of surface ''priming'' (53). All data obtained by the SFB technique refer to the condition of the adsorbed polymer still in contact with an aqueous solution.

6. Disclosing Methods

In these methods an agent is used to disclose the presence of the polycationic conditioning agent sorbed onto/into the keratin substrate. Three such agents are (1) dyes, (2) fluorescing agents, and (3) colloidal particles.

a. Use of Dyes. The dye generally carries a charge opposite in sign to the deposited conditioning agent, which draws the dye to the substrate and colors it; that is, for a cationic additive, a negatively charged dye would be employed. Within certain limits, the intensity of the coloration increases with increasing amounts of deposited agent. There are certain limitations: The color intensity may not be a simple function of the amount of conditioning agent. One of the contributing factors is the unknown number of sites on the deposited polymer that remain free to absorb the dye, and another is the extent of penetration of both agent and dye into the substrate. Also, the method works best on blonde (natural or bleached) hair. A limitation potentially more serious is mentioned below.

Despite its limitations the dye method has the advantage of being very simple and sensitive. In early work Scott et al. utilized the dye rubine to disclose the presence of the cationic surfactant cetyltrimethylammonium bromide (CTAB) on hair (56). Actually, the hair was sectioned and the dye was able to show the (considerable) penetration of the surfactant into the hair, especially under alkaline conditions. In a later paper, Crawford and Robbins demonstrated the potential of Red 80 as a replacement dye for rubine (57) in disclosing both cationic surfactants and polymers. Unilever scientists, among others, have reported the use of the dye, Fast Bordeaux Red, to disclose the presence of Polymer JR on hair (58).

Despite its convenience, today the dye method is seldom used for quantitative assessment of deposited polycation. It is suspected that one of the main reasons is that the presence of coadsorbed anionic surfactant (as would be the case in ordinary shampooing practice) could seriously affect the development of color.[This is a *possible* inference from the data registered for one such system (57).] However, it retains its usefulness as an indicator of polycation substantivity from simple aqueous solution (especially if coupled with hair fiber sectioning).

b. Use of Fluorescent Dyes. Fluorescence methods have the advantage of high sensitivity (and resolution when coupled with appropriate scanning and detection capabilities). The choice of actual fluorescing agent is governed to some extent by hair's being intrinsically fluorescent itself. Much work has been done on this substrate by the Textile Research Institute, Princeton, where the great utility of the method has been demonstrated. (See Chapter 12.) Generally, a negatively charged fluorescent dye, such as fluorescein, is added directly to model shampoos containing the polycation to be disclosed, and after a certain number of washing cycles, the hairs are scanned for fluorescence (59). Further details are provided in Chapter 12. (Note: It seems that the presence of anionic surfactant could again influence the results: this would also be the case if the fluorescing dye was postadded to treated fibers.)

c. Colloidal Particle Deposition. This method involves postexposure of hair, previously exposed to a conditioning polycation, to a fine particle colloid suspension. The principle is that if the adsorbed polymer is positively charged the hair surface will repel positively charged particles but attract negatively charged particles. Figure 25 is a schematic representation of the foregoing. Scanning electron microscopy is employed to record

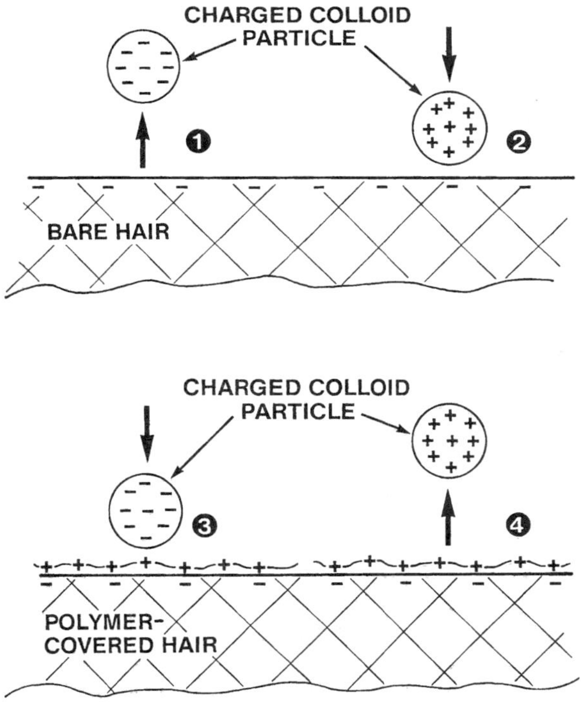

Figure 25 Schematic diagram of colloid deposition: a negatively charged surface (e.g., hair) will repel negatively charged particles (1) but attract positively charged particles (2). If the surface is positively charged due to adsorption of a polycation, the reverse sequence will obtain (3,4).

the particle deposition pattern (60,61). The method had previously been used for study of the surface of cellulose fibers (62), wool (63), and glass (64).

For their studies of the adsorption of polycations on hair Goddard and Schadt (60) used a negatively charged silica suspension, of particle size ~0.1 μ, prepared by the Stober method (65). Exposure of control hair to this suspension led to no deposition of particles (Fig 26). By contrast, following treatment with any of a number of different cationic polymers, and postrinsing, such exposure led to the deposition of a layer of silica particles, usually in the form of a close-packed monolayer (Fig 27). These results showed clearly the conversion of the surface of hair from its natural state of negative charge to one with a net positive charge.

The possibility of any critical influence of the exposure time upon the adsorption/deposition was examined (60) by varying conditions as shown in Table 6.

In all cases (a–d) a substantial layer of silica particles was seen to cover the hair fibers, showing that adsorption of both the polymer and the particles is fairly rapid. In the same way, the effect of reducing the concentration of the treating polymer solution from 0.1% to 0.01% was minimal, confirming the high substantivity of the two polymers (Polymer JR 400 and Quatrisoft LM 200) thus examined.

For all conditioning polymers investigated the level of silica deposition seemed roughly to parallel the cationic substitution level of the polymer, according to the following (60):

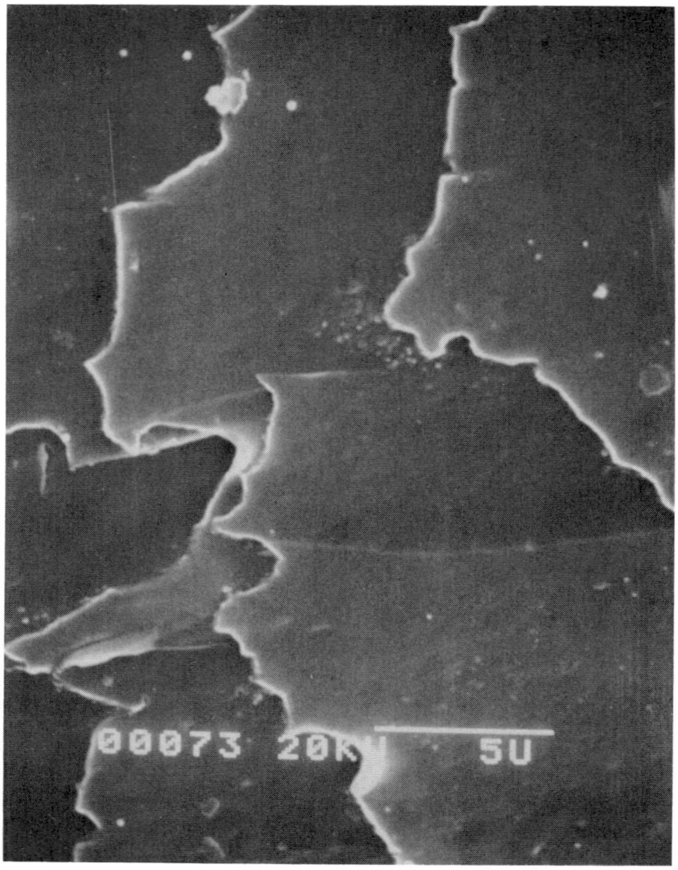

Figure 26 Scanning electron micrograph of clean hair that has been exposed to a negatively charged silica colloid: there is no evidence of any deposition of silica particles. (From Refs. 60, 61.)

Very heavy deposit (exceeding monolayer coverage),
  Merquat 100, Merquat 550
Heavy deposit (uniform, close-packed state),
  Polymer JR 400, Polymer LR 400, Gafquat 755
Medium-heavy deposit,
  Quatrisoft LM 200

In studies of a series of cationically derivatized protein hydrolysates, the level of observed silica deposition also seemed to parallel the level of cationic substitution (60).

Postexposure of polymer (Polymer JR, Quatrisoft, Reten 220)-treated fibers to SDS (1% solution, 30 min), prior to treatment with silica, led to virtual elimination of silica deposition (60). While this suggests complete removal of these polymers, caution in interpretation is needed as any adsorbed SDS could itself influence the ''charge driven'' deposition process. (See ESCA results.)

The influence of the nonionic surfactant, Tergitol (15-S-9, both as a cotreatment with the polymer and as a posttreatment, as above with SDS) was somewhat variable, affecting

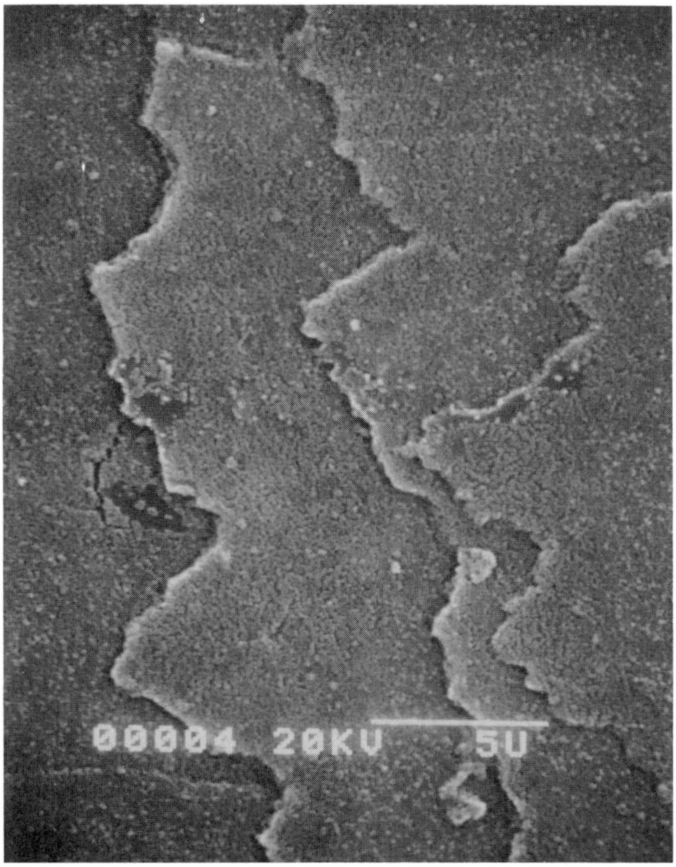

Figure 27 Scanning electron micrograph of hair exposed to 0.1% Polymer JR 400 solution, a rinse, and then to the silica colloid: a close-packed ''monolayer'' of silica particles can clearly be seen. (From Refs. 60, 61.)

Table 6 Exposure Details

Condition	Polymer solution[a] (exposure time, min)	Silica colloid (exposure time, min)
a (standard)	30	30
b	5	30
c	5	5
d	1	30

[a]0.1% Polymer JR 400.

deposition of some of the polymers, but not all. However, both procedures led to reduced adsorption of Quatrisoft LM 200 (by subsequent silica deposition criteria) showing the importance of hydrophobic effects in the case of this polymer (55,60).

7. *Solution Depletion Methods*

In this category the reliability of the results depends not only on the accuracy of the analytical method, but also on the extent of depletion, which is favored by higher-surface-area substrates (i.e., hair is more favorable than skin), and the relative mass of the substrate to the solution. At first sight, however, even hair would seem only marginally favorable in view of its low apparent surface area, but radiotracer studies referred to earlier proved otherwise. The substantial sorption observed was ascribed to a diffusion process into the water-swollen hair: this effect would be expected to be augmented by bleaching of the hair or raising of the temperature during the sorption process. It should be noted that, in general, in such experiments one studies the sorption for the polycation but not its retention, unless a prescribed rinse procedure, with collection of rinses, is included.

Several analytical procedures are available for assaying polyelectrolyte solutions, a selection of which is listed below.

a. Colloid Titration. This method is actually quite old (66,67) and it has been used (35,68) for studying the adsorption of polycations on fibers. In the case of a polycation, the solution is titrated against a standardized solution of a polyanion in the presence of a cationic dye, according to the following scheme:

$$\underset{\text{color 1}}{P^{n+} + \text{dye}^{+}} \xrightarrow{P^{m-}} (P^{n+})(P^{m-})_{n/m} + \underset{\text{color 2}}{(P^{m-})(\text{dye}^{+})_{m}}$$

Convenient choices for polyanion and dye are, respectively, polyvinylsulfate and toluidine blue, which undergoes a color change at the endpoint.

The method is convenient and easy to execute but has several disadvantages.

The stoichiometry of the polyelectrolyte complex may not correspond to charge neutralization as in the above equation; i.e., it is not independent of polycation structure.

The endpoint suffers from time effects.

The method is sensitive to ionic contaminants, especially surfactants.

Leached protein can affect the results.

In work reported by Hutter et al. (69) the method was applied to a study of the interaction of Polymer JR 400 with bleached hair at 40°C. By careful control of procedures and conditions they obtained consistent and reproducible results. (See Fig. 28.) From the estimated 60-min uptake value in this figure for lightly bleached hair one finds reasonably good agreement with a value (3.5 mg/g) interpolated from radiotracer data (7) for bleached hair but five times the radiotracer value for virgin hair (8). On the other hand, further bleaching of hair led to a tripling of Polymer JR uptake (Fig. 28), clearly showing the effect of such oxidation on the hair matrix (and, presumably, its swelling in water).

In a second publication Hutter et al. (70) examined the individual effects of adding various nonionic cellulosic polymers on the uptake of Polymer JR 400 by bleached hair. The effects observed were generally not major. Competitive effects may well have been stronger on virgin hair, which is more hydrophobic, and where hydrophobic effects with

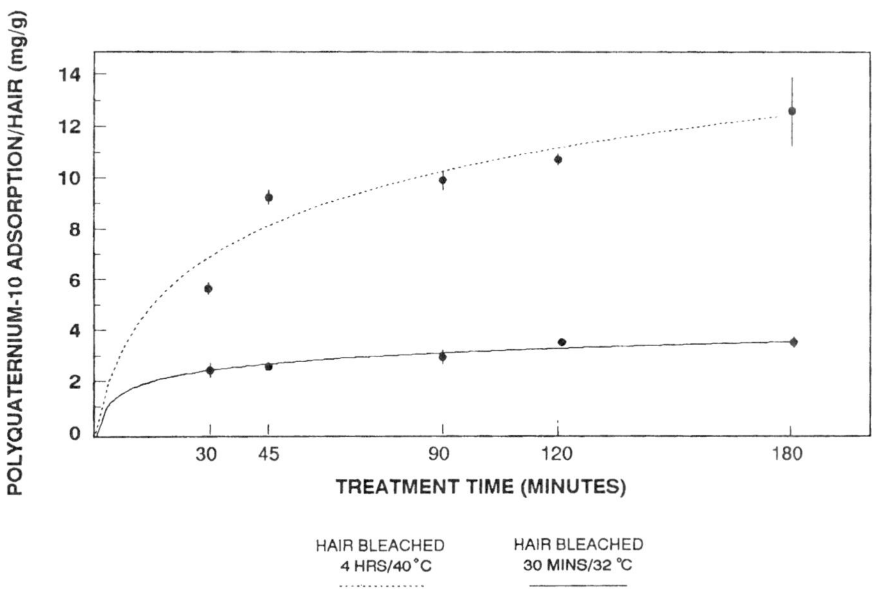

Figure 28 Uptake of Polymer JR 400 from 0.1% solution at 40°C onto bleached hair. (From Ref. 69.)

polymers such as HPC and HMHEC would be expected to compete more effectively with the electrostatic forces governing the adsorption of Polymer JR.

b. Potentiometric Titration.

Background. Another form of "colloid titration" for estimating cationic (quaternary ammonium) compounds is based on a potentiometric procedure and utilizes an electrode that is specific to the titrating anionic surfactant chosen. The theory is that the cationic material complexes stoichiometrically with the anionic surfactant.

Specific surfactant ion electrodes of this type have been known (71) for some time and, together with the knowledge that anionic surfactants generally form 1:1 (charge/charge) association complexes with cationic compounds, such as cationic surfactants and polycations, they allow determination of the latter from the potentiometric titration. (Performance of this type of electrode is generally checked by establishing conformance to the Nernst equation whereby a 10-fold change in concentration of the standard solution, e.g., SDS, should lead to an e.m.f. change of 59 mV. Endpoints in titration curves are, however, generally estimated empirically. See below.)

Much more work of this type, involving polyion/oppositely charged surfactant mixtures, has been carried out on polyanion/cationic surfactant systems (72,73), mainly because it was found easier to "home-make" cationic surfactant electrodes! Now that anionic-surfactant-specific electrodes are available commercially (e.g., Orion Research Model 93-42), this situation is likely to change, especially in the cosmetics field with its high interest in polycationic conditioning agents. In the case of ideal behavior, the electrode allows determination of the equivalent weight of the polycation.

Practical Results. Van Nguyen et al. (74) reported the use of the Orion anionic surfactant electrode to study the uptake of a variety of cationic agents by hair. Sorption was favored, as in the colloid titration studies just mentioned, by the use of bleached hair and

Table 7 Uptake of Celquat L-200; Bleached Hair, 35°C (74)

30-min exposure		0.1% polymer solution	
Sol'n conc'n	Uptake	Expos time	Uptake
0.05%	4.1%	5 min	2.7%
0.1%	5.9%	15 min	3.3%
0.2%	9.8%	30 min	5.7%

a slightly elevated temperature (35°C). Van Nguyen et al. obtained excellent linearity in their calibration plots of the concentration of cationic material versus the amount of SDS required for equivalence. While a number of cationic agents were examined, the results obtained for Celquat L-200 (a copolymer of starch and dimethyldiallylammonium chloride, National Starch) are most relevant for our present purpose (see Table 7).

It is evident, as has been pointed out several times in this chapter, that the uptake of polycation in such model studies can be appreciable—in this case up to 10% by weight, which is colossal by monolayer adsorption standards. Among a variety of other cationic agents examined were two hydrolyzed protein (HP) derivatives, viz. laurdimonium wheat HP and cocodimonium keratin HP (Croda). Uptake was again found to be substantial and to increase markedly with hair damage, namely perming and, especially, bleaching.

Limitations. A serious limitation of both of the preceding "titration" techniques is that the adventitious presence of other ionic agents, e.g., polyions or especially surfactants (as would be the case in complete formulations), could seriously affect the utility and precision of these methods.

c. Radiotracers: Residual Solution Activity. If a radiotagged version of the conditioning agent is available, it affords what is probably the most reliable of all solution analysis methods in view of its sensitivity and relative freedom from interference from other solution components.

d. Ultraviolet (UV) Spectroscopy. UV (or other) spectroscopy can be applied if the conditioning agent has a suitable UV-absorbing or other chromophoric group. One drawback is that natural keratins can release UV-absorbing material into solution during the adsorption step. In dealing with spectroscopic methods, one should be aware of the unusually high sensitivity of the fluorescence method, i.e., if it is feasible to introduce a fluorescing group into the adsorbing molecule.

e. Chromatography. The applicability of chromatographic methods for solution analysis depends on the particular conditioning agent being investigated; they have to be carefully standardized. Problems can be encountered, for example, with high-molecular-weight polymers, especially polycations, in gel or other chromatography because irreversible adsorption can occur during the determination. Also gel permeation chromatography (GPC) has traditionally been used to determine the molecular weight of polymers rather than for their quantitative assessment.

Despite these apparent limitations, considerable success in the use of GPC as a quantitative means of studying the adsorption of a number of polycations (and polyampholytes) on hair has recently been reported (75):

> Two injections of each treatment solution were made. Based on the polymer mass injected and the refractive index polymer peak area, the specific refractive index increment (dn/dc) of each sample was computed. The two dn/dc values were averaged. Two injections

of each post-treatment solution were made. The mass of the polymer injected was then determined based upon the refractive index polymer peak area and the dn/dc measured from the treatment solution. The same procedure was used to compute the mass of polymer in each rinse. The amount of polymer found in the rinses was negligible.

The method (GPC/RI) was checked by repeating an experiment done previously using the radiotracer technique (17), namely by measuring the uptake of Merquat 550 by heavily bleached hair. Under the conditions chosen (0.1% solution, 30-min exposure) excellent agreement was obtained between the results from the two methods (17,75).

Listed in Table 8 are data extracted from the paper of Blanco et al. (75) for a series of polycations. Regarding the data shown in Table 8:

1. There seems to be an optimal CS value for sorption (compare values for Merquat 100 and 550; Gafquat HS 100 and 755 N)
2. The value for Polymer JR 400 is in good agreement with a value that can be interpolated from radiotracer data (7).
3. The measured uptake of Celquat L-200 is less by an order of magnitude than that reported by Van Nguyen et al. (74) perhaps reflecting a higher level of hair bleaching in the latter case (as well as a higher temperature of exposure).

On the basis of the above results, much more inquiry into the use of the GPC method can be expected.

8. Ion Exchange

If the adsorbate is ionic, adsorption usually involves an ion exchange process and, in principle, the ions released into solution can be assayed to assess the adsorption. The process can be represented as

$$(Pr^{n-})X_n^+ + nY^+ \rightarrow (Pr^{n-})\,Y_n^+ + nX^+$$

where Pr^{n-} refers to the keratin substrate with attached X^+ counterions and Y^+ is the adsorbate (surfactant, polymer, etc.) written as a monomer for convenience.

The concentration of species X^+ released can be determined by a titration, electrometric, or other method. Ion exchange processes in aqueous systems are generally accompanied by a pH change, as hydrogen and hydroxyl ions redistribute during the interaction, and in principle, this change can be used to follow the adsorption (76). A general comment on ion exchange processes is that they are sensitive to the presence of ionic contaminants, which can obscure the endpoint. Another way to follow the course of the ion exchange

Table 8 Polymer Uptake: GPC/RI Method: Blond Bleached Hair: 0.1% Solution, 22°C

Polycation	30-min uptake (mg/g)
Celquat L-200	3.1
Merquat 100	1.0
Merquat 550	3.0
Polymer JR 400	2.2
Gafquat HS 100	0.1
Gafquat 755 N	1.0

process is to measure the change of electrical conductivity of the solution (77), but exact interpretation of the data can be difficult and the method suffers from the drawback just mentioned.

9. Direct Extraction Procedures

In principle, the extent of sorption of a material can be obtained by subjecting the exposed substrate (e.g., hair) to an extraction procedure involving a highly efficient solvent for the sorbate. In the present context, whereas this approach may not be realistic for the usual sorbates (based on C, H, O, and N) it may be feasible in certain cases. As an example, the work of Yahagi is referred to again. It involved the deposition of silicone on hair (26). In this case, the exposed hair was extracted with chloroform, the extract dissolved in methylisobutyl ketone, and analyzed by ICP emission spectroscopy. The method could, of course, be extended to aminosilicones.

V. PROTEIN HYDROYSATES

Reference has been made in several places in this chapter to studies on the sorption of a variety of derivatized protein hydrolysates. Although this is not a main theme of this chapter, which emphasizes high-molecular-weight polycation conditioning agents, it seems appropriate to include a brief summary of some of this work, especially as it represents some of the earliest investigations of macromolecule sorption by hair and skin.

Work from the Wilson/Inolex companies on collagen hydrolysates (78–80) utilized a staining procedure based on the ninhydrin test for hydroxyproline to demonstrate the adsorption (and penetration) of these materials on keratin substrates. This approach was reported in some detail by Stern and Johnsen (81), who demonstrated the highest substantivity for hydrolysates of molecular weight around 1000.

Maybrook scientists have reported the use of a radiotagging procedure (tritium labeling) to demonstrate the substantivity of collagen hydrolysates to hair (82).

The colloid heteroflocculation technique (see above) involving a disclosing silica suspension was used to monitor the adsorption of various derivatized proteins on hair (60,61).

Finally, an e.m.f. method using a surfactant electrode titration procedure was used to determine the sorption by hair of various protein hydrolyzates (74). (See above. For further information on proteins see Chapter 9.)

VI. FINAL COMMENTS

A variety of experimental techniques have been used to study the sorption of cationic polyelectrolytes by hair and skin. The results show that substantial sorption can occur, often vastly exceeding the requirement for simple monolayer coverage of the external geometric surface of these substrates. Early work (56) on the uptake of cationic surfactants, employing a staining procedure, had demonstrated definite penetration of hair fibers. Penetration is obviously facilitated by the swelling of the latter that occurs in water. The conclusion to be drawn is that similar penetration can also occur with polycations. The diffusion path has not yet been established. Certainly, the results presented seem to rule out a simple radial route. As with the case of wool recently discussed (83), an intercellular diffusion path seems most feasible. The most likely point of entry is the area of the edges of the surface cuticular cells. This route is strongly suggested in fluorescence patterns of hair exposed to (the cationic) Rhodamine G dye (84).

One can thus conclude that conditioning polycations can both adsorb onto and also penetrate a keratin substrate. At the molecular level the flat configuration of an adsorbed polycation depicted in Figure 1 is oversimplified: it is likely, as pointed out in Chapters 2 and 3, that there will be some level of "loopiness" of the adsorbed polymer molecule, (See also the sections in this chapter on the surface forces balance and atomic force microscopy). Flatter configurations will, however, be favored (85) when a polyion is adsorbed on an oppositely charged substrate, which is the situation usually encountered in practice. They would also be favored in polymers with a "stiffer" backbone, such as the cellulosics. In any event, the dimensions of the loops of adsorbed conditioning polymers will generally be small when measured on the scale of the natural rugosity of hair and skin surfaces at the molecular level.

Methods of evaluating such "conditioned" keratin (in particular, hair) are discussed in Chapter 12. While mechanisms are not fully understood, a very broad expectation might be that friction and static electrification would be influenced by surface adsorption, strength and bending modulus by bulk sorption, and abrasion resistance by both of the foregoing.

Most of the results reported herein on the sorption of polycations by natural keratins have been obtained on simplified model systems. The rationale behind such an approach was to seek to determine the fate of sorbing polymer under well-defined conditions and so to obtain mechanistic insight. The results have clearly indicated that both adsorption and absorption processes can occur. They have also shown that the nature, extent, and consequences of polycation sorption can all be influenced by the presence of surfactant. In general, nonionic surfactants have a small effect on sorption, because of low interaction while cationic surfactants can have a very large effect because of competition for the sorption sites. Because of interaction and complex formation with cationic polyelectrolytes anionic surfactants can exercise an intermediate, but potentially very important, influence.

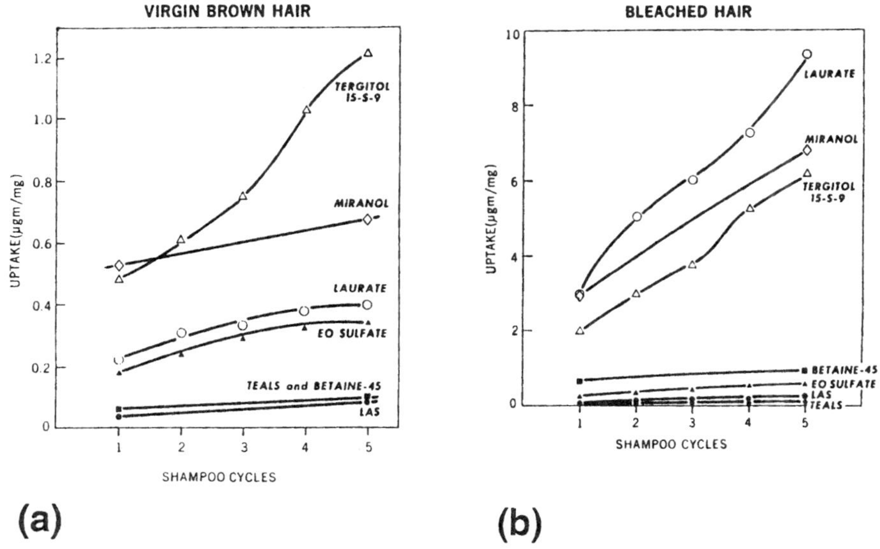

Figure 29 Deposition of Polymer JR 400 on (a) brown hair and (b) brown hair from model shampoos containing different surfactants. (From Ref. 6.)

A

Figure 30 Confocal micrographs of hair fibers (A) Control (B) Treated 30 minutes with 0.1% Polymer JR 400. (Paper presented at the 216th meeting, Am. Chem. Soc., Cellulose Division, Boston, August 1998.)

The latter category of surfactant is the most important and most interesting in the sense of its being the type most commonly employed in conditioning shampoos and body washes.

As stated earlier, some of the first experiments (6) using radiotagged polymer and employing *simulated shampooing* conditions had demonstrated substantial, but differing effects depending on the anionic surfactant chosen. (See Fig. 29.) Clearly, deposition under these conditions of simulated shampooing is a complicated phenomenon, involving not only the formation of (generally) soluble polycation complexes in the shampoo itself, but in all likelihood precipitation of complexes of different composition during some stage of the rinse. (See Chapter 5.) As an extreme example, the massive deposition observed by electron microscopy (and radioassay) on bleached hair shampooed in a potassium laurate/Polymer JR 400 system probably involved the codeposition of polymer, polymer-surfactant complex, and insoluble calcium laurate. While most synthetic anionic surfactants would not be expected to give such extreme effects, some degree of analogous behavior is a definite possibility. Today's practice of including an insoluble coconditioning compo-

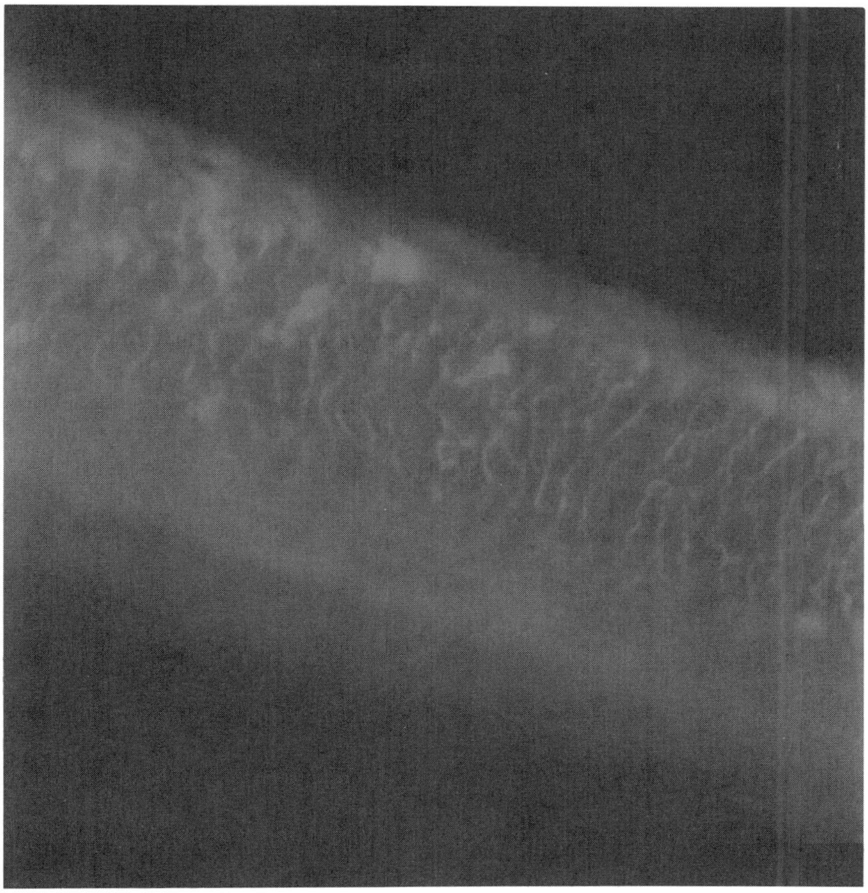

B

nent, such as silicone oil, in shampoos obviously makes determination of the exact process(es) of deposition a difficult, if challenging, exercise.

VII. WHAT OF THE FUTURE?

Because of the widespread and increasing use of polymeric conditioning agents it is desirable and necessary to have detection methods and analytical procedures for their determination on treated surfaces. The ideal method should be safe, sensitive, quantitative, and reliable, convenient to use, not impose any interference on the deposition process, and be free from interference from other formulation components. Radioassay satisfies all of these requirements—except, in today's climate, the first! Of other ''tagging'' procedures, fluorescence labeling would appear to have most promise, again because of high sensitivity of the measuring technique and the ability to satisfy most of the above criteria. Progress in this direction has been made recently (86). See Figure 30.

A wave of the future can be seen in the development and growing application of surface spectroscopic procedures. Reference has already been made to the use, for keratin surface analysis, of ESCA (essentially a surface technique) and ATR infrared analysis and EPMA (which sample a depth of ~1 μ). There has, however, been an explosive growth of surface analytical procedures. For example, a very recently compiled handbook (87), some 1000 pages in length, lists close to 100 spectroscopic procedures that are now in use for analyzing surfaces. Because of their proliferation these techniques are generally referred to in shorthand acronyms, such as ESCA, AES, EDS, EELS, and so on. While most applications to date have involved inorganic substrates, many would appear to be suitable for biological substrates such as hair. For example, a recent publication describes a study (88) using time of flight–secondary ion mass spectrometry (TOF-SIMS) on silicone deposition on hair. This, essentially surface technique gave clear evidence of the deposition of silicone and (by suitable manipulation) also of *penetration* of hair by silicone as supplied from an emulsion or, especially, a microemulsion.

It is to be expected that the use of instrumental surface analytical techniques on biosubstrates, including hair and skin, will grow substantially.

REFERENCES

1. Davies JT, Rideal EK. Interfacial Phenomena. New York: Academic Press, 1961:155.
2. Robbins CR. Chemical and Physical Behavior of Human Hair, 3rd ed. New York: Springer-Verlag, 1994.
3. Stam PB, White HJ Jr. Textile Res J 1954;24:785.
4. Chow CD. Textile Res J 1971; 41:444.
5. Woodard J. J Soc Cosmet Chem 1972; 23:593.
6. Goddard ED, Faucher JA, Scott RJ, Turney ME. J Soc Cosmet Chem 1975; 26:539.
7. Faucher JA, Goddard ED. J Colloid Interface Sci 1976; 55:313.
8. Goddard ED, Hannan RB, Faucher JA. Proc. VIII Int Congress Surface Active Agents, Moscow, Vol 2, 1977, 834.
9. Faucher JA, Goddard ED, Hannan RB. Textile Res J 1977; 47:616.
10. Hannan RB, Goddard ED, Faucher JA. Textile Res J 1978; 48:57.
11. Hunter RJ. Foundations of Colloid Science, Vol I. Oxford: Clarendon Press, 1991.
12. Goddard ED. Cosmet Toilet 1987; 102:71.
13. Hill AV. Proc Roy Soc Lond 1928; 104B:39.
14. Faucher JA, Goddard ED. J Colloid Interface Sci 1978; 65:444.
15. Faucher JA, Goddard ED. J Soc Cosmet Chem 1976; 27:543.
16. Goddard ED, Leung PS. Cosmet Toilet 1982; 97:55.
17. Sykes AR, Hammes PA. Drug Cosmet Ind 1980; 62.
18. Robbins CR, Bahl MK. J Soc Cosmet Chem 1984; 35:379.
19. Bahl MK. J Soc Cosmet Chem 1985; 36:287.
20. Goddard ED, Harris WC. J Soc Cosmet Chem 1987; 38:233.
21. Goddard ED, Harris WC. J Soc Cosmet Chem 1987; 38:295.
22. Goddard ED, Harris WC. Proc. XIV Congress IFSCC, Barcelona, 1986, p 1039.
23. Wendel SR, DiSapio AJ. Cosmet Toilet 1983; 98:103.
24. Band PA, Brode GL, Goddard ED, Barbone AG, Leschinger E, Harris WC, Pavlichko JP, Partain EM III, Leung PS. In: Gebelein CG, ed. Cosmetic and Pharmaceutical Applications of Polymers. New York: Plenum Press, 1991:129.
25. Baty AM, Leavitt PK, Siedlecki CA, Tyler BJ, Suci PA, Marchant RE, Geesey GG. Langmuir 1997; 13:5702.
26. Yahagi K. J Soc Cosmet Chem 1992; 43:275.
27. Harrick NJ. Phys Rev Lett 1960; 4:224.
28. Puttnam NA, Baxter BH. J Soc Cosmet Chem 1967; 18:469.
29. Potts RO. J Soc Cosmet Chem 1986; 37:9.

30. Signori V, Lewis DM. Int J Cosmet Sci 1997; 1.
31. Klimisch HM, Chandra G. J Soc Cosmet Chem 1986; 37:73.
32. Budrys RS. Ann Scientific Mtg Soc Cosmet Chem, New York, 1986.
33. Shaw DJ. Introduction to Colloid and Surface Chemistry. London: Butterworths, 1966:122, 132.
34. Davies JT, Rideal EK. Interfacial Phenomena. New York: Academic Press, 1961:76.
35. Jachowicz J, Berthiaume M, Garcia M. Colloid Polym Sci 1985; 263:847.
36. Norde W, Rouwendal E. J Colloid Interface Sci 1990; 139:169.
37. Jachowicz J, Maxey S, Williams C. Langmuir 1993; 9:3085.
38. Jachowicz J, Williams C. J Soc Cosmet Chem 1994; 45:309.
39. Jachowicz J. J Soc Cosmet Chem 1995; 46:100.
40. Goddard ED, Leung PS. Proc. XIII Congress IFSCC, Buenos Aires, 1984, p 79.
41. Goddard ED, Leung PS. Parfum Kosmet 1987; 68:546.
42. Somasundaran P, Kulkarni RD. J Colloid Interface Sci 1973; 45:591.
43. Kamath YK, Dansizer CJ, Weigmann H-D. J Appl Polym Sci 1984; 29:1011.
44. Goddard ED. Unpublished results.
45. Andrade JD, Hlady V. Adv Surf Sci 1986; 79:1.
46. Goddard ED, Schmitt RL. Cosmet Toilet 1994; 109(3):55.
47. Lea AS, Pungor A, Hlady V, Andrade JD, Herron JN, Voss EW. Langmuir 1992; 8:68.
48. Schmitt RL, Goddard ED. Cosmet Toilet 1994; 109(12):83.
49. Hössel P, Sander DIR, Schrepp W. Cosmet Toilet 1996; 111:57.
50. Tabor D, Winterton RHS. Proc Roy Soc Lond 1969; A312:435.
51. Israelachvili JN, Adams GE. J Chem Soc Faraday Trans I 1978; 74:975.
52. Anathapadmanabhan KP, Mao G-Z, Goddard ED, Tirrell M. Colloids Surfaces 1991; 61:167.
53. Dhoot S, Goddard ED, Murphy DS, Tirrell M. Colloids Surfaces 1992; 66:91.
54. Argillier J-F, Ramachandran R, Harris WC, Tirrell M. J Colloid Interface Sci 1991; 146:242.
55. Shubin V. Langmuir 1994; 10:1093.
56. Scott GV, Robbins CR, Barnhurst JD. J Soc Cosmet Chem 1969; 20:135.
57. Crawford RJ, Robbins CR. J Soc Cosmet Chem 1980; 31:273.
58. Unilever Ltd., US Patent 4,298,494.
59. Weigmann H-D, Kamath YK, Ruetsch SB, Busch P, Tessman H. J Soc Cosmet Chem 1990; 41:379.
60. Goddard ED, Schadt RL. Proc. XV Congress IFSCC, London, 1988, p 197.
61. Goddard ED, Chandar P. Colloids Surfaces 1988; 34:295.
62. Alince B, Robertson AA, Inoue M. J Colloid Interface Sci 1978; 65:98.
63. Haffey MJ, Watt IC. J Colloid Interface Sci 1986; 109:181.
64. Onoda G, Somasundaran P. J Colloid Interface Sci 1987; 118:169.
65. Stober W, Fink A, Bohn E. J Colloid Interface Sci 1968; 26:62.
66. Terayama H. Kagaku no Kenkyu 1948; 1:75.
67. Wang LK, Shuster WW. Ind Eng Chem Prod Res Dev 1975; 14:312.
68. Onabe F. Mokusai Gakkaishi 1982; 28:445.
69. Hutter JM, Clarke MT, Just EK, Lichtin JL, Sakr A. J Soc Cosmet Chem 1991; 42:87.
70. Hutter JM, Clarke MT, Just EK Lichtin JL, Sakr A. J Soc Cosmet Chem 1992; 43:229.
71. Birch BJ, Clarke DE. Anal Chim Acta 1973; 67:387.
72. Hayakawa K, Kwak JCT. J Phys Chem 1982; 86:3866.
73. Santerre JP, Hayakawa K, Kwak JCT. Colloids Surfaces 1985; 13:35.
74. Van Nguyen N, Cannell DW, Mathews RA, Oei HHY. J Soc Cosmet Chem 1992; 43:259.
75. Blanco B, Durost BA, Myers RR. J Soc Cosmet Chem 1997; 48:127.
76. Van den Berg JWA, Staverman AJ. Rec Trav Chim Pays-bas 1979; 16:1151.
77. Vanlerberghe G, Handjani-Vila RM, Poubeau MC. Proc. VII Int Congress Surface Active Agents, Moscow, 1977, p 791.
78. Karjala SA, Williamson JE, Karler A. J Soc Cosmet Chem 1966; 17:513.

79. Cooperman ES. Am Cosmet Perfum 1972; 87:65.
80. Cooperman ES, Johnsen VL. Am Cosmet Perfum 1973; 88:19.
81. Stern ES, Johnsen VL. Proc. IX Congress IFSCC, Boston, 1976, p 753.
82. Francis DH, Felson KK. Private communication, 1996.
83. Wortmann F-J, Wortmann G, Zahn H. Textile Res J 1997; 67:720.
84. Tate ML, Kamath YK, Ruetsch SB, Weigmann H-D. J Soc Cosmet Chem 1993; 44:347.
85. Fleer GJ, Cohen Stuart MA, Scheutjens JMHM, Cosgrove T, Vincent B. Polymers at Interfaces. London: Chapman & Hall, 1993:Chapter 7.
86. Winnik FM, Regismond STA, Heng -M, Goddard ED. Unpublished work.
87. Rivière JC, Myhra S. Handbook of Surface and Interface Analysis. New York: Marcel Dekker, 1998.
88. Berthiaume MD, Merrifield JH, Riccio DA. J Soc Cosmet Chem 1995; 46:231.

11

The Adsorptivity of Charged and Uncharged Cellulose Ethers

E. Desmond Goddard, R. B. Hannan, and J. A. Faucher
Union Carbide Corporation, Tarrytown, New York

I. INTRODUCTION

An overview of the field of polymer adsorption, including theoretical and general aspects, has been presented in Chapters 2 and 3. In historical terms it can be said that, while interest in the adsorption of polymers is now quite old (1), the development of interest in polyelectrolyte adsorption is more recent (2,3). This subject is treated in some detail (including the case where the adsorption interface is oppositely charged) in a recently published general treatise on the subject of polymer adsorption (3).

During the course of other work, we became interested in such studies involving a cationic derivative of hydroxyethyl cellulose, whose adsorption characteristics onto various keratinous substrates, such as bleached hair (4) [and also stratum corneum membranes (5)], were investigated. Chief features established were the relatively high uptakes observed, the pronounced time effects associated with them, and the appreciable influence of added salts and surfactants. The purpose of the present studies was to extend the investigation of the adsorption of this cationic polymer (and its uncharged parent molecule) to (1) the virgin natural fibers, hair and cotton, (2) the artificial fibers, rayon and nylon, and (3) the solid, nonporous substrates, glass and hydroxyapatite.

II. EXPERIMENTAL

Polymer JR (6) is a quaternary ammonium derivative of hydroxyethyl cellulose (HEC). The three grades of Polymer JR, -125, -400, and -30M, are estimated to correspond to molecular weights (MW) of 250,000, 400,000, and 600,000 respectively. The HEC utilized in these experiments has an estimated MW of 330,000. Radiotagged polymers were prepared by carrying out the polymer syntheses from cellulose with ^{14}C-tagged ethylene oxide. Brown hair was obtained from DeMeo Bros., Inc., New York. Fabrics were obtained

---

This chapter, a slightly modified version of a paper presented at the VIIth International Congress on Surface Active Agents, Moscow, 1976, is reprinted here because of virtual inaccessibility of the original article.

from Test Fabrics, Inc., as follows: unsized cotton, No. 400, viscose rayon, No. 226, and nylon 66, No. 306A. Hydroxyapatite was used as supplied by Calbiochem. The sodium dodecyl sulfate (SDS) was a pure sample from BDH. Cetyltrimethylammonium bromide (CTAB) was obtained from Fine Organics, and Barlox 12 amine oxide from Lonza. All other reagents were Fisher grade. The water used in all experiments was twice distilled, the second distillation being from alkaline permanganate.

Hair tresses (approximately 50 g each) were shampooed twice with the nonionic surfactant ''Tergitol'' 15-S-9 (Union Carbide Corp.) and rinsed thoroughly with running tap water. Each tress was then rinsed twice in 1 L of distilled water for 10 min, extracted in 500 ml ethanol at 30–40°C, and again rinsed twice in distilled water.

Cotton fabric as received was cut into rectangles approximately 4 cm × 5 cm, then dewaxed by Soxhlet extraction for 72 hr, first with toluene and then ethanol (3 A grade). Viscose rayon and nylon fabrics were washed in a 1.0% solution of ''Tergitol'' 15-S-9 for 30 min in a Terg-o-tometer and then thoroughly rinsed in distilled water. Samples 5 cm × 7 cm were then cut for use.

Polymer sorption was followed radiometrically, using ^{14}C-tagged polymers with specific activities of the order of 0.04 mCi/g, at room temperature (23 ± 2°C). Each sample of fabric or hair was placed in a 22-ml glass vial into which was poured 20 ml of sorbate solution. Agitation was provided for exposure times up to 120 min by means of an Eberbach 6460 platform shaker at 280 lateral excursions per minute and 3 cm amplitude per excursion. Samples employing longer exposure times were allowed to stand unagitated. At the appropriate time, the sorbate solution was decanted and the sample rinsed repeatedly with distilled water, dried, weighed, and oxidized in a Packard Sample Oxidizer, Model 306. The resultant cocktail was counted in a Packard Model 3300 Liquid Scintillation Spectrometer. Counting efficiencies were monitored by the automatic external standard method.

Sorption of polymer by powdered hydroxyapatite was accomplished similarly except that at the appropriate time, the powder was filtered from the sorbate solution onto a Millipore filter (EHWPO 4700) of refractive index equal to toluene. The filter and its contents were rinsed thoroughly with twice-distilled water and dried before being placed in a toluene-based counting cocktail. Appropriate backgrounds were determined for polymer that might have become entrapped in the filter. Sorption of polymer by glass was determined by exposing cleaned counting vials to the polymer solution for the appropriate time interval. The vials were rinsed thoroughly, dried, filled with scintillation solution from the sample oxidizer, and then counted as described above. The counting geometry was verified to be 2π.

III. RESULTS

A. Hair

Figures 1 and 2 present the adsorption data for brown hair, for a constant polymer concentration of 0.1%. Two features of Polymer JR adsorption are noteworthy. First, equilibrium sorption is not attained even after 2 days, whereas sorption of the uncharged HEC achieves a constant value in 5 min. Second, sorption of Polymer JR decreases markedly with increasing MW. If one converts the adsorption value of HEC (ca. 0.05 mg/g hair) to an area value per anhydroglucose residue (MW 250), one finds it corresponds to the value expected for a close-packed monolayer of the cellulose in flat orientation, viz., ~85 A^2

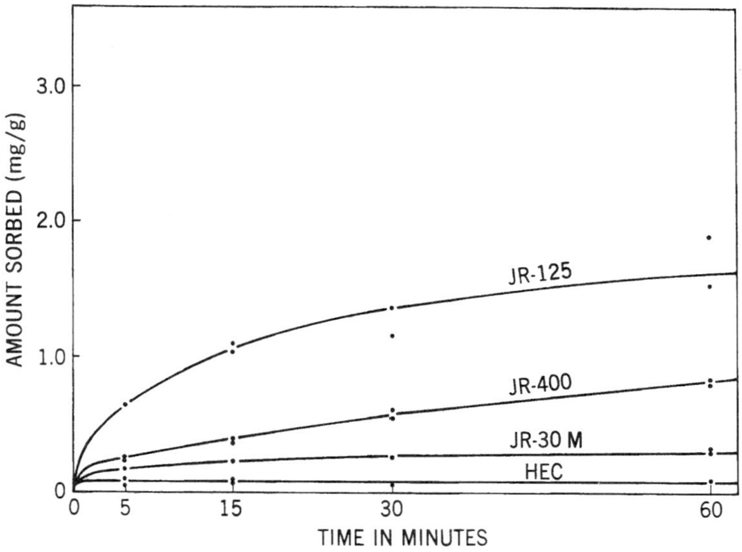

Figure 1 Sorption of polymers by hair; 0.1% polymer solution.

(7). Similar calculations for Polymer JR (residue MW per cationic group, 670) lead to a value of 0.06 mg/g for monolayer coverage of hair. The values in Figures 1 and 2 and Table 1 greatly exceed this figure. We have previously interpreted all data similar to the above, i.e., the kinetic effects, dependence on MW, and extent of sorption, as supporting a process of diffusion of the polycation into the keratinous substrate (4,5). Further evidence favoring a diffusion mechanism is obtained by plotting the sorption against the square

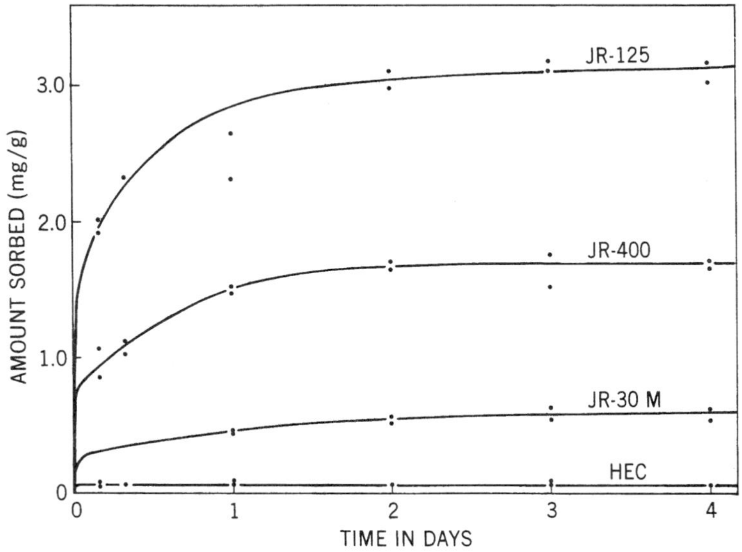

Figure 2 Sorption of polymers by hair; 0.1% polymer solution.

Table 1 Sorption Data

Substrate	Surface area (cm^2/mg)	Polymer	4-day uptake: μg polymer/mg	4-day uptake: Monolayers
Brown hair	0.40[a]	JR-125	3.12	53
		JR-400	1.70	28
		JR-30M	0.60	10
		HEC	0.05	1
Cotton	7.2[b]	JR-125	5.0	5
		HEC	0.70	0.7
Rayon	4.6[c]	JR-125	1.9	3
		JR-400	1.4	2
		JR-30M	0.5	0.7
		HEC	0.5	0.8
Nylon	2.0[c]	JR-125	0.14	0.5
		JR-400	0.14	0.5
		JR-30M	0.20	0.7
		HEC	0.17	0.7
Hydroxyapatite	500[d]	JR-400	14	0.2
Glass	38.5[c] cm^2	JR-400	6 μg	1

[a] BET area (10).
[b] BET area (16).
[c] Estimation based on geometric area.
[d] BET area.

root of time. (See Fig. 3.) The linear portions of these plots satisfy the equation for diffusion into a semi-infinite slab (4,8,9)

$$Q_t = 2C_o\,(Dt/\pi)^{1/2} \tag{1}$$

where Q is the amount sorbed per unit area in time t, C_o is the bath concentration, and D is the diffusion coefficient. The D values for Polymer JR-125, JR-400, and JR-30M are, respectively, 6.4×10^{-9}, 1.1×10^{-9}, and 1×10^{-10} cm^2/sec.

The difference in adsorption behavior between uncharged hydroxyethyl cellulose and the JR polymers, which have essentially the same structure with the exception of possessing a positive charge, implicates charge as the responsible factor. If this is true, then the sorption of the polycations would be expected to be strongly influenced by added salts. The data in Figure 4 confirm this expectation. Results after longer times of sorption exaggerate the effects. Sorption values after 4 days reveal that the presence of NaCl and $CaCl_2$ at 0.25 M reduces the uptake by approximately six-fold and 25-fold, respectively. Other work of the authors (10) shows that appreciable reductions in uptake can be effected by much lower concentrations of salt, e.g., 0.01 M, and that the trivalent lanthanum ion exerts an even more potent influence than calcium, in accordance with a Schulze-Hardy valence mechanism. It has also been established that the cation of the added salt determines the reduction in sorption.

A further anticipated consequence of the above mechanism would be an appreciable reduction in polycation sorption in the presence of a cationic surfactant. Not only would the latter species compete for the external anionic sites of the keratin, but it is known to penetrate into the body of the hair (11). Measurements in fact showed that the surfactant

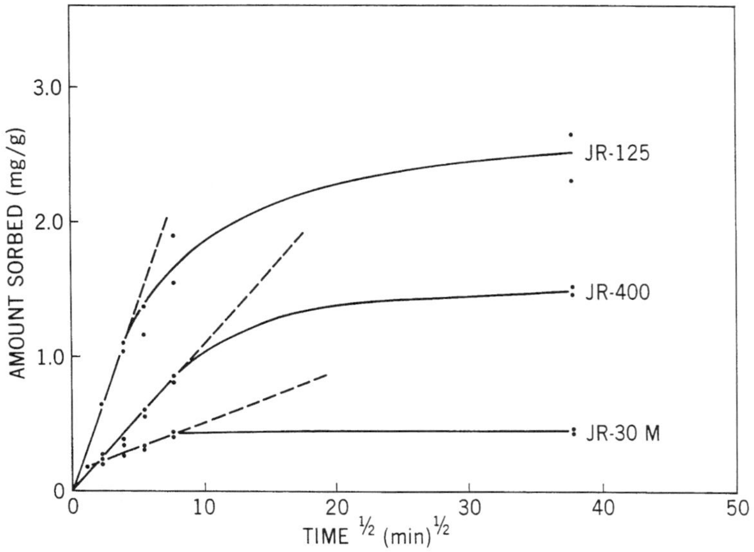

Figure 3 Sorption of Polymer JR by hair; 0.1% polymer solution.

CTAB sharply reduces sorption of Polymer JR-125. This is shown in Figure 5, which includes results for other surfactants. The nonionic surfactant Tergitol 15-S-9 has a comparatively minor influence on the sorption, as a result, presumably, of little interaction tendency of this surfactant (12) with either the polymer or the keratin. The reduction in sorption observed in the presence of the amine oxide Barlox 12 is ascribed to sorption of this material by the hair in view of the appreciable sorptive tendency of the related material

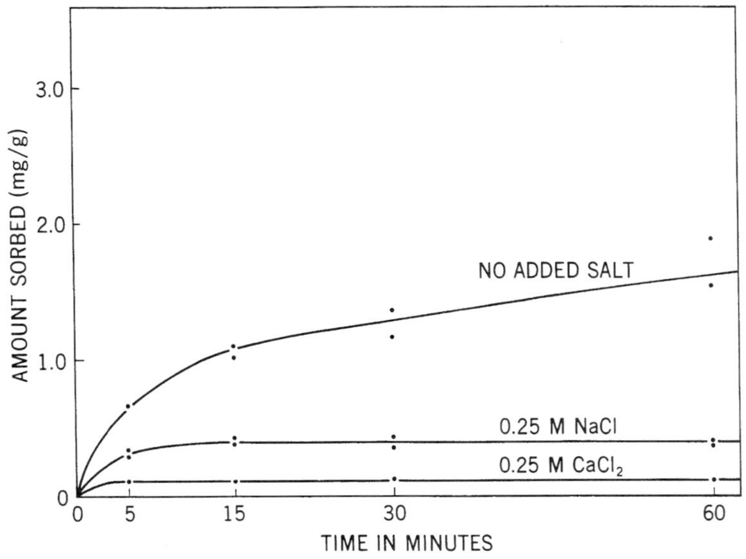

Figure 4 Effect of salts on the sorption of Polymer JR-125 by hair; 0.1% polymer solution.

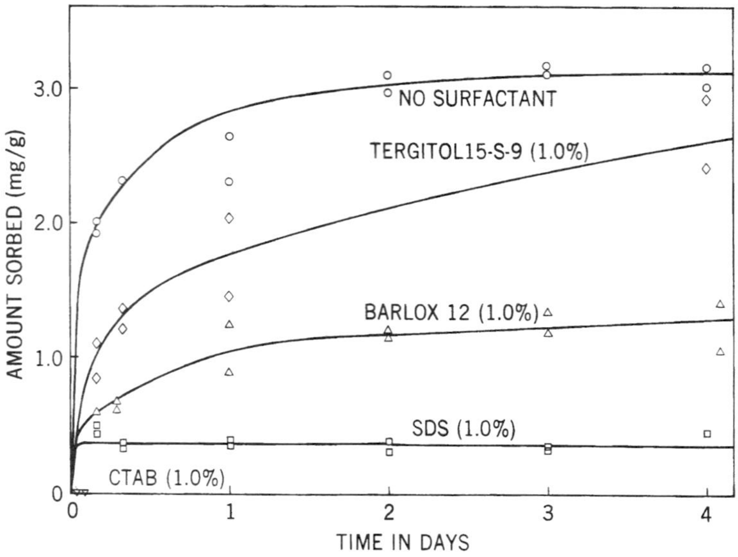

Figure 5 Effect of surfactants on the sorption of Polymer JR-125 by hair; 0.1% polymer solution.

dodecyldimethyl phosphine oxide (13). The pronounced reduction caused by SDS must result from two effects. First, it is known to react strongly with polycations; SDS precipitates Polymer JR from solution, but at high concentration solubilizes the complex and in the process transforms the polymer in effect into a polyanion (12). Second, SDS is sorbed strongly by various natural keratins (14,15). In this way, it could exert a blocking action upon the sorption of the polymer.

In Figure 6 a sorption isotherm for Polymer JR-400 on hair is presented. The data points represent values after contact times of 3 1/2 days. It should be pointed out that these measurements were carried out on a batch of hair different from that employed for the measurements of Figures 1, 2, etc., and somewhat higher sorptions were observed. The isotherm is typical of polymer sorption in the sense of possessing an apparent zero concentration adsorption intercept. However, a steady increase in sorption was observed with concentration, and no obvious plateau was evident (1).

The form of polymer sorption isotherms has received much attention and many adsorption equations have been proposed and employed. In the present case, conformance was found with an equation of the Freundlich type:

$$S = kC^n \tag{2}$$

but not with the Langmuir type:

$$S/S_\infty = bC/(1 + bC), \tag{3}$$

where S = the sorption, C = bulk "equilibrium" concentration, and k, n, b are constants.

B. Cotton

The second natural fiber investigated was cotton; sorption results for Polymer JR-125 and HEC are given in Figure 7. It is of interest that, although there was less reproducibility

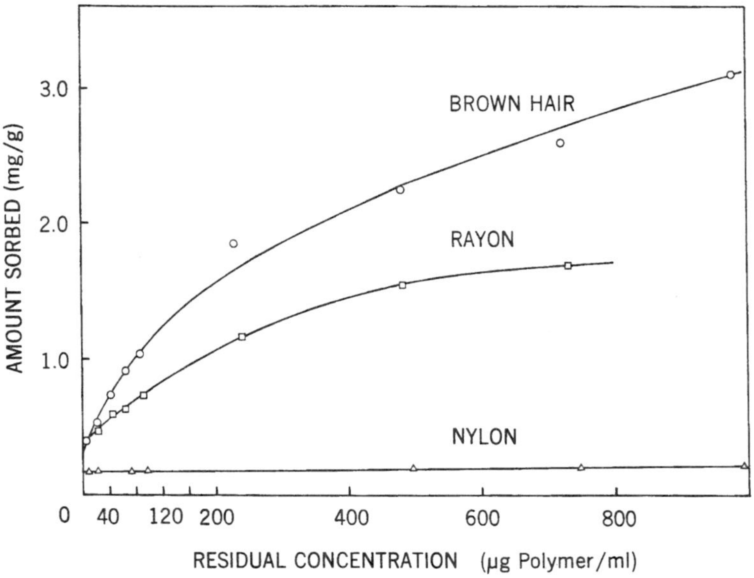

Figure 6 Sorption of Polymer JR-400 by hair, rayon, and nylon versus residual concentration.

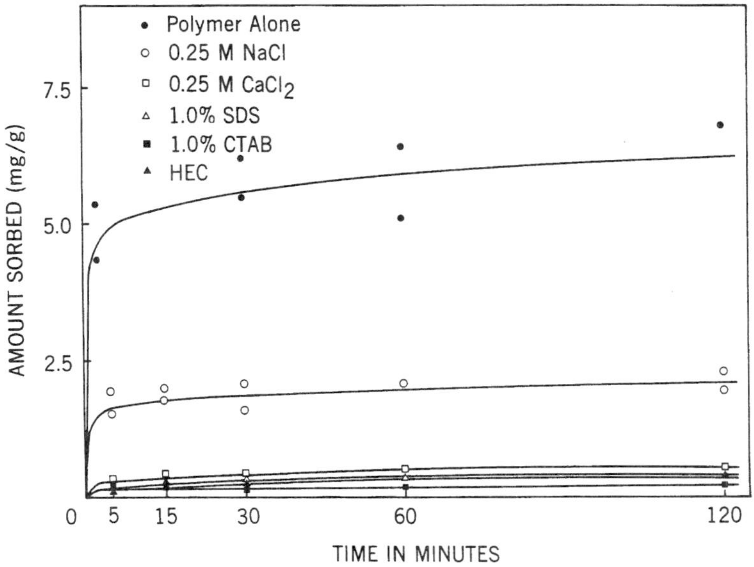

Figure 7 Effect of salts and surfactants on the sorption of Polymer JR-125 by cotton; 0.1% polymer solution.

of measurement for this substrate, the observed sorption values for JR-400 and JR-30M (not shown) are close to those for JR-125; i.e., there is little dependence on MW. Another point of interest is the relatively fast initial sorption of Polymer JR compared to that on hair. Both of these observations are likely to result from the ready tendency of cotton to imbibe water and hence create access routes for sorbing species. It is seen that sorption of uncharged HEC is again very limited, viz., 0.8 mg/g. This corresponds closely to monolayer coverage, if one accepts the BET surface area, viz., 0.72 m^2/g, for cotton (16). The much larger sorption of Polymer JR, viz., ~7 mg/g, corresponds to an apparent coverage of ~5 monolayers (Table 1), and, as with hair, implicates the negative sites on the cotton. In support of this, the addition of NaCl (0.25 M) led to a threefold reduction in uptake of Polymer JR, and of 0.25 M $CaCl_2$ to a 10-fold reduction (see Fig. 7). By contrast, addition of $CaCl_2$ scarcely affected the sorption of HEC. Likewise, addition of the cationic surfactant CTAB, which is known to adsorb strongly onto cotton (17), reduced the sorption of Polymer JR even more, whereas the anionic SDS (1%) led to about the same level of sorption reduction as 0.25 M $CaCl_2$. Since it is known (18) that clean cotton adsorbs virtually no SDS, the reduction in sorption of the polycation must be the result of modification of its properties by adsorption of a double layer of the DS anion (12).

C. Rayon

The high sorption values of Polymer JR on the natural fibers, hair and cotton, prompted us to investigate sorption onto fibers with simpler geometry, i.e., smoother surface topography. Data for rayon are presented in Figure 8. It is evident that sorption of the JR polymers, especially those of higher MW, is considerably less than on cotton. However, in the case of rayon, there is a pronounced reduction in uptake of the polymer with increased MW, as was observed for hair. As shown in Figure 9, addition of NaCl again leads to a marked reduction in uptake of the polycation. A larger reduction is effected by 0.25 M

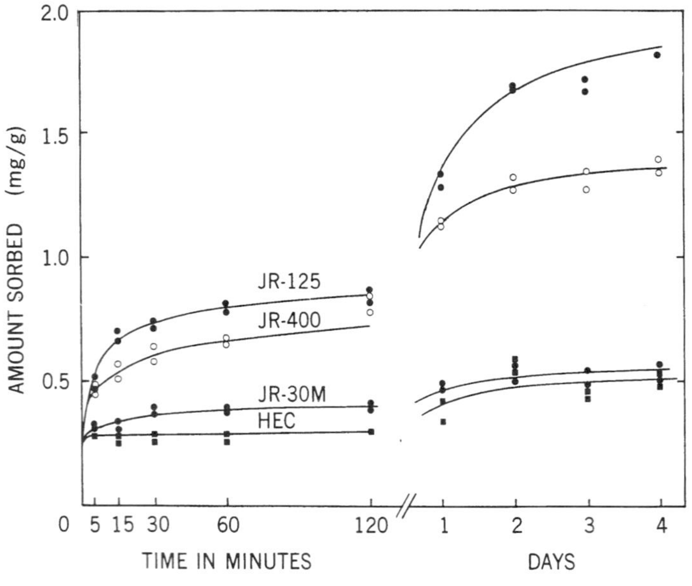

Figure 8 Sorption of polymers by rayon; 0.1% polymer solution.

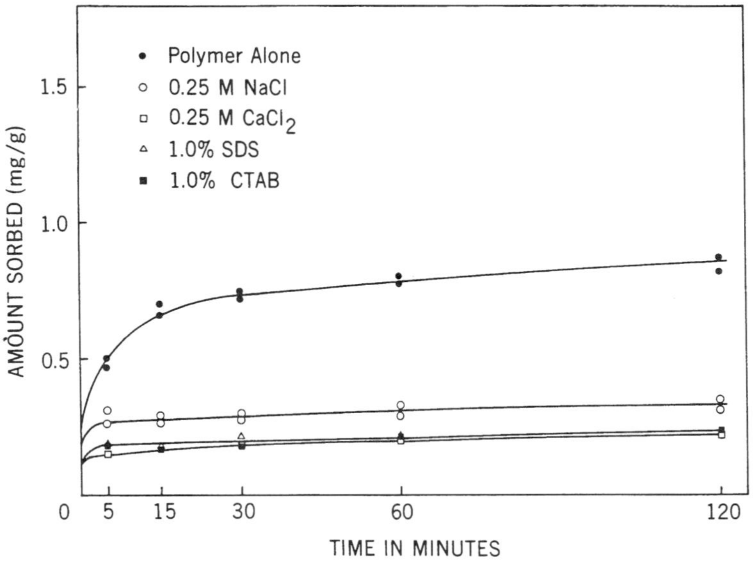

Figure 9 Effect of salts and surfactants on the sorption of Polymer JR-125 by rayon; 0.1% polymer solution.

$CaCl_2$: the resultant sorption value of JR-125 is close to that observed on addition of 1% SDS, which in this case leads to a drop in uptake equal to that caused by CTAB. It is of interest that sorption values of HEC, Polymer JR-30M, and Polymer JR-125 in 0.25 M NaCl are all close and approximate a value required for monolayer coverage. The sorption isotherm for Polymer JR-400 on rayon is included in Figure 6. As with hair, no evidence of a sorption plateau was obtained, and conformance with Freundlich behavior was found.

D. Nylon

Nylon was chosen as the fiber possessing a ''smooth'' surface, a very small or zero intrinsic charge, and very limited or zero porosity to sorbing macromolecules. Sorption data are presented in Figure 10. Several important aspects emerge. First, the sorption values are relatively low. Second, for the first time, sorption increases with MW, a pattern traditionally expected for polymers (19). Third, the sorption of uncharged HEC is similar to that obtained for the charged polymers. Interesting features emerge on introducing additives to the sorption bath, as shown in Figure 11. While the cationic surfactant CTAB virtually eliminates sorption, SDS and $CaCl_2$ appear, if anything, to exert a small positive effect on the sorption. Both SDS and CTAB are known (20) to be adsorbed by nylon. The reduction of polycation sorption by CTAB is ascribed to a charge repulsion effect, and the slight increase by SDS to charge attraction and competition by adsorbed DS anions for the polycation in solution. These effects, combined with the elevating influence of added $CaCl_2$, which is ascribed to an ion-shielding effect, point to a sorption mechanism for nylon that is different from that for the other fibers.

The sorption isotherm for Polymer JR-400 on nylon is given in Figure 6. Although the uptake is relatively small, it can be seen that the isotherm is typical of polymer adsorption in possessing a high-affinity characteristic and the appearance of a sorption plateau.

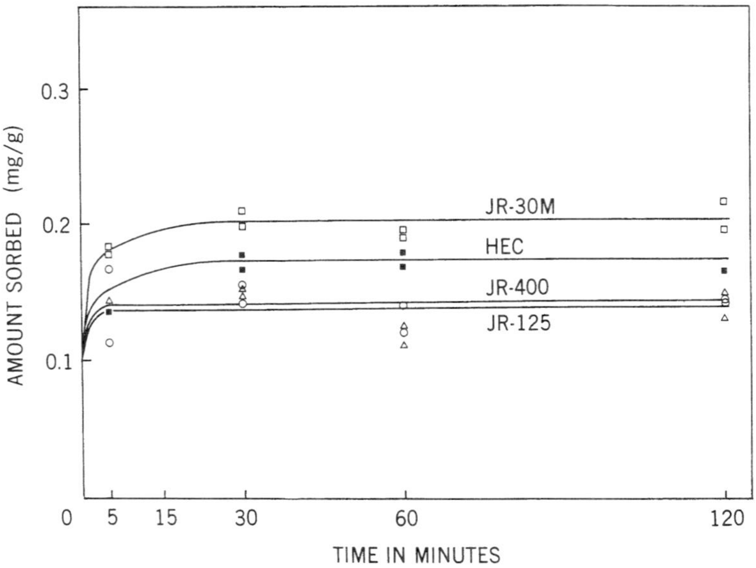

Figure 10 Sorption of polymers by nylon; 0.1% polymer solution.

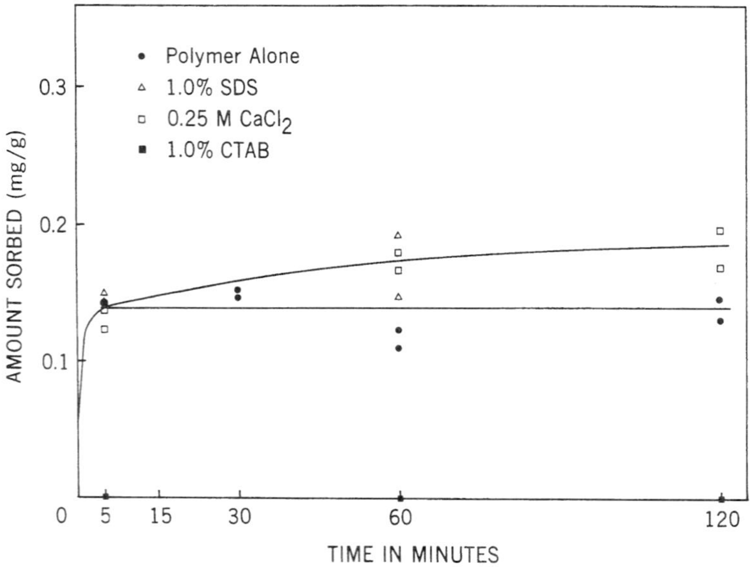

Figure 11 Effect of salt and surfactants on the sorption of Polymer JR-125 by nylon; 0.1% polymer solution.

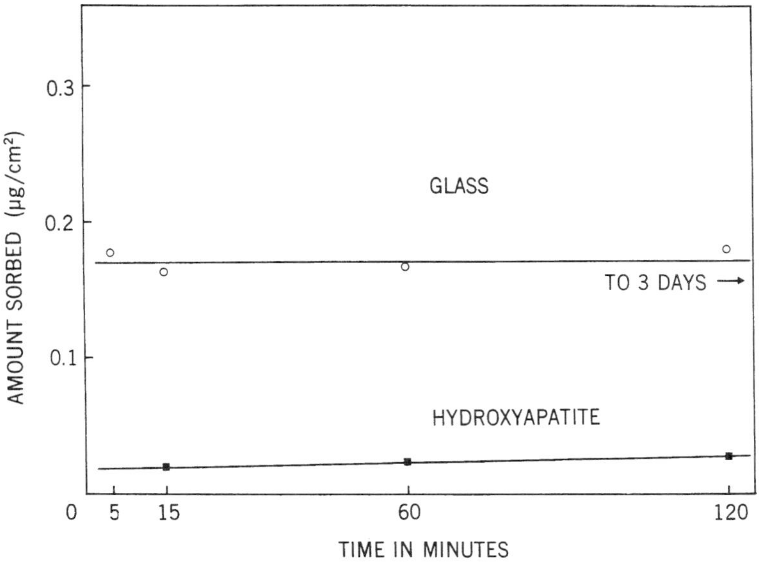

Figure 12 Sorption of Polymer JR-400 by glass and by hydroxyapatite; 0.1% polymer solution.

''Saturation'' sorption of Figure 6 corresponds approximately to monolayer coverage of the nylon by Polymer JR-400. (See Table 1.)

E. Glass and Hydroxyapatite

As examples of inorganic substrates, glass was chosen as a surface bearing a negative charge in water, and hydroxyapatite (p.z.c. = 7) as one being effectively uncharged in neutral aqueous fluids. Sorption data, presented in Figure 12, reveal that coverage of glass by JR-400 corresponds approximately to a single monolayer, whereas that on hydroxyapatite corresponds to only ~0.1 monolayer (Table 1). Glass attains adsorption equilibrium in about 5 min while adsorption onto hydroxyapatite proceeds very slowly.

IV. DISCUSSION

Much progress has been made in recent years in the understanding of polymer adsorption, the most recent theoretical treatments being due to Silberberg (1,21) and Hoeve (1,22). The generally accepted pattern is that polymer chains first adsorb through isolated contacts at adsorption sites on the surface, and this anchoring process is then followed by reorientation of the sorbed polymer with or without the creation of more anchored positions. Much of the sorbed polymer can actually be out of true contact with the surface, and in the form of loops emanating from the surface from the ''train'' segments attached to the surface. The model explains several well-known features of the adsorption of polymers, viz., their high affinity, and the irreversibility, time dependence, and molecular weight effects. Furthermore, in the present case, two other factors must be considered: first, being polyelectrolytes, the cationic derivatives of cellulose would have a very stiff, extended chain conformation; second, many of the fiber substrates are swellable and contain pores into which the polymer can migrate.

As mentioned in the introduction, very little published information exists on the adsorption of polyelectrolytes. We shall briefly review polymer sorption results that are relevant to the present work. Qualitative data have shown that a protein hydrolysate (23) and a polyethylenimine (24) penetrate human hair. More quantitative kinetic data were obtained for the penetration of polyethylenimine into hair (25) and cellulose (26) and some work on the influence of charge was included. Sorption studies on cellulose carried out by Robertson and his co-workers (27) with uncharged polymers emphasize the important role of solvent swelling of the cellulose on the extent of sorption. One of the most interesting papers for comparison with our work is that of Higuchi et al. (28) on the adsorption of amino derivatives of polyvinyl alcohol and cellulose onto rayon. Although charge attraction was found essential for adsorption, maximum adsorption was found at relatively low levels of amino substitution of the polymer and at a pH of 10.3, where much of the charged amino functionality would have been lost. The results were interpreted as showing flat orientation of the charged polymers and no penetration. A second paper of important significance to our work is that of Evans and Evans (29) on the sorption of the anionic cellulose polyelectrolyte sodium carboxymethyl cellulose (Na CMC) onto cotton. In this case *no* sorption of this polyanion onto negatively charged cotton was found unless extraneous salts were added; furthermore, added calcium ions *increased* the uptake more than added sodium ions.

A. Sorption as a Charge Attraction Process

Cotton and rayon, as well as hair, are water-swellable fibers that possess ionic sites. Their carboxyl content was determined by acid-base titration (30) to be, respectively, 5.46×10^4 and 4.23×10^4 g/eqt., corresponding to net Polymer JR uptakes of 12.3 mg/g and 15.8 mg/g of fiber for total charge neutralization by the polycation. Although the observed uptakes of the polycation in the most favorable case (JR-125) are somewhat less than these latter figures, they are comparable, at least for cotton; this lends support to a mechanism involving penetration of the polycation into pores of the fibers. The depressing influence of added electrolytes, in which the valence of the cation exerts a dominating influence, is in agreement with this postulate, and is a consequence of the more rapid diffusion of these inorganic ions into the fibers and consequent shielding of their anionic sites by the cations. An extreme case of this is the depression caused by a cationic surfactant, in which case shielding of the sites and stabilization of this sorbate at these sites will occur. Further evidence in support of an ionic mechanism comes from the results with nylon, where adsorption of a layer of CTAB, and consequent positive charging of the surface, eliminates the sorption of the polycation altogether. Again, the slight increase in sorption of Polymer JR by nylon in the presence of added salt is likely to be the result of charge shielding between adsorbed and adsorbing polycation molecules, or between the adsorbed polycation molecules themselves.

Two effects will prevail when SDS is present in the nylon/Polymer JR system. Since SDS is known to adsorb onto nylon, the latter will become negatively charged and hence tend to repel the SDS-modified polymer, itself therefore negative. Since a reduction in polymer adsorption is not in fact observed, it is likely that the SDS adsorbed onto the nylon actually competes with the SDS adsorbed onto the polymer for the polymer, and acts as a bridge to bind it to the nylon surface. Finally, the difference in adsorption upon the inorganic substrates glass and hydroxyapatite also supports a charge/charge attraction mechanism as the main driving force for adsorption.

B. Sorption as a Diffusion Process

Several features of the sorption of the polycation by brown hair and, to a lesser extent, rayon and cotton suggest diffusion of the polymer into the fiber. First, the level of polymer sorbed by hair corresponds to several monolayers. (See Table 1.) By contrast, sorption onto the glass substrate closely approximates monolayer coverage. Second, the decrease in polymer sorption by hair that accompanies an increase in polymer MW is the reverse of that which is normally observed for the adsorption of polymers on nonporous solid interfaces. Finally, evidence for diffusion is found in the dependence of polymer sorption (M_t) upon the square root of time (t) for values of M_t/M_∞ of up to 0.5 (Fig. 3). Crank (9) has shown that, in the simplest case where the sorption isotherm is linear, such a relationship always holds for diffusion of solute from an infinite bath.

Further evidence favoring a diffusion mechanism for polymer sorption is obtained from a consideration of the sorption isotherm on hair and rayon in Figure 6. The data do not conform to the Langmuir adsorption equation. Langmuirian behavior would imply that the adsorbing sites along the polymer act independently of one another, a situation that would be approached in the case of extensive looping of the polymer at the interface. The observed data are found, rather, to fit the Freundlich isotherm. Crank (9) has shown that diffusion accompanied by nonlinear adsorption is governed by the concentration of free diffusant, which is, in turn, governed by the total initial concentration of diffusant. In the case of the Freundlich isotherm ($n < 1$), when $\partial C/\partial t \ll \partial S/\partial t$, the effective diffusion coefficient, D_e, is given by

$$D_e = (D/n)\ (1/k)^{1/n} S^{(1-n)/n} \tag{4}$$

and increases as the sorbed concentration, S, increases. In such cases, the linear relationship between M_t and $t^{1/2}$ holds for values of M_t/M_∞ that exceed 0.5 (31). In Figure 3 it can be seen that this is indeed the case for the highest MW polycation.

The equation governing diffusion into a finite cylinder of radius r during short-time intervals for a constant value of D has been shown (9) to be

$$D = (\pi r^2/16t)\ (M_t/M_\infty)^2 \tag{5}$$

For diffusion of Polymer JR-400 into brown hair of radius 1.25×10^{-3} cm, at time 3600 sec., D takes on a value of 2.0×10^{-11} cm^2/sec. Since sorption is nonlinear, this is the effective diffusion coefficient, and insertion of this value into Eq. (4) yields an actual diffusion coefficient of approximately 2.0×10^{-9} cm^2/sec. This value is in excellent agreement with that provided by the more general relationship expressed by Eq. (1).

C. Orientation of the Sorbed Layers

Although much has been written about the configuration of adsorbed polymers, which, by virtue either of composition or of the bathing solvent, are unionized, much less information exists on the state of adsorbed polyions. However, Higuchi et al. have adduced evidence that amino derivatives of polyvinyl alcohol adsorb onto rayon in a flat, extended state at low pH values. Several pieces of information support a flat-without-looping configuration for sorbed Polymer JR: (1) Cellulose is known to possess a "stiff" backbone. Possession of positively charged sites along the backbone would augment this effect. (2) Many of the sorbents considered possess anionic adsorption sites. Since the energy of interaction between these and the positive sites of the chain would be high, that configuration, i.e., flat, which allows maximum ion/ion interaction would be favored. (3) For the impenetrable, negatively charged surface of glass, the extent of adsorption corresponds to monolayer coverage and is independent of MW. (4) For uncharged nylon, although the coverage also approximates that expected of one monolayer, there is a MW dependence, which in this case supports a small degree of looping as does the effect of adding salt. (5) Despite its very high MW, Polymer JR is able to penetrate the pores of several substrates. Such penetration would be facilitated if the penetrant had a small cross-sectional size, i.e., existed in rod form.

V. CONCLUSIONS

The high sorptivity of positively charged derivatives of hydroxyethyl cellulose (HEC) on hair, cotton, and rayon results from (1) the water swellability of, and diffusion of the polymer into, these fibers, and (2) the presence in them of negatively charged sites. On nylon, which is uncharged and less swellable, sorption is much lower and equal to that observed with uncharged HEC.

Sorption of the charged polymers onto glass corresponds to monolayer coverage: much lower adsorption is observed on hydroxyapatite.

VI. SUMMARY

A study, using radiotracer techniques, of the adsorption of positively charged and uncharged cellulose ethers, all of high MW, is reported. The absorbents include the fibers human hair, cotton, nylon, and rayon, and the inorganic solids glass and hydroxyapatite; the influence of added surfactants and salts on the adsorption is presented. The adsorption of the charged polymers is in general greater than that of the uncharged polymer, and this result plus the effect of salts confirms the importance of electrostatic forces. An interpretation is made of the high uptake of the charged polymer into the natural fibers, and of the pronounced effect of surfactants in reducing its uptake.

REFERENCES

1. Lipotov YS, Sergeeva LM. Adsorption of Polymers. New York: Halsted-Wiley, 1974.
2. Fontana BJ. In: Hair ML, ed. The Chemistry of Biosurfaces. New York: Marcel Dekker, 1971: 114.
3. Fleer GJ, Cohen Stuart MA, Scheutjens JMHM, Cosgrove T, Vincent B. Polymers at Interfaces. London: Chapman & Hall, 1993: Chapter 7.
4. Faucher JA, Goddard ED. J Colloid Interface Sci 1976; 55:313.
5. Faucher JA, Goddard ED. J Soc Cosmet Chem 1976; 27:543.
6. Stone FW, Rutherford JM. U.S. Patent 3,472,840,1969.
7. Saunders FL. J Colloid Interface Sci 1968; 28:475.
8. Hill AV. Proc Roy Soc (Lond) 1928; 104B:39.
9. Crank J. The Mathematics of Diffusion. London: Oxford University Press, 1956.
10. Faucher JA, Hannan RB, Goddard ED. Unpublished work.
11. Scott GV, Robbins CR, Barnhurst JD. J Soc Cosmet Chem 1969; 20:135.
12. Goddard ED, Phillips TS, Hannan RB. J Soc Cosmet Chem 1975; 26:461.
13. Mast RC, Benjamin L. J Colloid Interface Sci 1969; 31:31.
14. Griffiths JC, Alexander AE. J Colloid Interface Sci 1967; 25:317.
15. Harrold SP, Pethica BA. Trans Far Soc 1958; 54:1876.

16. Rowen JW, Blaine RL. Ind Eng Chem 1947; 39:1659.
17. Sexsmith FH, White HJ. J Colloid Sci 1959; 14:598.
18. Schott H. Textile Res J 1967; 37:336.
19. Kipling JJ. Adsorption from Solutions of Non-electrolytes. New York: Academic Press, 1965.
20. Weatherburn AS, Bayley CH. Textile Res J 1952; 22:797.
21. Silberberg A. J Phys Chem 1962; 66:1872.
22. Hoeve CA. J Chem Phys 1965; 43:3007.
23. Cooperman ES, Johnson VL. Cosmet Perfum 1973; 88:19.
24. Woodard J. J Soc Cosmet Chem 1972; 23:593.
25. Chow CD. Textile Res J 1971; 41:444.
26. Kindler WA, Swanson JW. J Polym Sci 1971; 9:853.
27. Chan FS, Minhas PS, Robertson AA. J Colloid Interface Sci 1970; 33:586.
28. Higuchi M, Koyakumara T, Senju R. Bull Chem Soc Jpn 1974; 47:2990.
29. Evans PG, Evans WP. J Appl Chem 1967; 17:276.
30. Neale SM, Stringfellow WA. Trans Faraday Soc 1937; 33:881.
31. Crank J, Park GS. Diffusion in Polymers. New York: Academic Press, 1968.

12

Evaluation Methods for Conditioned Hair

Hans-Dietrich Weigmann and Yashavanth Kamath
TRI/Princeton, Princeton, New Jersey

I. INTRODUCTION

In an effort to make the term ''conditioner'' more meaningful, Robbins (1) has proposed the following narrow definition: ''A hair conditioner is an ingredient or a product, that when applied to hair in its recommended use procedure and concentration improves the combability relative to appropriate controls.'' However, polymeric compounds are being incorporated into cosmetic products for a number of purposes with the major goal of improving the ''condition'' of hair, which in this discussion includes in the broadest terms its appearance and manageability. Properties such as combability, flyaway, body and curl retention, to name just a few, are affected by the deposition of polymers on the hair surface. The question as to what extent polymeric conditioners with their high molecular weight are deposited strictly on the fiber surface or can penetrate into the cuticula or even beyond it into the cortex surprisingly has been answered in the affirmative, at least for long treatment times. Goddard et al. (2), using radioactively labeled cationic quaternized cellulose derivatives, have shown such penetration for the well-known Polymer JR compounds. While the major effects of polymer-containing treatment formulations are associated with the modification of surface properties, there is nevertheless recent evidence from work at TRI/Princeton (3,4) that at least intercuticular cohesion is affected by such treatments.

The evaluation methods we will discuss in this chapter are instrumental methods that provide objective and quantifiable assessments of treatment effects. Such methods are critically important for claim substantiations and are currently or will in the future be required by governmental agencies in this country and abroad. We decided to leave out the subjective methodology used in panel evaluations and consumer testing, since all companies in the cosmetic field have their own in-house evaluation procedures, which unfortunately are not yet standardized throughout the industry. For the same reason, we have not included comparisons between objective instrumental methods and subjective evaluation procedures.

For the reader not familiar with keratin fiber morphology, we recommend the book by Robbins *Chemical and Physical Behavior of Human Hair* (8). However, it is useful to start this chapter with a summary of current concepts of the structure and properties of human hair fibers.

II. STRUCTURE AND PROPERTIES OF HUMAN HAIR

The complex morphology of hair, schematically shown in Figure 1, essentially consists of four components of different functionality. The bulk of the fiber consists of the cortex and, in some thicker fibers, the medulla in its center. On the outside, a thick covering of up to 10 layers of overlapping cuticle cells provides protection against mechanical and environmental stresses. All these cellular structures are held together by the cell membrane complex (5).

A. Cortex

The majority part of the interior of the fiber mass is the cortex, which, from the point of view of mechanical properties, is also the most important component. The cortex consists of elongated, spindle-shaped cells aligned in the direction of the fiber axis. Within these cells resides the major part of the keratinized protein in the form of macrofibrils, which in turn are formed by lower levels of organization, i.e., microfibrils and finally protofibrils. The latter two are low-sulfur proteins and more or less crystalline in nature with their α-helical parts as crystalline lattice components. They are embedded in a noncrystalline, nonfibrillar matrix of disulfide cross-linked, globular proteins.

Recently, the nomenclature in the field of fibrous keratin structure has been changed to take into account new knowledge developed over the last few years by various groups of protein chemists, cell biologists, and molecular biologists. Crewther and Fraser and their co-workers (6,7) developed models of molecular organization that can accommodate

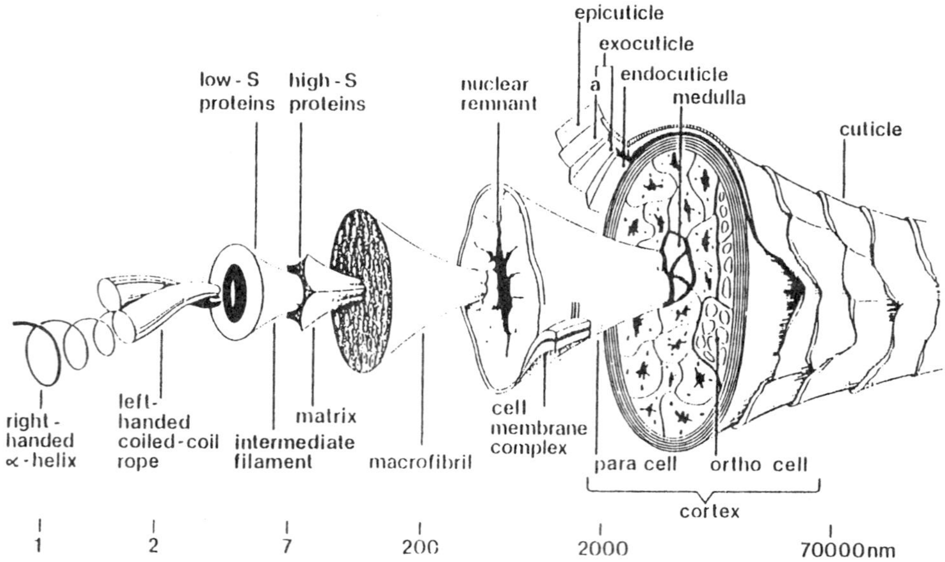

Figure 1 Schematic diagram of a human hair fiber showing the major structural features, except pigment granules, that are normally found in the cortical cells. (Adapted from Ref. 5.)

the chemical composition of low-sulfur filament keratins with sequences of helical and nonhelical domains of various lengths. They replaced the term ''microfibrils'' with the term ''intermediate filaments''(IF), which has its origin in cellular biology describing structural protein fibrils in the cytoskeleton of cells and is also being used to describe the nature of keratin filaments in the keratocytes of the epidermal stratum corneum. The *matrix* between the keratin intermediate filaments in the cortex consists of various families of *keratin-associated proteins* (KAP), which are mostly rich in cystine but also include various proteins rich in glycine and tyrosine. Zahn has been particularly active in promoting the general acceptance of this new nomenclature, and it has been incorporated by Robbins into the third edition of his book *Chemical and Physical Behavior of Human Hair* (8).

B. Medulla

The component of hair morphology located in the center of some thicker fibers and consisting of a loosely packed porous cellular structure is called the medulla. The medulla of human hair fibers apparently does not contribute to their mechanical properties, although occasionally fractures can initiate in the vicinity of medullary structures, which provide flaws for the initiation of cracks. Recent work at TRI/Princeton has also shown that the medulla does contribute to the optical properties of human hair fibers.

C. Cell Membrane Complex

The third component fulfills the vital function of cementing the various cells of the cuticula and the cortex together, thus making a fiber out of a conglomerate of cells. This intercellular cement, which together with the cell membranes forms the cell membrane complex (CMC) (see Fig. 2), is assumed to be the location of transport paths into the fiber,

Intercellular, as opposed to transcellular, transport is especially important for the incorporation of larger molecules such as polymeric materials into the cuticle, or even more so for diffusion into the cortex. The intercellular cement is thought to contain nonkeratinous, low-sulfur proteins, which are high in polar amino acids and are assumed to swell

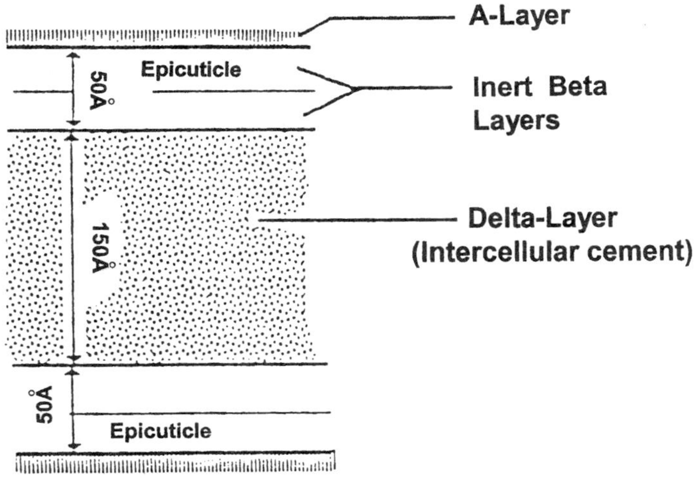

Figure 2 Schematic diagram of cell membrane complex in animal hairs. (From Ref. 5.)

extensively in water, thus opening passageways into the fiber. This so-called δ-layer lies between the inert β-layers, which consist of lipids covalently linked to neighboring protein and free fatty acids of various kinds.

D. Cuticle

As mentioned above, the cuticle of the human hair fiber consists of an array of flat cuticle cells, which are arranged in such a way that their free ends are oriented toward the tip of the fiber while their attached ends are always covered by overlapping cells. The cells form an angle of about three to five degrees to the fiber axis. This orientation gives rise to the differential frictional effect (DFE), which causes preferential movement of the fibers in the root direction and leads to felting. Felting is an industrially used property for wool (paper, felts, etc.), but occasionally can be a serious and irreversible problem for hair, especially if the scale edges are damaged and lifted by frequent cosmetic treatments. Individual cuticle cells are about 0.5–1 μm thick and are approximately 45 μm long. At the undamaged root end of the fiber scale edges are smooth with a distance between them of about 7–10 μm, while further away from the root end scale edges are ragged and nonuniform.

While at the root end up to 10 layers of cuticle cells are stacked over each other, this thickness of the cuticle layer decreases with increasing distance from the scalp as mechanical and environmental stresses cause ablation of cuticle fragments until occasionally the cuticle envelope has been totally worn away at the tips of long fibers. Since the cuticle envelope provides mechanical and chemical protection to the cortex, its absence can cause deterioration of the CMC between cortical cells leading to loss of intercellular cohesion and the formation of "split ends."

The cuticle cell itself is a multilayered structure as shown schematically in Figure 3.

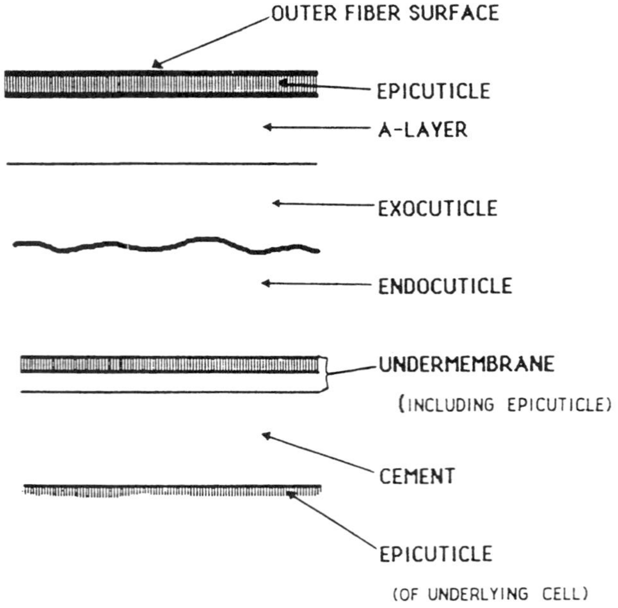

Figure 3 Schematic diagram of the proposed structure of a cuticle cell in cross-section. (From Ref. 8.)

Leeder et al. have proposed three proteinaceous layers surrounded by the epicuticle, a chemically resistant proteinaceous membrane of ~25 Å thickness covered by covalently bound structural lipids (9). These three layers differ in their amino acid composition, particularly in their cystine content. The outermost layer underneath the epicuticle is called the A-layer, which has the highest cystine content of about 35%, thus making it a highly cross-linked, mechanically tough layer. The next layer is the exocuticle with a cystine content of about 15%, followed by the endocuticle, which has only ~3% cystine and is highly swellable in water and mechanically weak. Swift and Brown (10) have shown that the swollen endocuticle is the weakest structural component during combing of wet hair and is the direct cause of cuticle fracture and ablation. Similarly, failure occurs in the endocuticle due to the generation of shear forces within the layered structure of the cuticle cell during extension of the fiber under ambient conditions (3,4).

The most important part of the cuticle from the point of view of polymer deposition is, of course, its outermost surface, i.e., the epicuticle. The epicuticle has been defined by Lindberg (11) as the membrane that contains sacs or bubbles raised upon immersion of wool fibers in chlorine water, i.e., the so-called Allwoerden reaction. It has been shown, however, that the removal of strongly bound surface lipids does not affect this phenomenon (12). It is assumed therefore, that the epicuticle, which is about 25 Å thick, is a residue of the cuticle cell membrane and is at least partly proteinaceous in nature and, together with surface-bound lipids (9), forms the F-layer. A recent model of the epicuticle membrane proposed by Negri and co-workers (13) incorporates new evidence and defines the epicuticle in terms of a membrane consisting of 25% lipids and 75% protein, the latter having an ordered, possibly β-pleated sheet structure with 12% cystine, as shown in Figure 4.

This structure could be arranged in such a way that it presents an abundance of cysteinyl groups toward the protein surface, where they are acylated by the fatty acids. The lipids are mainly 18-methyleicosanoic acid, which is about 28–30 Å long. They form the hydrophobic surface region, which has been known for some time. The total thickness of

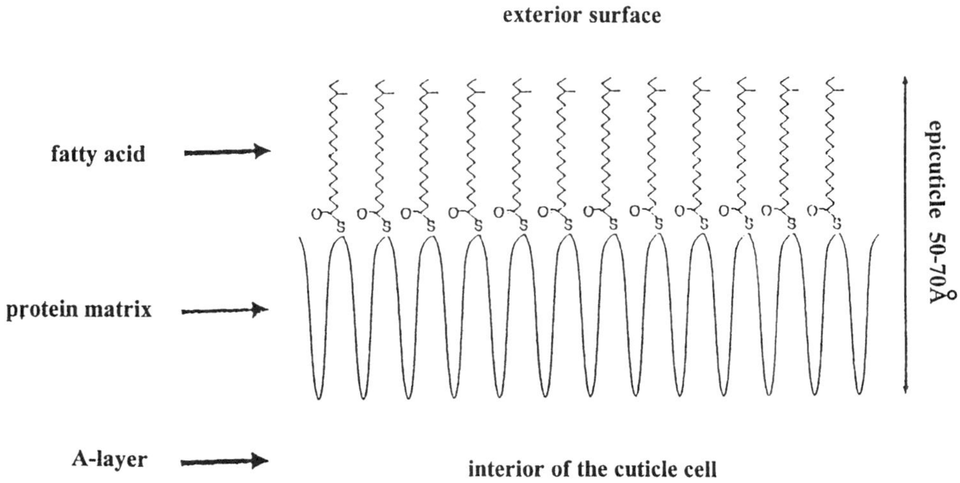

Figure 4 Model of the epicuticle of keratin fibers. Diagram represents a slice of the outer 100 Å of the cuticle cell. The protein matrix is heavily acylated with 18-methyleicosanoic acid, which forms a hydrophobic surface. (From Ref. 13.)

this layer is about 50–70 Å. Phan et al. (14), using transmission electron microscopy, on the other hand, could not find any evidence for the existence of such a layer and concluded that the Allwoerden membrane is not an additional morphological component but part of the cystine-rich A-layer.

III. EVALUATION METHODS FOR SINGLE HAIR FIBERS

In the following sections we will discuss methods for evaluating modifications of single-fiber properties by treatments with polymer solutions or dispersions of polymer-containing cosmetic formulations.

A. Surface Energy

As pointed out above, the surface energy of the intact human hair fiber is determined by the outermost layer of the epicuticle, which consists of covalently bound, long-chain fatty acids. This low-energy, hydrophobic surface is not uniformly wetted by high-surface energy liquids, such as water. In fact, the individual hair fiber will float on water, even though its density is considerably higher than that of water. The deposition of hydrophilic polymers on the hair fiber surface causes a significant increase in surface energy, which can be determined and quantified through wettability measurements.

1. Wetting Force Measurement—Immersion Method

TRI/Princeton has developed a method to determine wettability based on the Wilhelmy balance principle in which the force exerted on an individual fiber by a wetting liquid is determined (15–22). The experimental arrangement used in this method is shown schematically in Figure 5. It consists of a recording microbalance on which the fiber is mounted and a stage for raising and lowering the wetting liquid.

The forces acting on a counterbalanced single fiber immersed in water are schemati-

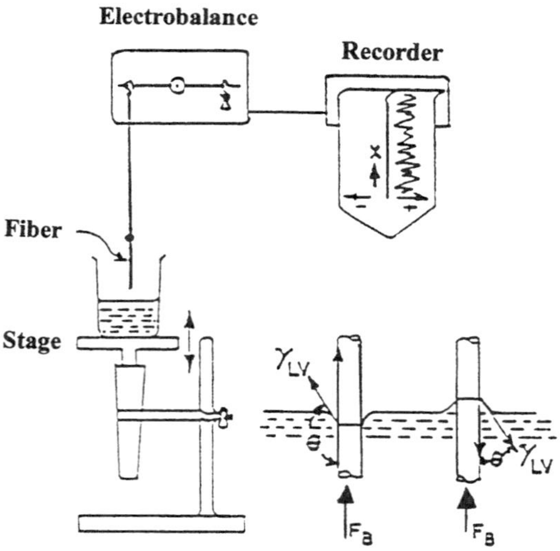

Figure 5 Apparatus for determining fiber wettability. Schematic representation of interactions between fiber and wetting liquid.

cally shown in Figure 5; two situations are shown here. In one case, corresponding to an untreated intact hair fiber, a contact angle θ larger than 90° produces a negative meniscus resulting in a negative wetting force w, which is given by

$$F_w = w - F_B$$

where F_w is the recorded force and F_B is the buoyancy force. In the second case, the contact angle is smaller than 90°, with a positive meniscus and wetting force corresponding to a high-energy surface like that of a hair fiber modified by deposition of a hydrophilic polymer. The buoyancy forces for the short immersion depths used in this method are negligible in comparison to the wetting force. If the wetted perimeter P at the line of contact between liquid and fiber is known, the wettability W is given by w/P, which is linked to the contact angle Θ through the Dupré equation:

$$W = \frac{w}{P} = \gamma_{LV} \cos\theta$$

where γ_{LV} is the surface tension of the wetting liquid.

The perimeter of the fiber is calculated from the approximate relation

$$P = 2\pi \left(\frac{A^2 + B^2}{2} \right)^{1/2}$$

where A and B are the major and minor half-axes of the fiber and can be determined by laser micrometry.

Another parameter that is frequently used is the work of adhesion A between the fiber and the liquid, which is given by

$$A = \gamma_{LV}(1 + \cos\theta) = W + \gamma_{LV}$$

The manner of deposition, the uniformity, and the substantivity of polymer deposits can be characterized by scanning the wettability along the length of the fiber before and after the treatment. Multiple immersions in the wetting liquid or in the other liquids intended to remove the deposits provide the required information. Typical wetting force curves after treatment (dip coating for 15 min without subsequent rinsing) with a 1% solution of the cationic Polymer JR-400 (a quaternized cellulose derivative, which is typical for polymeric compounds used in conditioner formulations) are shown in Figure 6.

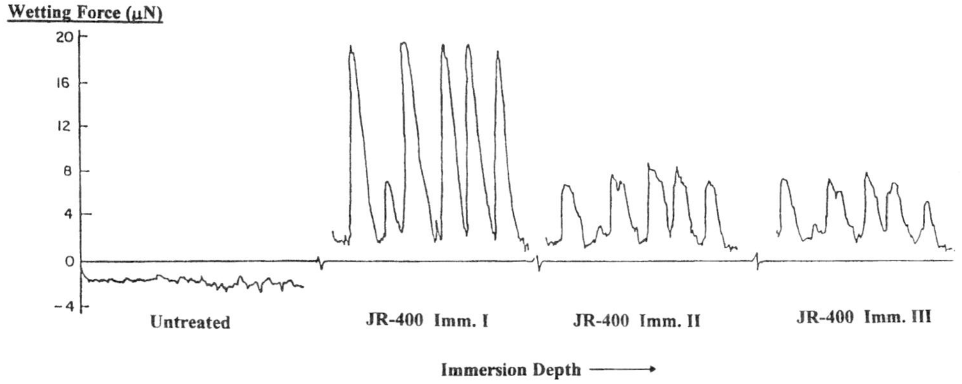

Figure 6 Advancing wetting force curves in successive immersions of untreated hair fiber and the same hair fiber treated with 1% JR-400.

The wetting force scan for the untreated fiber shows minor irregularites due to the scale structure and the usual chemical heterogeneity of the fiber surface. Immersion in the Polymer JR-400 solution has resulted in a very spotty deposition of the polymer, as can be seen in the wetting force curve during the first immersion in water. The second immersion in water of the same region of the fiber shows a significant reduction in the wetting force peaks, indicating a loss of hydrophilic material from the fiber surface and a reduction in the size of the hydrophilic domains. No further desorption appears to occur as indicated by the essentially unchanged scan during the third immersion.

Interactions between surfactant anions and the polymeric cation not only influence the solution properties of the two compounds, but also affect the nature of their deposition on the fiber surface. Averages (16 measurements each) of advancing wettabilities of fibers treated with 15 solutions of JR-400 containing increasing concentrations of sodium lauryl sulfate show high levels of deposition with low substantivity up to the critical micelle concentration (CMC) of the lauryl sulfate, at which point wettability decreases, especially after the third immersion. This decrease to values below that of the untreated fiber indicates a reorientation of the surfactant-polymer complex resulting in a hydrophobic fiber surface.

This phenomenon is even more pronounced for mixtures of JR-400 with Texapon N-25 (an anionic surfactant, PEG ether sulfate), which produce fibers with such hydrophobicity that at 2% Texapon N-25 they cannot be measured accurately, as indicated in Figure 7b by the dashed line.

2. *Wettability Measurement—Liquid Membrane Method*

Most studies of the surface wettability of fibers by the Wilhelmy balance method use relatively short specimens because of the difficulty of immersing long fibers vertically in the liquid. In an effort to overcome this disadvantage of the bulk immersion method, TRI has developed the liquid membrane method for the scanning of long filaments (23). The experimental arrangement for this method is shown schematically in Figure 8.

A stainless steel wire loop of 5–10 mm Ø is mounted on a stage that can be moved up or down at a given speed by a rack-and-pinion mechanism and a constant-speed motor. The fiber (up to 300 mm long) is taken through the ring and a wetting liquid (usually water, but other liquids or surfactant solutions can be used) is then introduced into the ring to form a film or membrane within its perimeter. As the ring moves up or down the fiber, the wetting force is continuously measured. In contrast to the immersion technique, liquid membrane scanning involves contact of the fiber with two liquid surfaces, and the force recorded is thus a function of both the advancing and receding wetting forces. The net force is given by

$$F = P\gamma_{LV}(\cos\theta_a - \cos\theta_r)$$

Assuming that $\cos\theta_r$, determined in a separate immersion experiment, does not vary along the fiber allows us to calculate $\cos\theta_a$ as a function of position along the fiber length. Typical scans along a hair fiber treated with a solution containing 0.5% cationic cellulose ether and 14% sodium laureth sulfate are shown in Figure 9 for oxidized and unoxidized hair (24).

These wettability methods can show that compounds have been deposited on the hair surface, providing information about surface coverage and substantivity, but they cannot quantify the amount of material that has been deposited, i.e., the film thickness of the deposit. For such a measurement, we can get help from an optical method, microspectrophotometry/microfluorometry, which will be discussed below.

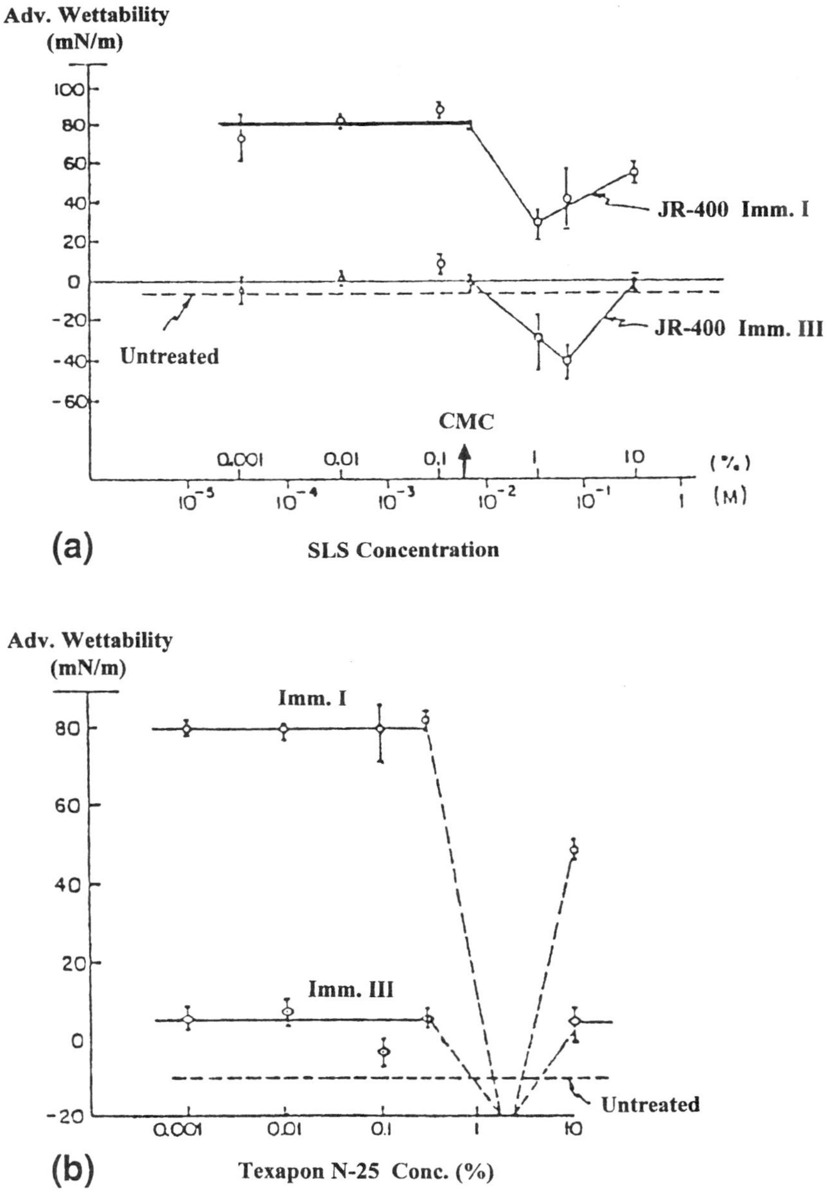

Figure 7 Advancing wettability of hair fibers treated with 1% JR-400 solutions containing various concentrations of (a) sodium lauryl sulfate, (b) Texapon N-25.

B. Dynamic Electrokinetic and Permeability Analysis (DEPA)

Streaming potential measurements have been used extensively to characterize surface properties of fibers (25), and this technique has been applied to analyze the effects of shampoos and conditioners on hair by a number of authors (26–28). Jachowicz and his co-workers developed new instrumentation for this purpose, which permits the simultaneous determination of electrokinetic and permeability parameters on hair fiber plugs. DEPA is

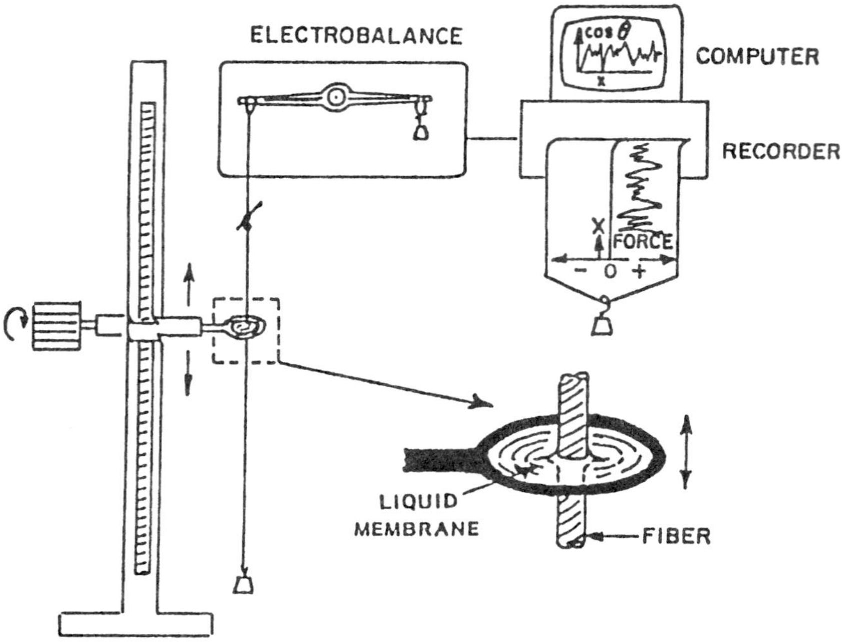

Figure 8 Experimental arrangement for fiber wettability scanning by the liquid membrane method.

a method that provides information about the interactions between the active components of shampoo and conditioner formulations and hair, and it is being used to "fingerprint" cosmetic formulations as a means of determining their ability to modify hair fiber surfaces. The instrument consists of a streaming potential cell, a conductivity meter, a pressure transducer, test and treatment solution reservoirs, a flow interruptor, an electronic balance, and several electric and manual valves for flow control through the measurement cell.

Jachowicz describes the key features of his instrument as follows: "a) on-line positioning of test and treatment-solution reservoirs, allowing fiber treatment within the streaming potential cell, b) the pulse method of measuring the streaming potential (the timing of the pulses is effected by the flow interruptors), c) simultaneous measurement of the streaming potential, conductivity, and the flow rate (permeability of the plug), d) special software allowing flexible design of the experiment, i.e., timing of treatment and test cycles, control of pressure, control of timing of the flow interruptor, forward and backward flow of the solutions through the plug, and data collection."

One gram of hair is packed into the cell, forming a plug with a density of 0.58 g hair/cm^3. The DEPA parameters of zeta potential, flow rate, and conductivity are determined by pulsing the test solution (dilute KCl) through the new hair plug prior to treatment in the cell, followed by five pulses with the treatment solution. The measurement phase of the treated hair plug consists of another series of pulses with the dilute KCl solution. On-line retreatment can be used to determine buildup or shampoo rinsing effectiveness.

The ζ-potential provides information about charges on the fiber surface, while conductivity depends on the presence of free ions in the test solution. Flow rate is a reflection of the permeability of the plug, which is affected by the swelling or shrinking of the fibers

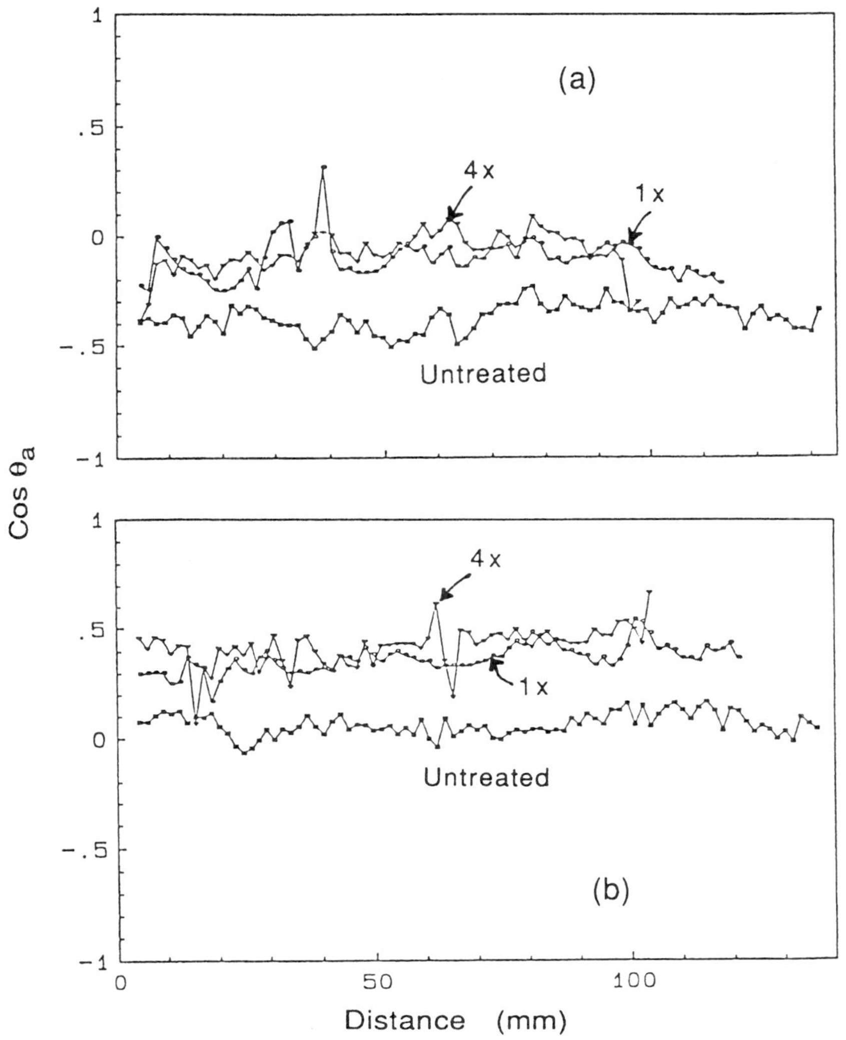

Figure 9 Typical wettability scans of (a) unoxidized and (b) oxidized hair fibers after single or multiple treatments with the formulation containing 0.5% CCE.

or by surfactant or polymer deposition on the fiber surface. A typical DEPA output for treatments with three different conditioners (28) is shown in Figure 10, where changes in the three parameters are shown as a function of time. The initial data points on these plots are the responses of the untreated hair plug to five pulses with the test solution.

The conditioner formulations C, D, and E are designed for damaged/dyed, regular, and fine hair, respectively. The most dramatic surface modification results from treatment with conditioner C, which precipitates a thick layer of conditioning agents on the hair fiber surface, as indicated by the large drop in flow rate, and also reverses the charge on the surface. This surface charge change to positive is maintained during prolonged rinsing. The flow rate increases slightly during rinsing, suggesting contraction of the adsorbed layer of the conditioner or possibly some desorption. Conditioner D also deposits a thick

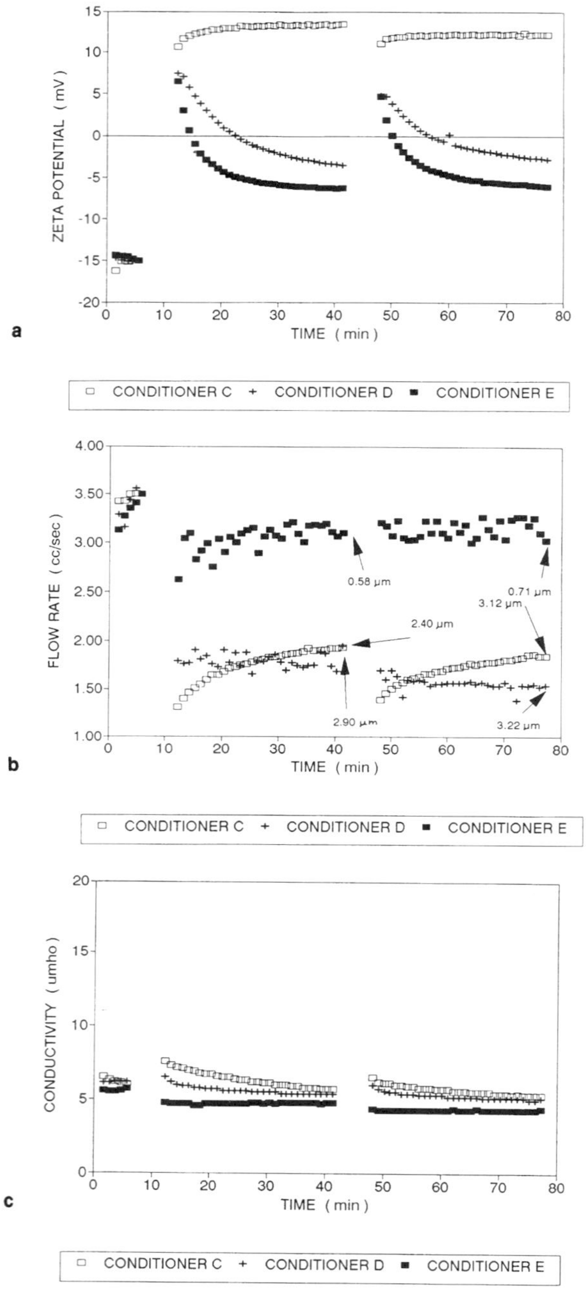

Figure 10 Zeta potential (a), flow rate (b), and conductivity (c) as a function of time for hair treated with 1.0% w/w solutions of conditioners F, G, and H. (From Ref. 28.)

layer on the fiber surface, which remains unaffected by rinsing even though the charge reverts back to negative during rinsing, suggesting some desorption. Conditioner E shows the least extent of surface modification. For detailed information of the composition of these three conditioners, see Ref. 28.

Frequent use of conditioners can lead to residual buildup of polymer or surfactant residues, which requires shampoos capable of removing them. DEPA experiments involving alternating treatments of conditioner and shampoo can establish the effectiveness of the shampoo designed for this purpose. Figure 11 shows an experiment in which the hair plug is first treated with a 1% solution of a conditioner containing various substantive ingredients such as behenyltrimethylammonium chloride (BTC), a cationic silicone emulsion, and polyquaternium-11; then, after the measurement cycle the plug is pulsed five times with a 5% solution of the shampoo. The process is repeated once to establish buildup after a conditioning/shampooing cycle.

The data show that the shampoo is capable of removing most of the deposited conditioner for which a film thickness of 3.56 μm was calculated after the first treatment. However, a residual film is left (0.71 μm) after shampooing. Adsorption of anionic moieties during shampooing, which gradually desorb during rinsing, contributes to the reversal of the positive charge after conditioning. These two examples of the application of DEPA clearly demonstrate the usefulness of the method in characterizing the interactions between various cosmetic formulations, specifically conditioners and hair.

C. Microfluorometry

Fluorescent reagents or dyes are employed as specific indicators for the presence of a charged or reactive group, or they are being used to determine the rate and extent of diffusion into fiber cross-sections where absorbence measurements are not sufficiently sensitive. Fluorescent tracers have also been used extensively for semiquanitative characterization of surface deposits on natural and synthetic fibers (29–39). This method is based on the observation that incorporation of a fluororescent compound into certain surface deposits, particularly of a micellar structure, protects it from deactivation processes and leads to an increase in quantum efficiency Φ. Quantum efficiency is defined in terms of the rate constants for fluorescence activation k_f and the combined rate constants for deactivation processes k_d:

$$\Phi = \frac{k_f}{k_f - k_d}$$

Deactivation processes are associated with the return of the excited molecule to the ground state without fluorescence emission. Any interactions with the environment that protect the excited molecules from deactivation, or at least decrease the rate at which deactivation occurs, increase quantum efficiency. On this basis we have incorporated fluorescent dyes to estimate the amount of polymer-containing complexes or their film thickness on the hair fiber surface, as will be discussed below.

1. Measurement Method

The instruments used for quantitative determinations of fluorescence on fiber surfaces are microspectrophotometers equipped for incident light illumination, such as the Zeiss UMSP-80 FL, whose light path is shown in Figure 12. The instrument has a monochromator for incident illumination and excitation of the fluorochrome. The emission spectrum

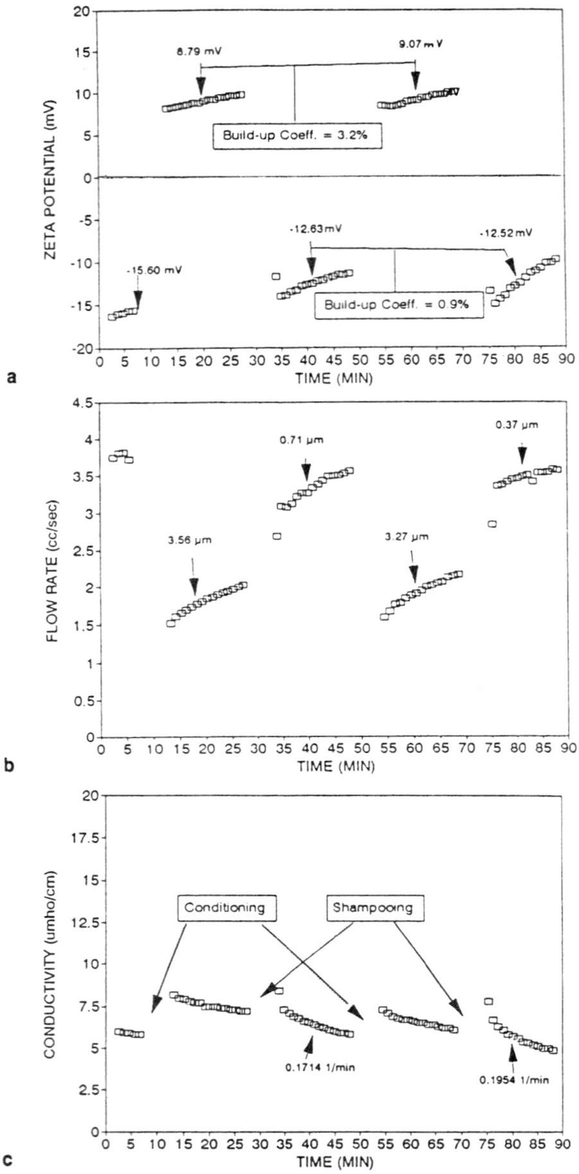

Figure 11 Zeta potential (a), flow rate (b), and conductivity (c) as a function of time for two consecutive applications of conditioner I and a shampoo. (From Ref. 28.)

resulting from the excitation at various wavelengths can be resolved by a monochromator on the image side.

The excitation beam is projected onto the specimen, which is mounted on a movable scanning stage. The size of the emission beam that enters the photometer is controlled by a variable measuring diaphragm, and its size and shape are determined by the available fluorescence intensity. The scanning mode across a longitudinally mounted fiber treated with a fluorochrome is shown in Figure 13, where a narrow slit parallel to the fiber axis

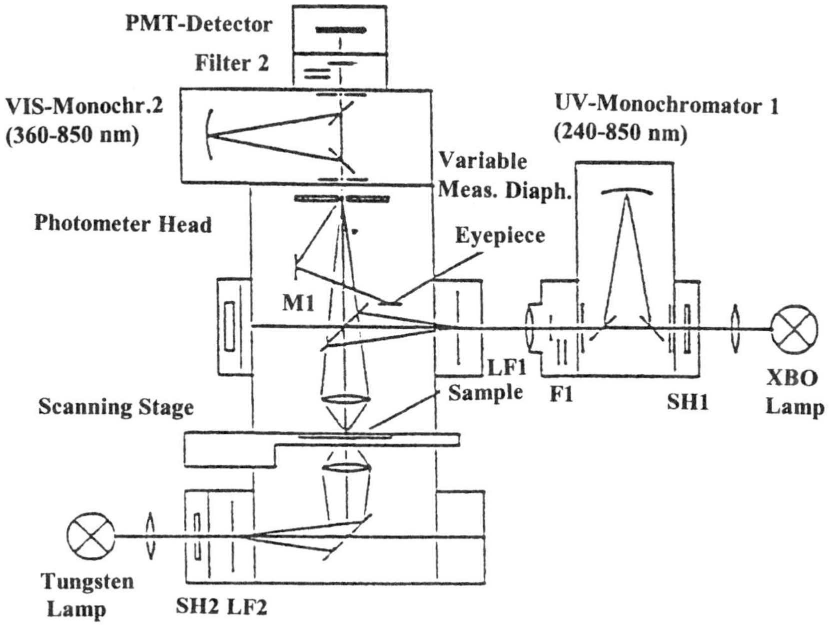

Figure 12 Schematic drawing of the Zeiss UMSP-80 microspectrophotometer for incident illumination and fluorescence intensity measurements. LF, luminous field stop; SH, shutter; F, filter.

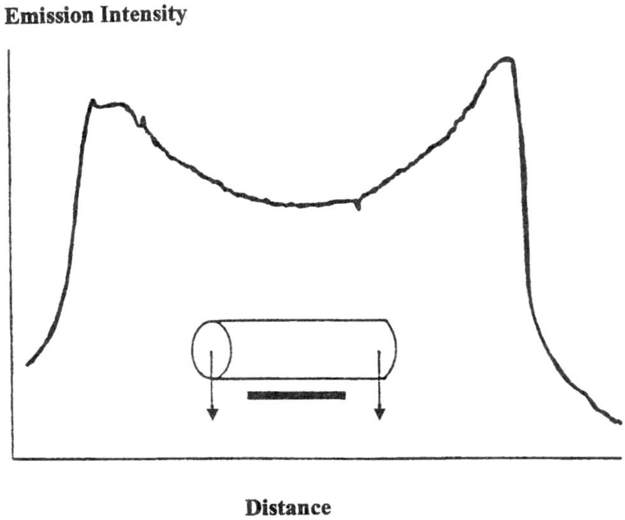

Figure 13 Microfluorometric scan, using a narrow slit parallel to the fiber axis, across a longitudinally mounted round nylon 66 fiber treated uniformly with CIFB-113. (From Ref. 37.)

is used. The scan shows a considerable increase of fluorescence near the edge of the fiber, as predicted by a theoretical analysis discussed by Kamath et al. (37).

Two different scanning modes are used for continuous measurements of fluorescence intensity along a fiber. For detailed information about the distribution of a substance deposited on the fiber surface a small beam is focused on the dome of the fiber. The fiber is moved through this beam providing a representative distribution pattern for that location on the fiber. The second scanning mode employs a slit of the measuring diaphragm wide enough to cover the diameter of the fiber; it yields an average fluorescence intensity profile as a function of position along the length of the fiber. With this procedure, focusing problems exist at higher magnification and the information is less accurate because of the edge distortion, discussed in more detail in Ref. 37 and 38. Another potential source of error in both scanning modes is the contribution of fluorescence from the opposite side of the fiber (32,39).

An example of the application of microfluorometry to the important question of polymer buildup in multiple treatments (24) is given in the following discussion. The hair was treated with the following formulation:

Cationic cellulose ether (CCE) 2%, 0.5%
Sodium laureth sulfate, 14%
Demineralized water
pH 6.3

The formulation was tagged by incorporating 0.1% uranine (sodium salt of fluorescein, CIAY-73). The fibers were scanned for a distance of 1.35 mm with a 5 μm × 5 μm beam focused on the dome of the fiber. Typical intensity scans are shown in Figure 14 after one and five applications with one or five rinses. The scans clearly indicate that the formulation

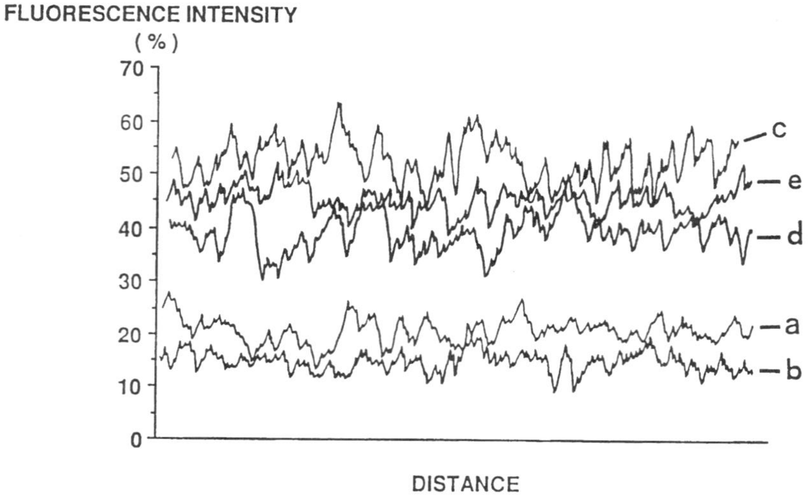

Figure 14 Typical fluorescence intensity scans of hair fibers after various treatment and rinsing procedures with the formulation containing 2% CCE: (a) one application, one rinse; (b) one application, five rinses; (c) five applications, one rinse; (d) five applications, five rinses; (e) five applications, five rinses, retagged (2. tag), rinsed. (From Ref. 24.)

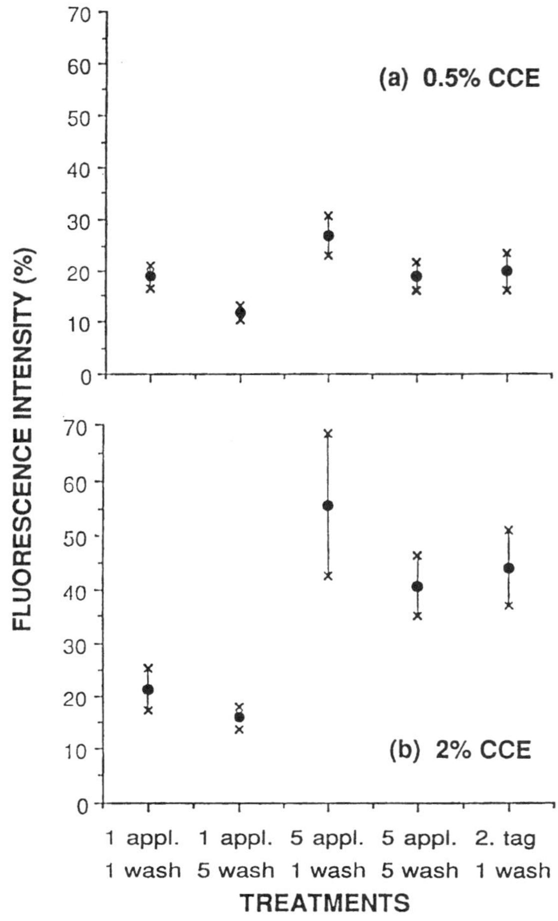

Figure 15 Average fluorescence intensities of hair fibers after treatment and rinsing procedures with the formulations containing (a) 0.5% CCE and (b) 2% CCE. (From Ref. 24.)

produces buildup in multiple applications with rinsing between treatments. Average values of fluorescence intensity are shown in Figure 15, comparing the effect of cationic polymer concentration.

D. Intercuticular Cohesion

Damage to the cuticular layer of the hair shaft due to various grooming processes is a well-known and rather common occurrence and can eventually lead to total loss of the cuticle, resulting in the formation of ''split ends.'' If it were possible to measure the intactness of the cuticle sheath, one could establish the extent of such damage and find a way to determine the effectiveness of potential treatments that might prevent further damage. We have developed a method to at least semiquantitatively measure intercuticular cohesion in the outermost cuticle layer (3,4). We could show that upon fiber extension scale-lifting phenomena occur at characteristic extension levels, which we feel result from unrelieved shear stresses that are building up as the fiber is being extended. These shear stresses develop owing to differences in the deformability of the various layers of each cuticle cell, leading to failure at the scale edge either in the endocuticular layer or in the intercuticular domain, i.e., in the cell membrane complex. As a result of this failure, the outermost scale lifts, and this phenomenon can be used as an indication of the extent of the relative intercuticular cohesion. Scale lifting is associated with increases in fluorescence upon UV excitation and can be directly observed under a fluorescence microscope.

1. Measurement Method

The fiber is mounted on an extension frame and slowly extended under ambient conditions (~50% RH, room temperature) while being observed in a fluorescence microscope with UV excitation (nonpolarized light, 340–380 nm). The extension level is determined at which certain ''stress release'' phenomena occur, such as: the onset of scale lifting, common scale lifting, extreme scale lifting, and finally, fiber failure. Comparisons between the scale-lifting behavior of the root and the tip ends of the fiber indicate that grooming and weathering have directly affected intercuticular cohesion, leading to shifts of scale-lifting phenomena to lower extension levels for the tip section of the fiber. While scale lifting as such can be reversed upon release of the fiber from extension and immersion in water, considerably lower extension levels at which various phenomena occur in a second extension reflect the extent of irreversible damage inflicted during the initial extension.

Deposition of polymeric or monomeric cationic conditioner ingredients on the fiber surface or conceivably their partial penetration into the surface layers of the fiber has a strong effect on intercuticular cohesion. For example, as shown in Figure 16b, 10 sequential 2-min treatments with a 0.5% solution of JR-400, with appropriate rinsing, virtually eliminate most scale-lifting phenomena or at least shift them to higher extension levels. In the fibers where scale lifting occurs, it now involves the intercuticular domains or the CMC as the weakest link during the shearing deformation in the cuticula. Alternatives to scale lifting as a means of stress release in the cuticula during fiber extension are radial cracks that form at very high extensions and penetrate the whole cuticular layer down to the cortex. SEM micrographs of extended fibers that have been transferred without release to metal stubs are shown in Figure 17 for some of the characteristic phenomena observed. However, semiquanitative comparisons between treated and untreated fibers or between treatments are based on real-time observations under ambient conditions in a fluorescence microscope.

E. Frictional Properties

One of the important properties that can be affected by topical treatments with polymer-containing formulations is friction. Both interfiber and fiber-comb friction play a major part in grooming and manageability considerations for human hair. It is not just the ease of combing or brushing that is important for consumer perception of a product, but also the secondary effects resulting from contact with grooming implements. Directly correlatable with combing forces are electrostatic charge buildup (flyaway), which will be covered in a different section, and cuticle abrasion or ablation. In other words, the ''health'' or intactness of the hair fibers and with it their lifetimes can be directly affected by polymer deposition. On the other hand, interfiber friction and adhesion are also important for hair body and volume and other aesthetic or ''psychophysical'' properties of hair. The distinction between these two frictional properties is to a considerable extent determined by the contact force between fiber and comb or fiber and fiber during measurement.

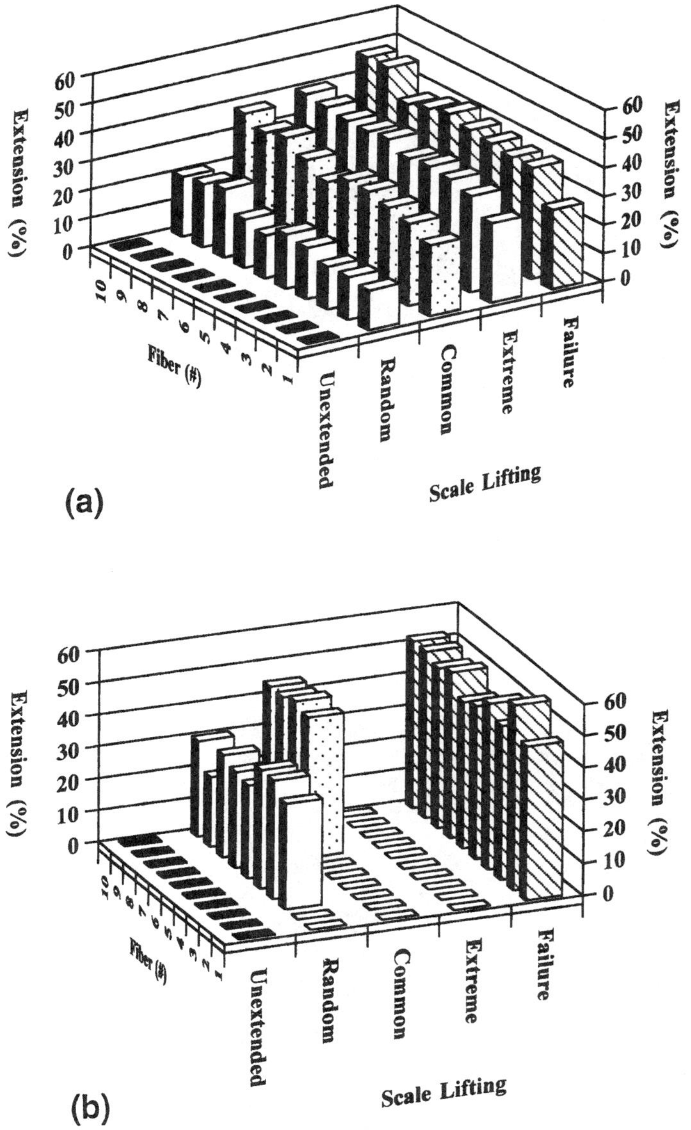

Figure 16 Distribution of extensions at which scale lifting is observed during longitudinal extension of (a) untreated hair fibers and (b) hair fibers exposed to 10 applications of JR-400.

1. Fiber-Capstan Friction

The fiber-capstan method involves draping or wrapping a weighted fiber over or around a reference rod as a means of increasing the contact area. In the method described by Scott and Robbins (40), the root end of the fiber is attached to the load cell of the Instron Tensile Tester; the fiber is then partially wrapped around two mandrels (one of which can be rotated) mounted on the Instron crosshead, as shown in Figure 18. A load of 1 g is attached to the tip end of the fiber. A similar version with a nonrotating mandrel is used at TRI, where the capstans are mounted on the Instron crosshead and can be

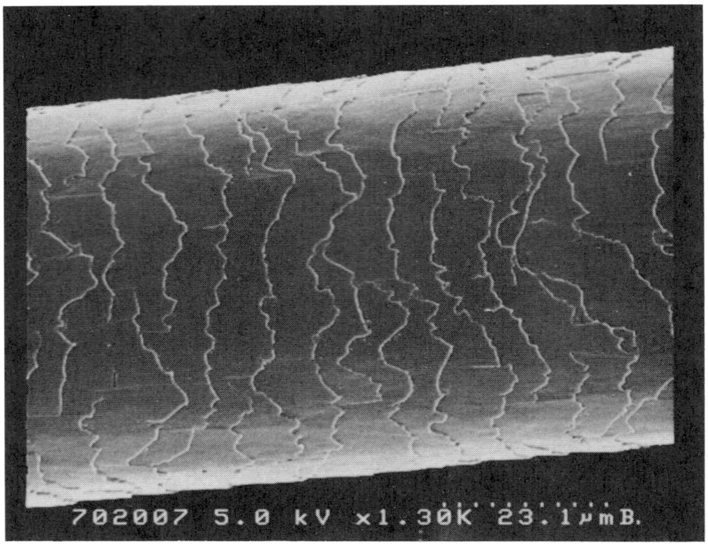

(a)

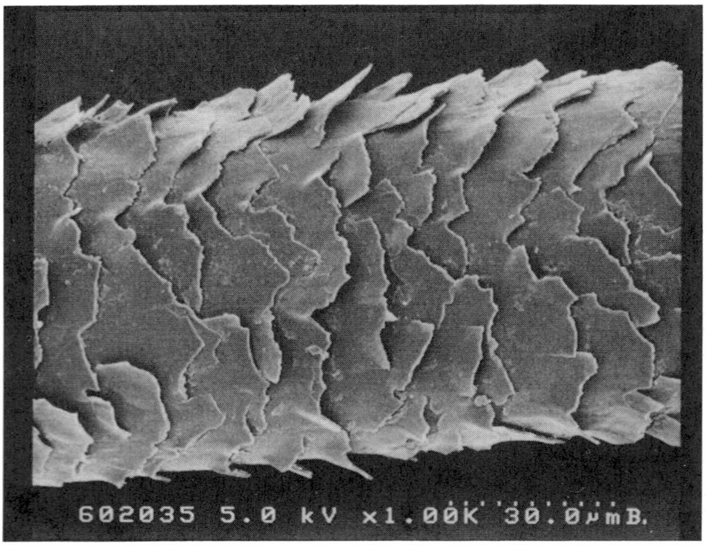

(b)

Figure 17 Scale lifting during extension of untreated hair fiber. (a) Unextended; (b) extended ~30%.

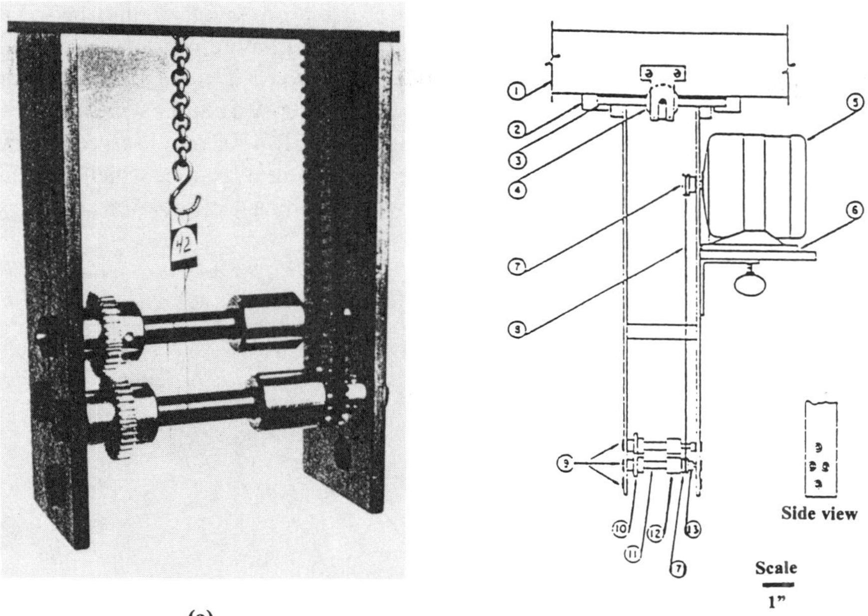

(a) (b)

Figure 18 (a) Photograph of apparatus; (b) schematic of apparatus. 1, Crosshead; 2, support blocks; 3, hanger plate; 4, screw assembly for positioning hanger plate; 5, motor; 6, hinged platform for tensioning belt; 7, geared pulleys; 8, drive belt; 9, flanged bearings; 10, geared couplings; 11, mandrels; 12, sleeve couplings; 13, set screw collars. (From Ref. 40.)

immersed in a liquid medium. As the crosshead moves downward, the frictional force is recorded.

The angle subtended by the line of contact is π for each capstan. The coefficient of friction μ can be calculated from

$$\mu = \frac{2.303}{2\pi \times \log T_1/T_2}$$

where T_1 is the frictional force and T_2 is the load on the fiber.

Frictional forces and coefficients of friction depend to a considerable extent on relative humidity, or in extreme cases on the presence of water. We are distinguishing between three conditions for frictional measurements: ambient (65% RH), wet-with-water (www, the fiber is taken directly from the bath to the friction measurement), and wet-in-water (wiw, friction measurement in a liquid bath). There is also a significant effect of the nature of the capstan material. Hard rubber produces a higher coefficient of friction than aluminium, an effect that is more pronounced in the wet state (41). Similarly, the surface of the hair, especially its hydrophilicity, affects its frictional behavior. Bleaching and permanent-waving treatments increase frictional forces (40). In both cases, scission of disulfide bonds in the outer layer of the cuticle leads to a softening of the surface, resulting in an increase in the area of real contact.

The deposition of polymeric materials on the fiber surface, e.g., in the form of creme rinses containing cationic polymer, lowers the coefficient of friction, especially for bleached hair. The latter observation is a reflection of the stronger interactions between cationic polymers and a fiber surface (42) that is progressively more negatively charged as bleaching levels increase. We made an interesting observation at TRI after the treatment with Polymer JR-400 (43). If a hair fiber treated with JR-400 was sliding in the www condition against a glass capstan that was also treated with JR-400, we observed a very pronounced stick-slip phenomenon in the against-scale-sliding direction, which we did not observe in the with-scale direction (Fig. 19). A ''ploughing'' effect of scale edges

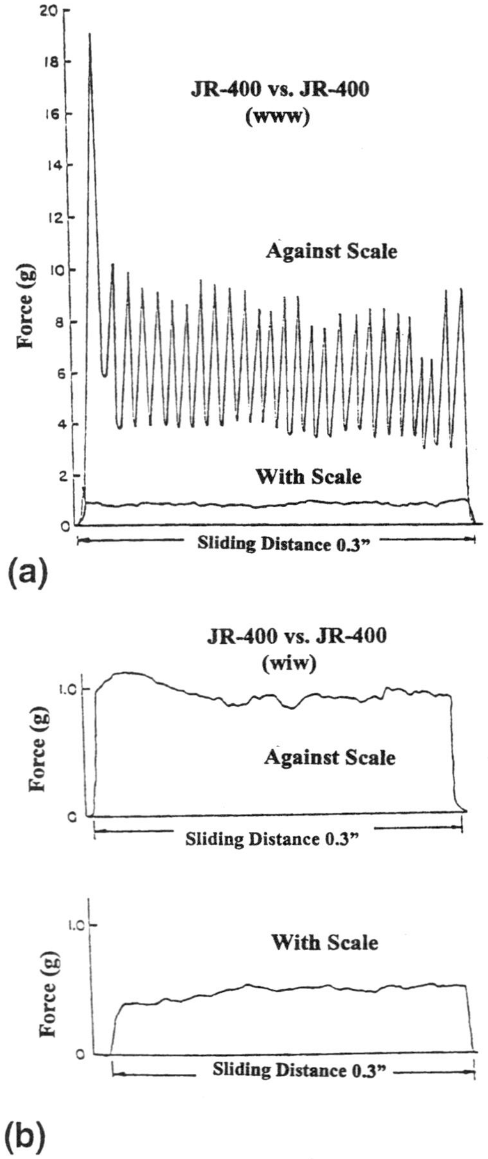

Figure 19 Frictional force curve of human hair treated with Polymer JR-400 against a capstan treated with the same polymer. (a) Wet with water (www); (b) wet in water (wiw).

into the water-swollen polymer film on the capstan may be involved. This seems to indicate that while polymer deposition on the fiber surface does lower friction against a hard surface, this may not necessarily be the case against soft surfaces with the appropriate implications for combability.

2. *Interfiber Friction at High Contact Force*

While fiber-capstan friction reflects the sliding of a comb through a hair mass, interfiber friction is actually the major contributor to the total combing force. Comb-hair friction is a major component to the ''midlength'' force but only a minor (~10%) component to the ''end-peak'' force that dominates the total combing force. The end-peak force arises from fiber entanglements that are removed by fibers sliding over each other, a process that is described by interfiber frictional behavior. The magnitude of the normal force acting at contact points between fibers within the entanglement is not known, and we have assumed an approximate value of ~100 mg per contact point.

Interfiber friction can be measured by the ''twist'' method of Lindberg and Gralen (44), which uses a twisted configuration as a means of increasing the contact area between two fibers. Fair and Gupta (45) developed a modification of that method by involving frictionless pulleys and a tensile tester; it showed good correlations with changes in hair morphology and various chemical treatments such as reduction, oxidation/bleaching, and dyeing.

An apparatus for measuring interfiber friction involving relatively well-defined contact forces in the range mentioned above for entanglements has been designed at TRI (43) and is shown in Figure 20. The method uses a fiber arrangement similar to that in a procedure reported by Pascoe and Tabor (46), consisting of a horizontal fiber mounted on a bow that slides against a vertical fiber mounted on the Instron crosshead with a 1-g weight and restrained laterally by a pulley.

The horizontal fiber is moved sideways to make contact with the vertical fiber, producing an angle of $\phi = 10°$. Under these conditions the force at the contact point can be calculated from $F = w \sin \phi$ to be ~100 mg. The frictional force is measured as the horizontal fiber is sliding down by moving the crosshead downward. Various configurations of fiber contact can be achieved by tilting the bow and reversing the orientation of the vertical fiber, as shown in Figure 20 (b), where the resulting frictional forces measured at 65% RH are indicated.

3. *Interfiber Friction at Low Contact Force*

Another very important frictional behavior at much lower contact forces measures fiber-fiber interactions associated with hair body and style retention. Robbins (47) discusses a method for determining dry static friction at low load (~1 mg) by using a modification of the incline plane fiber loop method of Howell and Mazur (48). In this procedure, the angle of slip is measured at which a small hair loop sitting on two parallel hair fibers begins to slide. At these low-contact loads, the interaction between deposited films on the fiber surface and the adhesive properties between them becomes important.

TRI has developed a different method for low-load friction (43), which uses a modification of the interfiber frictional apparatus mentioned above. In this instrument, the force-measuring device is a Kahn recording microbalance on which the vertical fiber is mounted. The horizontal fiber can be moved by a micrometer to establish the exact angle of deflection between the fibers. The system is shown schematically in Figure 21. The apparatus is an attachment to the TRI/SCAN surface force analyzer, which was described earlier in the discussion of wetting force measurements with the appropriate software.

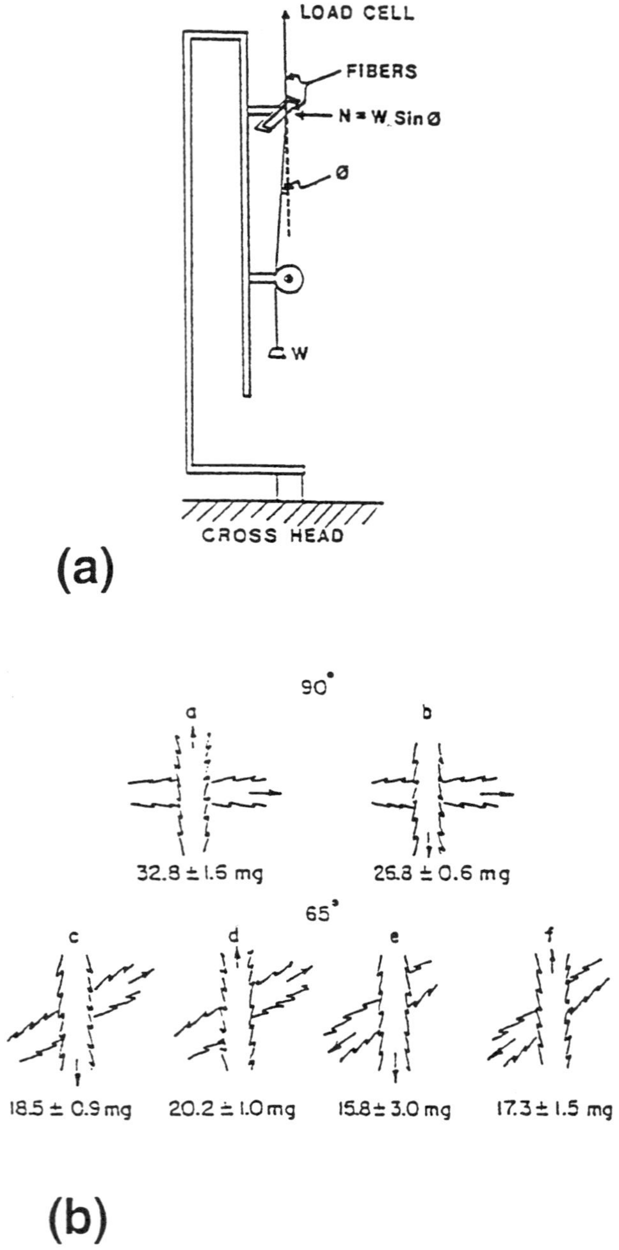

Figure 20 (a) Schematic drawing of apparatus for measuring interfiber friction. (b) Schematic drawing of different configurations of fibers used in the measurement of interfiber friction. Arrows point in direction of scales. Frictional force is the average of five measurements at the 95% confidence limit.

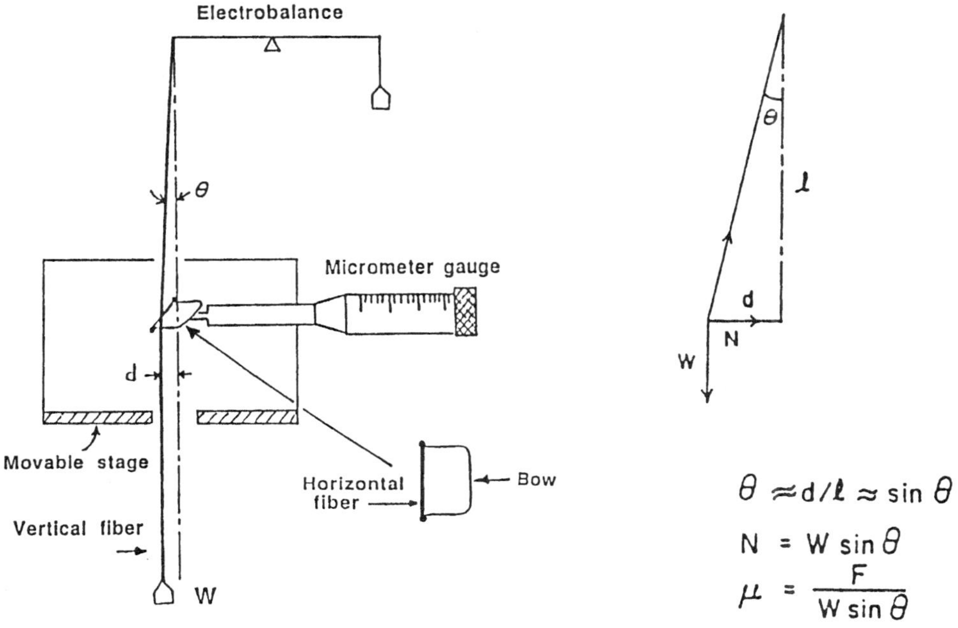

Figure 21 Apparatus for low-load friction measurements.

F. Interfiber Adhesion

Interfiber adhesive forces play an important role in various deformation modes of fiber assemblies, such as bending and compression. During such deformation fibers slip past one another at the points of contact to minimize the extent of deformation of individual fibers. The efficiency with which this is achieved depends on interterfiber adhesion forces at contact points. The apparatus developed at TRI for measuring interfiber adhesion is shown schematically in Figure 22. One of the fibers is fastened to a bow, which in turn is mounted on the weighing arm of a Kahn electrobalance, while the other fiber is hung over two glass rods with two equal weights at the ends to keep it taut. The fibers are brought in contact with each other with a predetermined contact load by raising the supporting platform. After a specific contact time, the platform is lowered until contact between the fibers is broken and the separation force is recorded.

While untreated hair fibers show no adhesion forces at contact forces of ~2 mg, treatment of both fibers with JR-400 produces high adhesion forces with considerable nonuniformity along their length, as shown in Figure 23. This nonuniformity with position must be attributed to the nonuniform distribution of the polymer on the fiber surfaces, which we have observed repeatedly in wettability measurements. Rinsing off the polymer again leads to a total lack of adhesive interactions, indicating almost complete removal of the polymer. The apparatus is another attachment to the TRI/SCAN Surface Force Analyzer.

Another method developed at TRI for interfiber adhesion is a pull-out technique in which a fiber is displaced for a distance of 5 mm within a hair fiber bundle of well-defined packing density. The pull-out technique utilizes another attachment to the TRI/SCAN surface force analyzer.

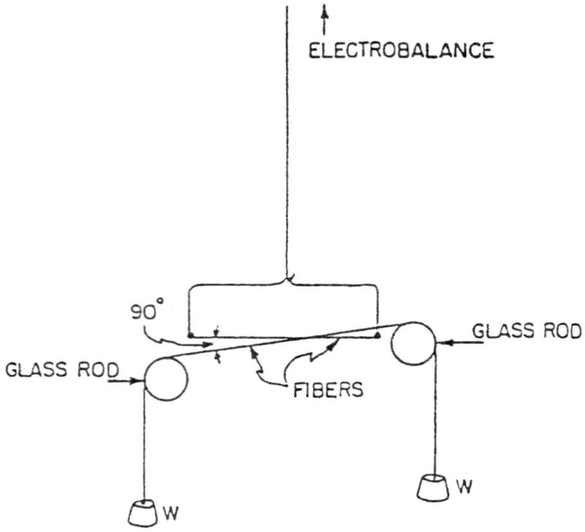

Figure 22 Apparatus to measure interfiber adhesion.

IV. EVALUATION METHODS FOR HAIR ASSEMBLIES

A. Hair Manageability

Polymer deposition is an important aspect of conditioner treatments as far as hair manageability is concerned. The effects of such treatments on a number of hair assembly properties determine "the ease of arranging hair in place and its temporary ability to stay in place," a definition of the term "hair manageability" introduced by Robbins (49). Based on this definition, Robbins et al. (50) postulate three assembly properties that are inherent in manageability: style arrangement, style retention, and flyaway hair. The appropriate methodology for evaluating these properties will be discussed in the following sections.

B. Combing Forces

One of the most frequently used grooming methods is combing, which is the most important aspect of "style arrangement"; it constitutes essentially an effort to render parallel hair fibers, and frequently involves a prior detangling process. During combing, the fibers are exposed to considerable frictional stresses, which can lead to surface abrasion and ablation of cuticle layers. In an extreme case, this results in the total loss of the cuticle, decrease of the intercellular cohesion within the cortex, and finally, split ends. Grooming aids are designed to facilitate combing by reducing frictional interactions and to prevent damage as a result of friction. Polymeric materials in conditioning formulations provide lubrication and thus fulfill the function of improved combability demanded by Robbins' definition (1) of a hair conditioner as "an ingredient or a product, that when applied to hair in its recommended use procedure and concentration improves the combability relative to appropriate controls."

A number of methods for determining combing forces that have been reported (51–57) are quite similar in their approach. In all cases, a comb is pulled through a hair tress and the forces or the work of combing is measured, usually with the load cell of the

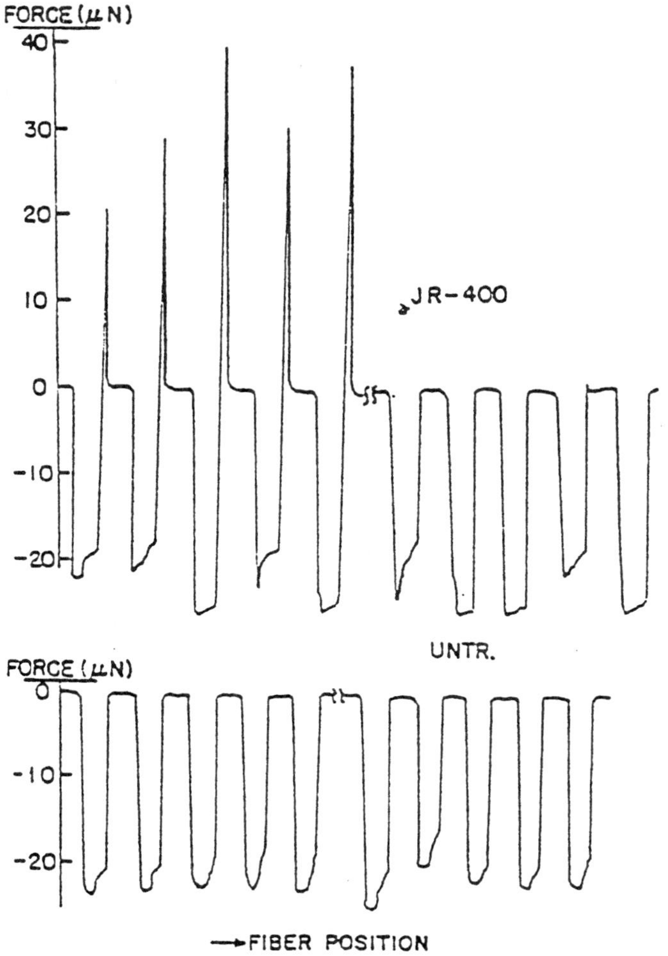

Figure 23 Adhesion force curves for untreated and JR-400-treated human hair fibers.

Instron tensile tester, although the use of a comb connected to a piezoelectric transducer (58) or a comb with a strain gauge in the handle (59) has been reported. Automation of the testing method involving robots has been reported with computerized data processing (60,61), sometimes attempting to simulate in vivo salon experiences of shampooing, rinsing, and tangling/detangling steps (62). An indirect method was developed by Waggoner and Scott (63), who pulled an electronic comb through the hair and measured the sound generated during passage as a relative measure of conditioning and combing ease. Robbins and Reich (64,65) related force and work of combing to single-fiber properties such as curvature, friction, stiffness, and diameter, using multiple regression analysis. Their analysis indicated that curvature is the most important property, whose effect increases with increasing curliness.

The parameters describing the forces encountered when a comb passes through a hair tress have been called "midlength force" (ML) and "end-peak force" (EP) by Tolgyesi et al. (52). The fundamental processes contributing to ML are interfiber friction and comb-hair friction, while EP is associated with the removal of entanglements of the free ends of the fibers and is notoriously irreproducible. Work at TRI (54) has explored the end-peak phenomenon and has established that entanglements in a hair tress that has been combed through occur during the springback of the hair tress when the tress leaves the comb and that the length of the hair tress is related to the extent of the entanglement. To overcome some of the irreproducibility we have developed the double-comb method shown schematically in Figure 24. The lower comb is not connected to the Instron load cell and serves merely as a prealignment tool. The free length of the hair tress that springs back when released from the prealignment comb is constant, which improves reproducibility of the end-peak force.

The introduction of more reproducible entanglements into the hair tress is the subject of a Dow Corning patent (66) in which the wet-combed, detangled hair is dipped into water to produce new entanglements of the free tip ends of the fibers. Another group (62) uses microprocessor-controlled robotic manipulations to entangle and disentangle hair tresses.

C. Body Evaluation

The apparent bulk that hair assumes after grooming is an important aesthetic characteristic often referred to as ''body,'' which can be considered a property associated with Robbins' term ''style retention.'' Tolgyesi and co-workers (67) proposed the following definition of this hair assembly property: ''Body is a measure of a hair mass's resistance to and recovery from externally induced deformation.'' This definition correlates well with the descriptive components ''springiness,'' ''volume,'' and ''stiffness'' that Wedderburn and Prall have obtained by applying statistical techniques to word association (58). The structural strength and resiliency of the hair mass are influenced by a number of independent parameters. Tolgyesi has identified the five most important parameters as fiber density

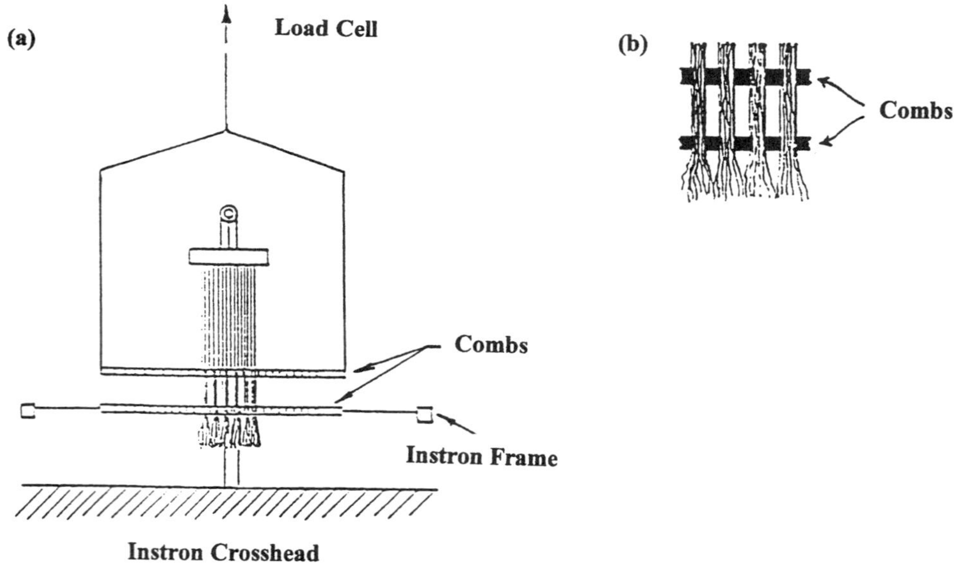

Figure 24 Schematic sketch of apparatus for measuring combing force (prealigning arrangement).

on scalp, bending and torsional stiffness and resiliency of fibers, fiber diameter, fiber configuration, and fiber-fiber interactions. Only the second, fourth, and fifth parameters can be affected by cosmetic treatments, so it is not surprising that most of the simulated tests that have been developed are sensitive to these three parameters.

1. *Omega (Ω) Loop Test*

Tolgyesi and co-workers (68) have developed a test procedure known as the ''omega'' loop test to study hair body. The test involves compressing a hair tress held in the form of the capital Greek letter omega ''Ω'' and measuring the compression forces using the Instron. This tress configuration appears to put too much emphasis on the bending of the hair mass and not enough on fiber-fiber interaction and fiber configuration. At TRI we have therefore attempted to develop a procedure giving a more balanced picture of the three parameters.

2. *TRI Radial Compression Method*

The radial compression of a hair tress entails frictional forces resisting the movement of fibers relative to each other, as well as bending deformations at a rather low level. Since the definition of the term ''body'' also contains the aspect of recovery from deformation, the hair mass has to be able to spring back under the influence of the bending modulus of the tress, overcoming any frictional resistance from fibers that have moved past one another. This recovery parameter can be measured conveniently by exposing the hair tress to multiple compression cycles. Since compaction or lack of recovery involves movement of fibers relative to each other, it is dependent on the rate of compression and especially on the time that the tress remains in the compressed state. The radial compression device used in this method (69) therefore has to be flexible in controlling these variables. As shown in Figure 25, it consists of a stand mounted on the Instron crosshead to which is connected a horseshoe bracket carrying two low friction pulleys on each end.

A hair tress of ~10 g and with a circular cross-section is clamped to the stand in such a way that it is supended between the pulleys. A string is looped around the tress above its free end, guided over the pulleys, and fastened to a rigid yoke connected to the load cell. The entire apparatus is placed in the environmental chamber of the Instron. The free end is protected from air currents by means of a cylinder that overlaps it by about 5 cm. A modification to the original apparatus takes into consideration that at low fiber densities frictional forces between string and pulley contribute significantly to the measured compression forces. In the modified version the hair tress is compressed between two semicircular brass plates, which are connected to the horseshoe bracket and pulled together by a Nomex braid (Fig. 26). The brass plates are held in the open position by two springs, so that after release of compression, the tress does not have to push back the plates and recovers without interference. The compression energy of the blank system (without a tress) is subtracted from the measurement.

The parameters that are determined by this method are sensitive to changes in tress configuration (waving) and topical treatments (conditioning, shampooing, rinsing, etc.). The term ΔE expresses the change in compression energy as the result of a treatment:

$$\Delta E_1 = (E_{1tr} - E_{1u})/E_{1u} \text{ and } \Delta E_2 = (E_{2tr} - E_{2u})/E_{2u},$$

where subscripts 1 and 2 refer to the first and second compression cycles, respectively. Multiple compression cycles are used to evaluate the ability of the tress to spring back from compression, which is an important characteristic of body. The effect of treatment

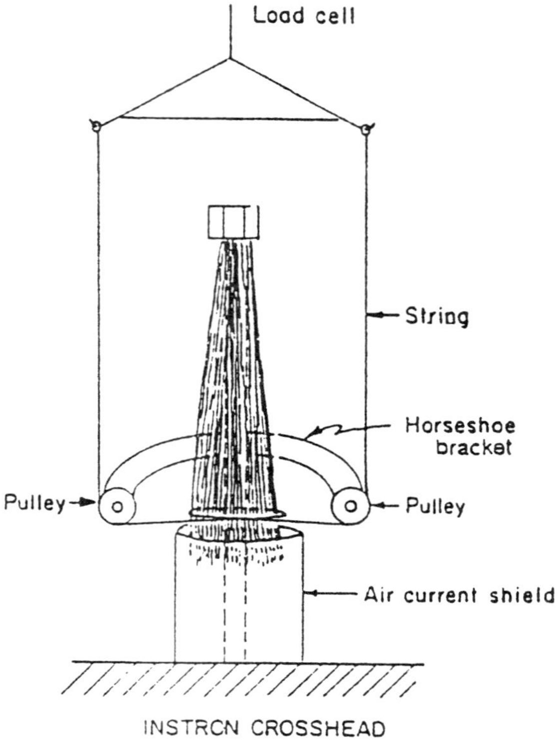

Figure 25 Apparatus for radial compression of a hair tress.

on this aspect of body is expressed by the relative energy dissipation (RED), which is defined as

$$\text{RED} = (\Delta E_1 - \Delta E_2)/(E_{1u} - E_{2u}),$$

or the fiber adhesion index (FAI), which does not relate to the behavior of the untreated tress

$$\text{FAI} = (E_{1tr} - E_{2tr})/E_{1tr}.$$

Correlations of body ratings predicted by such parameters with actual panel body ratings show a reasonable success (37).

3. Ring Compressiblity Method

Garcia and Wolfram (70) have developed a ring compression method in which a hair tress is pulled through an aluminum ring of a defined diameter and the forces generated are measured on the Instron. The ring compression apparatus is shown in Figure 27.

The recorded forces, or the "work of passage" (WP), are proportional to the resistance to radial compression. In addition, the proportionality factor depends on the shape or surface contour of the hair tress and on frictional interactions between the fibers and the inner surface of the ring. As a result of bundle compression, the contact force between fibers and ring increases continuously and with it the frictional component of WP. TRI has used a modification of this method in which a larger prealignment ring is positioned

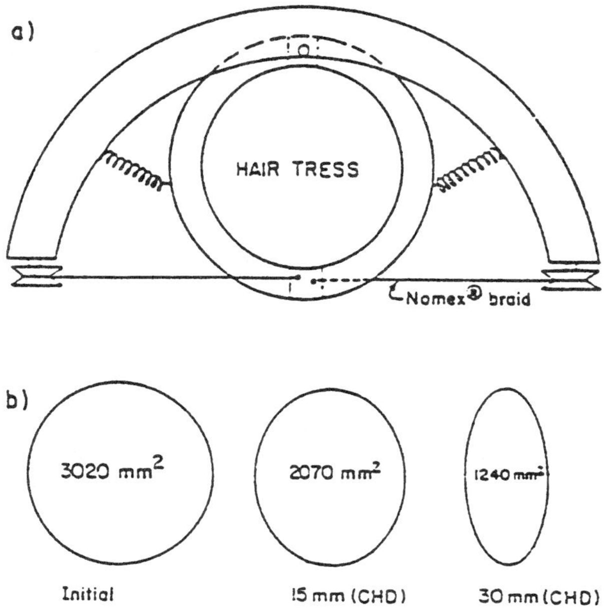

Figure 26 Modified compressibility apparatus. (a) Schematic diagram. (b) Cross-sectional shape of the tress in the plane of compression.

before the measuring ring, so that the angle of contact between fibers and measuring ring is always the same. A vibrator is used to eliminate some of the fiber-ring friction. Resilience of the hair tress is determined by measuring WP before and after multiple passes through the measuring ring. Treatment effects are established on the same hair tress before and after treatment. Garcia and Wolfram (70) pointed out the effect of geometry, which is demonstrated by measuring changes in work of passage and resiliency of waved hair (Table 1), the latter being determined by multiple passes through the ring. Hair-setting sprays produce a large increase in WP due to the formation of a network of bonded junction

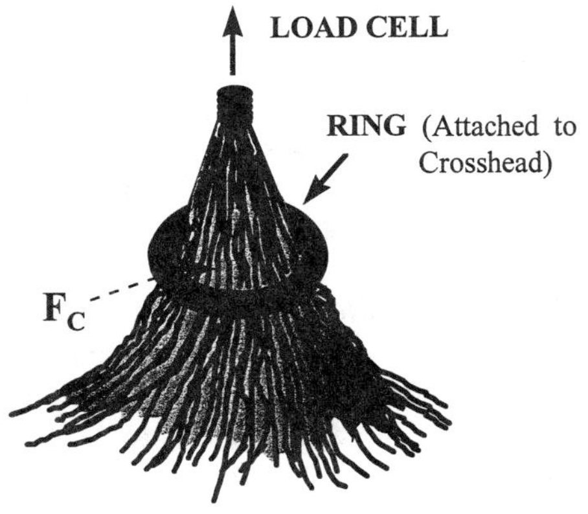

Figure 27 The ring method.

Table 1 Effects of Various Cosmetic Treatments on the Bulk Compressibility of Hair (70)

Treatment	% change in work of passage	% change in resiliency
Waving	+103	−23
Waving + conditioner	+89	−17
Hairspray	+540	−36

points between fibers. This network structure collapses to some extent upon compression, as indicated by the low resiliency.

Robbins and Crawford (71) discussed another modification of the Garcia-Wolfram method, in which the bulk of a hair tress is measured by determining the force required to pull it through a series of circular templates of decreasing diameter. The parameter "maximum tress diameter" is obtained by plotting work-of-passage values against template diameter and extrapolating to zero work. The authors measured the effects of various body-enhancing shampoos on the apparent tress bulk as determined by the maximum tress diameter. Other authors have used the template method to determine the effects of organosiloxanes as hair-body-enhancing ingredients. The German Wool Research Institute (72) has developed a similar approach based on the same principle.

4. *Volume of Hair Assemblies*

The apparent bulk of a hair tress has been used as a means of describing the body of a hair mass, especially with regard to the effects of conditioner treatments. Various methods based on optical measurements are being used in industry, and Clarke et al. (73) have described a technique involving image analysis. While hair volume may be an important parameter expressing hair appearance, it is not to be confused with the concept of hair body, which entails as its most important characteristic the resistance of a hair mass to tactile compression and its ability to recover from such compression.

D. Electrostatic Charge Generation

It is well known that when hair is combed, brushed, or blow-dried under low-humidity conditions, electrostatic charges build up that lead to difficulties in manageability associated with the third term of Robbins, i.e., flyaway. Charge buildup and flyaway produce entanglements and can severely damage hair in subsequent attempts at grooming. The "ballooning" effect resulting from fiber-fiber repulsion upon charge generation during dry combing was actually used in an attempt to estimate charge generation in hair (74). Since this is a very serious problem in the hair care industry, many efforts have been made to understand and overcome electrostatic charging and as a result a number of methods have been developed (59,74–78), some of which are discussed below.

The theoretical background of this phenomenon, which is also of considerable concern in the textile (79) and plastics industry, has been studied extensively and discussed relatively recently in papers by Lunn and Evans (76) and Jachowicz et al. (78). Triboelectric charging occurs upon contact between two materials that have different electrochemical surface potentials resulting in a transfer of electrons between them, thus generating charges of opposite sign but equal magnitude on their surfaces upon separation of the materials. The sign and magnitude of the charge depend on the relative positions of the two materials in the "triboelectric series." Lunn lists three principal factors contributing to the severity of flyaway during combing of human hair: the magnitude of the charge, its mobility and rate of dissipation, and its distribution along the length of the combed fibers. Modifying any one of these factors can result in the desired effect of reducing flyaway, and in an effort to establish the mechanism by which antistatic agents work, Lunn and Evans (76) developed three different methods.

1. *Charge Generation Methods*

The measurement of triboelectric charge generation is well known for its variability where relative humidity, surface contamination or abrasion, tress configuration, and other variables have to be strictly controlled. Even with the combing of up to five replicate tresses and five successive determinations, Lunn and Evans report a 95% confidence interval of ±15%. The apparatus that Lunn and Evans used is shown in Figure 28. The insulated tress is combed with a hand-held insulated test comb, and after the appropriate number of strokes, the tress is released into a Faraday cage connected to an electrometer. The whole setup is enclosed in a box in which temperature and humidity are controlled.

The apparatus developed by Jachowicz et al. (78) is based on the same principles, but it uses an exchangeable rotating half-cylinder at a rotation speed of 70 rpm instead of an insulated comb. Charge buildup is measured continuously by a static detector probe (Keithley 2503) as a function of time, and the apparatus is maintained at a constant relative humidity of 25–30% (Fig. 29).

These authors found that surface charge density is limited to values below 7×10^{-9} C/cm^2 due to electrical breakdown of the surrounding atmosphere. Typical charge buildup curves are shown in Figure 30, which indicates very fast positive charging with an electrical breakdown after three to four contacts (Fig. 30a). Figure 30c shows somewhat slower

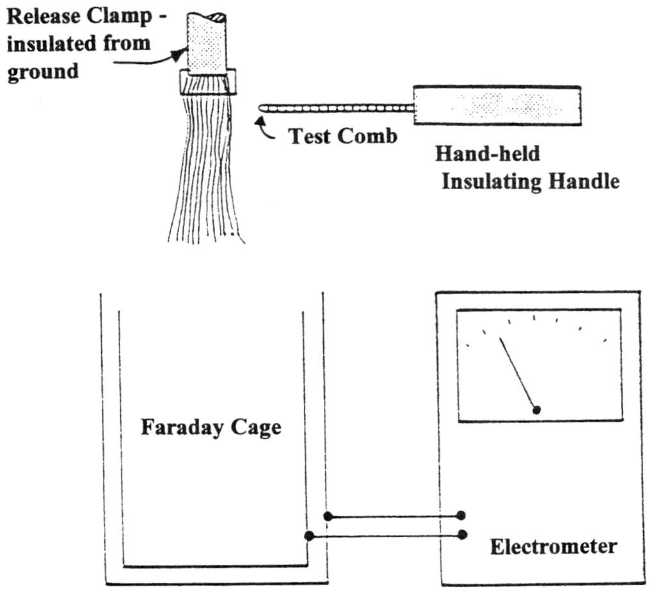

Figure 28 Apparatus used to measure electrostatic charges generated on hair tresses by combing. (From Ref. 76.)

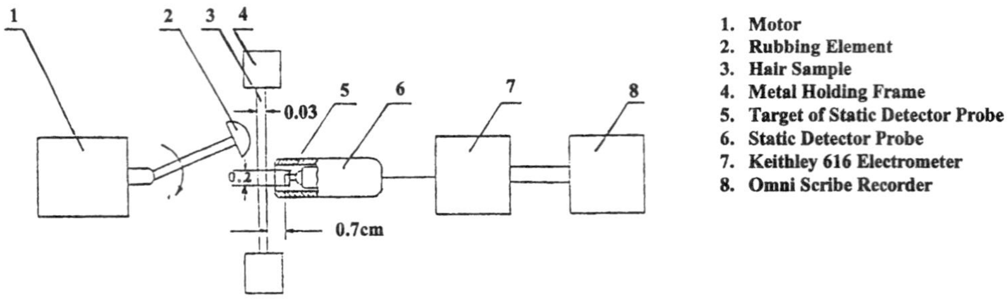

Figure 29 A device to study triboelectrification of keratin fibers. 1, Motor; 2, rubbing element; 3, hair sample; 4, metal holding frame; 5, target of static detector probe; 6, static detector probe; 7, Keithley 616 Electrometer; 8. Omni Scribe Recorder. (From Ref. 78.)

negative charging, but threshold charge densities are also reached. A slow charge buildup to below threshold values is seen in Figure 30d and occasionally such a buildup leads to a reversal in charge (Fig. 30b), suggesting changes in the nature of the contacting surfaces through mass transfer or surface abrasion.

Busch (80) used an automatic combing device with a pair of combs engaging the slowly rotating tress with a frequency of 16 rpm, while the tress was positioned in a conditioned double Faraday cage. In this approach the combs are discharged by means

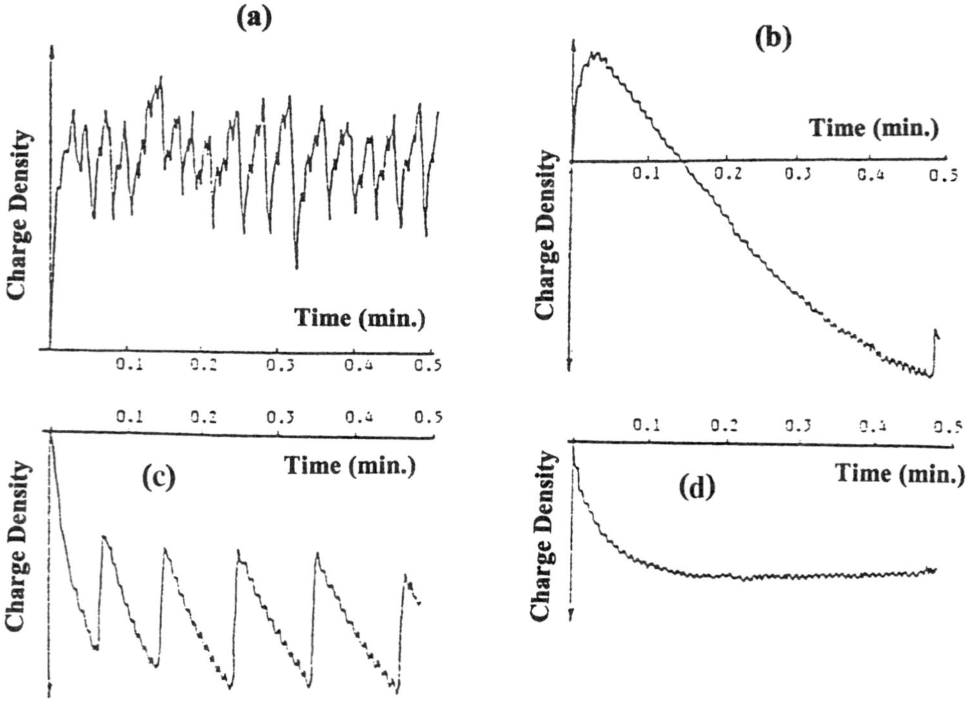

Figure 30 Examples of unsmoothed kinetic curves of charge buildup during rubbing of hair fibers. (From Ref. 78.)

of ionization rods each time they leave the cage, so that additional charging is always done by uncharged combs. Charge levels after 10 and 30 strokes are recorded.

2. Methods for Measuring Charge Mobility

As pointed out above, Lunn and Evans suggested that the mobility of the generated charge and its rate of dissipation from the fibers is another principal factor determining the extent of flyaway. The procedure used by Lunn and Evans (76) is a modification of the ASTM standard for measuring electrostatic charge mobility on flexible barrier materials used in the plastics industry (81). The apparatus, which Lunn and Evans call a Faraday shell, is shown in Figure 31 and consists of two cylindrical brass shells, each of which contains a circular electrode insulated from ground by Teflon spacers. The upper detector electrode is shielded from stray fields by placing a thin brass sheet over the lower shell with the exception of a 4-cm width in which the hair tress is mounted. The hair tress is spread uniformly between the electrodes by means of two combs that are used solely as spacers.

In operation, a high-voltage potential is applied to the lower electrode, which causes

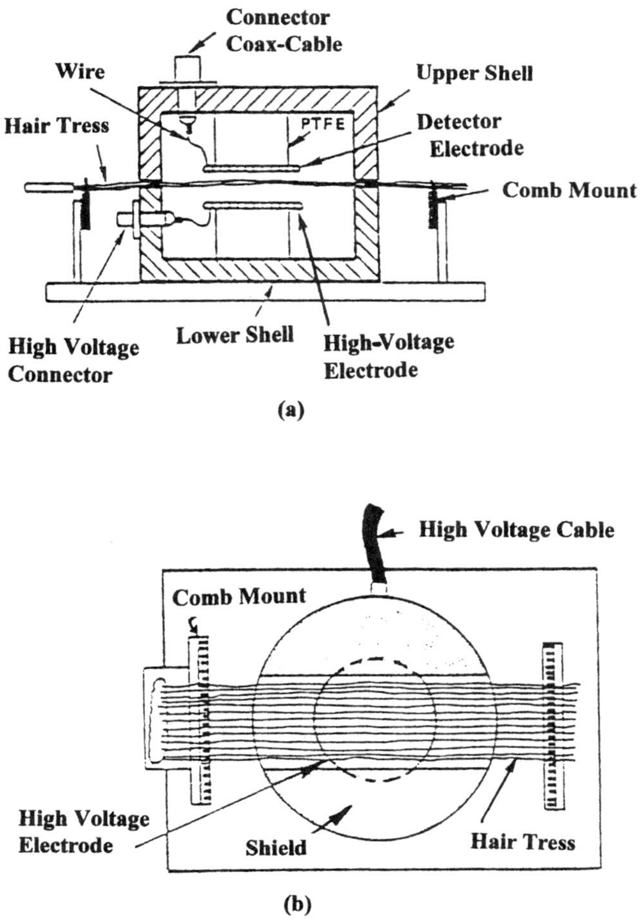

Figure 31 Faraday shell apparatus for measurement of charge mobility, with hair tress in position: (a) side view; (b) exposed top view, upper shell removed. (From Ref. 76.)

an instantaneous charging of the detector electrode. As the charge slowly builds up on the hair, the charge on the detector electrode decreases correspondingly until it reaches zero when the hair is fully charged. To measure charge decay from the hair the charging electrode is disconnected from the high-voltage source and is grounded. The half-lives of induction and charge decay are determined as indicated in Figure 32 and are identical. The logarithm of the root mean square values (τ_{RMS}) varies linearly over a relative humidity range from 20 to 50% and is used as a means to establish the effects of various treatments on charge mobility.

3. Charge Density Distribution Method

The third principal factor contributing to the severity of flyaway discussed by Lunn and Evans (76) is the nonuniform distribution of charge density along the length of the hair tress. The apparatus used to determine this parameter is shown in Figure 33. Using an Instron tensile tester, the hair tress is pulled through a set of two combs; the upper one is grounded while the lower comb acts as a charge-generating device. The charge is measured by a detector electrode, which is shielded by grounded guard electrodes.

By recording the electrometer output as a function of time as the tress is pulled through the comb, the charge distribution along the length of the combed hair is determined. A comparison of charge density distribution with combing forces shows that a high charge density is generated when the tress end moves through the comb, leading to the so-called end-peak force.

Based on this work Lunn and Evans propose a theory for the action of quaternary ammonium antistatic agents; they attribute their effectiveness not to increased conductiv-

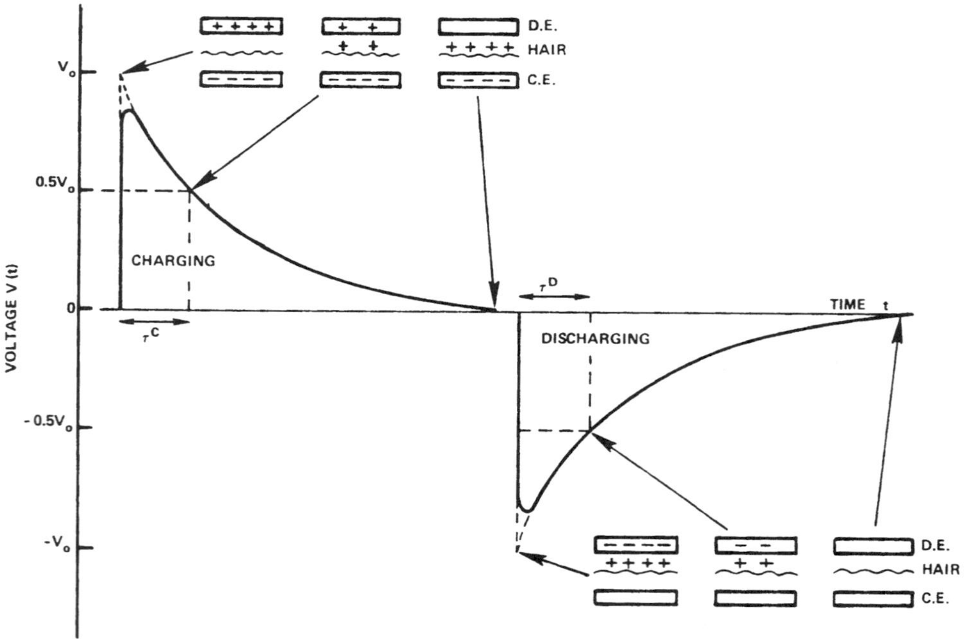

Figure 32 Voltage on detector electrode V(t) during charging and discharging of the hair (schematic). State of charge on charging electrode (C.E.), hair fibers, and detector electrode (D.E.) at various times is also shown. (From Ref. 76.)

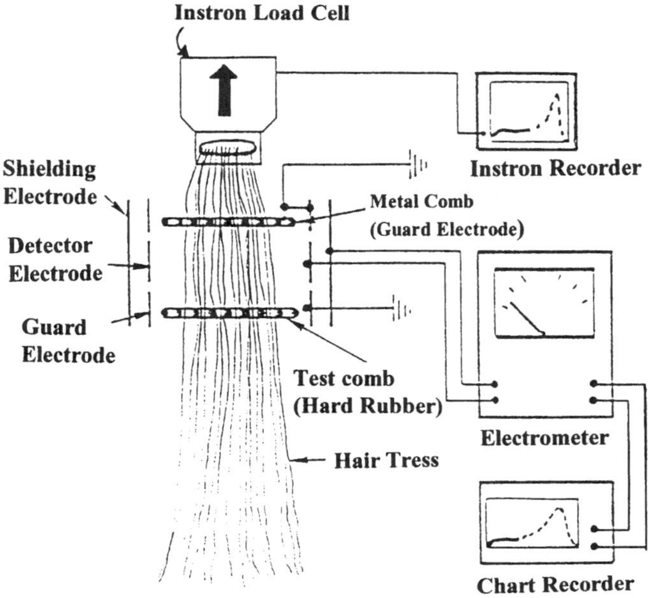

Figure 33 Apparatus used to measure distribution of charge density along length of hair as it is combed. (From Ref. 76.)

ity, but to their lubricating action and the concomitant decrease in normal contact force between hair and comb. The decrease in contact force leads to a decrease in contact area and thereby a reduction in the static charge generated.

Jachowicz et al. (78) use charge decay measurements from charges generated in their apparatus as a means of getting information on the mechanism of fiber conductivity. They conclude from their studies that the effective work functions and charge decay are strongly affected by fiber surface modification and are the controlling factors in the effectiveness of an antistatic agent. Modification of the hair fiber surface by adsorption of cationic polymers and the formation of polymer-detergent complexes changes both its effective work function and its conductivity, but in practice, static charge generation cannot be controlled by these compounds. However, Jachowicz et al. concede that during combing, parameters such as fiber elongation, stress, and magnitude of frictional forces result in nonuniform distribution of triboelectric charge densities along the length of the hair tress, which might lead to quantitatively different results than those presented in their paper (78).

E. Luster or Shine of Hair

The subjective terms "luster," "gloss," and "shine" of hair are being used interchangeably in the literature, although shine is most meaningful to consumers (82). Subjective panel evaluations of this property can be quite accurate, if care is taken to keep fiber alignment, lighting, and certain panel considerations constant. However, to be able to make quantitative statements about the effectiveness of various treatments, efforts have been made to develop instrumental, objective methods of shine evaluation. All these methods (83–87) are based on the contrast between the intensity of the specularly reflected light and that of the diffusely scattered light, measured either at specific angles or by scanning the reflected light envelope over a certain range of angles using goniophotometry. The alignment of fibers within a tress is one of the major variables that makes reproducible luster perception and measurement so difficult. Goniophotometric assessments of hair tresses have to consider the potential effects treatments can have on the alignment of fibers, even if measurements are made on the same tress before and after treatment.

A typical schematic diagram of a goniophotometric experiment (83) is shown in Figure 34, where the hair fiber is illuminated by the incident beam at a fixed angle i and the scattered light is scanned from 0 to 90 degrees by a photomultiplier tube. This goniophotometric approach for single fibers, which avoids problems of fiber alignment, has been discussed in two fundamental papers by Stamm and co-workers (85,86). The reflection of a light beam from an ideal cylindrical fiber is shown in Figure 35, where reflection from the front surface and the back surface appear at the same angle and cannot be distinguished. In a real hair fiber with a scale angle of ~3–4 degrees the back reflection is clearly shifted and appears as a separate peak in the light intensity scan shown in Figure 36, provided the light beam is not absorbed during its passage through the fiber by pigmentation or dissipated by medullar structures.

1. Luster Measurement

Integrated areas of the goniophotometer curve yield numerical values for specular reflection (S) and diffuse scattering (D). Following the approach of Nickerson (88) for contrast gloss of cotton yarns and fabrics, Stamm et al. used the following function to evaluate luster (L):

$$L = \frac{S - D}{D}$$

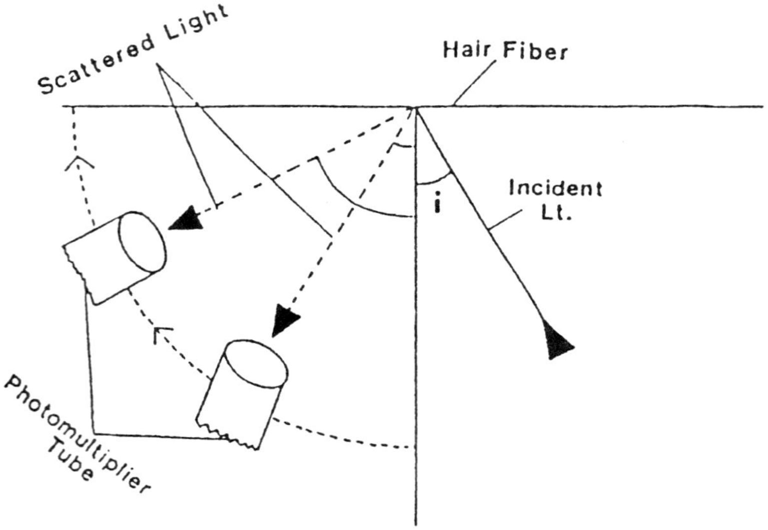

Figure 34 Rudimentary diagram of a goniophotometer experiment. A hair fiber is illuminated by incident light at angle i. Scattered light is then detected by rotating a photomultiplier tube from 0 to 90 degrees with respect to the perpendicular to the fiber. Two of the photomultiplier positions are shown. (From Ref. 83.)

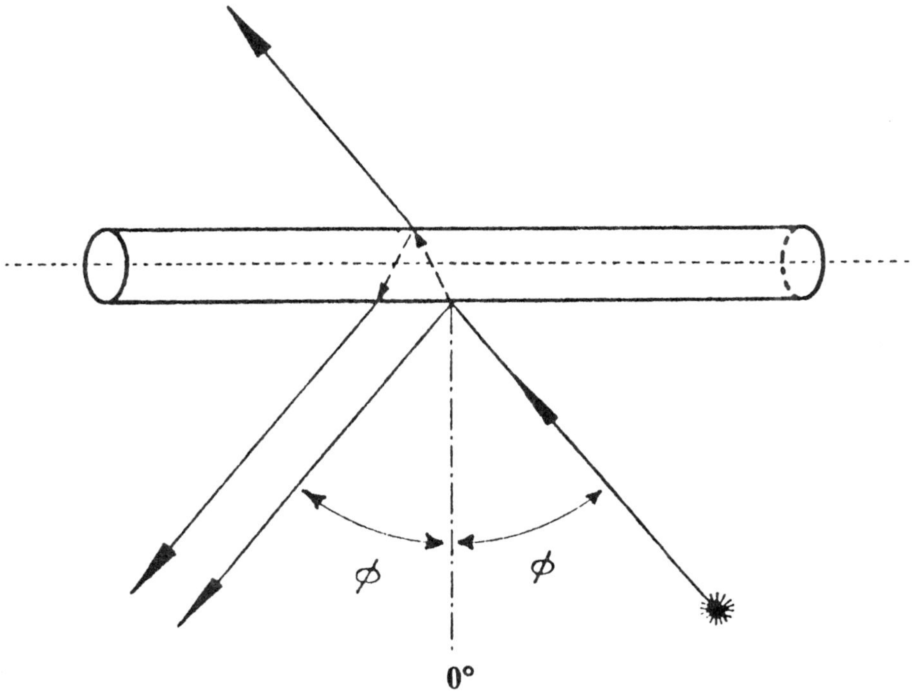

Figure 35 Reflection of light from near and far sides of idealized cylindrical fiber. Rays reflected from both sides are observed at the same angle and are indistinguishable from one another. This is in marked contrast to fibers with scales (see Fig. 36). (From Ref. 85.)

One of the other definitions of luster or gloss (G), which has been proposed by Schulze zur Wiesche and Wortmann (89) and has also been explored at TRI (87), uses the ratio of the specularly reflected to the total reflected light:

$$G \text{ or } L = \frac{S}{S + D}$$

Reich and Robbins (83) explored a number of other luster functions and found that the introduction of the width at half-height ($W_{1/2}$) of the specular reflection yields a function that agrees best with subjective evaluations:

$$L = \frac{S}{DW_{1/2}}$$

Clean hair has high luster, and deposition of compounds on the hair surface usually reduces luster. This is clearly shown in Figure 37, which compares the effects of washing with various shampoos (83). Shampoo B1 contains Polyquaternium-10, a polycationic compound known to be substantive to hair. A subsequent rinse with a shampoo containing sodium myristate produces a large decrease in luster, possibly due to complex formation between the polycation and the myristate anion. A rinse with 20% sodium lauryl sulfate, on the other hand, removes the polycation and restores the original luster of the fiber.

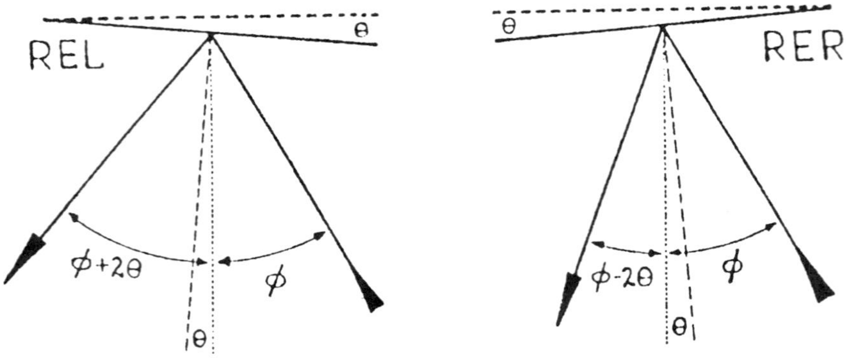

Figure 36 Method for illuminating planar array of parallel-oriented hair fibers in obtaining goniophotometer curves. Angle of incidence is fixed at 30° to fiber axis. Inclination of scales relative to fiber axis (dotted line) with a scale angle of Θ is shown, with orientation of fibers indicated by REL (root-ends-left) and RER (root-ends-right). Light reflected specularly from front end of the cuticle is observed at $\Phi + 2\Theta$ for the REL orientation and at $\Phi - 2\Theta$ for the RER orientation. (From Ref. 86.)

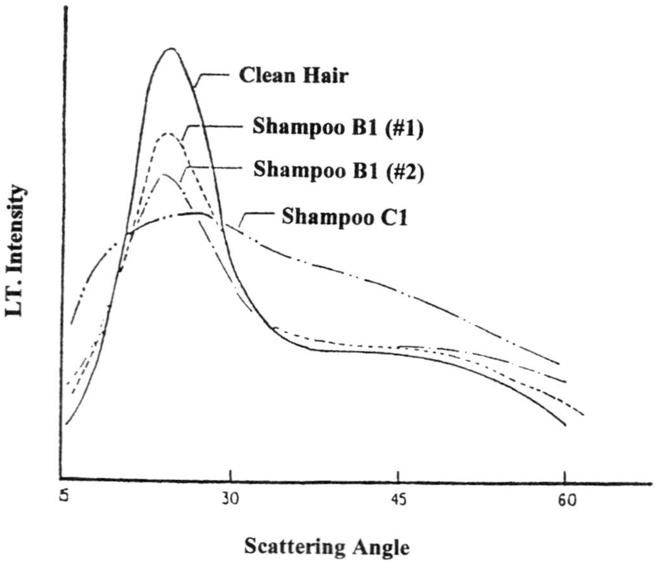

Figure 37 A single-fiber experiment measuring the effect of washing with two different shampoos. Note the huge increase in diffuse scattering and the great decrease in shine after the hair was treated with shampoo C1. (From Ref. 83.)

These observations show that goniophotometry on single fibers can provide comparative, objective information on the effects of polymer deposition on hair fiber surfaces.

Image analysis techniques have been used in recent years to measure luster by determining the contrast between areas of high reflection and the surrounding darker areas (90–92). Correlations between color image analysis data and visual subjective evaluations and also goniophotometry have been shown to exist (90,91).

F. Scale Angle Measurement

As pointed out earlier, the cuticle scales form an angle (Θ) of 3–4 degrees with the fiber axis, and this angle can be determined with reasonable accuracy from goniophotometric measurements (Fig. 38). The difference between specular reflection maxima measured in the root-to-tip and the tip-to-root orientation of the fiber is equal to 4Θ, as shown in the schematic drawing in Figure 36. Measurements at TRI (93) have shown that combing in the TRI combing machine under dry conditions produces surface abrasion preferentially at the surface scale edge leading to a significant decrease in scale angle (Fig. 39).

Under wet conditions, an ablative process is operative with scale fragmentation and gradual loss of the cuticula, but without any change in scale angle (Fig. 40). Deposition of a polymeric compound such as Polymer JR-400 totally eliminates the abrasive process as indicated by the lack of change in scale angle during dry combing (Fig. 41), which is probably due to decreased friction between comb and fibers. These conclusions can be

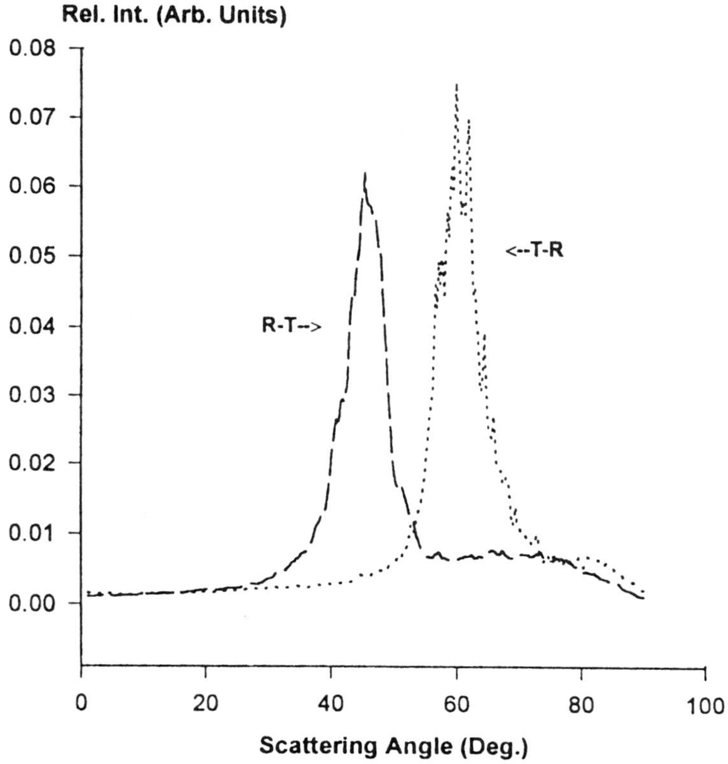

Figure 38 Light scattering from a control; hair fiber in the R-T and T-R orientations.

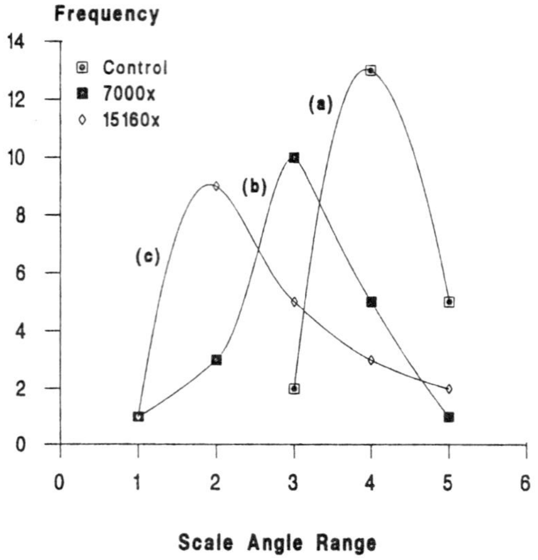

Figure 39 Frequency distribution of scale angles in the (a) control and after (b) 7000 and (c) 15,160 combings (population size 20).

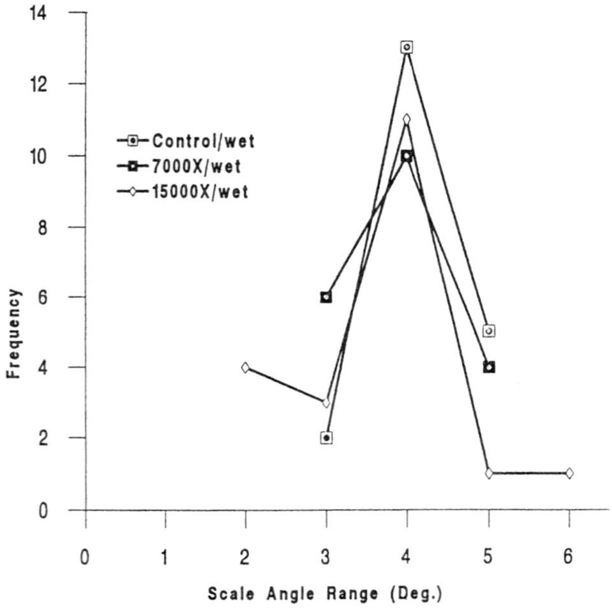

Figure 40 Change in the scale angle distribution with extent of wet combing of hair (control, 7000× and 15,000×; sample size: 20).

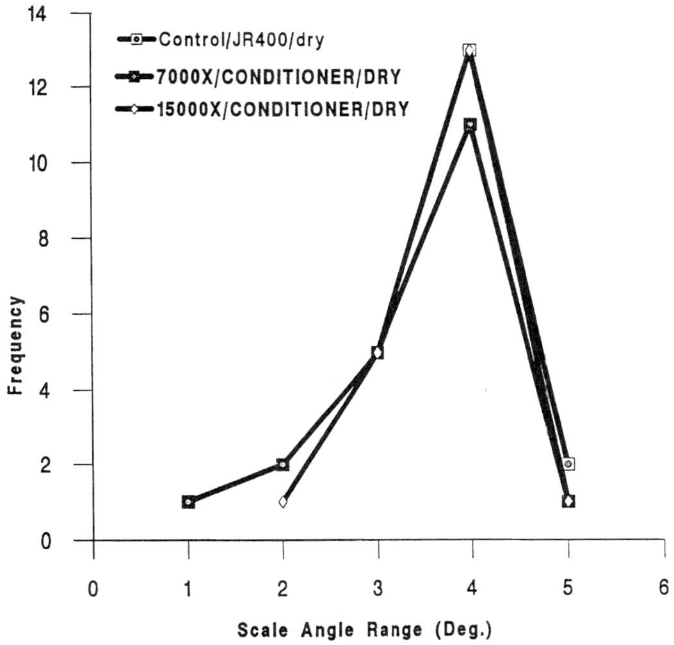

Figure 41 Change in the scale angle distribution with extent of dry combing of conditioner-treated hair (control, 7000× and 15,000×; sample size: 20).

substantiated by scanning electron microscopy, but lubrication effects resulting in decreased abrasion due to conditioner treatments are quantified by measuring scale angles.

V. CONCLUDING REMARKS

Within the limited context of this chapter, only a selection of methods for evaluating conditioned hair and specifically hair treated with polymeric conditioners can be covered, and the reader is encouraged to further explore the numerous publications on this topic, especially the often-quoted book *Chemical and Physical Behavior of Human Hair*, by Robbins. A number of authors have written about the importance of recognizing the limits as well as the interrelationships of subjective and objective evaluations of hair. Busch (94) in particular has discussed aspects of aesthetics and emotionalism as being intrinsic concepts in cosmetics and thereby making subjective evaluations deeply individualistic. While subjective statements of members of an evaluation panel are certainly close to their own perception of reality, they have to be carefully screened to ascertain their "intersubjectivity." Language is critical in reducing the number of individual statements to generally acceptable concepts. Language is also critical in bridging the gap between subjective and objective methods by formulating and defining a number of terms that are close to consumer perception and at the same time lend themselves to instrumental measurements. The literature points out again and again that there is a general interdependence of objectively measurable hair properties and that most, if not all, methods measure more than one aspect of hair properties without any sharply defined borders. It is therefore usually necessary to employ a number of objective methods to move the overall statement closer to the consumer-perceived reality. Statistical analysis of subjective as well as objective data is critical to establish the significance of the measured data, and modern robotics makes it possible to gather the necessarily large number of measurements and also to eliminate operator bias.

Research will continue to develop better methods for quantifying cosmetic effects and will ensure that these methods are both scientifically well based and as close to reality as possible.

REFERENCES

1. Robbins CR. Private communication.
2. Goddard ED, Hannan RB, Faucher JA. Proc VII Int Congress Surface Active Agents, Mocow USSR 1977; 2:834.
3. Ruetsch SB, Kamath YK, Weigmann H-D. 10th Int Hair Science Symp, Rostock/Warnemuende, Germany, 1996.
4. Ruetsch SB, Weigmann H-D. J Soc Cosmet Chem 1996; 47:13.
5. Fraser RDB, Gillespie JM, MacRae TP, Marshall RC. Internal Report CSIRO, Division of Protein Chemistry, Parkville, Vic. Australia, 1981.
6. Crewther WG, Dowling LM, Steinert PM, Parry DAD. Int J Biol Macromol 1982; 5:267.
7. Fraser RDB, MacRae LP, Sparrow LG, Parry DAD. Int J Biol Macromol 1988; 10:106.
8. Robbins CR. Chemical and Physical Behavior of Human Hair, 3rd ed. New York: Springer-Verlag, 1994:27.
9. Leeder JD, Rippon JA, Rivett DE. Proc 7th Int Wool Text Res Conf, Tokyo, Vol IV, 1985: 312.
10. Swift JA, Brown AC. J Soc Cosmet Chem 1972; 23:695.
11. Lindberg J Textile Res J 1949; 19:43.
12. Leeder JD, Rippon JA. J Soc Dyers Col 1985; 101:11.
13. Negri AP, Cornell HJ, Rivett DE. Textile Res J 1993; 63:109.
14. Phan KH, Thomas H, Heine E. Proc 9th Int Wool Text Conf, Biella, Italy, Vol II, 1995:19.
15. Miller B, Young RA. Textile Res J 1975; 45:359.
16. Kamath YK, Dansizer CJ, Weigmann H-D. J Soc Cosmet Chem 1977; 28:273.
17. Kamath YK, Dansizer CJ, Weigmann H-D. J Appl Polymer Sci 1978; 22:2295.
18. Kamath YK, Dansizer CJ, Weigmann H-D. J Appl Polymer Sci 1984; 29:1011.
19. Kamath YK, Dansizer CJ, Weigmann H-D. J Coll Interface Sci 1984; 102:164.
20. Kamath YK, Dansizer CJ, Weigmann H-D. Proc 6th Int Wool Text Res Conf, Pretoria, South Africa, Vol II, 1980: 507.
21. Kamath YK, Dansizer CJ, Weigmann H-D. J Appl Polym Sci 1985; 30:937.
22. Weigmann H-D, Kamath YK. Cosmet Toilet 1986; 101:37.
23. Kamath YK, Dansizer CJ, Hornby S, Weigmann H-D. Textile Res J 1987; 57:205.
24. Weigmann H-D, Kamath YK, Ruetsch SB, Busch P, Tesmann H. J Soc Cosmet Chem 1990; 41:379.
25. Jacobasch H, Baubock G, Schurz J. Colloid Polym Sci 1985; 263:834.
26. Jachowicz J, Maxey S, Williams C. Langmuir 1993; 9:3085.
27. Jachowicz J, Williams C. J Soc Cosmet Chem 1994; 45:309.
28. Jachowicz J. J Soc Cosmet Chem 1995; 46:100.
29. Kokot S, Matsuoka M, Meyer U, Zuercher J. Textilveredl 1975; 10:127.
30. Gottschalk H, Hohm G, Kaminski H. Proc 5th Int Wool Text Res Conf, Aachen, Germany, Vol II, 1975:349.
31. Garcia-Dominguez J, Julia MR, de la Maza A. J Soc Dyers Col 1976; 92:433.
32. Meyer U. Textilveredl 1982; 17:440.
33. Weigmann H-D, Steenken I, Moore RAF, Ruetsch SB. Proc 7th Wool Text Res Conf Tokyo, Japan, Vol V, 1985:141.

34. Greaves PH. J Soc Dyers Col 1985; 101:359.
35. Schaefer K, Hoecker H. Melliand Textilber 1991; 72:213.
36. Schaefer K. Melliand Textilber 1993; 74:1138.
37. Kamath YK, Ruetsch SB, Weigmann H-D. Textile Res J 1993; 63:19.
38. Weigmann H-D, Kamath YK, Ruetsch SB. Microspectrophotometry. In: Peters AT, Freeman HS, eds. Analytical Chemistry of Synthetic Colorants. Glasgow: Blackie Academic and Professional, 1995.
39. Zuercher-Vogt J. Chemiefaser/Textilind 1991; 41:93.
40. Scott GV, Robbins CR. J Soc Cosmet Chem 1980; 31:179.
41. Schwartz A, Knowles D. J Soc Cosmet Chem 1963; 14:455.
42. Scott GV, Robbins CR, Barnhurst JD. J Soc Cosmet Chem 1969; 20:135.
43. Kamath YK, Weigmann et al. Unpublished results.
44. Lindberg J, Gralen N. Textile Res J 1948; 18:287.
45. Fair NB, Gupta BS. Proc 14th IFSCC Congress, Barcelona, Spain, Vol 2, 1986:1113.
46. Pascoe MW, Tabor D. Res Lond 1955; 8:515.
47. Robbins CR. 3rd Int Hair Science Sympos, Syburg, Germany, 1984.
48. Howell HG, Mazur J. J Text Inst 1952; 43T:59.
49. Robbins CR. Chemical and Physical Behavior of Human Hair, 3rd ed. New York: Springer-Verlag, 1994:343.
50. Robbins CR, Reich C, Clarke J. J Soc Cosmet Chem 1986; 37:489.
51. Newman W, Cohen GL, Hayes C. J Soc Cosmet Chem 1973; 24:773.
52. Tolgyesi WS, Cottington E, Fookson A. Mechanics of hair combing. Presented at Symposium on Mechanics of Fibrous Structures, Fiber Society, Atlanta, GA, May 14, 1975.
53. Garcia ML, Diaz J. J Soc Cosmet Chem 1976; 27:379.
54. Kamath YK, Weigmann H-D. J Soc Cosmet Chem 1986; 37:111.
55. Bauer JP, Beck C, Monnais C, Vayssie C. Int J Cosmet Sci 1983; 5:113.
56. Epps J, Wolfram LJ. J Soc Cosmet Chem 1983; 34:213.
57. Naik A, Vives RJ, Cot J. Proc 14th IFSCC Congress, Barcelona, Spain, Vol 2, 1986:993.
58. Wedderburn DC, Prall JK. J Soc Cosmet Chem 1973; 24:561.
59. Sakamoto K, Tanaka M, Ide N, Yokata H, Takahara M. Fragrance J 1984; 8:330.
60. Busch P, Grundmann H. Proc 14th IFSCC Congress, Barcelona, Spain, Vol 2, 1986:991.
61. Busch P. Unpublished results.
62. Zviak C, Camp M. In: Zviak C, ed. The Science of Hair. New York: Marcel Dekker, 1986: 332.
63. Waggoner WC, Scott GV. J Soc Cosmet Chem 1966; 17:171.
64. Robbins CR, Scott GF. J Soc Cosmet Chem 1978; 29:783.
65. Robbins CR, Reich C. J Soc Cosmet Chem 1986; 37:141.
66. Chandra G, Kohl GS, Tassoff JA. Dow Corning Corp, US Patent 4,559,227, 1985.
67. Hough P, Huey H, Tolgyesi W. J Soc Cosmet Chem 1976; 27:571.
68. Yin NE, Kissinger RH, Tolgyesi WS, Cottingham EM. Proc 9th IFSCC Congress, Boston, MA, 1976:587.
69. Kamath YK, Weigmann H-D. Preprints of 1996 Annual Scientific Meeting, 1996, New York. J Soc Cosmet Chem 1996; 47:256.
70. Garcia ML, Wolfram LJ. Presented at 10th IFSCC Congress, Sydney, Australia, 1978.
71. Robbins CR, Crawford RJ. J Soc Cosmet Chem 1984; 35:369.
72. Blankenburg G, German Wool Research Institute, Aachen. Private communication.
73. Clarke J, Robbins CR, Reich C. J Soc Cosmet Chem 1991; 42:341.
74. Mills CM, Ester VC, Henkin H. J Soc Cosmet Chem 1956; 7:466.
75. Barber RG, Posner AM. J Soc Cosmet Chem 1959; 10:236.
76. Lunn CA, Evans RE. J Soc Cosmet Chem 1977; 26:549.
77. Jachowicz J, Wis-Surel G, Wolfram LJ. Textile Res J 1984; 54:492.
78. Jachowicz J, Wis-Surel G, Garcia ML. J Soc Cosmet Chem 1985; 36:189.
79. Hersh SP, Montgomery DJ. Textile Res J 1956; 26:903.

80. Busch P. Presented at Annual SCC Technical Meeting, New York, 1984.
81. American Society for Testing and Materials, Ann Book ASTM Stand, Part 21, Method 365-75T, 1975.
82. Thompson W, Mills C. Proc Sci Section TGA No. 15, May 1951.
83. Reich C, Robbins CR. J Soc Cosmet Chem 1993; 44:221.
84. Czepluch W, Hohm G, Tolkiehn K. J Soc Cosmet Chem 1993; 44: 299.
85. Stamm RE, Garcia ML, Fuchs JJ. J Soc Cosmet Chem 1977; 28:571.
86. Stamm RE, Garcia ML, Fuchs JJ. J Soc Cosmet Chem 1977; 28:601.
87. Ramaprasad K, TRI/Princeton. Unpublished results.
88. Nickerson D. Textile Res J 1957; 27:111.
89. Schulze zur Wiesche E, Wortmann FJ. 10th Int. Hair Science Symp, Rostock/Warnemuende, Germany, 1996.
90. Zviak C, Boullion C. In: Zviak C, ed. The Science of Hair Care. New York: Marcel Dekker, 1986:136.
91. Maeda T, Hara T, Okada M, Watanabe H. Proc 16th IFSCC Congress, New York, Vol I, 1990:127.
92. Maeda T, Okada M, Hara T. Cosmet Toilet 1992; 107(2):53.
93. Ramaprasad K, Kamath YK, Weigmann H-D. Presented at SCC Annual Scientific Meeting, New York, December 1995.
94. Busch P. Aertzl Kosmetol 1989; 19:270.

Appendix: Encyclopedia of Polymers and Thickeners for Cosmetics

Robert Y. Lochhead
University of Southern Mississippi, Hattiesburg, Mississippi

James V. Gruber
Amerchol Corporation, Edison, New Jersey

This encyclopedia of polymers and thickeners has been reorganized and expanded from the May 1993 issue of *Cosmetics & Toiletries.* A detailed questionnaire was sent to each supplier of polymers and thickeners. When a supplier provided limited information, the entry was expanded as much as possible from information in the public domain.

Entries are categorized as natural and modified natural polymers and thickeners and their derivatives' and synthetic polymers and thickeners.

The first category includes many polysaccharides. In this Appendix, we have used Haworth structures for these polysaccharides.

Within each category, entries are listed alphabetically according to CTFA nomenclature. If a CTFA[1] name was not available, a USP/NF[2] name was adopted, and if this was not available, either the IUPAC[3] or a manufacturer's preferred name was entered.

Only primary thickeners are listed. Thickeners that depend on interaction with another component of a formulation are excluded. Thus, cosurfactants, such as lauric diethanolamide, are not listed because these should be categorized as cosurfactants that alter micelle structure. They are not primary thickeners.

The information contained in this encyclopedia should be used only as a guide. The information should not be construed as specifications for these raw materials. Interested users are advised to contact the relevant supplier(s) for detailed guidance in the use of these raw materials. The author and editors of *Cosmetics & Toiletries* provide this information without warranty, expressed or implied, regarding its correctness or accuracy.

---

[1] Cosmetics, Toiletries and Fragrance Association
[2] United States Pharmacopeia/National Formulary
[3] International Union of Pure and Applied Chemistry

I. NATURALS AND MODIFIED NATURALS

Algin/Alginic Acid

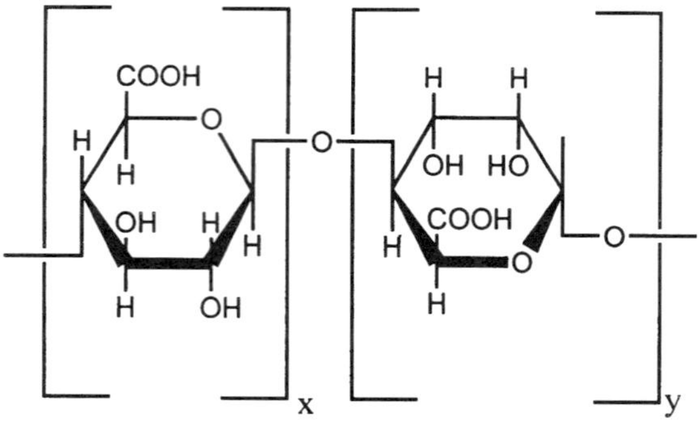

Chemical Names: Sodium alginate, potassium alginate, alginic acid
Chemical Description: Alginic acid is the carbohydrate obtained by alkaline extraction of various species of brown seaweed. Algin is the sodium salt of a copolymer of mannuronic acid and glucuronic acid, represented schematically as shown in the structure.
Trade Names: Texamid 558, Texamid 778 (Henkel), Keltone, Kelmar, Kelacid (Kelco)
Function in Formula: Thickener, stabilizer, gelling agent
Use Concentration: 0.2–2% in creams and gels; 0.1–1% in facial masques, gels; 1% in toothpastes
Solubility Characteristics: Soluble in water, cold water soluble, solvent-soluble. Forms slightly turbid viscous solutions in water.
Formulating Considerations: Compatible with anionic and nonionic surfactants. Incompatible with polyvalent cations. Premix with parts of the water phase and pour into the water with good agitation
Form Supplied: Powder, granules
Microbial Considerations: Below 1000 germs/g, maximum 10,000 TPC
Suppliers: Henkel, Kelco Division; Merck

Alumina

Chemical Names: Boehmite alumina, alumina monohydrate, aluminum oxide hydroxide
Trade Name: Dispal Alumina
Function in Formula: Thickener
Use Concentration: 0.5–5%, water-based systems; 0.5–5%, water-miscible organic solvent systems
Solubility Characteristics: Insoluble, but forms colloidal dispersions in water
Formulating Considerations: Disperse in water first, thicken by changing pH or by adding salt (e.g., NaCl, $CaCl_2$, etc.), add other components, mix until smooth
Form Supplied: Water-dispersible powder or concentrated liquid dispersion
Microbial Considerations: Will not support microbial growth
Regulatory Status: Generally recognized as safe (GRAS) per **21** CFR 182.90. Dispal Alumina satisfies the language at **21** CFR 176.170(a)(2) and is considered FDA-allowed as a component on paper and paperboard in contact with aqueous and fatty foods
Special Comments: Synthetic, white, colloidal alumina, average dispersed particle size 40–70 nm
Supplier: VISTA

AMP Isostearoyl Hydrolyzed Collagen

Chemical Description: Aminomethylpropanol salt of isostearoyl hydrolyzed collagen
Trade Name: Crotein AD Anhydrous
Function in Formula: Conditioner
Use Concentration: 0.1–2% in alcoholic aerosol hair sprays, setting lotions, and aftershave lotions
Solubility Characteristics: Alcohol-soluble
Formulating Considerations: Do not heat above 40°C. May partially neutralize acid resins—adjustment of base amount may be necessary
Form Supplied: Clear yellow liquid
Supplier: Croda

AMP Isostearoyl Hydrolyzed Wheat Protein

Chemical Description: Aminomethylpropanol salt of isostearoyl hydrolyzed wheat protein
Trade Name: Crotein ADW
Function in Formula: Conditioner
Use Concentration: 0.1–2% in alcoholic hair sprays, setting lotions, aftershave lotions, nail preparations, quick-breaking foams
Solubility Characteristics: Alcohol-soluble
Formulating Considerations: Do not heat above 40°C. May partially neutralize acid resins—adjusting amount of base used may be necessary
Form Supplied: Clear yellow liquid
Supplier: Croda

Bentonite

Chemical Description: Native hydrated colloidal alumina silicate clay
Trade Names: Bentonite (Southern Clay), Bentonite USP/NF (Kraft)
Function in Formula: Thickener/suspending agent
Use Concentration: 0.5–5% in emulsions or suspensions
Solubility Characteristics: Highly swellable in water
Formulating Considerations: Pregel in water preferred, compatible with most ingredients, wide pH range performance, synergism with organic gums
Form Supplied: Powder
Microbial Considerations: Can be bacteria-controlled
Regulatory Status: FDA status confirmed as GRAS
Suppliers: Southern Clay; Kraft Chemical

Carrageenan (Kappa, Iota, Lambda)

Kappa

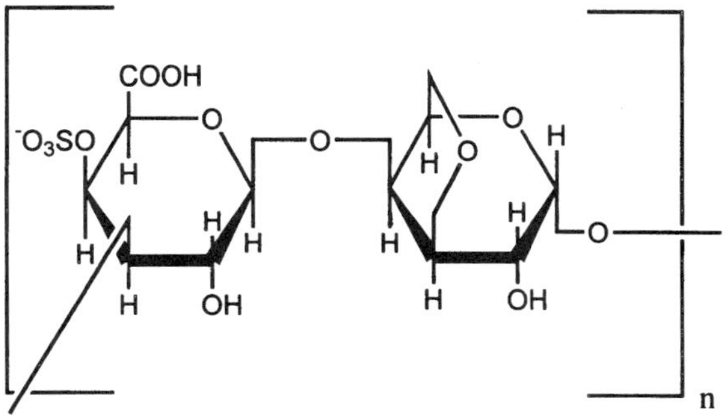

Iota

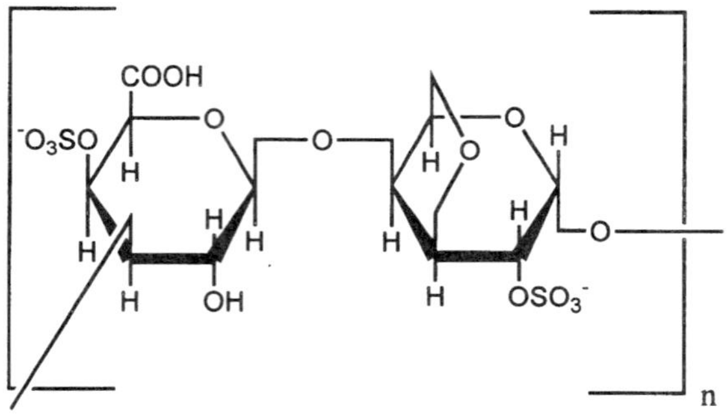

Lambda

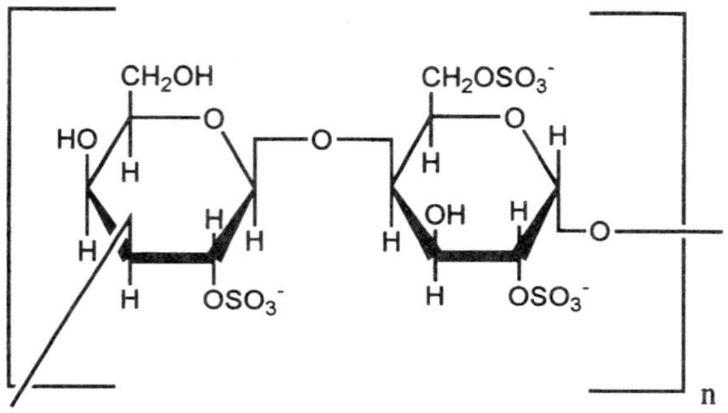

Chemical Definition: Water extract from various members of the Gigartinaceae or Solieriaceae families of red seaweed. Sulfated linear polysaccharide of D-galactose and 3,6 anhydro-D-galactose, both sulfated and nonsulfated

Trade Names: Gelcarin (FMC), Viscarin (FMC), Colloid 710H (Kappa-carrageenan, TIC)

Function in Formula: Gelation, thickening

Use Concentration: 0.4–1% in skin creams and lotions, 0.6–1.2% in toothpaste, 0.25–0.75% in aloe vera gels/lotions

Solubility Characteristics: 10% max. solubility in H_2O, weight %

Formulating Considerations: Compatible with other anionic and nonionic compounds at normal use levels. Carrageenan will precipitate with cationic compounds. It disperses in water more readily if first moistened with alcohol or glycerin

Form Supplied: Free-flowing powder

Microbial Considerations: Standard specification—less than 5000/g TPC

Regulatory Status: GRAS; comply with **21** CFR 172.620, 172.626

Suppliers: FMC, Marine Colloids Division; TIC Gums

Cellulose Gum

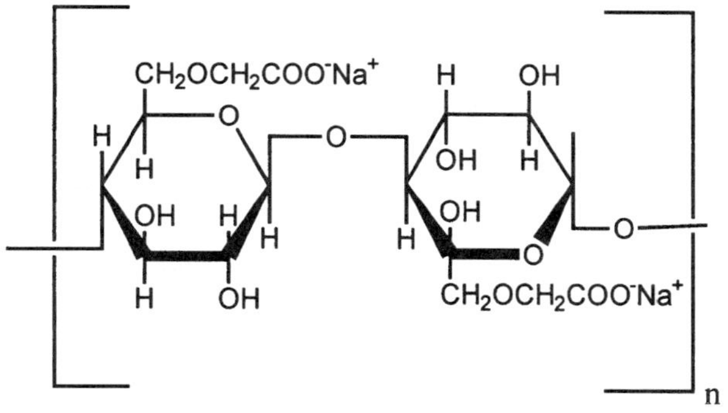

Chemical Name: Sodium carboxymethylcellulose

Trade Names: Aqualon Cellulose Gum(Aqualon), Walocel CRT (Miles), Dehydazol 7000 (Henkel), Ticalose (TIC)

Function in Formula: Thickener, gelling agent, stabilizer, rheology modifier, water binder

Use Concentration: 1.0% in shampoos and lotions, 0.5% in liquid makeup, 0.5–1.0% in toothpaste, 1% in linaments, 30–50% in denture adhesives

Solubility Characteristics: Complete in hot or cold water, insoluble in most organic solvents, but will tolerate small amounts of organic solvents. Compatible with anionic and nonionic surfactants

Formulating Considerations: High-DS types more compatible in surfactant systems

Form Supplied: Free-flowing powder, granular powder, fine powder, coarse powder

Microbial Considerations: Solutions and finished products must be preserved

Regulatory Status: GRAS. Food Chemicals Codex and United States Pharmacopeia. Meets standards set by **21** CFR, Sections 121.101 (d). Meets requirements of Food Chemicals Codes, National Formulary, and U.S. Pharmacopeia

Special Comments: Four different DS grades, three different viscosity types

Suppliers: Aqualon; Henkel; TIC Gums

Cellulose Gum

Chemical Name: Sodium carboxymethyl cellulose crosslinked

Trade Name: Aquasorb

Function in Formula: Absorbent fiber or powder

Use Concentration: Varies widely depending on need

Solubility Characteristics: Insoluble, but swellable

Form Supplied: Fiber or powder

Supplier: Aqualon

Cetyl Hydroxyethylcellulose

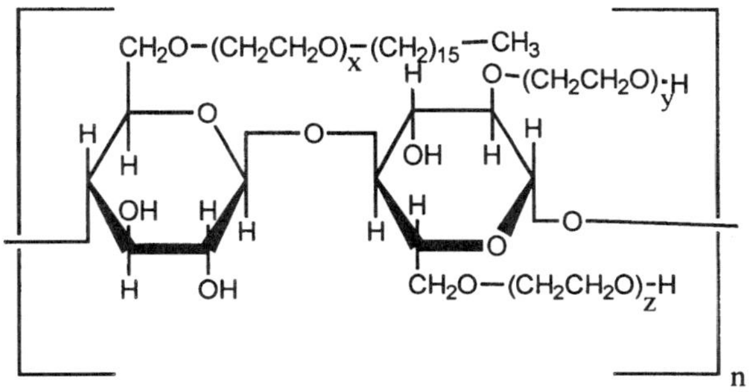

Chemical Name: Hexadecyl-2-hydroxyethylcellulose
Trade Names: PolySurf cetyl hydroxyethylcellulose, Natrosol Plus
Function in Formula: Rheology modifier
Use Concentration: <1% in hair care products, <1% in skin care products
Solubility Characteristics: Water-soluble
Form Supplied: Powder
Microbial Considerations: Preserve solution and finished products appropriately
Special Comments: Gives superior rheological properties than conventional hydroxyethylcellulose. True yield value and excellent suspension stability. Desirable shear-thinning rheology and outstanding rub-out properties on skin. No tack. Stable in aqueous solution from pH 3 to 10.5. Compatible with electrolyte
Supplier: Aqualon

Chitosan PCA

Chemical Name: Chitosonium pyrrolidone carboxylic acid salt
Trade Name: Kytamer PC
Function in Formula: A multifunctional ingredient that provides substantive moisturization to the skin and hair in a uniform film. Also shown to work as a water-based fixative in hair products
Use Concentration: 0.25–1.0% in water and up to 50% aqueous alcohol blends
Solubility Characteristics: Soluble in water and up to 50% aqueous alcohol blends
Formulating Considerations: Compatible with nonionic, cationic, and amphoteric systems
Form Supplied: Off-white powder
Microbial Considerations: Does not contain an antimicrobial as sold. Formulations must be preserved
Regulatory Status: Demonstrated to be safe for use, sold in North America, Europe, and other major markets. Currently approved for use in skin care products in Japan
Special Comments: Highly substantive to negatively charged protein substrates. The films that are formed are highly resistant to being rinsed off. These films, however, remain semipermeable and do not allow for transmission of oxygen and moisture through the barrier
Supplier: Amerchol

Chondroitin Sulfate (and) Hydrolyzed Protein

Chondroitin Sulfate A

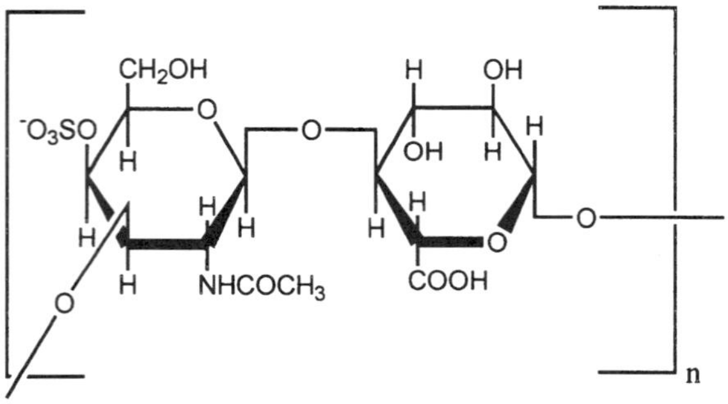

Chondroitin Sulfate B

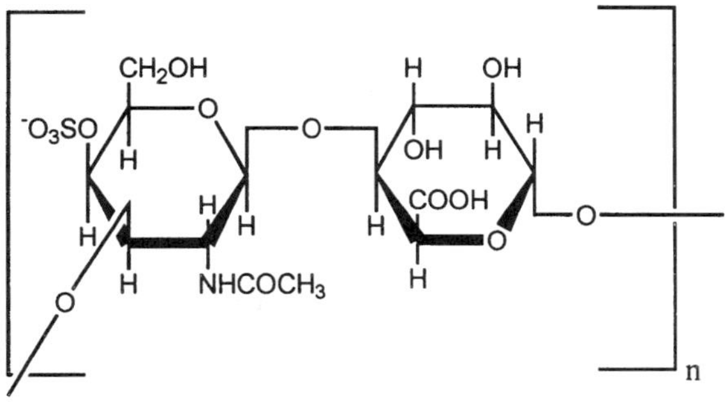

Chondroitin Sulfate C

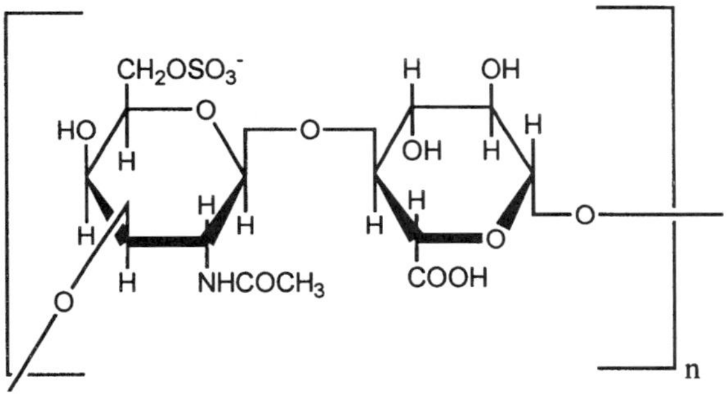

Chemical Description: Biological complex of acetylated galactosamine and iduronic acid with hydrolyzed proteins
Trade Name: Cromoist CS
Function in Formula: Skin moisturizer
Use Concentration: 0.5–5% in skin creams and lotions
Solubility Characteristics: Water-soluble
Formulating Considerations: Do not heat above 40°C
Form Supplied: Clear to slightly hazy amber liquid
Microbial Considerations: Standard for proteins
Supplier: Croda

Cocoamidopropyldimethylamine C_{8-16} Isoalkysuccinyl Lactoglobulin Sulfonate

Trade Name: Polymer SBOCP
Function in Formula: Absorbing oil and emulsification
Use Concentration: 1–5% in skin cleansers and shampoos; 0.1–0.5% in toners
Solubility Characteristics: Soluble in water
Formulating Considerations: Add last
Form Supplied: Liquid
Microbial Considerations: Must be preserved
Supplier: Brooks

Cocodimonium Hydroxypropyl Hydrolyzed Collagen

Chemical Description: Cocodimethylammonium salt of hydrolyzed collagen
Trade Name: Croquat M

Function in Formula: Substantive conditioner
Use Concentration: 0.5–2.5% in shampoos, conditioners, conditioning perms, relaxers
Solubility Characteristics: Water-soluble
Formulating Considerations: Do not heat above 40°C
Form Supplied: Amber viscous liquid
Microbial Considerations: Standard for proteins
Special Comments: Quaternizing confers higher substantivity than parent protein
Supplier: Croda

Cocodimonium Hydroxypropyl Hydrolyzed Hair Keratin

Chemical Description: Cocodimethylammonium salt of hydrolysate of human hair keratin
Trade Name: Croquat HH
Function in Formula: Substantive permanent conditioning
Use Concentration: 1–5% in conditioning perms, relaxers, posttreatment products, shampoos, conditioners
Solubility Characteristics: Water-soluble
Formulating Considerations: Do not heat above 40°C
Form Supplied: Amber viscous liquid
Microbial Considerations: Standard for proteins
Supplier: Croda

Cocodimonium Hydroxypropyl Hydrolyzed Keratin

Chemical Description: Cocodimethylammonium salt of hydrolyzed keratin
Trade Name: Croquat WKP
Function in Formula: Permanent conditioning protein
Use Concentration: 0.25–2% in shampoos, conditioners, and cream rinses, conditioning perms, relaxers, nail care products
Solubility Characteristics: Water-soluble
Formulating Considerations: Do not heat above 40°C. Should be added between reduction and oxidation steps when used in permanent waves
Form Supplied: Clear amber liquid
Microbial Considerations: Standard for proteins
Special Comments: Provides immediate and perceptible effect in salon hair care
Supplier: Croda

Cocodimonium Hydroxypropyl Hydrolyzed Wheat Protein

Chemical Description: Cocodimethylammonium salt of hydrolysate of wheat protein
Trade Name: Hydrotritium QM
Function in Formula: Substantive conditioner
Use Concentration: 1–5% in shampoos, conditioners, and other hair care products
Solubility Characteristics: Water-soluble
Formulating Considerations: Do not heat above 40°C
Form Supplied: Clear liquid

Microbial Considerations: Standard for proteins
Special Comments: Carries positive charge up to its isoionic point (pH 10). Natural vegetable-derived source
Supplier: Croda

Cocodimonium Hydroxypropyloxyethyl Cellulose

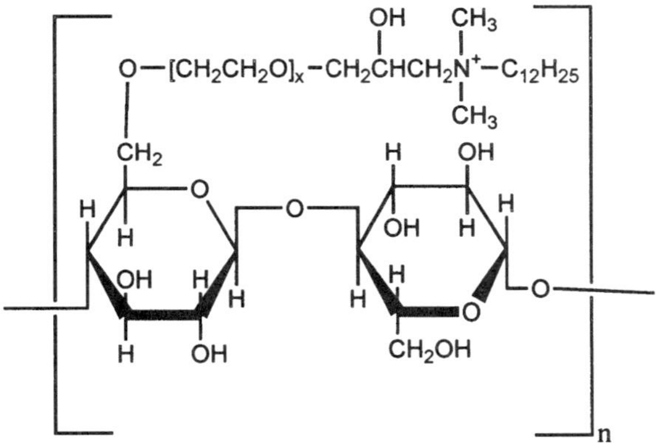

Trade Name: Crodacel QM
Function in Formula: Conditioning agent
Use Concentration: 1–4% in shampoos, conditioners, and cream rinses, skin care products
Solubility Characteristics: Water-soluble
Formulating Considerations: Compatible with anionic surfactants
Form Supplied: Clear pale-yellow, viscous liquid
Special Comments: Quaternizing gives material high substantivity
Supplier: Croda

Cornstarch

Amylose

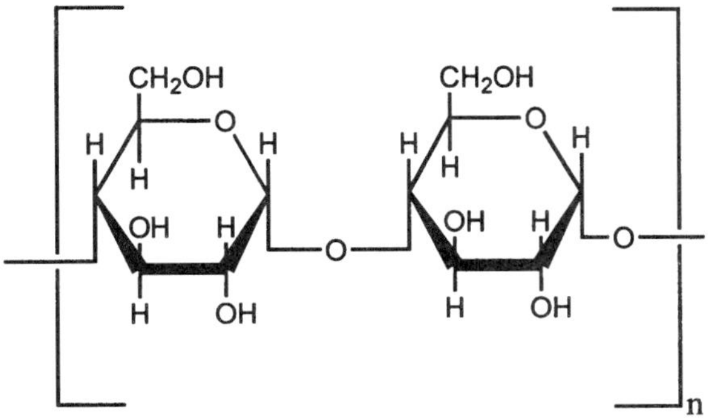

Amylopectin

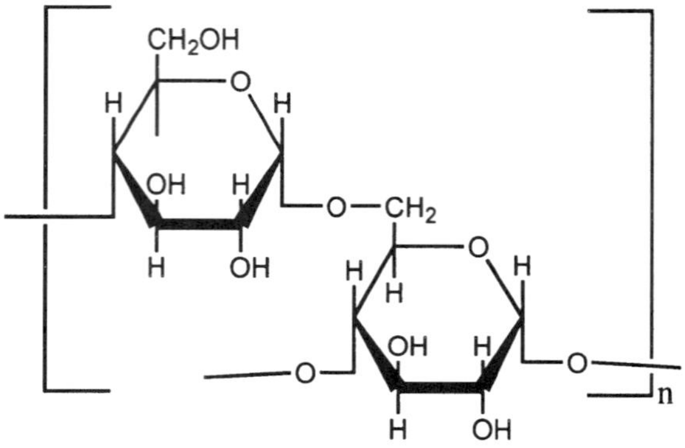

Chemical Description: Natural material obtained from the grain of corn, *Zea mays*; a mixture of two polymeric forms known as amylose and amylopectin
Trade Name: Purity-21
Use Concentration: 1–50% in powders
Solubility Characteristics: Soluble in water when cooked
Form Supplied: White powder
Microbial Considerations: Will support microbial growth. Needs preservation
Supplier: National Starch

Dextrin

Chemical Description: Gum produced by the incomplete hydrolysis of starch by the enzyme amylase to maltose and the high-molecular-weight residue known as dextrin
Trade Name: Nadex 360
Function in Formula: Binder
Use Concentration: 1–10% in soaps
Solubility Characteristics: Soluble in water
Form Supplied: Tan powder
Microbial Considerations: Will support microbial growth
Suppliers: National Starch

Distarch Phosphate

Chemical Description: Material produced by crosslinking starch with sodium metaphosphate
Trade Name: National 78-1898
Function in Formula: Oil and water adsorbent
Use Concentration: 1–50% in powders
Solubility Characteristics: Insoluble in water and alcohol
Form Supplied: White powder
Microbial Considerations: A crosslinked starch. Will support growth of bacteria, etc.
Supplier: National Starch

Ethyl Ester of Hydrolyzed Animal Protein

Chemical Description: Ethyl ester of the hydrolysate of collagen
Trade Names: Crotein ACS

Function in Formula: Conditioner and film modifier
Use Concentration: 0.1–0.5% in alcoholic and hydroalcoholic hair care products and skin care lotions
Solubility Characteristics: Alcohol- and water-soluble
Formulating Considerations: Compatible with most hairspray resins
Form Supplied: Clear amber liquid
Microbial Considerations: Standard for proteins
Supplier: Croda

Ethyl Ester of Hydrolyzed Keratin

Chemical Description: Ethyl ester of the acid hydrolysate of keratin
Trade Name: Crotein ASK
Function in Formula: Conditioner and film modifier
Use Concentration: 0.1-0.5% in alcoholic and hydroalcoholic lotions and hair care setting products
Solubility Characteristics: Alcohol- and water-soluble
Formulating Considerations: Do not heat above 40°C
Form Supplied: Clear amber liquid
Microbial Considerations: Standard for proteins
Supplier: Croda

Gelatin

Chemical Description: Form of partially hydrolyzed collagen that lacks triple helical structure of soluble collagen
Trade Name: Crodyne B419
Function in Formula: Protein conditioner
Use Concentration: 1–5% in skin creams and lotions, hair care products, shaving creams and mousses, soap formulations
Solubility Characteristics: Water-soluble
Formulating Considerations: Dissolve in water before addition. Do not heat above 40°C
Form Supplied: Buff crystalline powder
Microbial Considerations: Standard for proteins
Regulatory Status: NF grade
Supplier: Croda

Trade Name: Cosmetic Gelatin
Function in Formula: Thickening agent, film former, humectant, emulsion stabilizer, skin protectant, antiirritant
Use Concentration: 3% in nail polish or nail hardener, conditioner; 2% in moisturizers as a humectant skin protectant; 1% in emulsions to thicken and stabilize
Formulating Considerations: Add to water, heat to 80°C to dissolve—thickens as it cools
Form Supplied: Crystalline powder
Microbial Considerations: Store in cool, dry area
Regulatory Status: Cosmetic grade
Special Comments: Naturally derived, amphoteric, provided in various gel strengths
Supplier: Hormel

Glycerin (and) Glyceryl Polyacrylate

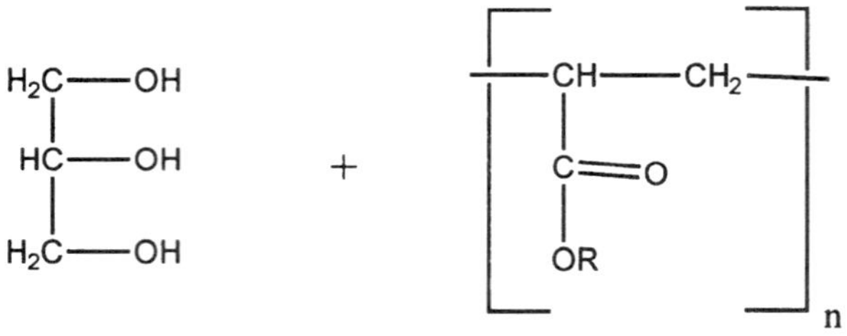

Trade Name: Hispagel 100
Function in Formula: Thickener (gellant), stabilizer, humectant
Use Concentration: 10–30% in flowable to stiff gels, 3–20% in emulsion products (moisturizers), 1–5% in toners/astringents
Solubility Characteristics: Fully miscible in water/polar liquids
Formulating Considerations: Add to water/polar liquid phase with sufficient agitation to fully disperse. Material is not overly shear-or heat-sensitive. Minimize ionic concentration
Form Supplied: Gel concentrate
Microbial Considerations: Material as supplied is highly stable from a microbiological point of view. Dilutions need preserving
Regulatory Status: Approved for use in Japan
Special Comments: Gel structure is destabilized by ionic interactions (avoid salts)
Supplier: Centerchem

Glyceryl Tribehenate (and) Calcium Behenate

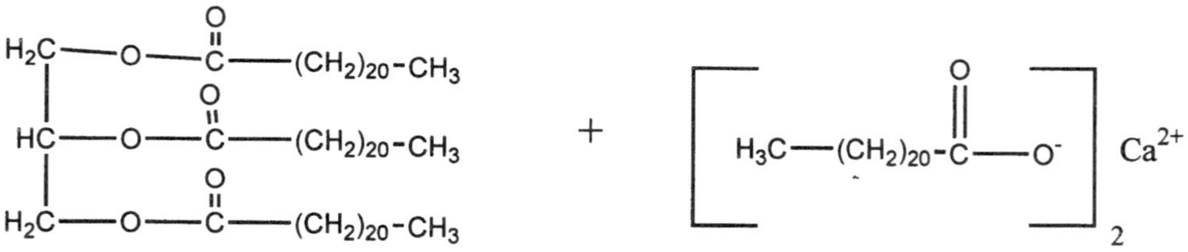

Trade Name: Syncrowax HRS-C
Function in Formula: Gellant
Use Concentration: 2–10% in oils/triglycerides/volatile silicones
Solubility Characteristics: Volatile silicone/oils
Formulating Considerations: Add to oil phase in emulsion systems. Heat until dissolved
Form Supplied: Pale cream flakes
Microbial Considerations: None for special storage–standard emulsion preservative systems
Supplier: Croda

Guar Gum

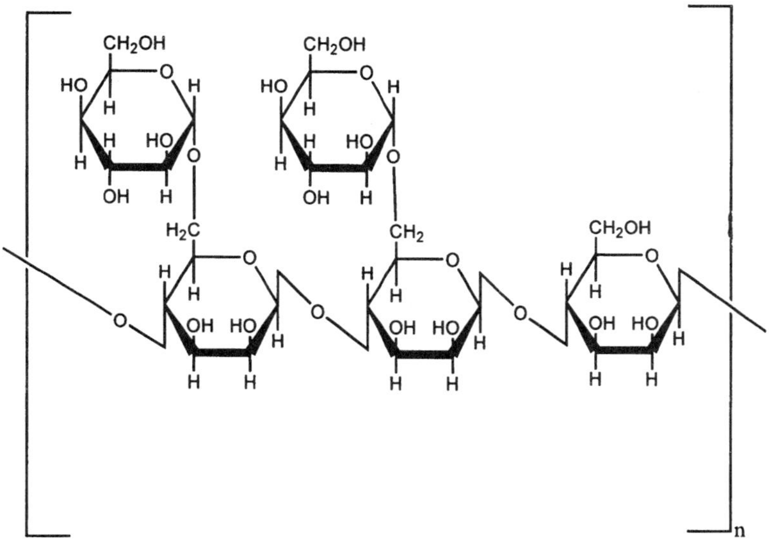

Chemical Description: Backbone of D-mannopyranose units with D-galactopyranose branches
Trade Name: N-Hance 3000 Guar
Function in Formula: Thickener, binder, rheology modifier, substantive polymer
Use Concentration: <1% in hair conditioners, <0.5% in conditioning shampoos, <0.3% in aerosol shave creams
Solubility Characteristics: Soluble in hot and cold water
Form Supplied: Free-flowing powder
Microbial Considerations: Solutions and finished products need to be preserved
Regulatory Status: GRAS
Supplier: Aqualon

Guar Hydroxypropyltrimonium Chloride

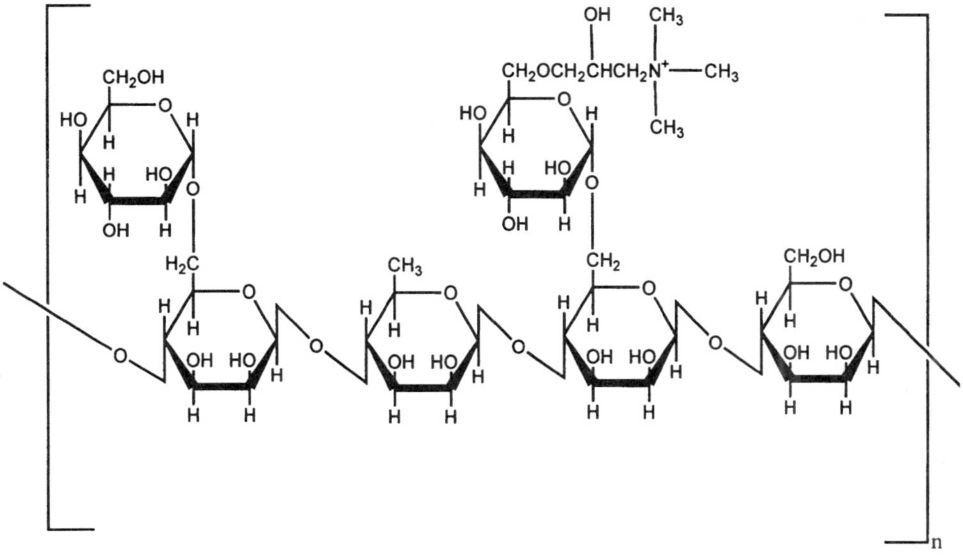

Chemical Name: Depolymerized guar gum, 2-hydroxy-3-(trimethylammoniun) propyl ether chloride
Trade Names: Hi-Care 1000, Jaguar C-135, C-162, C-17 (Rhone-Poulenc); Cosmedia Guar C 261 N (Henkel); NHANCE 3000 Cationic Guar (Aqualon)
Function in Formula: Smooths and protects, is substantive, adds lubricity on skin. Thickening, conditioning, and antistatic agent
Use Concentration: 0.8% in creams; 0.1–1.0% in lotions, shampoos, conditioners, mousses; 0.1–0.3% in o/w skin emulsions; 0.2–0.6% in skin cleansers and liquid soap
Solubility Characteristics: Completely soluble in water and aqueous alcohols. Forms slightly turbid, viscous solutions in water
Formulating Considerations: (1) Add directly to water with agitation, solubilizes immediately, and becomes clear and hydrated with addition of acid (ex. Citric acid) for pH adjustment; or (2) slurry with a nonsolvent such as isopropanol or propylene glycol and add slurry to vigorously agitated water. Compatible with anionic surfactants
Form Supplied: Powder, 100% active
Microbial Considerations: Aerobic plate count: 1000/g max; gram-negative bacteria 0.g: *S. aureus, P. aeruginosa, E. coli, Salmonella*; negative; aerobic organisms <1000 colony-forming units/g; fungi < 100 colony-forming units/g; yeasts < 100 colony-forming units/g
Regulatory Status: Listed on the TSCA inventory, CAS number 65497-29-2
Special Comments: Product is substantive to hair and skin, D.S. = 0.13. Cationic polymer compatible with common anionic surfactants
Suppliers: Rhone-Poulenc, Henkel, Aqualon

Gum Arabic/Gum Acacia

Trade Name: Arabic FT
Function in Formula: Adhesive in lotions, facial masks
Use Concentration: 10–15%
Solubility Characteristics: Water-soluble
Form Supplied: Powder
Microbial Considerations: *Salmonella*-negative, *Staphlococus*-negative
Regulatory Status: No volatile organics
Supplier: TIC Gums

Hectorite

Chemical Name: Sodium magnesium fluorolithosilicate
Chemical Description: One of the montmorillonite minerals that are the principal constituents of bentonite clay
Trade Names: Macaloid and Bentone EW (Rheox); Hectabrite (American Colloid)
Function in Formula: Thickener, suspending agent in water-based systems or o/w emulsions
Use Concentration: 2% in creams and lotions; 2% in antidandruff shampoos
Solubility Characteristics: Disperses in water
Formulating Considerations: Compatible with most cosmetic raw materials. New materials give compatibility with high-cationic loadings. Must be hydrated in water phase prior to addition to formulation
Form Supplied: Flake and powder
Microbial Considerations: Meets ZUSP/NF requirements
Special Comments: Free of crystalline silica
Suppliers: Rheox, American Colloid

Hydrolyzed Collagen

Chemical Description: Hydrolysate of animal collagen
Trade Names: Crotein SPA, Crotein SPO, Crotein SPC

Function in Formula: Conditioner
Use Concentration: 0.2–2% in skin creams and lotions, shampoos, conditioners
Solubility Characteristics: Soluble in cold water or hydroalcoholic systems up to 50% alcohol
Formulating Considerations: Do not heat above 40°C. Dissolve in water before addition
Form Supplied: White powder
Microbial Considerations: Standard for proteins
Regulatory Status: NF grade
Special Comments: Crotein SPC can be used as pharmaceutical binder, excipient, and encapsulant
Supplier: Croda

Hydrolyzed Elastin

Chemical Description: Hydrolysate of elastin
Trade Name: Crolastin
Function in Formula: Skin moisturizer and conditioner
Use Concentration: 1–5% in creams and lotions, hair care products
Solubility Characteristics: Water-soluble
Formulating Considerations: Do not heat above 40°C
Form Supplied: Clear yellow liquid
Microbial Considerations: Standard for proteins
Special Comments: High moisture-binding capacity
Supplier: Croda

Hydrolyzed Fibronectin

Chemical Description: Hydrolysate of fibronectin
Trade Name: Cronectin H
Function in Formula: Humectant and moisturizer
Use Concentration: 0.5–6% in skin creams and lotions
Solubility Characteristics: Water-soluble
Formulating Considerations: Do not heat above 40°C
Form Supplied: Opalescent low-viscosity liquid
Microbial Considerations: Standard for proteins
Supplier: Croda

Hydrolyzed Keratin

Chemical Description: Hydrolysate of keratin
Trade Names: Crotein K, Crotein WKP
Function in Formula: Permanent conditioning protein
Use Concentration: 0.5–3% in shampoos, conditioners, cream rinses, permanent waves, relaxers, nail care products
Solubility Characteristics: Water-soluble
Formulating Considerations: Do not heat above 40°C. Dissolve in water before addition
Form Supplied: Light tan powder (Crotein K), pale yellow liquid (Crotein WKP)
Microbial Considerations: Standard for proteins
Special Comments: Contains cystine. Crotein WKP is derived from wool and has a low salt content
Supplier: Croda

Hydrolyzed Milk Protein

Chemical Description: Hydrolysate of milk protein
Trade Name: Hydrolactin 2500
Function in Formula: Skin conditioner

Use Concentration: 0.2–2% in creams and lotions, especially cleansing creams, eye wrinkle creams
Solubility Characteristics: Water-soluble
Formulating Considerations: Heat-stable, forms clear solutions even at acid pH
Form Supplied: Cream-colored powder
Microbial Considerations: Standard for proteins
Supplier: Croda

Hydrolyzed Protein (and) Hyaluronic Acid

Chemical Description: Complex of hydrolyzed collagen proteins and hyaluronic acid mucopolysaccharide formed from *N*-acetyl-D glucosamine and glucuronic acid
Trade Name: Cromoist HYA
Function in Formula: Skin conditioner
Use Concentration: 0.5–2% in creams and lotions, especially facial creams
Solubility Characteristics: Water-soluble
Formulating Considerations: Do not heat above 40°C
Form Supplied: Clear yellow liquid
Microbial Considerations: Standard for proteins
Special Comments: Can increase moisture retention by 33%
Supplier: Croda

Hydrolyzed Silk

Chemical Description: Hydrolysate of silk protein
Trade Name: Crosilk 10,000
Function in Formula: Skin moisturizer, hair conditioner
Use Concentration: 0.5–2% in creams, lotions, shampoos, and conditioners
Solubility Characteristics: Water-soluble
Formulating Considerations: Do not heat above 40°C
Form Supplied: Clear amber liquid
Microbial Considerations: Standard for proteins
Supplier: Croda

Hydrolyzed Soy Protein

Chemical Description: Hydrolysate of soya flour
Trade Name: Hydrosoy 2000/SF
Function in Formula: Moisturizer
Use Concentration: 0.2–3% in skin care preparations
Solubility Characteristics: Water-soluble
Formulating Considerations: Do not heat above 40°C
Form Supplied: Clear amber liquid
Microbial Considerations: Standard for proteins
Special Comments: Naturally derived from vegetable source; salt-free
Supplier: Croda

Hydrolyzed Wheat Protein (and) Wheat Oligosaccharides

Chemical Description: Hydrolysate of wheat proteins containing oligosaccharides
Trade Name: Cropeptide W
Function in Formula: Moisturizer
Use Concentration: 1–5% in shampoos, conditioners, styling aids especially for damaged hair

Solubility Characteristics: Water-soluble
Formulating Considerations: Do not heat above 40°C; product may show slight precipitate on aging
Form Supplied: Clear amber liquid
Microbial Considerations: Standard for proteins
Special Comments: Increases relaxation of hair at low humidity, decreases it at high humidity
Supplier: Croda

Hydrolyzed Wheat Protein Polysiloxane Copolymer

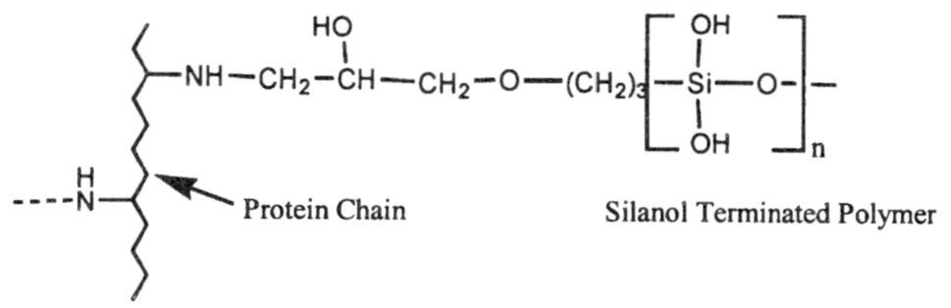

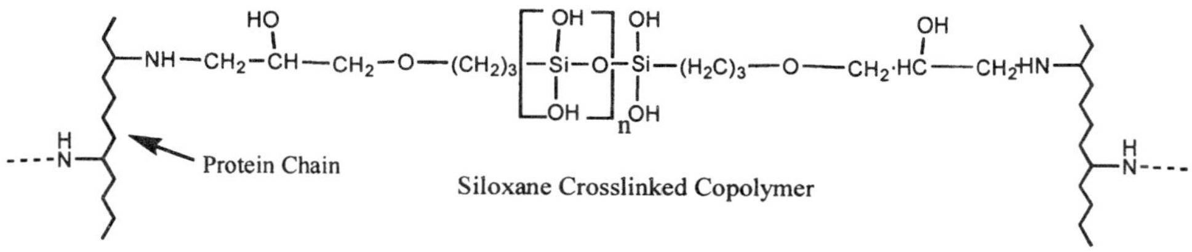

Trade Name: Crodasone W
Function in Formula: Forms conditioning network on hair
Use Concentration: 1–5% in shampoos and conditioners, also used in styling aids
Solubility Characteristics: Water-soluble above pH 5.5, soluble in aqueous surfactant systems at all pHs
Formulating Considerations: To obtain clear solutions, adjust pH above or turbidity (pH 4–6) or add to surfactant solution
Form Supplied: Amber liquid
Microbial Considerations: Standard for proteins
Special Comments: Has ability to cross-link with itself on drying or at ambient conditions of dehydration
Supplier: Croda

Hydrolyzed Whole Oats

Chemical Description: Hydrolysate of whole oats containing oligosaccharides and protein
Trade Name: Cromoist O-25
Function in Formula: Skin conditioner, moisturizer
Use Concentration: 1–5% in creams and lotions
Solubility Characteristics: Water-soluble
Formulating Considerations: Do not heat above 40°C
Form Supplied: Mobile amber liquid
Microbial Considerations: Standard for proteins
Special Comments: Can enhance feel of properties of emulsions
Supplier: Croda

Hydrolyzed Whole Wheat Protein

Chemical Description: Hydrolysate of wheat protein
Trade Name: Hydrotritium 2000
Function in Formula: Conditioner
Use Concentration: 1–5% in shampoos, conditioners, creams and lotions
Solubility Characteristics: Water-soluble
Formulating Considerations: Do not heat above 40°C
Form Supplied: Yellow to light amber clear liquid
Microbial Considerations: Standard for proteins
Special Comments: Contains cystine, provides permanent conditioning
Supplier: Croda

Hydroxyethylcellulose

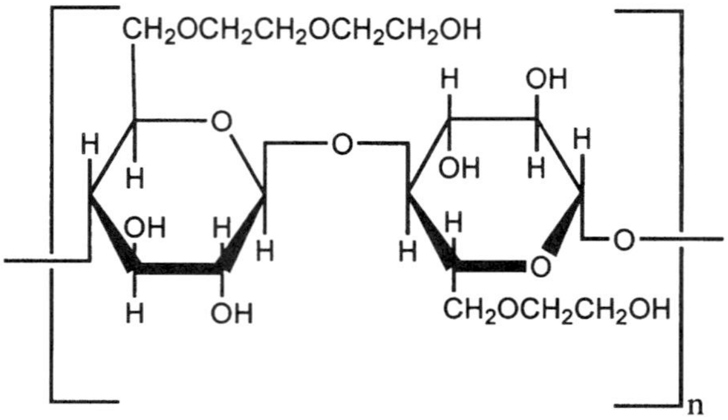

Trade Names: Natrosol (Aqualon); Cellosize (Amerchol); Viscontran HEC (Henkel); Liporamnosan, Alcoramnosan, Idraramnosan (Vevy)
Function in Formula: Thickener and stabilizer; rheology modifier
Use Concentration: 0.5–1% in conditioning products; 1% in shampoos; 1% in toothpastes, 1% in vaginal lubricants; 0.5–1.5% in shaving gels
Solubility Characteristics: Complete in hot and cold water, will tolerate small amounts of some organic solvents
Formulating Considerations: Dissolve in water first and then add remaining ingredients; excellent tolerance to salts and pH variation. Cosmetic grades are usually surface-treated to simplify solution preparation
Form Supplied: Free-flowing granular powder
Microbial Considerations: Solutions and finished products require preservation
Regulatory Status: Complies with FDA regulation (**21** CFR), for adhesives in packaging. Listed on EPA/TSCA inventory. Grades that conform to National Formulary requirements are available. Reviewed and approved for use by CTFA's CIR panel. Approved for use by MHE in Japan. CIR: *JACT* 5(3), 1986
Special Comments: Available in 10-molecular weight grades. Both surface-treated and non-treated forms are available. A nonionic polymer that functions as a highly efficient thickener of aqueous solutions. The solutions are pseudoplastic. It has a high tolerance for dissolved electrolytes/salts
Suppliers: Aqualon, Henkel, Amerchol, Kraft Chemical, Vevy

Hydroxypropyl Guar

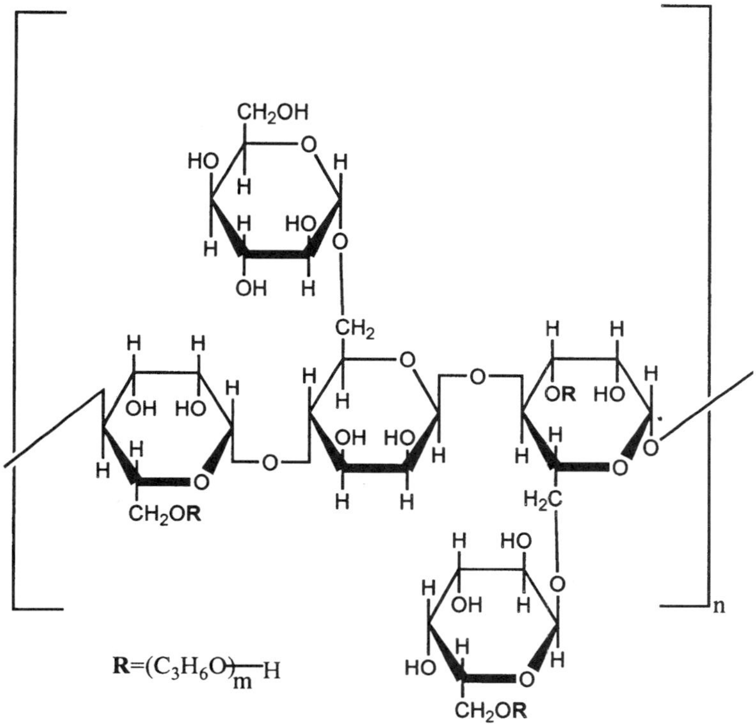

Trade Names: Jaguar HP 8, HP 60, HP 120
Function in Formula: Viscosity building, emulsion stabilizer, foam stabilizer, lubrication
Use Concentration: 1–3% in toiletry products, creams and lotions, shave gels, astringents, and shampoos
Solubility Characteristics: Soluble in water
Formulating Considerations: Disperse in water phase, adjust pH to 4–6 with acid. Once hydrated, pH can be adjusted as desired
Form Supplied: Free-flowing powder
Microbial Considerations: Total plate count 1000 max
Regulatory Status: TSCB inventory CAS no. 3941-75-5
Special Comments: Nonionic polymer compatible with all surfactant types
Supplier: Rhodia

Hydroxypropylmethyl Cellulose

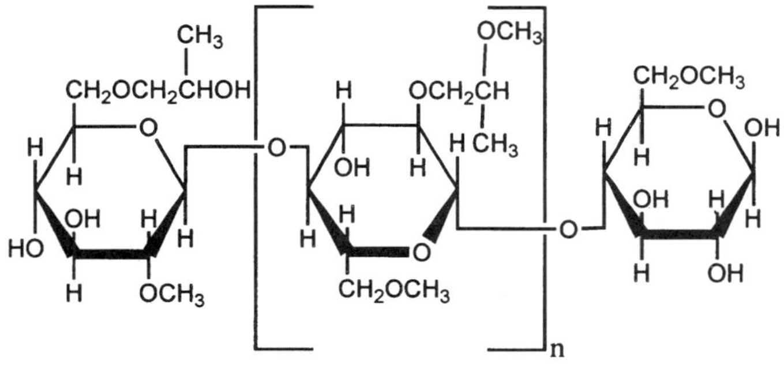

Trade Names: Methocel (Dow), Viscontran (Henkel)
Function in Formula: Thickens, improves later, emulsion stabilizer
Use Concentration: 0.5–8% in shampoos, 0.3–0.5% in liquid hand soap; 0.8% in cleansing gels, 0.5% in hair conditioners; 0.4% in cosmetic emulsions; 0.4–2% in linaments; 0.2–2% in creams
Solubility Characteristics: Cold-water-soluble
Formulating Considerations: Some grades of Methocel are efficient, good-clarity thickeners that are surface-treated to enable direct addition to tap water of pH ≤ 7.5. Good electrolyte tolerance stable over pH range 3–11. Some grades are dispersible in alcohols and glycols
Form Supplied: Powder; granulated
Microbial Considerations: Is manufactured under nearly sterile conditions, not readily degraded by bacteria, is attacked by cellulase enzymes
Regulatory Status: No special rules apply
Special Comments: A polymeric surfactant and thickener. Methocel F4MP is often used in tandem with magnesium aluminum silicate
Suppliers: Dow Chemical, Henkel

Hydroxypropylcellulose

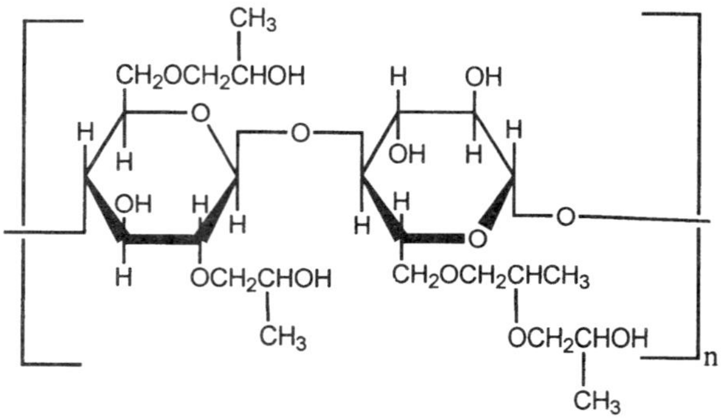

Trade Name: Klucel
Function in Formula: Thickener, foam stabilizer, rheology modifier, film former
Use Concentration: <1% in shaving creams, <1% in hair-styling products
Solubility Characteristics: Insoluble in water hotter than 45°C. Soluble in many polar organic solvents, including ethanol
Formulating Considerations: Disperse in water at 60°C and cool to hydrate
Form Supplied: Free-flowing powder, granular powder
Microbial Considerations: Subject to microbiological degradation. Needs to be preserved
Regulatory Status: Grades designated ''F'' comply with U.S. Code of Federal Regulations Title 21, Section 172-870—for food use. Conforms with Food Chemical Codex
Special Comments: Six viscosity ranges available
Supplier: Aqualon

Isostearoyl Hydrolyzed Collagen

Chemical Description: Condensate of isostearic acid chloride and the hydrolysate of collagen
Trade Name: Crotein IP
Function in Formula: Conditioner
Use Concentration: 0.1–0.5% in nail care products
Solubility Characteristics: Oil-soluble, solvent-soluble
Formulating Considerations: Add to oil phase; do not heat above 40°C

Form Supplied: Clear viscous liquid
Microbial Considerations: Standard for proteins
Supplier: Croda

Karaya Gum

Trade Name: Gum Karaya
Function in Formula: Thickener
Solubility Characteristics: Soluble in water
Microbial Considerations: *Salmonella*-negative, *Staphylococcus*-negative
Supplier: TIC Gums

Lauryldimonium Hydroxypropyl Hydrolyzed Wheat Protein

Chemical Description: Lauryl dimethylammonium salt of hydrolysate of wheat protein
Trade Name: Hydrotritium QL
Function in Formula: Substantive conditioner
Use Concentration: 1–5% in shampoos, conditioners, and other hair care products
Solubility Characteristics: Water-soluble
Formulating Considerations: Do not heat above 40°C
Form Supplied: Clear liquid
Microbial Considerations: Standard for proteins
Special Comments: Carries positive charge up to isoionic point (pH = 10)
Supplier: Croda

Laurdimonium Hydroxypropyl Oxyethyl Cellulose

Trade Name: Crodacel QL
Function in Formula: Conditioner
Use Concentration: 1-4% in shampoos, conditioners, and cream rinses, skin creams and lotions
Solubility Characteristics: Water-soluble
Form Supplied: Clear, pale yellow, viscous solution
Special Comments: High substantivity due to quaternization
Supplier: Croda

Magnesium Aluminum Silicate

Chemical Description: A complex silicate refined from naturally occurring minerals
Trade Names: Veegum F, HS, HY, K, Regular, T (Vanderbilt); Gelwhite MAS-H, Gelwhite MAS-L (Southern Clay)
Function in Formula: Thickener/suspension aid
Use Concentration: 0.5–5% in aqueous systems
Solubility Characteristics: Insoluble, easily dispersible in water to form thixotropic gels
Formulating Considerations: Activated by shear and heat. Hydrate in water before adding other ingredients. Functions over a wide pH range. Synergistic with organic polymers
Form Supplied: Flake, powder
Microbial Considerations: Inert. All major indicator organisms are absent
Regulatory Status: CIR reviewed and safe. GRAS listed. N. F. Monograph
Suppliers: Vanderbilt, Kraft Chemicals, Southern Clay

Maltodextrin

Chemical Description: Saccharide material obtained by hydrolysis of starch
Trade Name: Maltrin Maltodextrin

Function in Formula: Moisturizer, thickener
Solubility Characteristics: Soluble in cold water
Formulating Considerations: Compatible with gums and other hydrocolloids
Form Supplied: Spray-dried powder or agglomerated particles
Microbial Considerations: Complex carbohydrate, very fermentable
Regulatory Status: GRAS, **21** CFR 184.1444
Special Comments: Grain processing

Melanin

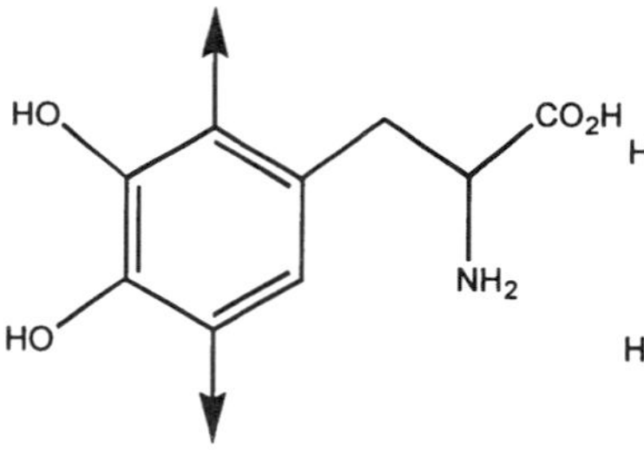

uncyclized units

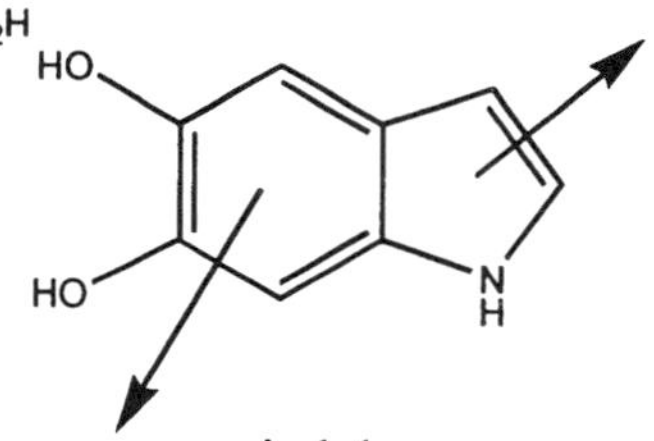

indoles

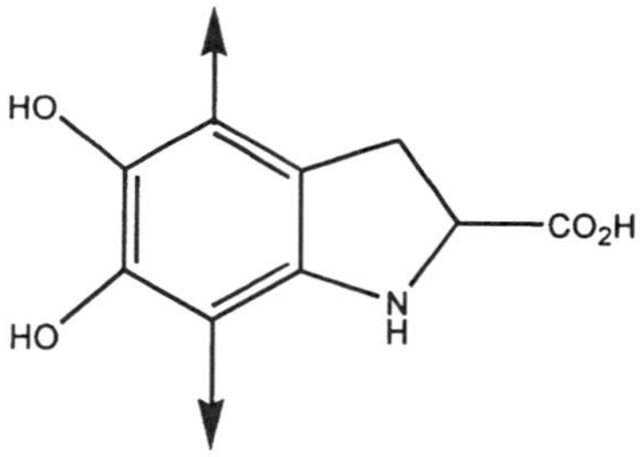

indolines

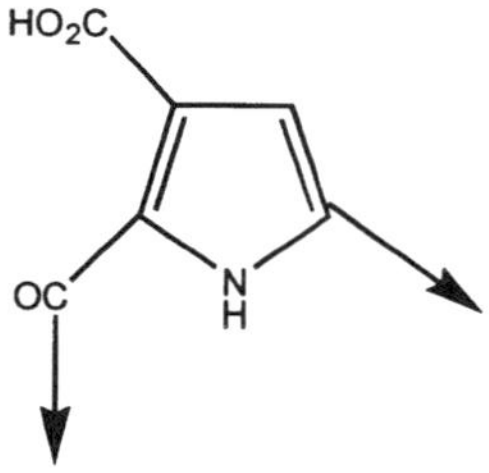

pyrroles

Chemical Name: Melanin
Chemical Descriptions: A nanoparticulate suspension that imparts a natural color to formulae, hair, and skin. Melanin is composed of four major monomeric units: uncyclized units; indoles; indolines; and pyrroles. It has an empirical formula of $C_{7.4\text{-}7.8}$ $H_{4.5\text{-}6.2}$ N $O_{3.6\text{-}3.8}$. Both the fractional nature and range of the empirical formula reflect the fact that melanin is a polymer composed of various percentages of more than one type of monomeric unit
Trade Names: MelanInk, SepiaMelanInk, All Natural Melanin
Function in Formula: Free-radical neutralization, adjuvant for boosting SPF
Use Concentration: 0.1–10% in skin care formulations; 0.1–10% in hair care formulations
Solubility Characteristics: Sparingly soluble in dilute alkali; insoluble in other solvents
Formulating Considerations: Compatible with gels and creams; incompatible with acidic pH (i.e., below 4); best results when added with aqueous phase
Form Supplied: Aqueous suspension (10% solids wt/wt) or dry, free-flowing powder
Microbial Considerations: None
Regulatory Status: None
Supplier: Mel-Co

Methylcellulose

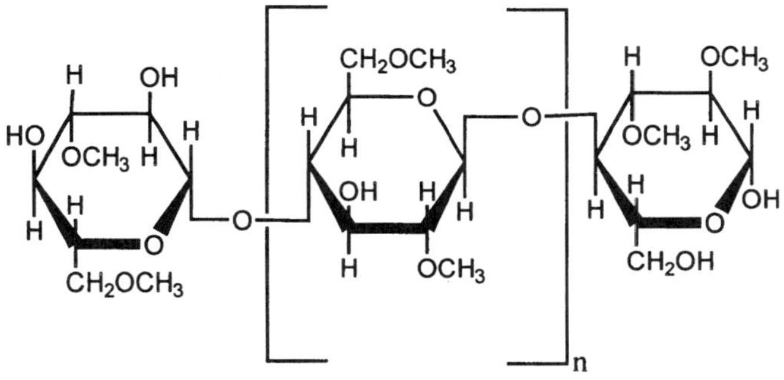

Trade Name: Viscontran
Function in Formula: Thickener and stabilizer
Use Concentration: 1–2% in linaments; 1–2% in toothpaste; 1–2% in creams
Solubility Characteristics: Soluble in water
Formulating Considerations: Generally unaffected by salts in solution or by wide changes in pH
Form Supplied: Granulated or powder. Not readily degraded by bacteria; is attacked by cellulase enzymes
Microbial Considerations: Below 1000/g
Regulatory Status: Free from solvents
Special Comments: Viscosity 2% (20°C): ~3000 mPa
Supplier: Henkel

Microcrystalline Cellulose and Carboxymethyl Cellulose Sodium, N. F

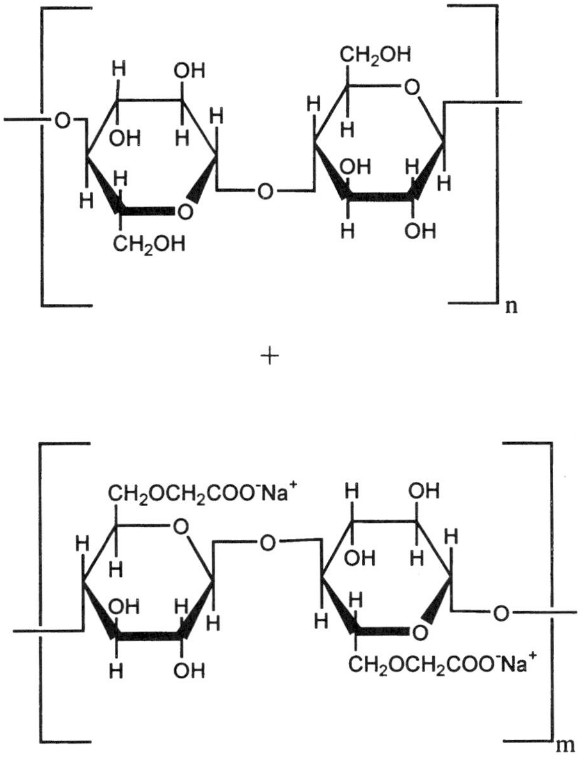

Chemical Name: Cellulose
Trade Name: Avicel
Function in Formula: Suspending, thickening agent, colloidal thixotrope
Use Concentration: 1.2% in cosmetic, personal care suspensions; 2% in reconstitutable suspensions; 1–2% in pharmaceutical suspensions; 1.5–2.5% in cosmetic creams and lotions
Solubility Characteristics: Water-dispersible
Formulating Considerations: Always add first to water with good mixing. Compatible with other hydrocolloids and some hydroalcoholic liquids
Form Supplied: White powder, odorless
Microbial Considerations: Total plate count, not more than 100/pg. Total yeasts and molds, not more that 20/g
Regulatory Status: GRAS
Supplier: FMC, Food and Pharmaceutical Products Division

Montmorillonite

Structure: Refined complex silicate clay mineral with a general composition of: $Al_2O_5 \cdot 4\ SiO_2 \cdot 4\ H_2O$
Trade Names: Gelwhite or Mineral Colloid
Function in Formula: Suspending/thickening agent
Use Concentration: 0.5–5% in suspensions of emulsions
Solubility Characteristics: Easily dispersible in water to form thixotropic gels
Formulating Considerations: Hydrate in water before adding other ingredients. Functions over a wide pH range. Provides synergism with organic polymers
Form Supplied: Powder
Microbial Considerations: Can be bacteria-controlled
Regulatory Status: FDA status-GRAS
Supplier: Southern Clay

Nitrocellulose

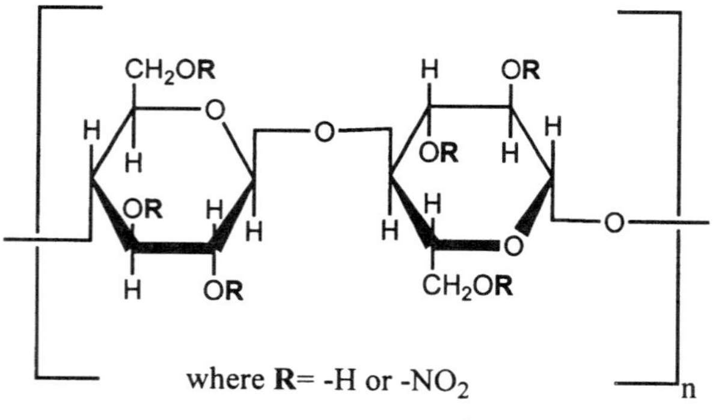

Chemical Name: Cellulose nitrate
Trade Names: Nitrocellulose RS 1/4 Sec., Isopropyl Wet, RS1/2 Sec., Isopropyl Wet
Function in Formula: Film former in nail lacquers
Solubility Characteristics: Soluble in esters, ketones, ether/alcohol mixtures, glycol ethers. Excellent tolerance for aromatic diluent (toluene), less tolerant for aliphatic diluents
Formulating Considerations: Avoid drying out during processing
Supplier: Aqualon

Nonoxynyl Hydroxyethylcellulose

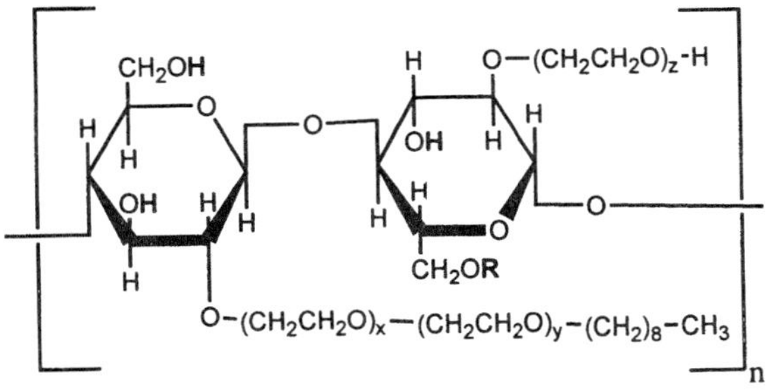

Chemical Name: Hydrophobe modified hydroxyethyl cellulose
Trade Name: Amercell Polymer HM-1500
Function in Formula: Primary thickener
Use Concentration: 0.5–1.5% in lotions and creams, 0.1–0.5% in liquid makeup, 0.1–1.5% in shampoo
Solubility Characteristics: Readily soluble in water and water/alcohol mixtures
Formulating Considerations: A nonionic polymer that enables it to be widely compatible with most standard personal care ingredients
Form Supplied: Off-white, free-flowing, granular powder
Microbial Considerations: Does not contain an antimicrobial as sold. Formulations must be preserved
Special Comments: An associative thickening without the tacky feel usually associated with high-molecular-weight polymers
Supplier: Amerchol

Pectin

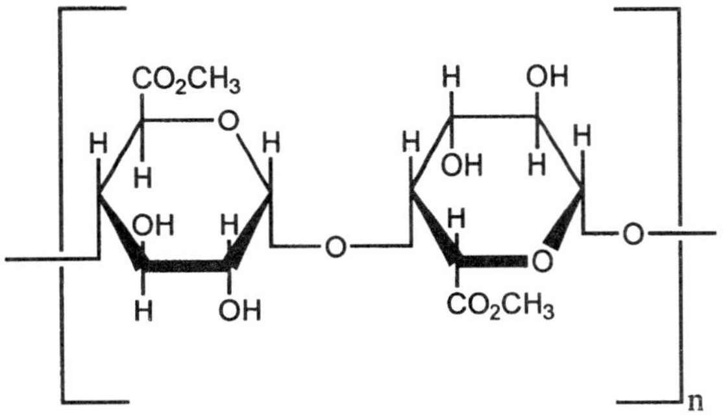

Trade Name: Pectin HM Slow (Cesapectin)
Function in Formula: Gel former
Solubility Characteristics: Soluble in boiling water
Formulating Considerations: Optimum percent solids and pH
Form Supplied: Powder
Microbial Considerations: *Salmonella*-negative, *Staphylococcus*-negative
Supplier: TIC Gums

Polyquaternium-4

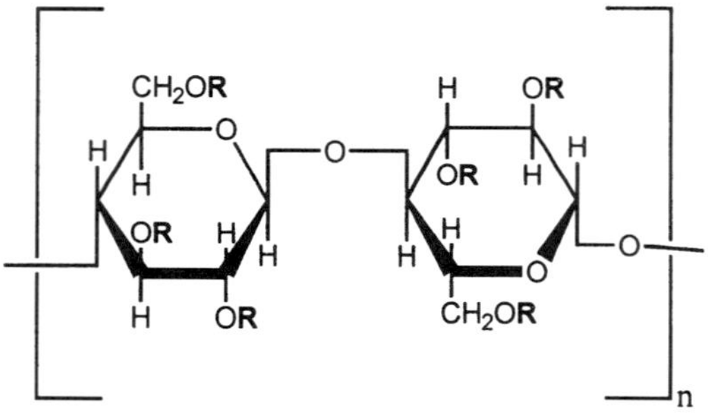

R= -H, or -$(CH_2CH_2O)_n$-H, or

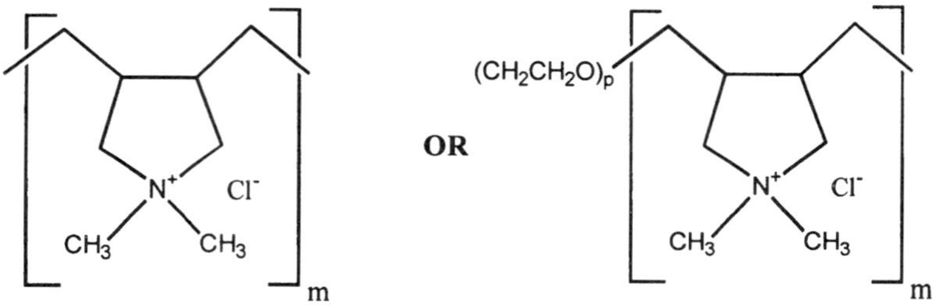

Chemical Description: Copolymer of hydroxyethylcellulose and dimethyldiallyl ammonium chloride

Trade Names: Celquat-L200, 14-100, 5C-240

Function in Formula: Hair fixative/conditioning agent

Use Concentration: 0.5% in shampoo; 1–3% in water for use in hair lotion, mousse; 1–3% in skin care products

Solubility Characteristics: Soluble in water

Form Supplied: Tan granular powder

Microbial Considerations: Can be bacteria-controlled

Special Comments: Polymer in cationic. Contains 2% nitrogen

Supplier: National Starch

Polyquaternium-10

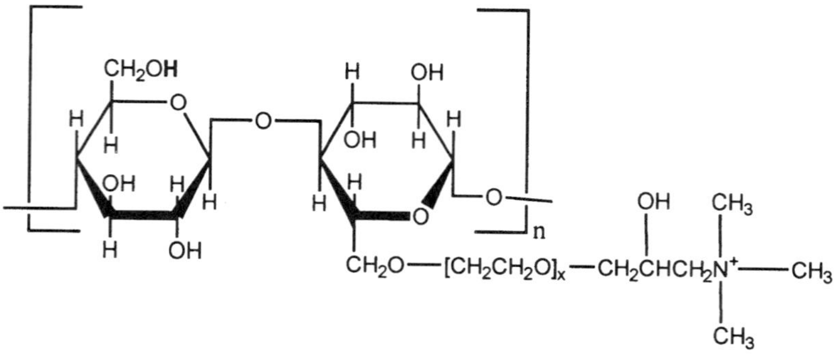

Chemical Description: Polymeric quaternary ammonium salt of hydroxyethylcellulose and a trimethyl ammonium substituted epoxide

Trade Names: Ucare Polymers JR, SR, SK and LR (Amerchol); Celquat 5C-240 (National Starch)
Function in Formula: Substantive conditioning agent for hair and skin
Use Concentration: 0.3–1% in shampoos; 0.3–1% in hair care lotions, gels, mousses; 0.2–1% in skin care products; 0.3–1% in cleansers
Solubility Characteristics: Soluble in water and 50% aqueous ethanol
Formulating Considerations: Compatible in anionic, amphoteric, nonionic, or cationic systems and is formulation flexible to suit any conditioning requirement
Form Supplied: Powder
Microbial Considerations: Free of bacteria contamination, does not contain an antimicrobial as sold. Formulations require preservation
Regulatory Status: Reviewed and approved by CIR panel. Reviewed and approved by MHW for use in Japan. Approved for use in Europe and all major markets throughout the world
Special Comments: Substantive to protein substrates
Supplier: Amerchol, National Starch

Polyquaternium-24

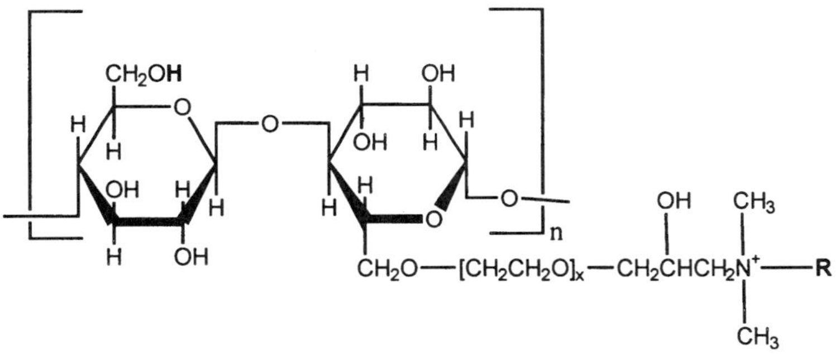

Chemical Description: Alkyl-modified hydroxyethyl cellulose quaternary
Trade Name: Quatrisoft Polymer LM-200
Function in Formula: Multifunctional substantive conditioner for skin and hair products. Adds mild surfactancy. Efficient thickener
Use Concentration: 0.2–0.5% in skin lotions/creams, 0.5–1.0% in shampoo, 0.5–1.0% in conditioning mousse products
Solubility Characteristics: Soluble in water, soluble in hydroalcoholic systems to 50% ethanol
Formulating Considerations: Compatible with most standard personal care ingredients
Form Supplied: Powder
Microbial Considerations: Product does not contain an antimicrobial
Special Comments: Substantive to protein substrates, forms a uniform film on hair and skin as a result of its balanced hydrophobic/hydrophilic structure. Has associative thickening properties that can generate desired solution rheology
Supplier: Amerchol

Polyquaternium-24 and Hyaluronic Acid

Chemical Description: Association complex of an alkyl-modified quaternized hydroxyethylcellulose and hyaluronic acid
Trade Name: BioCare Polymer HA-24
Function in Formula: A substantive complex that greatly enhances the durability of hyaluranonic acid on protein substrates

Use Concentration: 1.0–5% in moisturizing lotions, 1.0–3% in cleansers, 0.5–3% in moisturizing gels
Solubility Characteristics: Readily soluble in water
Formulating Considerations: Widely compatible with most standard personal care ingredients
Form Supplied: 2.6% active association complex in water
Microbial Considerations: Contains a preservative and should be handled accordingly
Special Comments: The substantivity has been demonstrated by a number of sophisticated techniques, including radiolabeling. Additionally, the material has excellent hydrating and skin-smoothing properties
Supplier: Amerchol

Quaternium-18 Bentonite

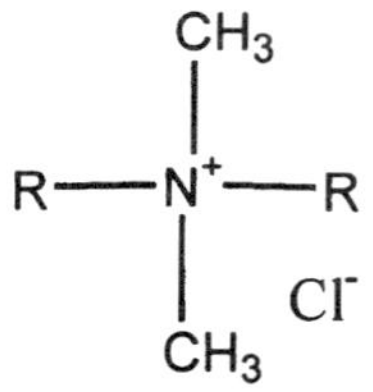

Chemical Description: Reaction product of bentonite and quaternium-18
Trade Name: Claytone
Function in Formula: Thickener/suspending agent
Use Concentration: 0.5–5% in organic solvent systems
Solubility Characteristics: Designed for solvent systems such as cyclomethicone
Formulating Considerations: Disperse under high shear prior to adding other ingredients
Form Supplied: Powder
Microbial Considerations: Can be bacteria-controlled
Supplier: Southern Clay

Quaternium-18 Hectorite

Chemical Description: Reaction product of hectorite and the quaternary salt that conforms to the structure shown, where R represents hydrogenated tallow free radicals
Trade Name: Bentone 38
Function in Formula: Thickener/suspending agent, thixotrope
Use Concentration: 1.5% in hair grooming products; 1.5% in suntan products; 1.5% in eye products
Solubility Characteristics: Disperses in oils
Formulating Considerations: Needs activation and high shear for dispersion
Form Supplied: Powder or predispersed gels
Regulatory Status: CIR approved
Special Comments: Free of crystalline silica, also available in minneral oil, petroleum distillates and volatile silicon
Supplier: Rheox

Sclerotium Gum

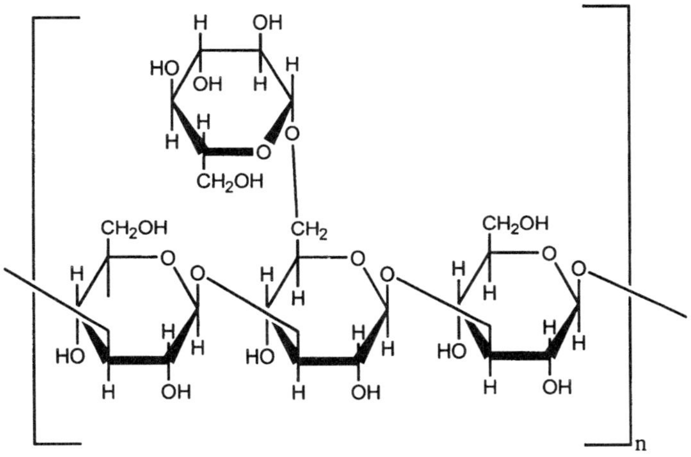

Trade Name: AMIGEL
Function in Formula: Gelling agent
Use Concentration: 1% in gel, 0.02% in emulsion as a thickener
Solubility Characteristics: Soluble in water (up to 4%)
Formulating Considerations: Compatible with oils, surfactants, electrolytes
Microbial Considerations: Aerobic germs < 100/g
Supplier: Alban Muller

Silk Powder

Chemical Description: Undenatured protein of pulverized silk
Trade Name: Crosilk Powder
Function in Formula: Modifies application, leveling, and oil adsorbancy in solid makeup systems
Use Concentration: 1.5% in solid makeup systems
Solubility Characteristics: Insoluble
Formulating Considerations: Can tolerate temperatures as high as 100°C for 5 hr
Form Supplied: Milky white, crushed powder
Microbial Considerations: Standard for proteins
Supplier: Croda

Sodium C_{8-16} Isoalkylsuccinyl Lactoglobullin Sulfonate

Trade Name: Biopol OE
Function in Formula: Oil-absorbing polymer
Use Concentration: 1.5% in foundations and cleansers, 0.5–1% in toners/fresheners
Solubility Characteristics: Water dispersible
Formulating Considerations: Add last
Form Supplied: Liquid
Microbial Considerations: Will support microbial growth—must be preserved
Supplier: Brooks Industries

Sodium Hyaluronate

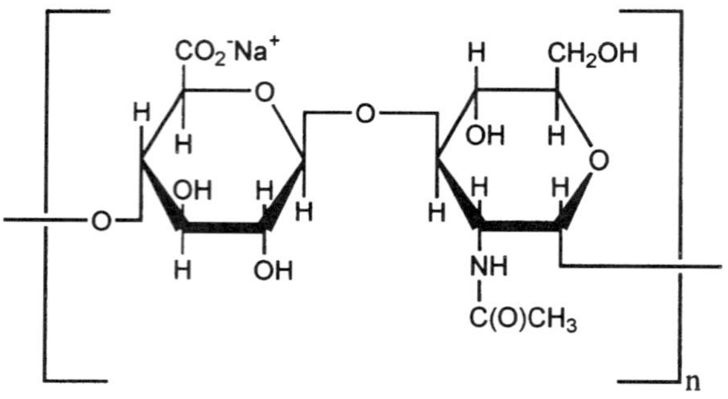

Trade Name: Hyalure
Function in Formula: Moisturizer, viscosifier, emulsifier
Solubility Characteristics: Very soluble in water. Gel will form at higher concentrations
Formulating Considerations: Compatible with aqueous solutions, low alcohol aqueous systems, oil systems
Form Supplied: Aqueous solution with Germaben II7 as a preservative
Microbial Considerations: Rich nutrient source, must be preserved
Supplier: Life Core Biomedical

Sodium Lignosulfonate

Chemical Structure: This product is a mixture of polymeric species; no distinct chemical structure can be drawn
Trade Name: DARVAN No. 2
Function in Formula: Dispersing agent
Use Concentration: 0.5–4% of the weight of the material to be dispersed
Solubility Characteristics: Soluble in water
Form Supplied: Dark brown powder, 84.5% min. Active
Microbial Considerations: Susceptible to microbial attack, requires preservation
Supplier: Vanderbilt

Sodium Magnesium Silicate

Trade Name: Laponite
Function in Formula: Thickener/suspension aid
Use Concentration: 0.2–2%
Solubility Characteristics: Disperses in water to form clear thixotropic gels
Formulating Characteristics: Disperse in water prior to addition of other ingredients. Gives synergistic effect with organic polymers
Form Supplied: Powder
Microbial Considerations: Can be bacteria-controlled
Supplier: Southern Clay

Sodium Collagen

Chemical Description: Nonhydrolyzed native protein of collagen consisting of precursors of mature collagen
Trade Names: Collasol, Clearcol

Function in Formula: Skin moisturizer and conditioner
Use Concentration: 2–10% in creams and lotions
Solubility Characteristics: Water-soluble
Formulating Considerations: Do not heat above 35°C
Form Supplied: Off-white dispersion (Collacol), clear to slightly hazy viscous liquid (Clearcol)
Microbial Considerations: Standard for proteins
Supplier: Croda

Sodium Keratin

Chemical Description: Keratin protein in soluble form
Trade Name: Kerasol
Function in Formula: Permanent conditioning protein
Use Concentration: 1–10% in conditioning perms, relaxers, shampoos, and conditioners
Solubility Characteristics: Water-soluble
Formulating Considerations: Do not heat above 40°C; add to permanent waves at reduction stage
Form Supplied: Clear to slightly hazy viscous amber liquid
Microbial Considerations: Standard for proteins
Supplier: Croda

Sodium Reticulin

Chemical Description: Reticulin in soluble form
Trade Name: Reticusol
Function in Formula: Film-forming moisturizer
Use Concentration: 0.5–2% in creams and lotions
Solubility Characteristics: Water-soluble
Formulating Considerations: Do not heat above 40°C
Form Supplied: Pale straw liquid
Microbial Considerations: Standard for proteins
Supplier: Croda

Sodium Wheat Protein

Chemical Description: Wheat protein in soluble form
Trade Name: Tritisol
Function in Formula: Film-forming conditioner (permanent)
Use Concentration: 1–5% in creams and lotions, especially moisturizing creams and antiwrinkle creams, conditioners, shampoos
Solubility Characteristics: Water-soluble
Formulating Considerations: Do not heat above 40°C
Form Supplied: Amber viscous liquid
Microbial Considerations: Standard for proteins
Special Comments: Contains cystine, shows perceptible, temporary skin-firming effect

Stearalkonium Bentonite

Chemical Description: Reaction product of bentonite and stearalkonium chloride
Trade Name: Claytone
Function in Formula: Thickener/suspension aid
Use Concentration: 0.5–5%
Solubility Characteristics: Designed for solvent systems such as cyclomethicone, mineral oil, and toluene

Formulating Considerations: Disperse under high shear prior to adding other ingredients
Form Supplied: Powder
Microbial Considerations: Can be bacteria-controlled
Supplier: Southern Clay

Stearalkonium Hectorite

Chemical Description: Reaction product of hectorite clay and stearalkonium chloride
Trade Name: Bentone 27
Function in Formula: Thickener, suspension agent, thixotrope
Use Concentration: 1.5% in nail polish; 1.5% in antiperspirants; 1.5% in lip products
Solubility Characteristics: Disperses in oils and solvents
Formulating Considerations: Compatible with most cosmetic raw materials. Needs activation and high shear for dispersion
Form Supplied: Powder or predispersed gels
Special Comments: Free of crysalline silica, also available predispersed in IPM, lanolin oil, castor oil, and Finsolve TN
Supplier: Rheox

Steardimonium Hydroxyethyl Cellulose

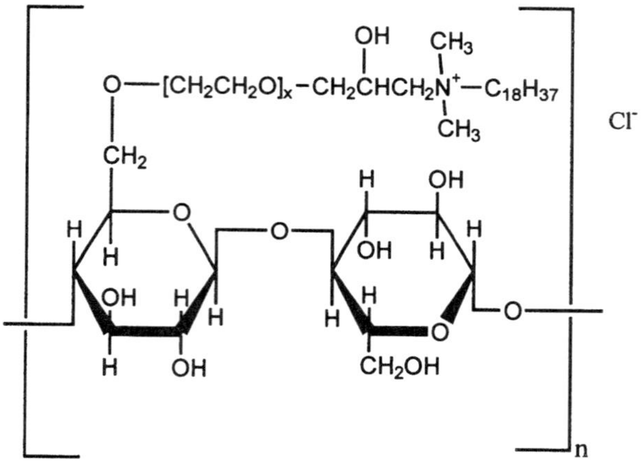

Trade Name: Crodacel QS
Function in Formula: Conditioning agent
Use Concentration: 1–4% in creams, lotions, hair conditioners, shampoos
Solubility Characteristics: Water-soluble at low concentrations
Formulating Considerations: Heat to 50°C and stir well before using to ensure homogenicity
Form Supplied: Pale yellow solution
Microbial Considerations: Use a standard preservative system
Supplier: Croda

Stearyldimonium Hydroxypropyl Hydrolyzed Collagen

Chemical Description: Stearyldimethylammonium salt of hydrolysate of collagen
Trade Name: Croquat S
Function in Formula: Substantive conditioner
Use Concentration: 0.5–2.5% in cream rinses and conditioners

Solubility Characteristics: Partially water-soluble with slight haze
Formulating Considerations: Do not heat above 40°C
Form Supplied: Amber viscous liquid/semisolid
Microbial Considerations: Standard for proteins
Supplier: Croda

Stearyldimonium Hydroxypropyl Hydrolyzed Wheat Protein

Chemical Description: Stearyl dimethylammonium salt of hydrolysate of wheat protein
Trade Name: Hydrotritium QS
Function in Formula: Substantive conditioner
Use Concentration: 1–5% in shampoos, conditioners, cream rinses
Solubility Characteristics: Essentially water-soluble
Formulating Considerations: May require warming to achieve homogeneity. Do not heat above 40°C
Form Supplied: Opaque viscous dispersion
Microbial Considerations: Standard for proteins
Supplier: Croda

Stearyldimonium Hydroxypropyl Oxyethyl Cellulose

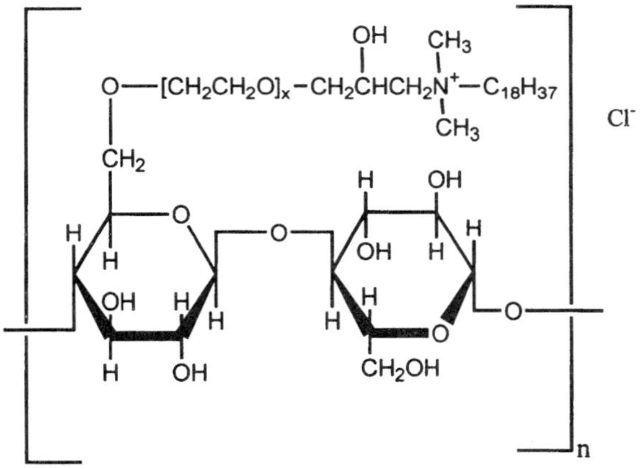

Trade Name: Crodacel QS
Function in Formula: Conditioning agent
Use Concentrations: 1–4% in hair care, skin care products
Solubility Characteristics: Water-soluble at low concentrations
Formulating Considerations: To ensure homogeneity, heat to 50°C and stir well before using; some phase separation of product may occur
Form Supplied: Pale yellow, opaque viscous liquid
Microbial Considerations: Standard for proteins
Supplier: Croda

Stearyltrimonium Hydroxyethyl Hydrolyzed Collagen

Chemical Description: Stearyl trimethylammonium salt of hydrolysate of collagen
Trade Name: Crotein Q
Function in Formula: Substantive conditioner
Use Concentration: 0.5–2.5% in shampoos and conditioners

Solubility Characteristics: Water-soluble
Formulating Considerations: Do not heat above 40°C. Dissolve in water before addition
Form Supplied: White to off-white powder, free-flowing
Microbial Considerations: Standard for proteins
Supplier: Croda

Tragacanth Gum

Chemical Description: Dried gummy exudate obtained from *Astragatus gummifer*
Function in Formula: Effective emulsifying agent, stabilizer in lotions
Use Concentration: 1.0–1.5% in shampoo; 1.0–2.0% in toothpaste
Solubility Characteristics: Cold-water-soluble
Formulating Considerations: To maximize hydration, always add gum to water before adding any other ingredients with water under vigorous agitation
Form Supplied: Powder
Microbial Considerations: *Salmonella*-negative, *Staphylococcus*-negative
Regulatory Status: **21** CFR 184.1351
Supplier: TIC Gums

Xanthan Gum

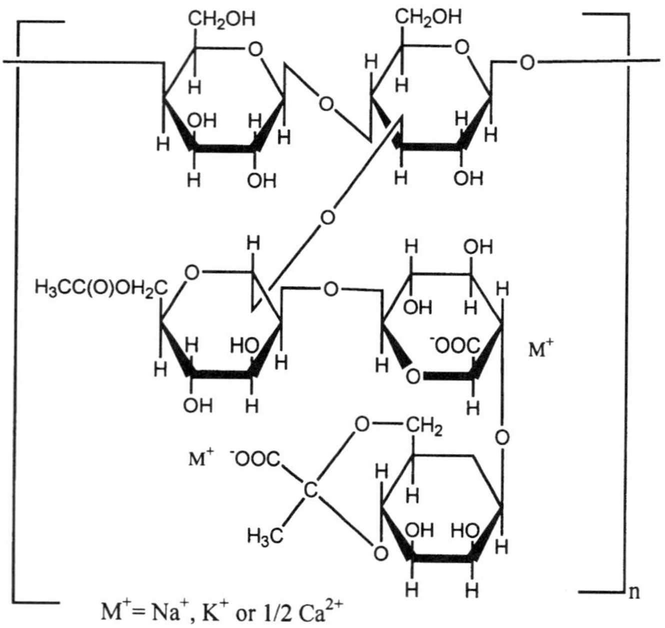

$M^+ = Na^+, K^+$ or $1/2\ Ca^{2+}$

Trade Names: Keltrol CG (Calgon), Tixaxan (TIC), Rhodigel (Rhodia and Vanderbilt)
Function in Formula: Stabilizer, thickener, enhances mouthfeel, is an excellent suspension agent, pumpability, stabilizes emulsions, creamy consistency, controls rheology
Use Concentration: 0.1–3% in creams and lotions; 0.1–3% in shampoos and conditioners, 0.1% in mascaras, 0.1–3% in toothpaste, 0.1–1% in suspensions
Solubility Characteristics: Cold-water-soluble; it is readily dispersed in cold and hot water to form colloid solutions, insoluble in most organic solvents
Formulating Considerations: For best results, always add gum to water before adding any other ingredient with water under vigorous agitation. Compatible with cellulose derivatives, starch,

pectin, gelatin, dextrin, alginates, carrageenan, and stable in solutions containing mono- and divalent salts. Incompatible with cationics

Form Supplied: Cream to white powder or fine powder, 95% min. through 80 mesh

Microbial Considerations: Highly resistant to enzymatic degradation. Total plate count 2000 max. Susceptible to microbial attack. Preservation required

Regulatory Status: **21** CFR 172.695, Food Chemicals Codex and National Formulary. TSCA registered. CAS No. 11138-66-2

Special Comments: Excellent stability in the presence of acids and salts and at low pH. Excellent pseudoplastic rheology. Anionic polysaccharide

Supplier: Calgon, TIC Gums, Rhone-Poulenc, Vanderbilt

Xanthan Gum/Locust Bean Gum Blend

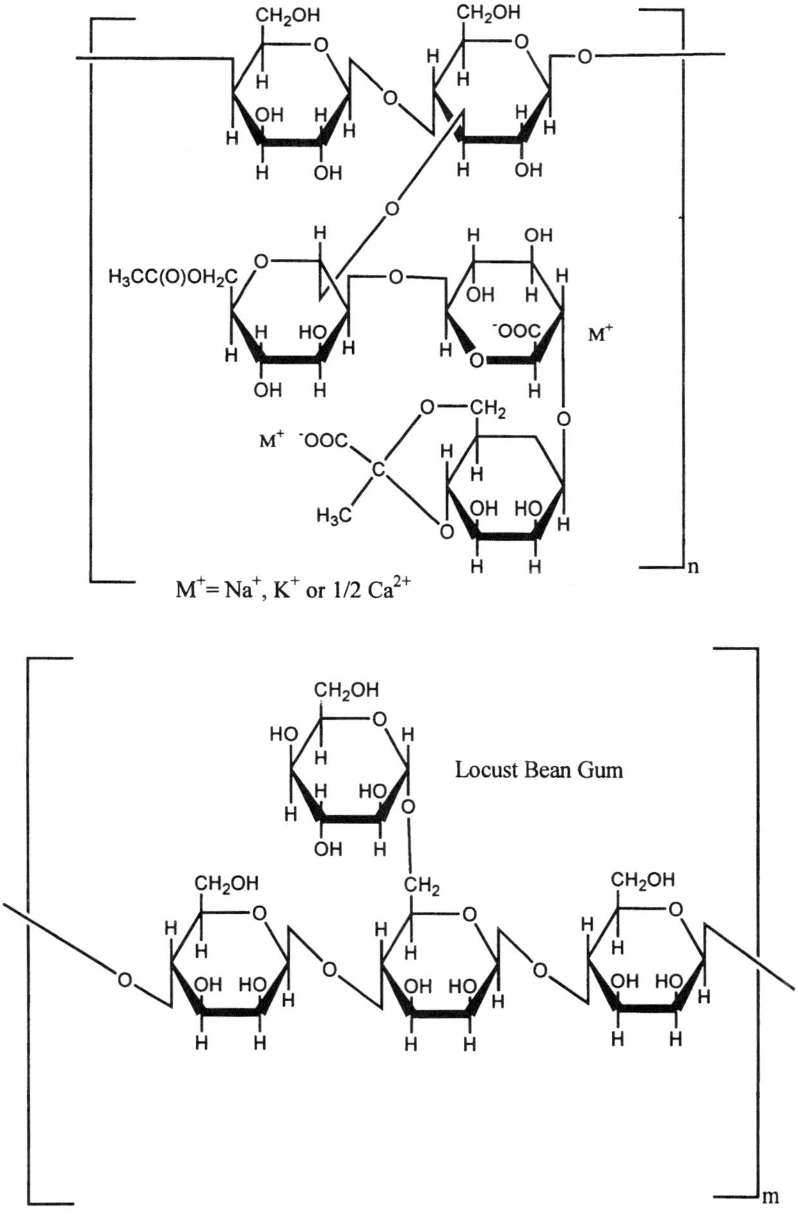

Trade Name: Kelgum CG
Function in Formula: Thickening/gelling agent, suspension and emulsion stabilizer
Use Concentration: 0.2–0.5% in creams and lotions
Solubility Characteristics: Soluble in hot water
Formulating Considerations: For best results, should be hydrated in hot water, preferably above 80°C. Thermo-reversible gels melt and reset at 50–55°C
Form Supplied: White to tan powder
Regulatory Status: Locust bean gum meets FDA regulations 186.1343. It is also accepted as a food additive by the WHO and the Codex Alimentarius. **21** CFR 172.695, Food Chemical Codex and National Formulary
Supplier: Calgon

II. SYNTHETICS

Acrylamide/Sodium Acrylate Copolymer

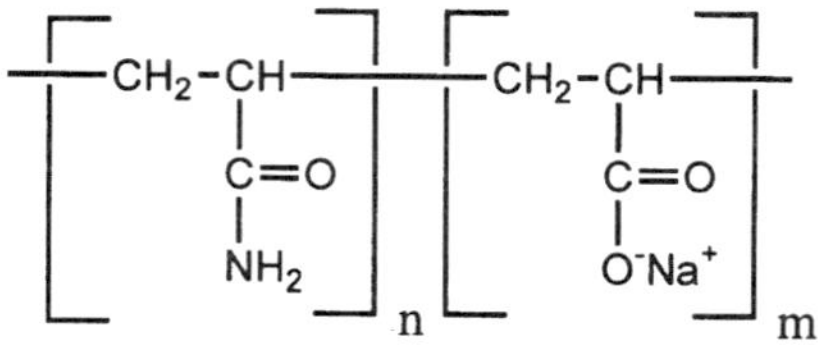

Chemical Name: Poly(acrylamide-co-sodium acrylate)
Trade Name: Hostacerin PN 73
Function in Formula: Thickener
Use Concentration: 0.5–1.0% in emulsions
Solubility Characteristics: Soluble in water
Form Supplied: Powder
Regulatory Status: Benzene-free
Supplier: Hoescht

Acrylate/Acrylamide Copolymer

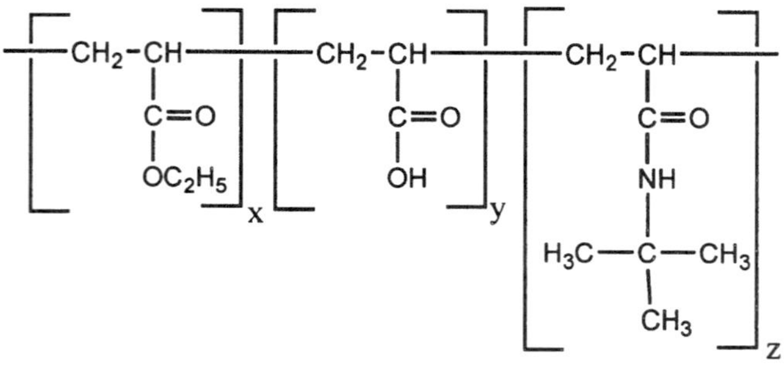

Chemical Description: Terpolymer of acrylic acid, ethyl acrylate, and *N*-t-butyl acrylamide
Trade Names: Ultrahold 8, Ultrahold Strong
Function in Formula: Hair resin, fixative, film former
Use Concentration: 2–4% in hair fixatives
Solubility Characteristics: Soluble in alcohols and alkalies

Formulating Considerations: Must be neutralized to approximately 75–80% for best results. 100% neutralization confers water solubility
Form Supplied: Powder
Special Comments: Solubility can be controlled by pH adjustment
Supplier: BASF

Acrylate Copolymer

Trade Name: ANTIL 208
Function in Formula: Thickening agent for surfactant solutions
Use Concentrations: 0.5–2% in shampoos, shower gels, etc.
Form Supplied: Liquid
Supplier: Goldschmidt

Acrylate/C10-30 Alkyl Acrylate Crosspolymer

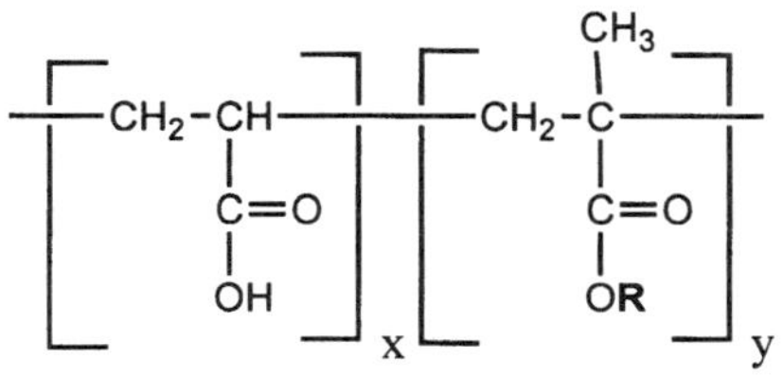

R = long chain alkyl group

Chemical Description: Copolymers of acrylic or methacrylic acid and a long-chain alkyl acrylate cross-linked with an allyl ether pentaerythritol or sucrose
Trade Names: Carbopol 1342, 1382 resins; Pemulen TR-1 TR-2 resins
Function in Formula: Carbopol 1342 and 1382 resins are thickening/gelling and suspending agents for surfactant systems; Pemulen TR-1 and TR-2 resins are primary emulsifiers for lotions and creams
Use Concentration: 0.5–1.5% in shampoos, shower gels, and sanitizing gels (Carbopol 1342 and 1382); 0.1–0.2% in creams, lotions, and low to high viscosity emulsions (Pemulen TR-1 and TR-2)
Solubility Characteristics: Appreciable solubility in water, alcohol, and polar solvents
Formulating Considerations: Pemulen resins are mostly easily handled by dispersing the resins in the oil phase, preparing a slurry in the oil, and adding the slurry to the water phase with mixing. Heat is not necessary for emulsification unless the oil phase contains solid waxy materials. Carbopol resins are most easily dispersed into ambient temperature water with rapid agitation and then combining with the surfactant, alkali, or amine solution to neutralize Carbopol for maximum gel strength. Thickening efficiency is reduced in the presence of electrolytes
Form Supplied: White, fine amorphous powders
Microbial Considerations: Resists bacterial attack and does not support mold growth. Preservation recommended for dispersions that will be stored for several weeks and for other components in the final formulations
Regulatory Status: Carbopol 1382 and Pemulen TR-1 and TR-2 are manufactured without benzene. Carbopol 1342 and Pemulen TR-1 and TR-2 are approved by Japanese MHW
Special Comments: If higher-viscosity emulsions are required, Carbopol resins may be used in combinations with Pemulen TR-1. Pemulen TR-2 is effective where the mode of emulsion applications is via spray mechanism
Form Supplied: Powder
Supplier: BF Goodrich

Acrylates/Copolymer

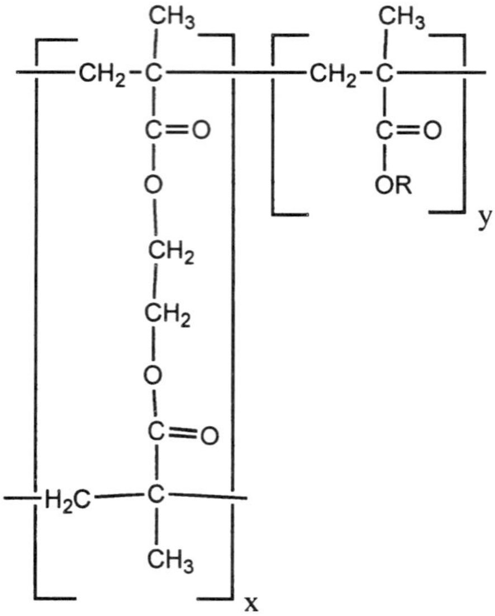

Chemical Description: Copolymer of methylmethacrylate and ethylene glycol dimethacrylate
Trade Name: Polytrap Q5-6603, Microsponge Delivery System
Function in Formula: Controlled delivery of silicones, esters, mineral oils, solvents, waxes, glycerols, glycols, water, perfumes to the skin. Allows formulator to combine incompatible materials in same formula. Reduces comedone formation. Absorbs excess oil and sebum from the skin. Used in pigmented makeup, sun care products, skin creams, and lotions, antiperspirants and deodorants, body powders, perfumes, pressed powders, facial cleansers
Solubility Characteristics: Insoluble, cross-linked polymer
Formulating Considerations: Adsorption of actives is achieved by simply folding the active ingredient into the polymer powder with good mixing. Adsorption capacity can be modified by use of surfactants or coupling agents. Do not use at pH greater than 10 or less than 2
Form Supplied: Free-flowing powder
Microbial Considerations: Preservatives should be added after the addition of acrylates copolymer
Supplier: Dow Corning

Acrylates/Octylacrylamide Copolymer

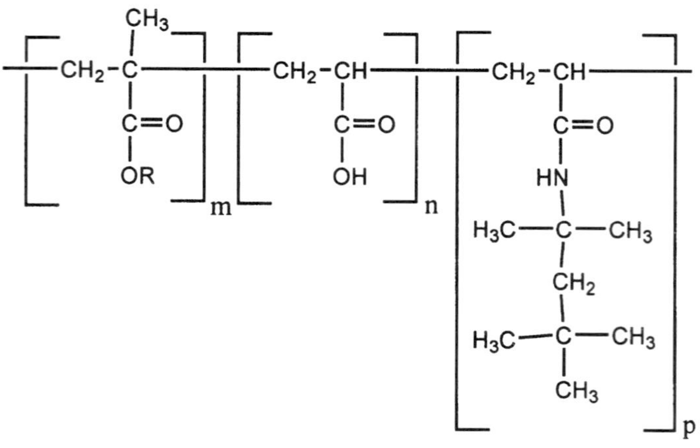

Trade Name: Versatyl-42
Function in Formula: Hair fixative
Use Concentration: 3–5% in hairspray, 5% in styling lotion
Solubility Characteristics: Soluble in ethanol and isopropanol
Formulating Considerations: Must be neutralized when formulated. AMP is most commonly used
Form Supplied: White powder
Regulatory Status: Benzene-free
Special Comments: Acidity = 3.2 mEq/g. Hard holding with good tactile properties
Supplier: National Starch

Acrylates/Steareth-20 Methacrylates Copolymer

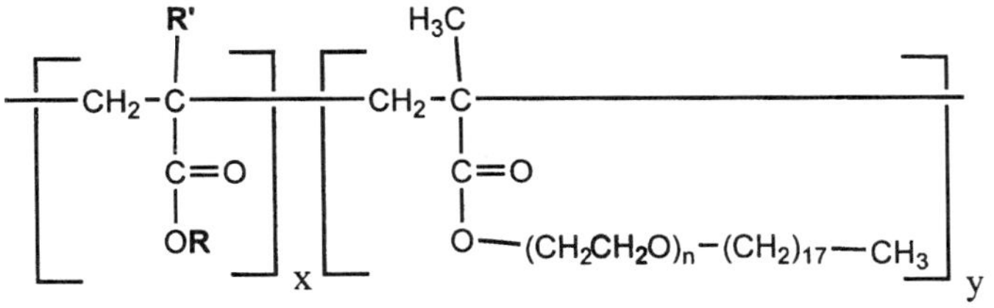

where **R** = alkyl; n has average value of 20
R′ = H or CH_3

Chemical Name: Acrylic polymer
Trade Name: Acrysol ICS-1
Function in Formula: Thickener
Use Concentration: 1.5% in shampoos; 1.0% in hand creams; 3.5% in free-standing gels
Solubility Characteristics: Yields clear formulations, highly soluble
Formulating Considerations: Can be added directly to aqueous formulation
Form Supplied: 30% active aqueous emulsions
Special Comments: Works in formulations with a pH > 7.0
Supplier: Rohm and Haas

Acrylic Acid/Acrylonitrogens Copolymer

Trade Name: Hypan SA-100H, SR-150H
Function in Formula: SA-100H is an emulsifier, viscosifier, and tactile modifier; SR-150H builds viscosity in presence of electrolytes
Use Concentration: 0.05–1% in gels and emulsions
Solubility Characteristics: Hydrogel insoluble in all solvents. Swells in water
Formulating Considerations: Compatible in all aqueous systems. Always added to the water phase
Form Supplied: Powder
Regulatory Status: Contains no organic volatiles. OTC drug master file available
Special Comments: SA-100H forms continuous film on skin. Produces waterproofing emulsions. Detacktifies other polymers. SR-150H tolerates high electrolytes concentrations
Supplier: Lipo

Acrylic/Acrylate Copolymer

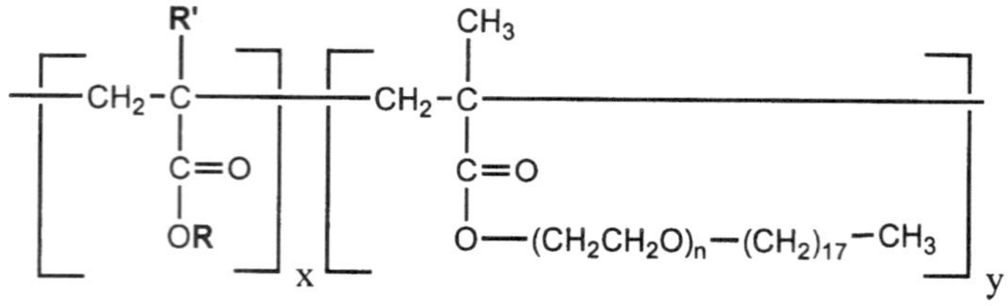

where **R** = alkyl; n has average value of 20
R′ = H or CH_3

Chemical Description: Copolymer of acrylic acid and a monomer consisting of methacrylic acid or a simple ester of acrylic acid or methacrylic acid
Trade Name: Carboset 514, 515, 525, XL-19, XL-19X2, XL-40;526
Function in Formula: Film former, waterproofing agent
Use Concentration: 1–25% in waterproof sunscreens; 1–10% in waterproof mascara
Solubility Characteristics: Soluble in ethanol, isopropanol ethyl acetate. Soluble at 10% solids in ammonia water, pH 7–8.5
Form Supplied: 515—syrup; 525, 526—flake; 514, XL-19, XL-28, XL-40—30–40% dispersions in ammonia water
Microbial Considerations: Preservation required in contact with water. 515, 525, 526 stable as supplied. XL-19X2, XL-28 are preserved with Dowicil 200. XL-40 is preserved with methylparaben plus propylparaben
Supplier: BF Goodrich

Acrylic Esters and Methacrylics Esters Copolymer

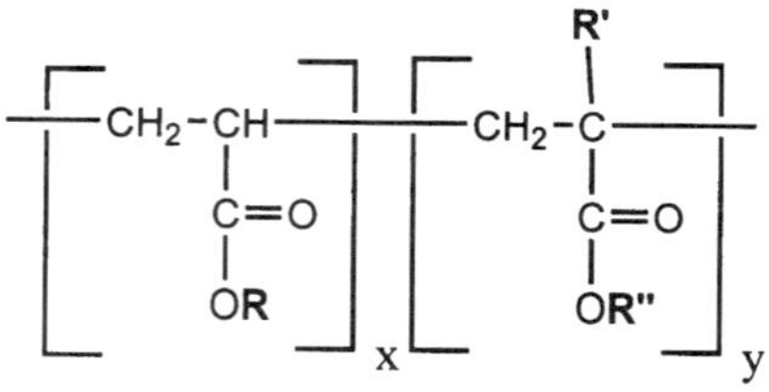

R = H or lower alkyl

Trade Name: Diahold EX-55
Function in Formula: Anionic hair fixative resin
Solubility Characteristics: Soluble in water and alcohol
Formulating Considerations: Compatible with most propellants and additives
Form Supplied: 55% SD-alcohol solution
Supplier: Mitsubishi Yuka

Adipic Acid/Dimethylaminohydroxypropyl Diethylenetriamine Copolymer

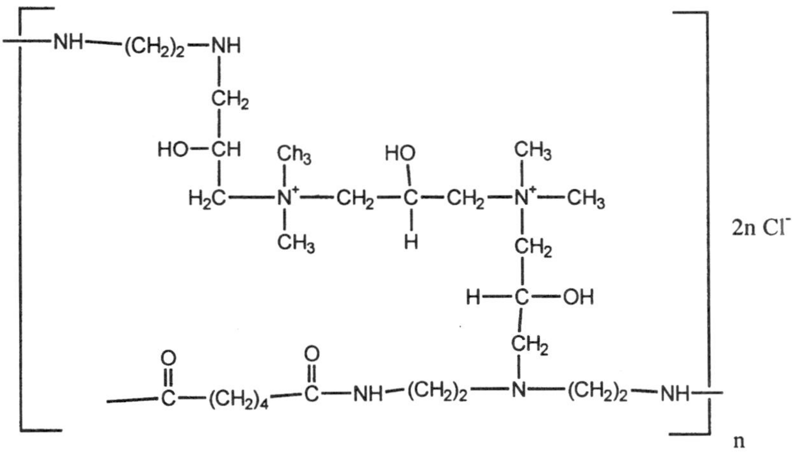

Trade Names: Cartaretin F-4 Liquid, Cartaretin F-23 Liquid
Function in Formula: Hair conditioner and bodifier
Use Concentration: 1–3% in shampoos; 3–10% in hair conditioners, rinses; 3–20% in hair-setting lotions, gels, sprays
Solubility Characteristics: Miscible in water, ethanol
Formulating Considerations: Compatible with cationics and most anionics, can be compatibilized with strongly anionic surfactants
Form Supplied: 30% active liquid in H_2O (F-4); 23% active liquid (F-23)
Microbial Considerations: No microbial problems experienced
Regulatory Status: No known hazardous components, nonirritant, not CIR reviewed
Supplier: Sandoz

Aluminum Starch Octenyl Succinate

Chemical Description: Aluminum salt of the reaction product of octenylsuccinic anhydride with starch
Trade Name: Dry Flo
Function in Formula: Active ingredient in powders and lotions
Use Concentration: 1–5% in powders; 1–20% in gels; 1–10% in lotions
Solubility Characteristics: Insoluble in water and alcohols
Formulating Considerations: Free-flowing, not wetted by liquid water
Form Supplied: Fine, white powder
Microbial Considerations: A starch derivative, will support growth of bacteria, etc.
Supplier: National Starch

Ammonium Acrylates/Acrylonitrogens Copolymer

Trade Name: Hypan SS-201
Function in Formula: Detackifier, thickener
Use Concentration: 0.05–1% in gels and emulsions
Solubility Characteristics: Hydrogel-insoluble in all solvents. Swellable in water
Formulating Considerations: Compatible in all aqueous systems. Always added to water phase

Form Supplied: Powder
Regulatory Status: Contains no organic volatiles. OTC drug master file available
Supplier: Lipo

Amodimethicone

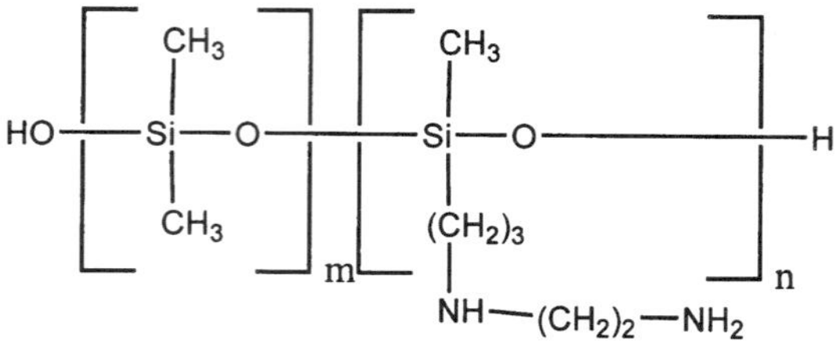

Chemical Description: Silicone polymer end-blocked with amino functional groups
Trade Name: 929 Cationic Emulsion
Function in Formula: Hair conditioning agent. Especially effective for damaged hair to give durability without buildup
Use Concentration: 2% in hair conditioners
Formulating Considerations: Excellent compatibility with cationic surfactants, glycol ethers, nonionic surfactants and anionic surfactants, at low concentrations. Amodimethicone emulsion should be added to anionic surfactants with continuous stirring to minimize chances of precipitation
Form Supplied: Water-thin emulsion
Special Comments: During formulation and processing, like other cationic emulsions, this product should be kept away from the face and eyes
Supplier: Dow Corning

AMP-Acrylated Copolymer

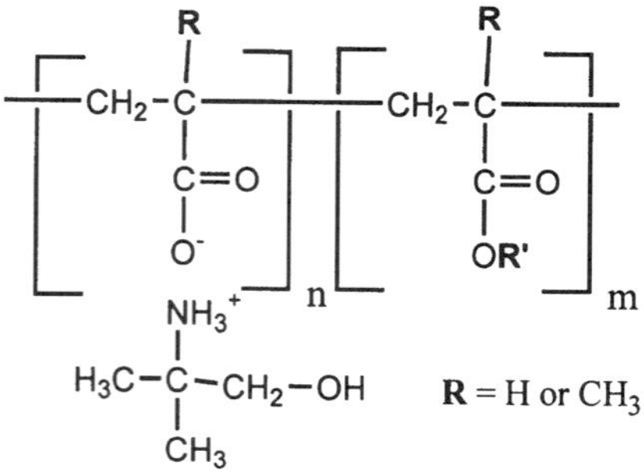

R = H or CH_3

Chemical Description: Copolymer of methacrylic acid and methacrylate neutralized with 2-amino-2-methylpropanol
Trade Name: Diahold A-503
Function in Formula: Fixative and film former
Use Concentration: 4–7% in hair sprays (actives basis); 4% in setting lotion (actives basis)
Solubility Characteristics: Water-soluble as supplied
Formulating Considerations: Supplied preneutralized with AMP. Good propellant compatibility
Form Supplied: 40% actives in ethanol
Supplier: Sandoz

Behenoxy Dimethicone

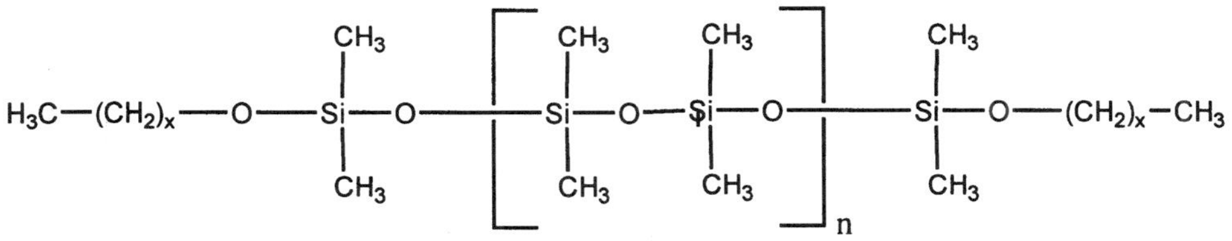

x = 21

Chemical Name: Dialkoxy dimethyl polysiloxane
Trade Name: Abil Wax 2440
Function in Formula: Emollient, pigment disperser, moisture barrier properties, lubricant
Use Concentration: 1–5% in deodorant roll-ons
Solubility Characteristics: Soluble in oils
Formulating Considerations: Add to oil phase, melting point 30–35°C. Warm to liquify before grinding pigments
Form Supplied: Solid wax, 100% active
Supplier: Goldschmidt

$C_{24\text{-}28}$Methicone

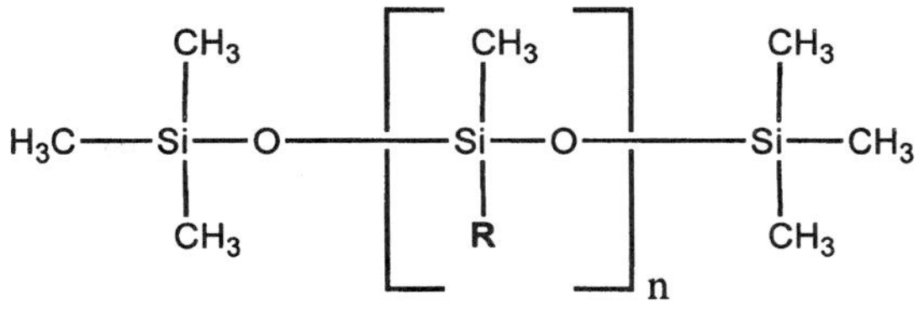

R = $C_{24\text{-}28}$

Chemical Name: Polymethylalkyl siloxane
Trade Name: Abil Wax 9810
Function in Formula: Emollient and barrier properties, nonionic
Use Concentration: 2–8% in eye makeup removers
Solubility Characteristics: Soluble in mineral oil, emollients, and esters
Formulating Considerations: Add with oil or wax phase. Melting point is 70°C
Form Supplied: Solid wax
Special Comments: Reduces greasiness or oils, soft emollient afterfeel, gels mineral oil
Regulatory Status: Nonhazardous
Supplier: Goldschmidt

Carbomer

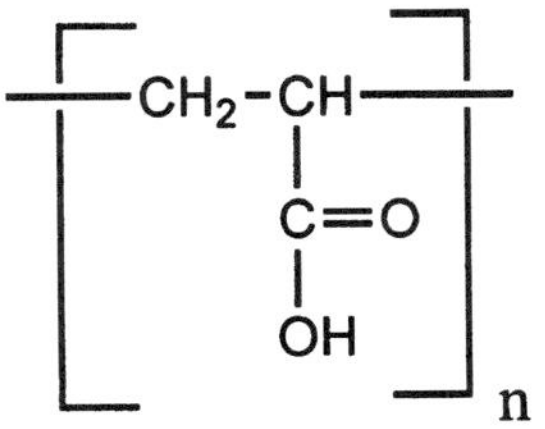

Chemical Description: Poly(acrylic acid) cross-linked with allyl ethers of pentaerythritol or allyl ethers of sucrose

Trade Names: Carbopol resins: 907, 910, 934, 934-P, 940, 941, 954, 980, 981, 2984, and 5984 (BF Goodrich); Acritamer 934, 934-P, 940, and 941 (R. I. T. A.); Synthalen K, Synthalen M, Synthalen N (3-V)

Function in Formula: Thickening/gelling agent. Suspension and emulsion stabilizer

Use Concentration: 0.3–1% in gels; 0.2–0.6% in creams; 0.0–0.5% in lotions

Solubility Characteristics: Very hydrophilic; highly swellable in water, alcohol, and polar solvents

Formulating Considerations: Highly efficient thickener needs care in dispersing in liquid. Swells rapidly in water upon neutralization with suitable base (no heat required). Effective thickeners in pH range 5–10. Thickening efficiency is reduced in presence of electrolytes. Incompatible with some cationic surfactants and some cationic polymers

Form Supplied: White, fine amorphous powder

Microbial Considerations: Resists bacterial attack and does not support mold growth. Preservation required for other components in the final formulation and for dispersions that will be stored for several weeks

Regulatory Status: Ultrapure and benzene-free grades are available. Carbomers 954, 980, 981, 2984, and 5984 are not synthesized in benzene. CIR Final Safety Assessment has been published. These materials have been determined to be safe. Carbomer resin are approved by the Japanese MHW

Special Comments: Carbomers 940 and 980 give highest clarity for gels. Carbomers 934, 941, 954, 981, 2984, and 5984 preferred for emulsion stabilization

Suppliers: BF Goodrich; 3-V; R. I. T. A

Carbomer

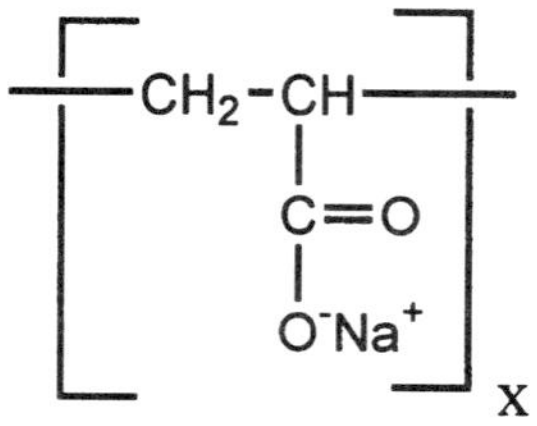

Chemical Description: Sodium salt of cross-linked poly(acrylic acid)

Trade Names: PNC 430, PNC 410, PNC 400

Function in Formula: To provide viscosity, stabilization, and rheology

Use Concentration: 0.1–1% in water-based gels; 0.1–0.3% in emulsions

Solubility Characteristics: Soluble in water

Formulating Considerations: Requires no neutralization. Should be added after all water-soluble materials are homogeneous, or dispersed in the oil phase prior to emulsification

Form Supplied: Fine white powder

Microbial Considerations: Does not support microbial growth and not does not prevent the growth of microorganisms

Regulatory Status: Benzene-free

Special Comments: Easy to use, offers all of the attributes of traditional carbomers

Suppliers: 3-V

Cetyl Dimethicone

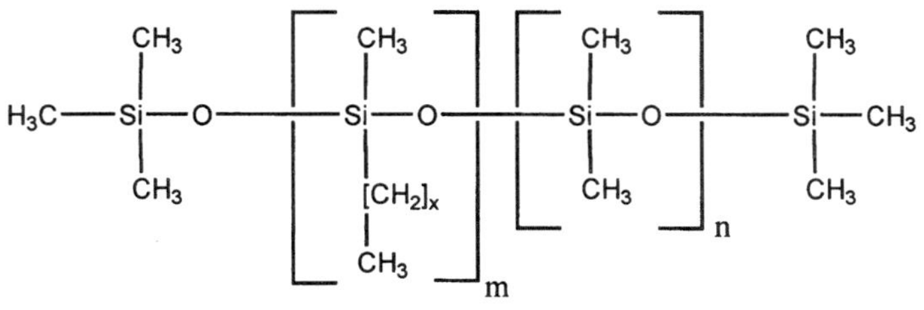

x = 15

Chemical Name: Polysiloxane polyalkylene copolymer
Trade Name: Abil Wax 9801D
Function in Formula: Emollient
Use Concentration: 1.5% in creams and lotions; deodorant sticks, roll-ons; skin care emulsions; lipsticks, pressed powders
Solubility Characteristics: Soluble in oils, insoluble in water
Formulating Considerations: Add in oil phase of emulsions, disperse into oils/waxes in pigmented products and antiperspirants
Form Supplied: Liquid
Special Comments: Improves the application of solid antiperspirants, improves the color of decorative cosmetics
Suppliers: Goldschmidt

Cetyl Dimethicone Copolyol

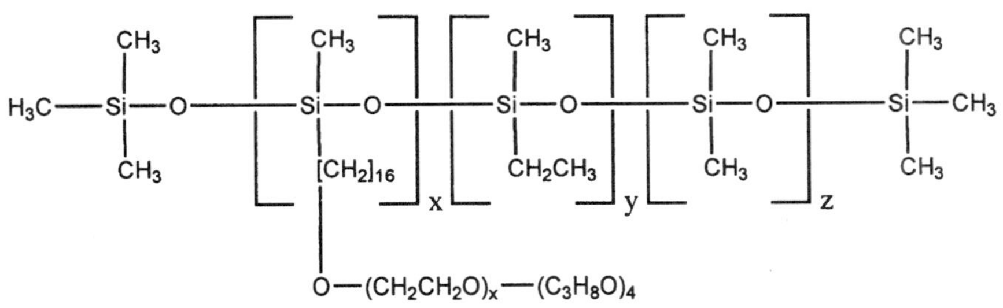

Chemical Name: Polysiloxane polyalkyl polyether copolymer
Trade Name: Abil EM 90
Function in Formula: Emulsifier, emollient
Use Concentration: 2% w/o in creams and lotions; 0.05% in conditioning shampoos for gloss, body, and combability
Solubility Characteristics: Soluble in oils, insoluble in water
Form Supplied: 100% active liquid
Special Comments: Provides emolliency in personal care products
Suppliers: Goldschmidt

Cyclomethicone

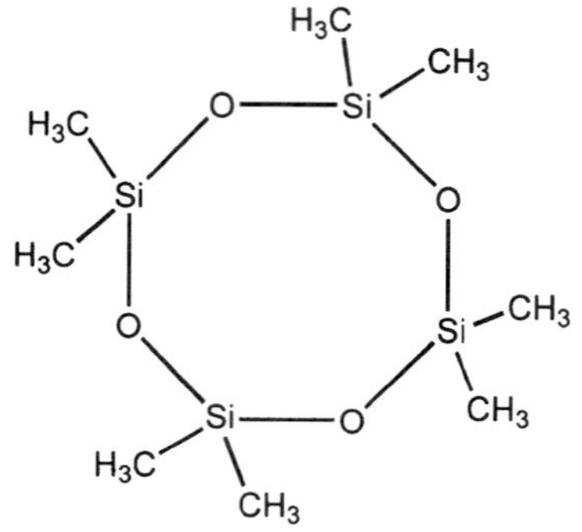

Chemical Name: Octamethylcyclotetrasiloxane
Trade Name: Abil K4
Function in Formula: Gives smoothness and silky sheen to hair
Use Concentration: 1–10% in hair sprays; 1–10% in skin care emulsions; up to 50% in deodorants
Solubility Characteristics: Soluble in ethanol and cosmetic oils
Suppliers: Goldschmidt

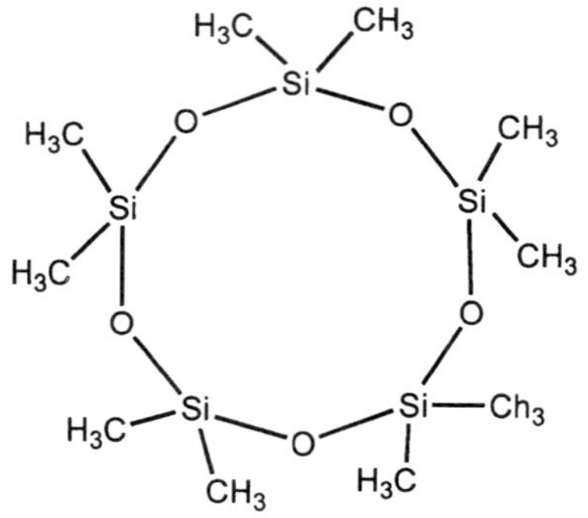

Chemical Name: Decamethycyclopentasiloxane
Trade Name: Abil B 8839
Function in Formula: Gives smoothness and silky sheen to hair
Use Concentration: 1–10% in hairsprays; 1–10% in skin care emulsions; up to 50% in deodorants, antiperspirants
Suppliers: Goldschmidt

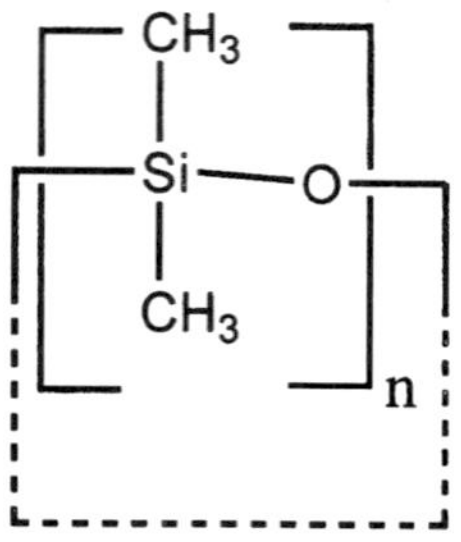

where n averages between 3 and 6

Chemical Name: Cyclic poly(dimethylsiloxane)
Trade Names: Silicone Fluids 244, 245, 344, 345 (Dow Corning); Silicone Fluids VS-79207, VS-7349, VS-7158 (Union Carbide)
Function in Formula: Reduces tackiness, conditions hair, lubricates, dry feel, aids gloss, emollient, carrier for actives
Solubility Characteristics: Soluble in ethanol, cetyl alcohol, aliphatic solvents, isopropyl myristate
Form Supplied: Liquid
Special Comments: Volatile emollient, wide range of solubility, nonstaining, low heat of vaporization
Suppliers: Union Carbide, Dow Corning

Diglycol/Cyclohexanedimethanol/Isophthalates/Sulfoisophthalates

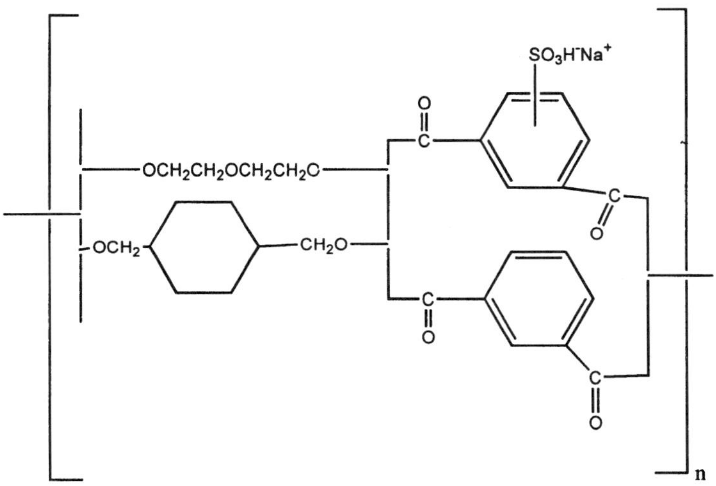

Chemical Description: Copolyester of diethylene glycol, 1,4-cyclohexanedimethanol, dimethyl isophthalate, and dimethyl sodiosulfoisophthalate
Trade Name: AQ 55S Polymer
Function in Formula: Film former, dispersant
Solubility Characteristics: Disperses in hot water
Formulating Considerations: Not compatible with cationics. Generally compatible with nonionics and anionics. Disperse in water first.
Form Supplied: Solid pellets
Microbial Considerations: Microbicide needed to stabilize aqueous dispersions
Regulatory Status: Included in TSCA inventory
Supplier: Eastman

Diglycol/Isophthalates/Sulfoisophthalates Copolymer

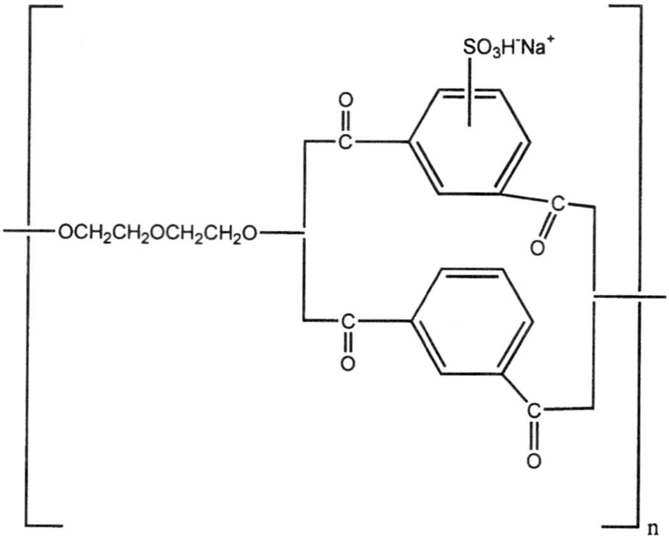

Chemical Description: Copolyester of diethylene glycol, dimethyl isophthalate, and dimethyl sodiosulfo isophthalate
Trade Name: AQ 29S Polymer
Function in Formula: Film former, dispersant
Solubility Characteristics: Disperses in hot water
Formulating Considerations: Not compatible with cationics. Generally compatible with nonionics and anionics. Disperse in water first or separately
Form Supplied: Solid pellets
Microbial Considerations: Microbicide needed to stabilize aqueous dispersions
Regulatory Status: Included in TSCA inventory
Supplier: Eastman

Dimethicone

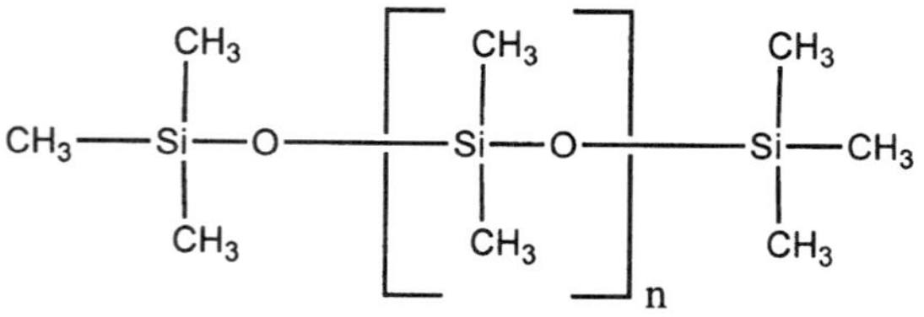

Trade Names: Abil 10-10 000 (Goldschmidt); Silicone Fluid SWS-101 (SWS Silicones); Dimethyl Silicone Fluids L-45, 200, 225 (Union Carbide); Silicone Fluids 200, 225 (Dow Corning); SE-30, Viscasil, SF-96 (GE)
Function in Formula: Elimination of ''whitening effect.'' Emollient, lubricant, and water repellent for hair and skin care products

Use Concentration: 0.5–5% in skin care emulsions. SE-30: 8–10% in hair cuticle laminate, 8–10% in skin preparations, 0.5–1% in shampoo/conditioner. Viscasil: 1–4% in shampoo/conditioner and soaps. SF-96: 0.5-7% in skin care. 5–10% in AP
Solubility Characteristics: Insoluble in polar media
Formulating Considerations: Solubilize first in cyclomethicone; for shampoo, use low-viscosity dimethicone
Form Supplied: Liquid/gum. Fluids range in viscosity from 0.65 to 60,000 centistokes
Supplier: Goldschmidt; Dow Corning; Wacker; GE Silicones

Dimethicone (and) Trimethylsiloxysilicate

Trade Name: SS-4267
Function in Formula: 3–5% in sunscreen formulations, 1–5% in hand lotions
Solubility Characteristics: Disperses in hot water
Formulating Considerations: Best used with anionic emulsifiers, avoid common organic esters
Form Supplied: Fluids
Microbial Considerations: Microbicide needed to stabilize aqueous dispersions
Supplier: GE Silicones

Dimethicone Copolyol

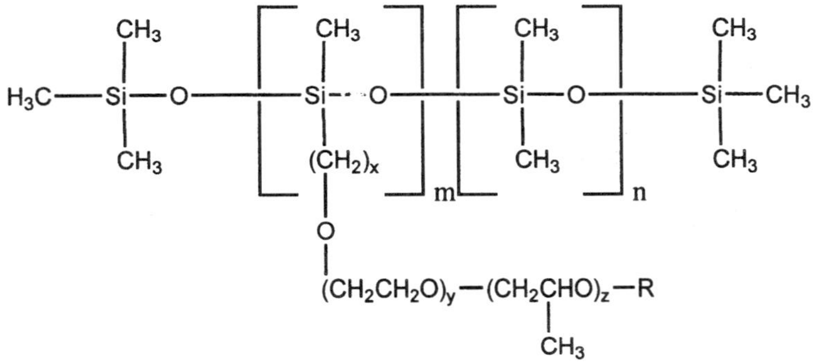

Chemical Name: Polysiloxane polyether copolymer
Trade Names: Abil B 8843D, B 8851D (Goldschmidt); Silwet L- Series (Union Carbide); SF-1188 (GE); Silicone Fluids 190, 193, Q2-5520 (Dow Corning)
Function in Formula: Refatting agents, smoothness, softness, shine hair products. Wetting, foaming, lubricant
Use Concentration: 0.5–3% in hair care; 0.5–3% in creams and lotions; 0.5–3% in antiperspirants; 0.2–1% in shaving foams; 0.2–1% in aftershaves/facial cleansers, shampoos, hair rinses, hair gels; 2–4% in conditioning shampoos; 1–3% in shaving cream; 0.1–0.5% in styling products
Solubility Characteristics: Water, lower alcohols, propylene glycol soluble
Formulating Considerations: Add to water phase
Form Supplied: 100% liquid
Regulatory Status: Nonhazardous
Special Comments: Contributes to gloss, sheen and combability. Contributes to skin feel
Supplier: Goldschmidt; Union Carbide; GE Silicones, Dow Corning

Dimethicone Copolyol Phosphate

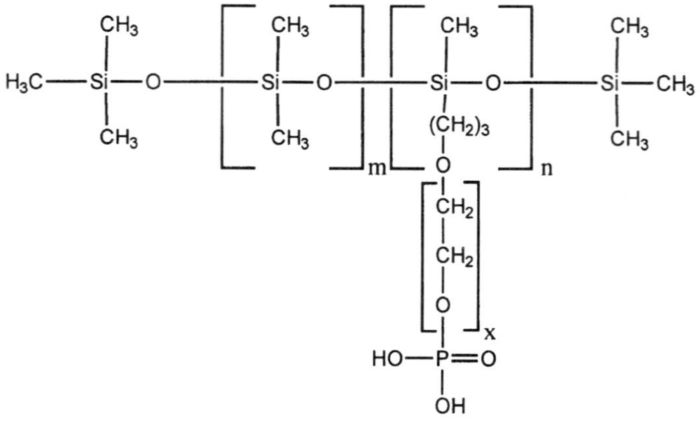

Trade Name: PECOSIL PS-100
Function in Formula: Emulsifier/gloss/substantivity
Use Concentration: 3% in body cream, 5% in sunscreen, 3% in conditioner
Solubility Characteristics: Soluble in water
Form Supplied: Liquid
Regulatory Status: Benzene-free
Supplier: Phoenix

Dimethicone/Disodium PG-Propyldimethicone Thiosulfate Copolyol

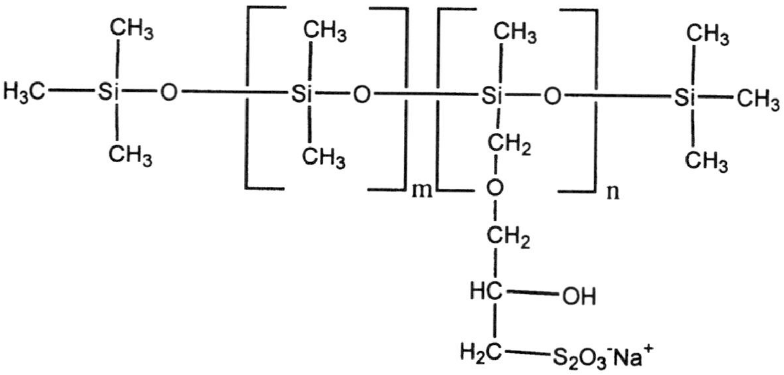

Chemical Name: Polysiloxane polyorgano thiosulfate
Trade Name: Abil S 255
Function in Formula: Conditioning agent
Use Concentration: 5–15% in permanent waves; 0.2–1% in hair conditioners; approx. 0.2% in hairsprays
Solubility Characteristics: Soluble in water
Form Supplied: Liquid
Supplier: Goldschmidt

Dimethicone Propyl PG-Betaine

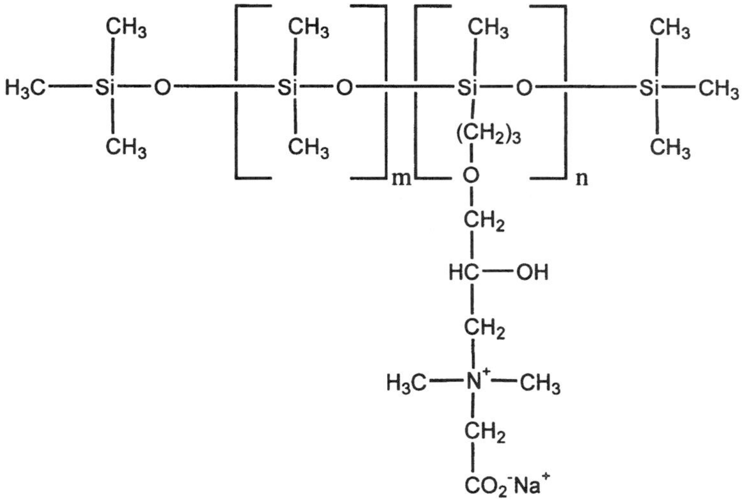

Chemical Name: Polysiloxane polyorganobetaine copolymer
Trade Name: Abil B 9950
Function in Formula: Substantive to hair; conditioner
Use Concentration: 0.5–1.5% in shampoos, shower and foam baths, hair gels and leave-on conditioners
Solubility Characteristics: Soluble in water
Form Supplied: Liquid
Supplier: Goldschmidt

Dimethicone/Sodium PG-Propyldimethicone Thiosulfate Copolyol

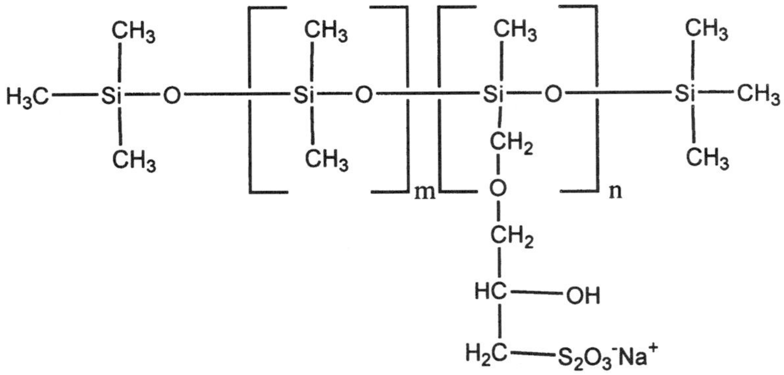

Chemical Name: Polysiloxane polyorgano thiosulfate
Trade Name: Abil S 201
Function in Formula: Conditioning agent
Use Concentration: 5–15% in permanent waves; 0.2–1% in hair conditioners, approx. 0.2% in hairsprays
Solubility Characteristics: Soluble in water
Form Supplied: Liquid
Supplier: Goldschmidt

Dimethiconol (and) Cyclomethicone (and) Dimethicone

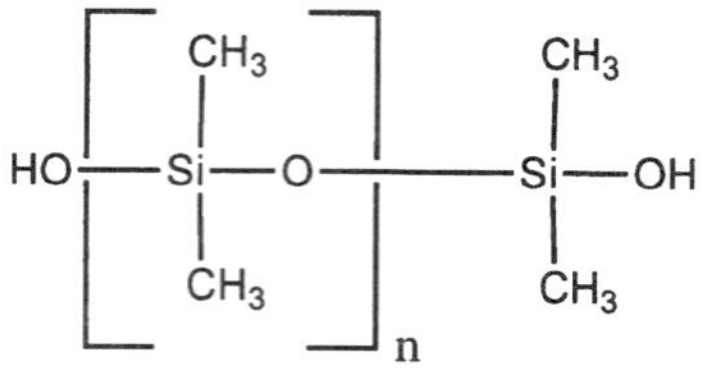

Trade Names: Abil OSW 12, Abil OSW 13
Function in Formula: Film former
Use Concentration: 100% as hair treatment fluid
Form Supplied: Liquid
Supplier: Goldschmidt

Ethylene/Acrylate Copolymer

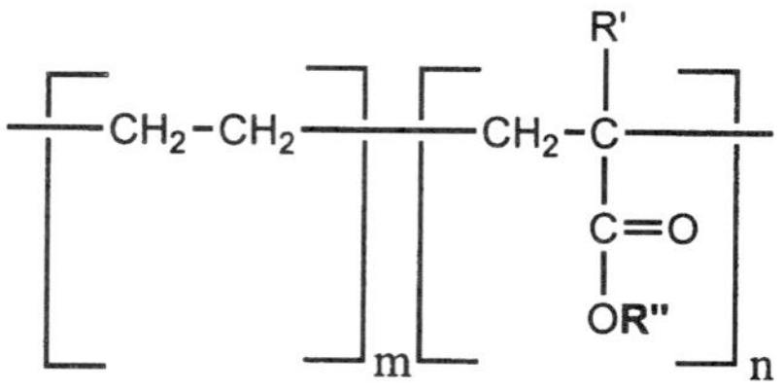

Chemical Description: Copolymer of ethylene and a monomer consisting of acrylic acid, methacrylic acid, or one of their simple esters
Trade Names: A.C. Copolymer 540, 540A
Function in Formula: To gel solvent, especially mineral oil in lipstick gloss, stick products, cleansing creams, hand creams; film former in waterproof sunscreen
Use Concentration: 5–10% in solvent phase; ~1% in finished product; 1–2% in waterproof sunscreen
Solubility Characteristics: Insoluble in water, insoluble in alcohol. Insoluble at room temperature in all solvents, flocculated dispersion when heated above the cloud point and allowed to cool
Form Supplied: Powder or prill
Microbial Considerations: Formulation needs to be preserved. The polymer itself is biologically inert
Regulatory Status: CIR reviewed and deemed safe
Supplier: Allied-Signal

Ethylene/Vinyl Acrylate Copolymer

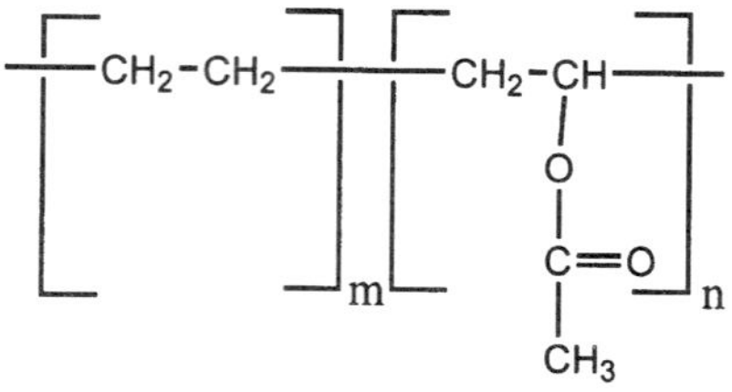

Chemical Name: Poly (ethylene-co-vinyl acetate)
Trade Names: A.C. Copolymer 400, 430
Function in Formula: Gellant for antiperspirants and gels
Use Concentration: 5–10% in solvent
Solubility Characteristics: Insoluble in water, insoluble in alcohol. Insoluble at room temperature in all solvents. Forms flocculated dispersion when heated above the cloud point and allowed to cool
Form Supplied: Powder or prill
Microbial Considerations: Formulation requires preservation. The polymer itself is biologically inert
Regulatory Status: CIR reviewed
Supplier: Allied-Signal

Glycerin and Diglycol/Cyclohexanedimethanol/Isophthalated/ Sulfoisophthalates Copolymer

Trade Name: Lipo PE Base G-55
Function in Formula: Thickening, waterproofing
Use Concentration: 30–55% in emulsions, gels, and makeup
Solubility Characteristics: Water-soluble, insoluble in organic solvents
Formulating Considerations: Used as a film former. Leaves a tack-free, flexible, water-resistant film that can be removed with soap and water
Form Supplied: Viscous liquid
Supplier: Lipo

Graft-copoly(dimethylsiloxane/t-butyl methacrylate)

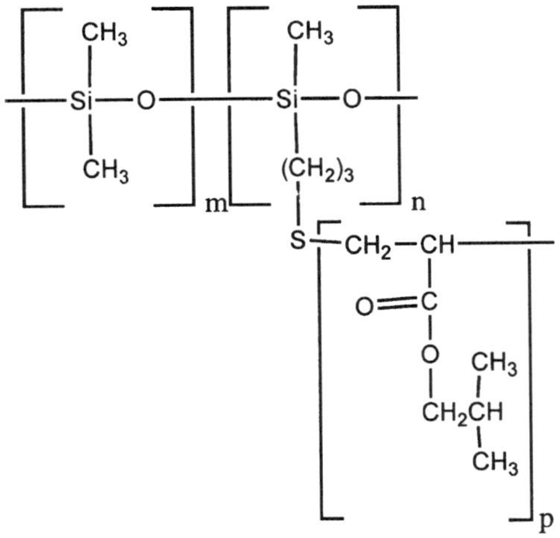

Chemical Name: Poly(dimethylsiloxane)-g-poly(isobutylmethacrylate)
Trade Names: 3M Brand Silicones "Plus" VS-70-IBM
Function in Formula: Lubricating, water-resistant, durable film former with good bioadhesion
Use Concentration: 1–5% in cosmetically acceptable solvents, e.g., Finsolv cyclomethicones, etc.
Solubility Characteristics: Soluble in alcohol, ketones, esters, glycol ethers, etc.
Formulating Considerations: Polymer solution can be mixed or diluted with other organic fluids or be converted into other solvents by standard solvent exchange processes
Form Supplied: Polymer solution in Finsolv (25% solids)

Special Comments: One part graft polymer combines silicone and acrylic benefits in cosmetics and toiletries
Suppliers: Encapsulated Products, 3M

Graft-copoly(IBMA; MeFOSEA/PDMS)

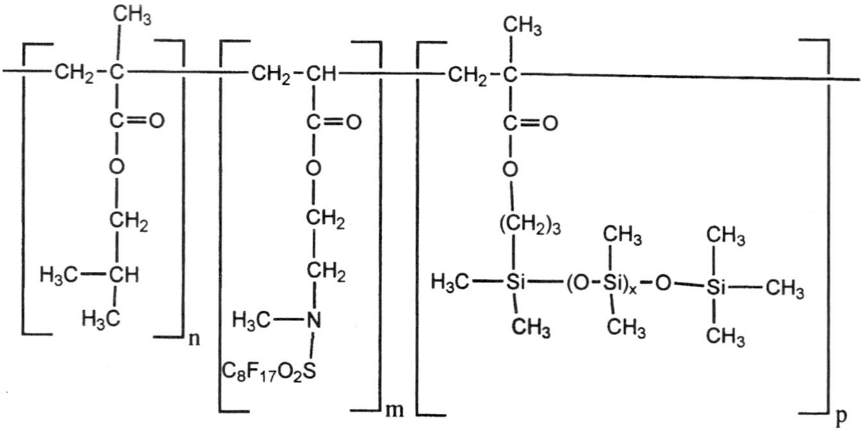

Chemical Name: [Poly(isobutylmethacrylate-co-methylFOSEA)]-g-poly(dimethylsiloxane) (70:5:25 mass%)
Trade Names: 3M Brand Silicones ''Plus'' SA-70-5-IBMMF
Function in Formula: Lubricating, water-resistant, durable film former with good bioadhesion
Use Concentration: 1–5% in cosmetically acceptable solvents, e.g., Finsolv cycomethicones, etc.
Formulating Considerations: Polymer solution can be mixed or diluted with other organic fluids or be converted into other solvents by standard solvent exchange processes
Form Supplied: Polymer solution in Finsolv (25% solids)
Special Comments: One part graft polymer combines silicone and acrylic benefits in cosmetics and toiletries
Supplier: Encapsulated Products, 3M

Hydrogenated Polyisobutenes

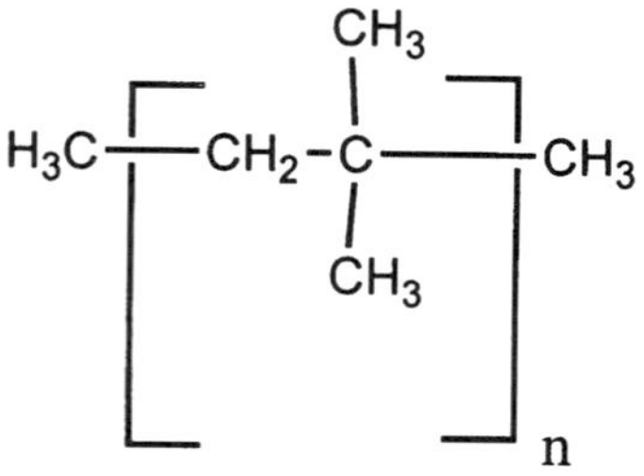

Trade Name: Panalane L-14E
Function in Formula: Oil
Solubility Characteristics: Hydrophobic
Form Supplied: Liquid polymer
Regulatory Status: Nontoxic meets FDA Title **21** *CFR* 178.3740
Supplier: Amoco

Hydrolyzed Soy Protein/Dimethicone Phosphocopolyol Copolymer

Chemical Description: Polymer hydrolysate of soy protein reacted with dimethicone copolyol phosphate via an alkyl chloride bridge to form a copolymer
Trade Name: PECOSIL SSP
Function in Formula: Conditioner/film former
Use Concentrations: 5% in hair styling gels, hair conditioners and shampoos
Solubility Characteristics: Soluble in water
Form Supplied: 35–38% in aqueous solution
Regulatory Status: Benzene-free
Supplier: Phoenix

Hydrolyzed Wheat Protein/Dimethicone Phosphocopolyol Copolymer

Chemical Description: Hydrolysate of wheat protein reacted with dimethicone copolyol phosphate polymer form a copolymer
Trade Name: PECOSIL SWP-83
Function in Formula: Conditioner/film former
Use Concentration: 5% in hair styling gels, hair conditioners and shampoos
Solubility Characteristics: Soluble in water
Form Supplied: 35–38% in aqueous solution
Regulatory Status: Benzene-free
Supplier: Phoenix

Methacryloyl Ethyl Betaine/Methacrylates Copolymer

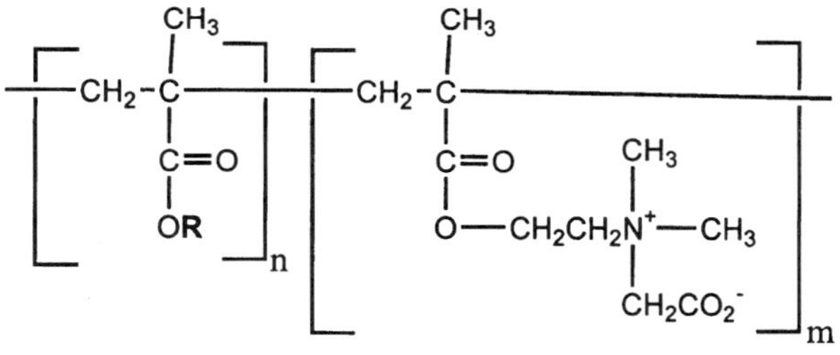

where **R** = $C_1 - C_{18}$ alkyl group

Chemical Description: Betaine-type methacrylate polymer
Trade Name: Z-W, A-301, Z-AT, Z-400, Z-A, Z-5M
Function in Formula: Fixative resins and film former. Z-W is a conditioning polymer
Use Concentration: 0.5–1% (actives) in shampoos; 1–3% (actives) in conditioners and rinses; 1–5% in gels; 4–7% (actives) in hairsprays; 2–4% (actives) in mousses; 4–5% (actives) in setting lotions
Solubility Characteristics: Z-W soluble in water, Z-310 is compatible with carbomer gels; Z-AT, Z-400, Z-A, and Z-SM are soluble in ethanol and hydroalcoholic solutions
Formulating Considerations: Compatible with commonly used propellants and most additives, at both acidic and basic pH ranges. Water-soluble grades are easily added to the formulation. No predispersion is required
Form Supplied: Z-W as 30% actives in water/8% ethanol solution. Z-301 as 30% actives in ethanol. Z-AT, Z-400, Z-A, and Z-SM do not require neutralization, they have good propellant com-

patibility, and they may be used in formulations containing up to 90% water. They are supplied in solution and do not need to be predispersed
Microbial Considerations: Free of bacterial contaminations
Regulatory Status: TSCA registered
Special Comments: Z-W has substantivity to hair and provides excellent antistatic properties in the formulation
Supplier: Sandoz

N-Dodecylamidopropyl-N′, N′-dimethyl-N″-dimethicone Copolyolphospho-2 Propanol Ammonium Chloride

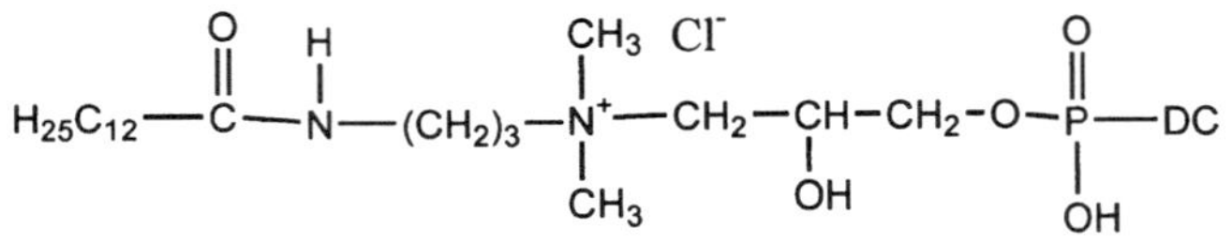

DC = dimethicone copolyol copolymer

Trade Name: PECOSIL CAP-1240
Function in Formula: Conditioner
Use Concentration: 5% in hair conditioner, shampoo, and hand lotion
Solubility Characteristics: Soluble in water
Form Supplied: Liquid
Regulatory Status: Benzene-free
Supplier: Phoenix

Octyldodecyl Dimethicone Copolyol Citrate

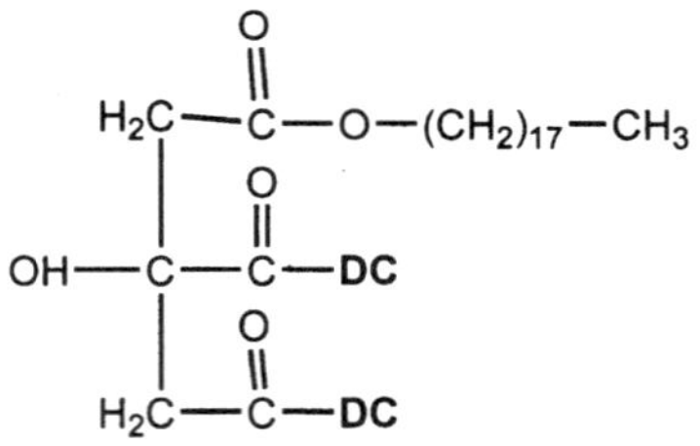

DC = dimethicone copolyol copolymer

Trade Name: PECOSIL CAS -55
Function in Formula: Pigment wetter and dispersant, emollient
Use Concentration: 3–5% in makeup products, lipsticks, creams, and lotions
Solubility Characteristics: Oil-soluble
Form Supplied: Liquid
Regulatory Status: Benzene-free
Supplier: Phoenix

Octylacrylamide/Acrylates Copolymer

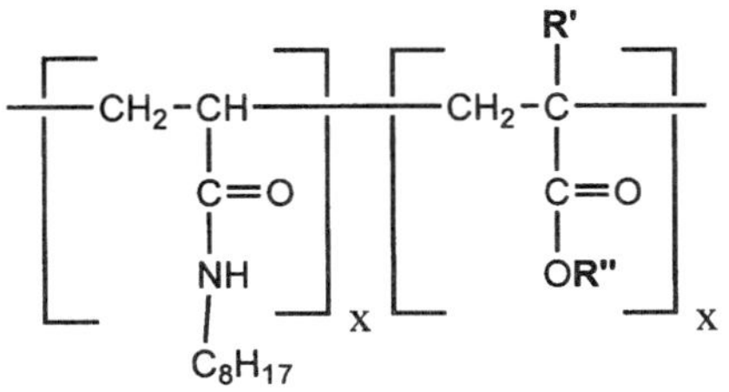

Chemical Description: Copolymer of octylacrylamide and two or more monomers consisting of acrylic acid, methacrylic acid, or any of their simple esters
Trade Name: Versacryl-40
Function in Formula: Binder/hair fixative
Use Concentration: 1–8% in ethanol for hairspray
Solubility Characteristics: Soluble in ethanol and isopropanol
Formulating Considerations: For optimum properties, suggest 90–95% neutralization with potassium hydroxide
Form Supplied: Fine white powder
Supplier: National Starch

Octylacrylamide/Acrylates/Butylaminoethylmethacrylate Copolymer

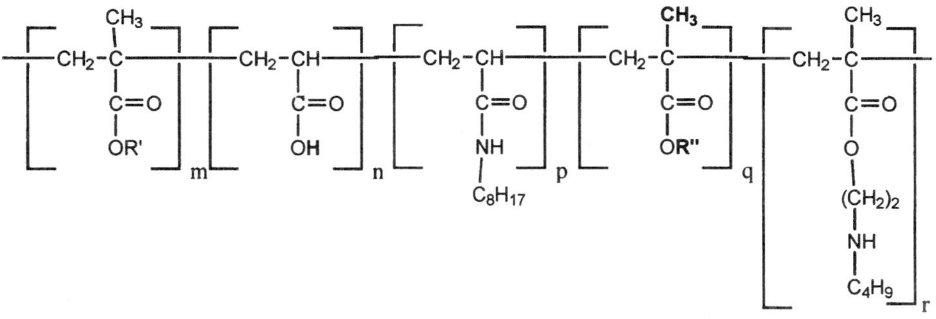

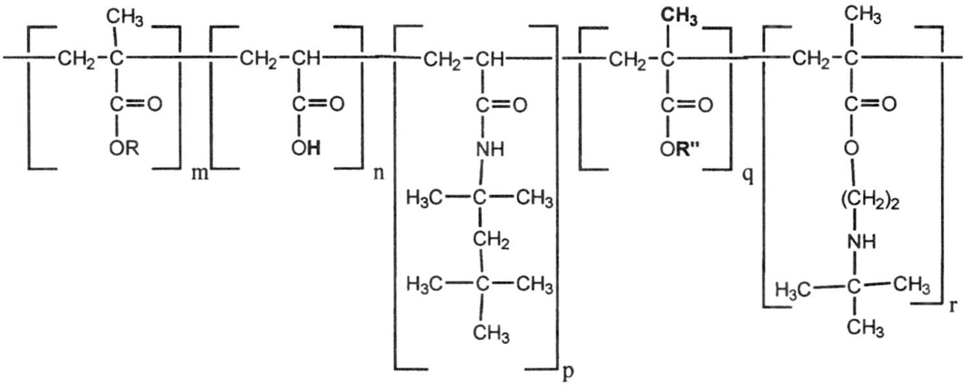

Chemical Description: Copolymer of octylacrylamide, *t*-butylaminoethyl methacrylate, and two or more monomers consisting of acrylic acid, methacrylic acid, or any of their simple esters
Trade Name: Amphomer 28-4910, Amphomer LV-71
Function in Formula: Binder/hair fixative
Use Concentration: 3–5% in hairspray; 5% in styling lotions
Solubility Characteristics: Soluble in ethanol and isopropanol
Formulating Considerations: Must be neutralized when formulated. Aminomethylpropanol (AMP) is most commonly used neutralizer. Normally 90% with AMP for use in hairspray. Becomes water-soluble when 100% neutralized
Form Supplied: Fine white powder
Regulatory Status: Benzene-free
Special Comments: 28-4910 acidity = 2.05 mEq/g; LV-71 acidity = 2.45 mEq/g
Supplier: National Starch

Oxidized Polyethylene

Chemical Name: Poly(ethylene)
Trade Name: A.C. Polyethylene 629, 680
Function in Formula: Gellant for anhydrous esters and oils. Emulsifiable polyethylene for creams and lotions
Use Concentration: 8–10% in solvent
Solubility Characteristics: Insoluble in water and short-chain alcohols
Formulating Considerations: Can be emulsified with anionic, cationic, or nonionic emulsifiers, soluble hot in fatty acids, fatty alcohols, fatty esters, petrolatum, mineral oil. Forms a flocculated dispersion upon cooling. Stable gels or dispersions form at 6–15%
Form Supplied: Prill or fine powder
Supplier: Allied-Signal

Oxy(methyl-1-1,2-ethanediyl) a-Hydro-w-hydroxy polymer with 1,1′-methylenabis(4-isocyanatocyclohexane)

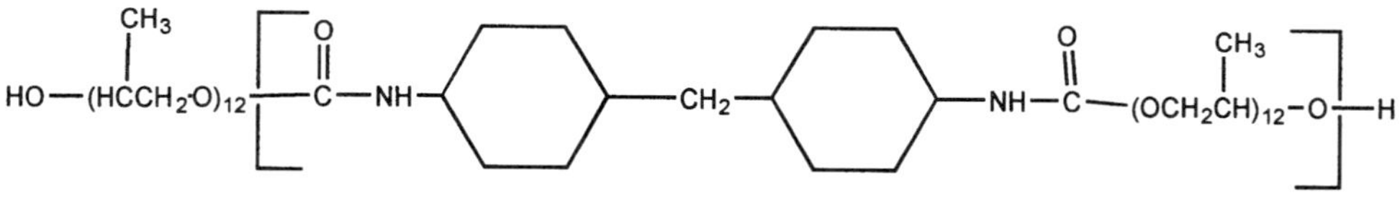

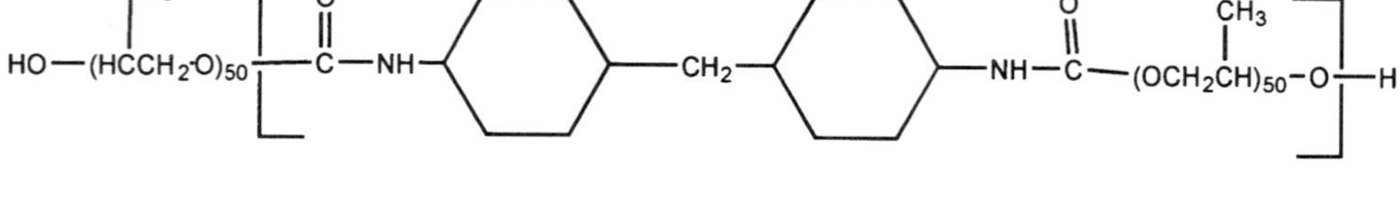

Trade Name: Polyolprepolymer-2
Function in Formula: Skin conditioning agent, delivery and deposition of active ingredient
Use Concentration: 0.5–2% in personal care formulations
Solubility Characteristics: Insoluble in water, soluble in alcohol

Formulating Considerations: Compatible with most personal care formulation ingredients
Form Supplied: Viscous liquid
Microbial Considerations: Does not support microbial growth
Regulatory Status: Cosmetic and pharmaceutical excipient
Supplier: Barnet

PEG-N where *N* = 4, 6, 8, 12, 20, 32, 75, 100, and 150

$HO—(CH_2CH_2O)_n—H$

n = 4-150

Chemical Name: Polyethylene glycol 200, 300, 400, 600, 1000, 1450, 3350, 4600, and 8000
Trade Name: Carbowax Polyethylene Glycols
Function in Formula: Solvent, carrier, humectant, lubricant, binder, base, coupling agent, solvent
Use Concentration: 5–30% in toothpaste, dentifrices; 5–15% in bar soap; 1–10% in shampoo
Solubility Characteristics: Water-soluble, soluble in ethanol
Formulating Considerations: Add directly to formulation; dissolve in water and add to formulation; compatible with cosmetic ingredients. Water-soluble but will precipitate near 100°C
Form Supplied: Liquid (200–600), soft solid (1000–1450), flake or powder (3750–8000)
Microbial Considerations: Does not support microbial growth
Regulatory Status: PEG-6 to PEG-150 are USP/NF/FCC; listed in the *Handbook of Pharmaceutical Excipients* and in the *Handbook of Food, Drug, and Cosmetic Excipients*; not reviewed by CIR
Special Comments: Low volatility; wide range of viscosity and melting point
Supplier: Union Carbide

PEG-2M, PEG-5M, PEG-7M, PEG-14M, PEG-9M, GEG-20M, PEG-23M, PEG-45M, PEG-90M

$HO—(CH_2CH_2O)_n—H$

Chemical Description: High-molecular-weight polymer of poly(ethylene oxide)
Trade Name: Polyox Water Soluble Resins
Function in Formula: Depending upon the concentration and grade, can provide lubricity or tack to a formulation
Use Concentration: 0.5–1% in shave cream/gel; 0.1–0.5% in shampoo; 0.1–0.3% in liquid/bar soap systems
Solubility Characteristics: Soluble in water
Formulating Considerations: Nonionic polymer, which ensures wide compatibility with most personal care ingredients
Form Supplied: White powder
Microbial Considerations: Does not contain an antimicrobial as sold. Normal precautions need to be followed to include a preservative in a formulation containing Polyox
Regulatory Status: Three grades have been approved for use and sale by MHW in Japan (PEG-9M. PEG-14M, PEG-90M). All grades have been shown to be safe and are sold in the other major markets, including North America and Europe
Special Comments: Impart a great deal of lubricity to a solution. They are extremely mild and are excellent film formers. At high concentrations, Polyox resins can add adhesive properties to a product
Supplier: Amerchol

PEG-N-Methyl Ether where *N* = 6.10, 16.40, or 100

$H_3CO—(CH_2CH_2O)_n—H$

n = 6-100

Chemical Names: Methoxy polyethylene glycols 350, 550, 750, 2000, and 5000
Trade Name: Carbowax Methoxy Polyethylene Glycols
Function in Formula: Solvent, carrier, lubricant
Use Concentration: 5–15% in nail polish remover; 5–10% in hand cleaner; 5–15% in bar soap
Solubility Characteristics: Soluble in water, soluble in ethanol
Formulating Considerations: Dissolve ingredients in MPEG, add to formulation; dissolve in water and add to formulation
Form Supplied: Liquid (350–550), soft solid (770), flake or powder (2000–5000)
Microbial Considerations: Resists microbial growth
Special Comments: Low volatility, wide range of viscosity and melting point
Supplier: Union Carbide

PEI

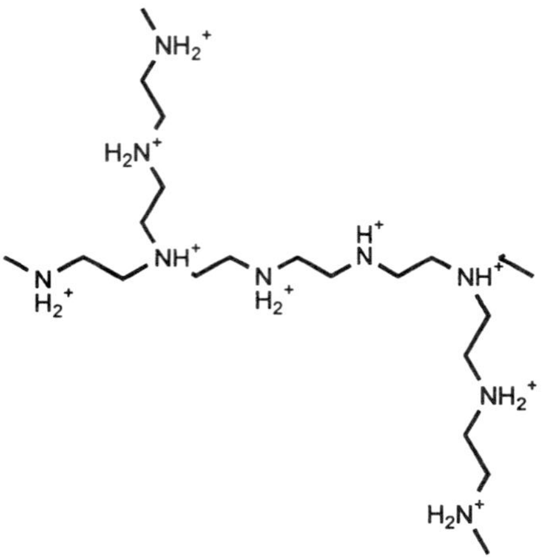

Chemical Name: Polyethylenimine
Trade name: Polymin
Function in Formula: Carrier for active, tie coat, solubilizer
Solubility Characteristics: Water-soluble
Formulating Considerations: Order of addition important to control ionic reactions
Form Supplied: Aqueous and liquid
Special Comments: High cationic density, high substantive to skin, hair, and nails
Supplier: BASF

Perfluoropolymethylisopropyl Ether

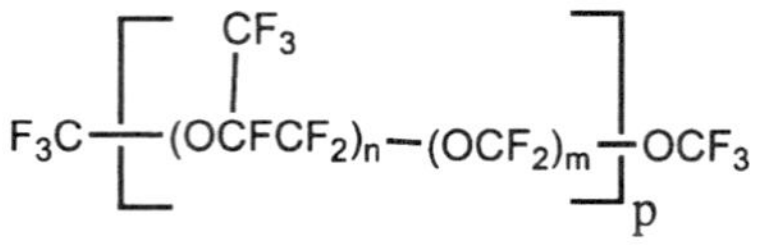

n/m = 20/40
Avg. MW = 1500–6250

Chemical Name: Perfluoropolyether
Trade Name: Fomblin HC (grades: HC/04, HC/25, and HC/R)
Function in Formula: Skin protectant, emollient, coemulsifier
Use Concentration: 1–3% in barrier creams and lotions; 0.2–1.0% in moisturizing creams and lotions; 0.05–0.3% in emulsion stabilizer
Solubility Characteristics: Completely insoluble in any cosmetic ingredient
Formulating Considerations: Fomblin HC can be pre-emulsified with glycerin; Fomblin HC can be added either to water or oil phase before emulsification
Form Supplied: 100% pure liquid material
Microbial Considerations: Absolutely inert from the biological point of view
Regulatory Status: Approved in Japan (up to 5%) by the MHW
Supplier: Ausimont (Brooks Industries, U.S.)

Phenyl Dimethicone

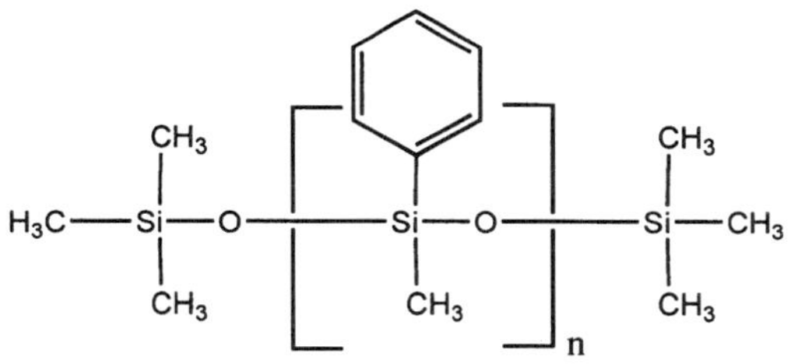

Chemical Name: Phenylmethyl polysiloxane
Trade Name: Abil AV8853
Function in Formula: Improves spreadability of emulsions; solubilizer
Use Concentration: 2–20% in deodorants
Solubility Characteristics: Soluble in ethanol and cosmetic oils. Chemically stable compounds that are not attacked by reagents. Excellent surface binding and very good spreading properties
Form Supplied: Clear odorless and tasteless liquids. Noncorrosive. Inert in the presence of metals and plastics
Supplier: Goldschmidt

Phenyl Trimethicone

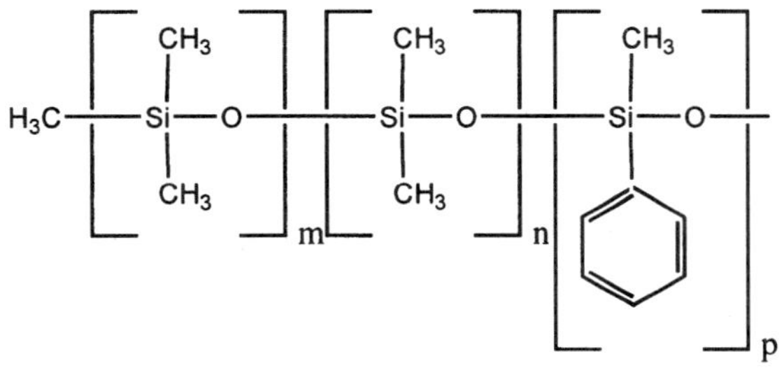

Trade Names: Abil AV 20, Abil AV 1000 (Goldschmidt); Phenyltrimethicone (Dow Corning)
Function in Formula: Improvement of spreadability; film-forming properties
Use Concentration: 0.5–5% in skin care and skin-protecting emulsions; 0.5–5% in deodorants, antiperspirants; 0.5–5% in decorative cosmetics
Solubility Characteristics: Soluble in ethanol as well as in cosmetic oils

Form Supplied: Liquid
Suppliers: Goldschmidt; Dow Corning

Poloxamer 407

$$HO{-}[CH_2CH_2O]_x{-}[CH_2\overset{\overset{CH_3}{|}}{C}HO]_y{-}[CH_2CH_2O]_x{-}H$$

Chemical Name: Polyethylene glycol/polypropylene glycol block copolymer
Trade Name: Pluronic F-127
Function in Formula: Thickener, gelling agent for aqueous systems
Use Concentration: Use up to 20% in water
Solubility Characteristics: Soluble in water
Formulating Considerations: Should be added to cold water, mixed thoroughly, and then allowed to warm to room temperature for best results
Form Supplied: Prill
Suppliers: BASF

Polyacrylamidomethylpropane Sulfonic Acid

Chemical Name: Polysulfonic acid polymer
Trade Name: Kraft Polymer 80-11
Function in Formula: Thickener, lubricity, friction reducer, emollient
Form Supplied: Clear, viscous liquid (17–18% active in water)
Special Comments: An anionic polymer supplied in 17% active solution in water. Special ''smooth feel'' agent for creams, lotions, liquids and bars, shaving creams, etc. Provides a pleasant slip during application and leaves a talc-like feel. Neutralization of this polymer has no effect on the rheology of the product
Supplier: Kraft Chemical

Poly(acrylic acid)

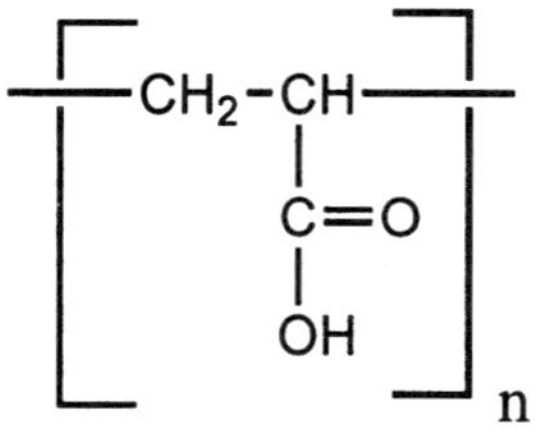

Trade Name: Carbopol 400 series (BF Goodrich); Aquatreat (Alco)
Function in Formula: Thickener, pigment disperser, calcium soap disperser
Use Concentration: 0.1–2.0% in pigment dispersions, soaps
Solubility Characteristics: Soluble in water
Form Supplied: Aqueous and isopropanol solution, flake, powder
Suppliers: BF Goodrich; 3-V

Polydecene/Polybutene Copolymer

Trade Name: Polyfix 106
Function in Formula: Film former, water resistance

Use Concentration: 4% in creams and lotions, 6% in foundations, 4% in silicone-based hair products
Solubility Characteristics: Oil-soluble
Formulating Considerations: Miscible with volatile silicones, mineral oil, most vegetable oils, esters, and sunscreens. Not miscible with water, alcohol, glycerin, or propylene glycol. Can be emulsified
Form Supplied: 100% active moderately viscous clear liquid
Microbial considerations: Does not support microbial growth
Regulatory Status: No known constraints under TSCA, SARA, OSHA, RCRA
Supplier: Collaborative Laboratories

Polyethylene

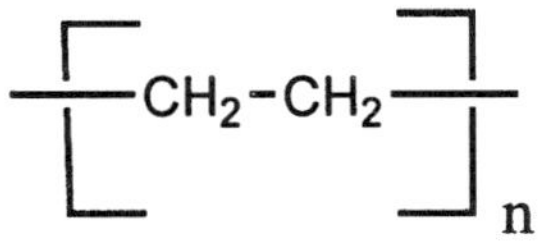

Chemical Name: Poly(ethylene)
Trade Name: A. C. Polyethylene 6A, 617A, 9A, 316A
Function in Formula: Abrasive in acne scrub and hand scrub products
Solubility Characteristics: Insoluble
Form Supplied: Powder
Microbial Considerations: Microbiologically inert
Supplier: Allied-Signal

Trade Name: A. C. Polyethylene 617, 6, 7, 8, 9
Function in Formula: Gellant for anhydrous hydrocarbon oil and fatty esters in eye shadow, medicated gels and ointments, pomades. Binder for pressed powders, eye shadow
Use Concentration: 5–10% in solvent
Solubility Characteristics: Insoluble in short-chain alcohols and water
Formulating Consideration: Soluble in hot petrolatum, mineral oil, fatty acids, fatty alcohols, fatty esters. Forms a flocculated dispersion on cooling
Form Supplied: Pellets, prills, or fine powder
Microbial Considerations: Microbiologically inert
Supplier: Allied-Signal

Trade Name: A. C. Polyethylene-9F
Function in Formula: Gellant in denture adhesive
Form Supplied: Prills or fine powder
Microbial Considerations: Microbiologically inert
Supplier: Allied-Signal

Trade Name: Acumist Products
Function in Formula: Binder for pressed powders, eye shadow
Form Supplied: Powder
Microbial Considerations: Microbiologically inert
Supplier: Allied-Signal

Polymethacrylamidopropyl Trimonium Chloride

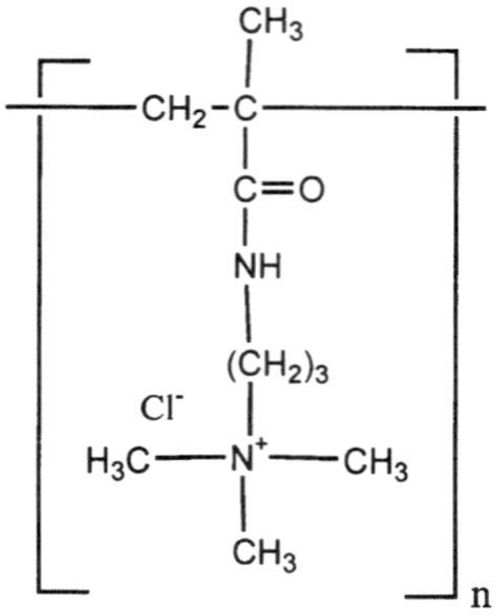

Chemical Name: Polymethacrylamidopropyltrimethylammonium chloride
Trade Name: Polycare 133
Function in Formula: Substantive to skin, clear, imparts softness to hair, styling aid
Use Concentration: 0.5–5% in hair-styling aids and skin care products
Solubility Characteristics: Completely soluble in water, aqueous alcohol, and other polar solvents
Formulating Considerations: Immediate water solubility at room temperature and high temperatures
Form Supplied: 33% polymer solids in water
Microbial Considerations: Aerobic plated count: 500 g max.; gram-negative bacteria: 0/g; *Staphylococcus aureus, Pseudomonas aeruginosa, Escherichia coli, Salmonella*: *negative*
Regulatory Status: It is on the TSCA inventory, CAS number 68039-13-4
Special Comments: Highly charged cationic homopolymer, which displays flexible hold properties on hair
Supplier: Rhone-Poulenc

Polyquaternium-2

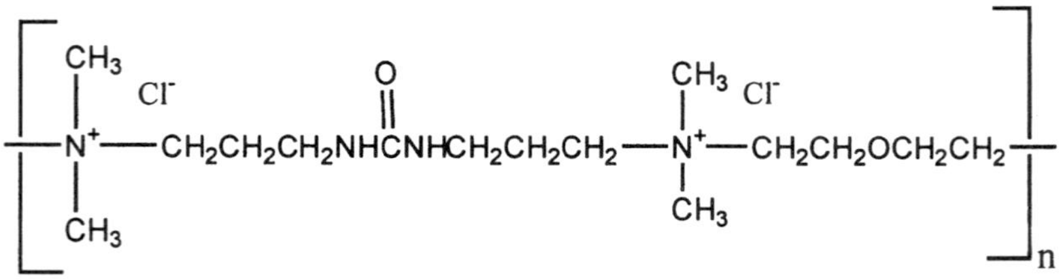

Trade Name: Mirapol A-15
Function in Formula: Conditioning agent for hair and skin. Reduces ''flyaway''
Use Concentration: 0.6–2.5% in conditioning shampoos, creams and lotions, skin cleansers
Solubility Characteristics: Completely soluble in water and lower alcohols
Formulating Considerations: Disperse in water prior to addition of surfactants
Form Supplied: Aqueous concentrate (62% active)
Regulatory Status: CAS number: 68555-32-2: TSCA registered
Special Comments: Highly substantive
Supplier: Rhone-Poulenc

Polyquaternium-6

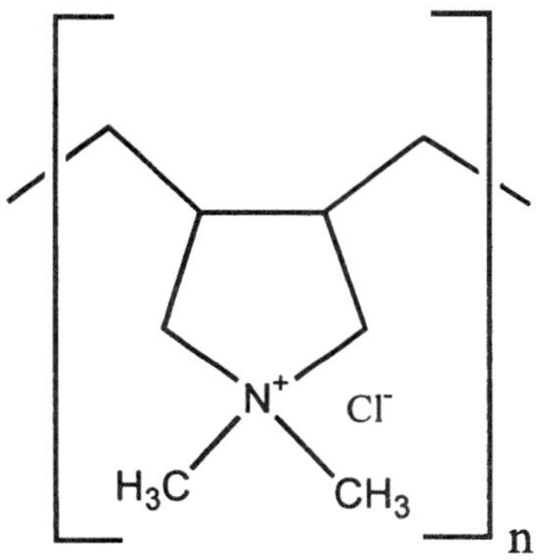

Chemical Name: *N,N*-Dimethyl-*N*-2-propen-1-aminium chloride homopolymer
Trade Name: Merquat 100 (Calgon); Conditioner P6 (3V)
Function in Formula: Conditioner, moisturizer
Use Concentration: 0.1–0.5% polymer solids in conditioners, shampoos, perms, hair dyes, hair relaxers, and rinses; 0.5–2% polymer solids in moisturizing creams, bath products, and shaving creams
Solubility Characteristics: Soluble in water in all proportions soluble in hyroalcoholic solutions containing up to 90% ethanol
Formulating Considerations: Limited compatibility with anionic surfactants and anionic polymers. Should be added to amphoteric or nonionic surfactants or to the water phase
Form Supplied: Viscous aqueous solution
Microbial Considerations: Self-preserving (Merquat). Does not support microbial growth or inhibit microorganism growth (3V)
Special Comments: High-charge-density polymer available for use in personal care products. Excellent substantivity to hair
Suppliers: Calgon, 3V

Polyquaternium-7

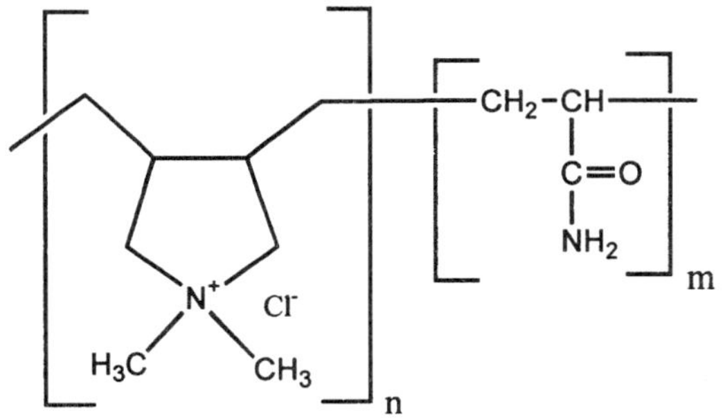

Chemical Name: Copolymer of acrylamide and *N,N*-dimethyl-2-propen-1 ammonium chloride
Trade Names: Merquat 550, Merquat S, Merquat 2200 (Calgon); Conditioner P7 (3V); Mirapol 550 (Rhone-Poulenc)
Function in Formula: Condition, moisturize, smooth; rheology builder
Use Concentration: 0.5–1.0% polymer solids in hair shampoos, conditioners, and rinses; 1–2% polymer solids in hair-styling products; 0.5% polymer solids in skin care products

Solubility Characteristics: Merquat S and Merquat 550 are soluble in water in all proportions and soluble in hydroalcoholic solutions containing up to 40% ethanol. Merquat 2200 is soluble in water in all proportions, in glycerin, and in propylene glycol. Conditioner P7 shows compatibility with anionic and cationic surfactants. Soluble in water in all proportions.
Formulating Considerations: In most formulations, should be added to the water before other ingredients. Predisperse in water phase
Form Supplied: Merquat S, Merquat 550, Conditioner P7, and Mirapol 550 are viscous aqueous solutions; Merquat 2200 is a dry powder
Microbial Considerations: Merquat polymers are preserved with methyl- and propylparabens. Conditioner P7 does not support or inhibit microbial growth
Regulatory Status: TSCA registered; CAS number 265-90-05-6
Special Comments: Highly substantive to skin and hair compatible with common anionic surfactants
Suppliers: Calgon, 3V, Rhone-Poulenc

Polyquaternium-11

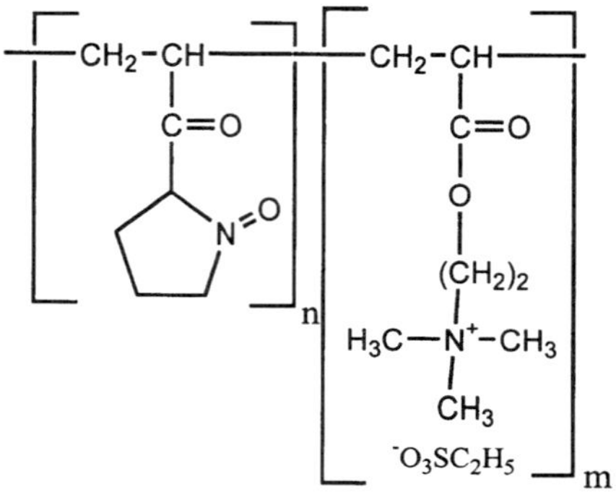

Chemical Name: Quaternized poly(vinylypyrrolidone/dimethylaminoethyl methacrylate)
Trade Name: Gafquat 755, 755N, 734
Function in Formula: Hair conditioner/fixative resin
Use Concentration: 2–10% in mousse and gel formulations; 2–5% in conditioners and shampoos
Solubility Characteristics: Water- or alcohol-soluble
Formulating Considerations: When making carbomer gels with polyquaternium-11, always maintain pH greater than 5 to prevent incompatibilities
Form Supplied: Water or alcohol solution
Regulatory Status: Determined to be safe by CIR
Supplier: ISP

Polyquaternium-16

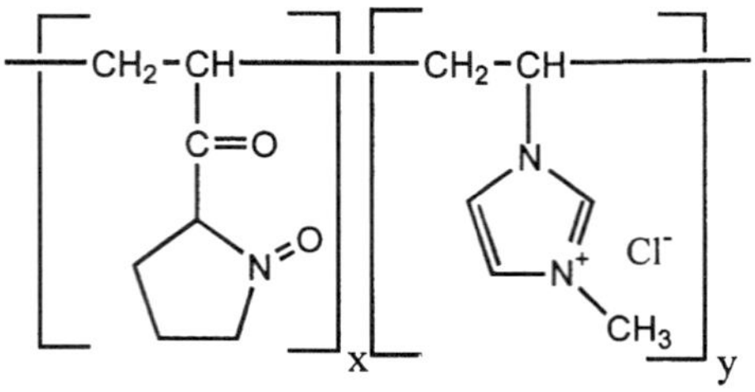

Chemical Description: Copolymer of polyvinyl pyrrolidone and imidazolinium methochloride
Trade Name: Luviquat FC, Luviquat HM
Function in Formula: Substantive conditioner, film former
Use Concentration: 3–4% in conditioners and shampoos
Solubility Characteristics: Water- or alcohol-soluble
Formulating Considerations: Add to water
Form Supplied: Aqueous solutions of 40% solids except Luviquat HM-552, which is 20%
Special Comments: High cationic density. Anionic surfactant compatible; available in varying PVP and PVI ratios: 70:30, 50:50, 95:5
Supplier: BASF

Polyquaternium-17

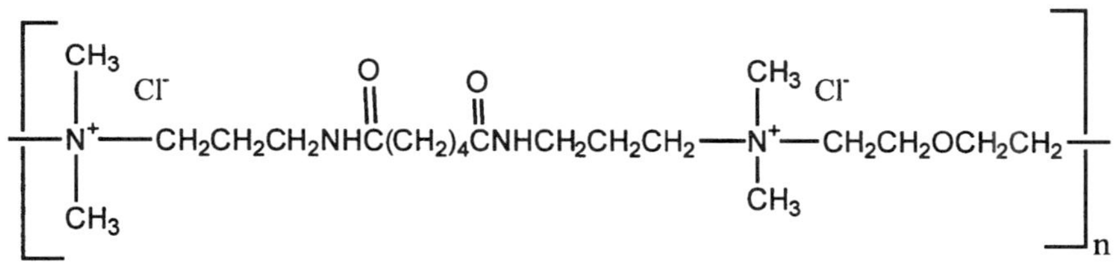

Trade Name: Mirapol AD-1
Function in Formula: Hair and skin conditioner, antistat
Use Concentration: 0.6–2.5% in shampoos, liquid skin cleansers
Solubility Characteristics: Completely soluble in water and lower alcohols
Formulating Considerations: Can be added to finished shampoo or soap. Readily dispersed in water and surfactant solutions
Form Supplied: Aqueous concentrate (62% active)
Regulatory Status: TSCA registered
Special Comments: Cationic polymer. Compatible with common anionic surfactants. Average molecular weight 50,000
Supplier: Rhone-Poulenc

Polyquaternium-18

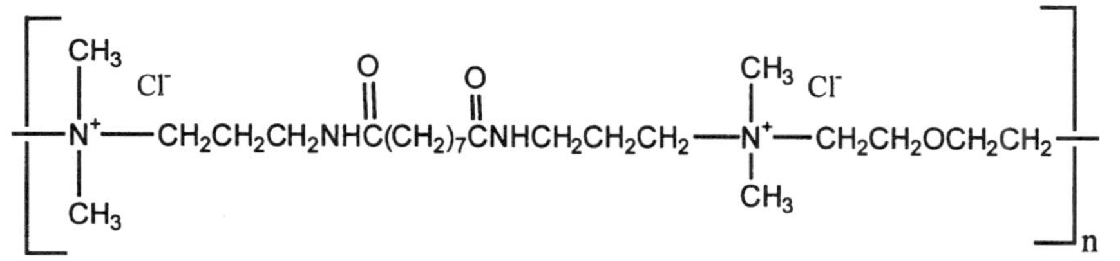

Trade Name: Mirapol AZ-1
Function in Formula: Conditioner and thickener with smectite clays
Use Concentration: 1.0–2.5% in conditioning shampoos; 1.0–2.5% in liquid soaps; 1.0–2.0% in creams and lotions (with 2–5% smectite clay)
Solubility Characteristics: Completely soluble in water and lower alcohols
Formulating Considerations: Can be added to finished shampoo or soap. With clays, add to clay dispersed in water and mix homogenizer for best results
Form Supplied: Aqueous concentrate (62% active)

Microbial Considerations: Bacteriostatic
Special Comments: Low degree of substantivity. Antistat. Remains clear in anionic systems
Suppliers: Rhone-Poulenc

Polyquaternium-22

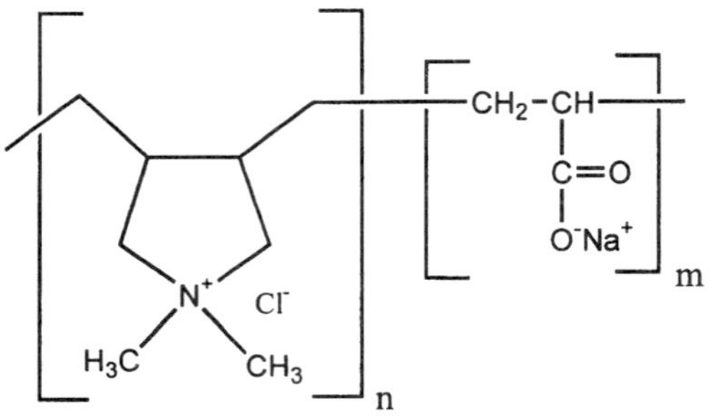

Chemical Description: Copolymer of sodium acrylate and dimethyl diallyl ammonium chloride
Trade Name: Merquat 280, 295
Function in Formula: Conditioner, moisturizer
Use Concentration: 0.5–2% in polymer solids in hair products including perms and hair dyes; 0.5–1% polymer solids in skin care products
Solubility Characteristics: Soluble in water in all proportions; soluble in hydroalcoholic solutions up to 60% ethanol
Formulating Considerations: In most formulations, should be added to water before other ingredients
Form Supplied: Viscous aqueous solution
Microbial Considerations: Merquat 280 is preserved with methyl- and propylparabens
Special Comments: Highly substantive to skin and hair
Supplier: Calgon

Polyquaternium-27

Chemical Description: Block copolymer of polyquaternium-17 and polyquaternium-2
Trade Names: Mirapol 9, Mirapol 95, Mirapol 175
Function in Formula: Conditioner and thickener with smectite clays
Use Concentration: 1.0–2.5% in conditioning shampoos; 1.0–2.5% in liquid soaps; 1.0–2.0% in creams and lotions (with 2–5% smectite clay)
Solubility Characteristics: Completely soluble in water and lower alcohols
Formulating Considerations: Same formulating procedure as for polyquaternium-2. With clays, same procedure as for polyquaternium-17 or -18
Form Supplied: Aqueous concentrate (62% active)
Microbial Considerations: Bacteriostatic
Supplier: Rhone-Poulenc

Polyquaternium-28

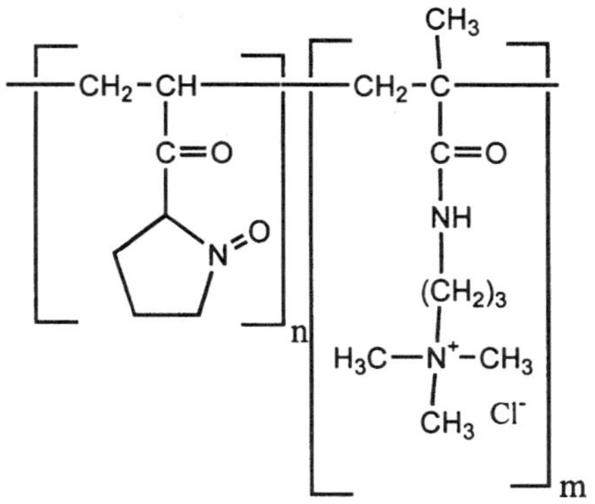

Chemical Description: Copolymer of vinyl pyrrolidone and methacrylamidopropyl/trimethylammonium chloride
Trade name: Gafquat HS-100
Function in Formula: Hair conditioner/fixative resin
Use Concentration: 2–10% in mousse and gels; 2–5% in conditioners and shampoos; 5% in permanent wave solutions
Solubility Characteristics: Water- and alcohol-soluble
Form Supplied: Aqueous solution
Special Comments: Polymer possesses excellent hydrolytic stability at pH extremes
Supplier: ISP

Polyquaternium-28 (and) Dimethicone

Chemical Description: Dimethicone encapsulated by poly(vinylpyrrolidone methacrylamidopropyl trimethyl ammonium chloride), dispersed in an aqueous solution of poly(vinylpyrrolidone methacrylamidopropyl trimethyl ammonium chloride)
Trade Name: Polymer ACP-104
Function in Formula: Conditioning and moisturizing agent
Use Concentration: 2–8% in conditioners and shampoos; 2–8% in styling products; <2% in creams and lotions
Solubility Characteristics: Encapsulates not soluble in water or oil
Formulating Considerations: In creams and lotions, add at 60–65°C after neutralization and emulsion is made
Form Supplied: Aqueous solution
Supplier: ISP

Polyquaternium-39

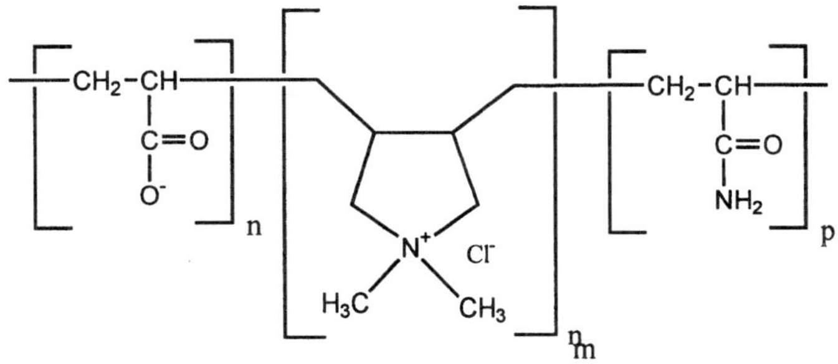

Chemical Description: Terpolymer of dimethyldiallyl ammonium chloride and sodium acrylate and acrylamide
Trade Name: Merquat Plus 3330
Function in Formula: Conditioner, moisturizer, static flyaway reduction
Use Concentration: 0.5% polymer solids in shampoos, shower gels, and liquid hand soap; 0.1–0.2% polymer solids in creams and lotions; 0.1–0.4% polymer solids in hair-styling products
Solubility Characteristics: Soluble in water in all proportions; soluble in hydroalcoholic solutions containing up 40% ETOH
Formulating Considerations: In most formulations should be added to the water before other ingredients. Good anionic surfactant compatibility
Form Supplied: Viscous aqueous solution
Microbial Considerations: Preserved with methyl- and propylparabens
Special Comments: Substantive to skin and hair
Supplier: Calgon

Polyquaternium-41

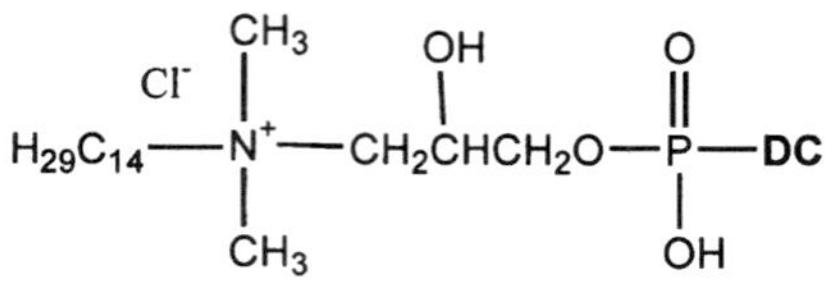

DC = dimethicone copolyol copolymer

Chemical Name: *N*-Tetradecyl-*N′*,*N′*-dimethyl-*N‴*-dimethiconecopolyolphospho-2-propanolammonium chloride
Trade Name: PECOSIL SMQ-40
Function in Formula: Conditioner
Use Concentration: 5% in conditioners, shampoos, hair-styling gels
Solubility Characteristics: Soluble in water
Form Supplied: 35–38% in aqueous solution
Regulatory Status: Benzene-free
Supplier: Phoenix

Polyquaternium-42

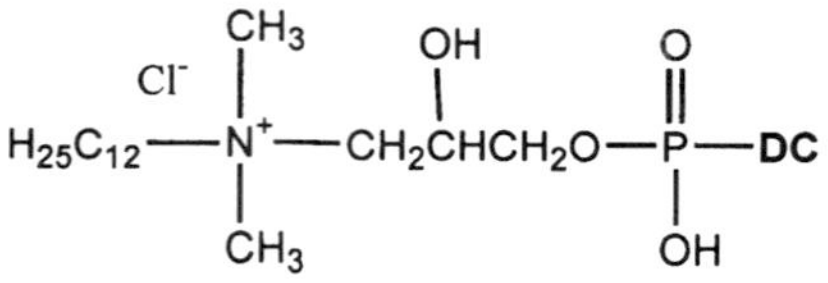

DC = dimethicone copolyol copolymer

Chemical Name: *N*-Lauryl-*N′*,*N′*-dimethyl-*N″*-dimethiconecopolylphosho-2-propanolammonium chloride
Trade Name: PECOSIL SPB-1240
Function in Formula: Conditioner
Use Concentration: 5% in conditioners, shampoos, hand lotions
Solubility Characteristics: Soluble in water
Form Supplied: 35–38% in water

Regulatory Status: Benzene-free
Supplier: Phoenix

Potassium Dimethicone Copolyol Panthenyl Phosphate

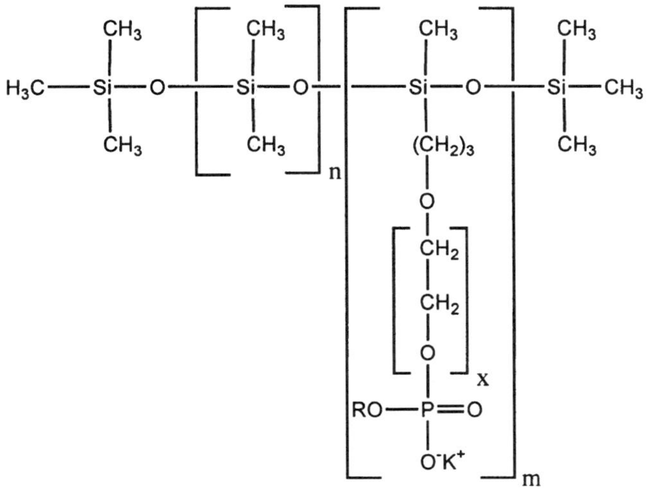

Chemical Name: Poly(dimethylsiloxane copolyol phosphonopanthenoate)
Trade Name: PECOSIL SPP-100
Function in Formula: Conditioner
Use Concentration: 3–5% in conditioners, shampoos, hair-styling gels
Solubility Characteristics: Soluble in water
Form Supplied: Paste
Regulatory Status: Benzene-free
Supplier: Phoenix

PVM/MA Copolymer

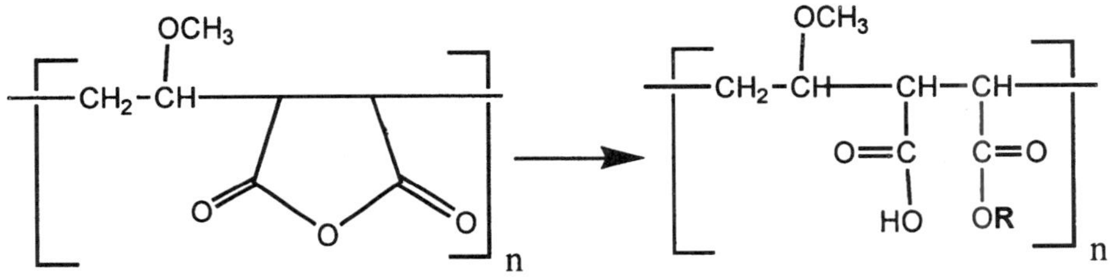

Base Polymer

where **R** = C_2H_5, C_3H_7, C_4H_9
Esterified Derivative

Chemical Name: Poly(methyl vinyl ether-co-maleic anhydride)
Trade Names: Gantrez ES-225, Gantrez V-225, Gantrez SP-215, Gantrez V-215 (ISP), UCARSET Resin (Amerchol), *Isopropylester*; Gantrez ES-334 (ISP); Gantrez ES-425, Gantrez V-425 (ISP), *Butylester*
Function in Formula: Hair fixative resin
Use Concentration: 4–12% in hairspray; 5–8% in mousse

Solubility Characteristics: Soluble in alcohol and hydroalcoholic solutions
Formulating Considerations: Compatible with commonly used propellants and solvents. V polymers for 80% VOC compliance
Form Supplied: Alcoholic solution
Microbial Considerations: Free of bacterial contaminations
Regulatory Status: Not reviewed by CIR
Suppliers: ISP, Amerchol

PVM/MA Decadiene Crosspolymer

Chemical Description: Copolymer of methyl vinyl ether/maleic anhydride, which has been crosslinked
Trade Name: Stabileze 06
Function in Formula: Thickener and stabilizer
Use Concentration: 0.25–2.0% in styling gels; 1–2% in shampoos and conditioners; <1% in skin creams and lotions
Solubility Characteristics: Hydrophilic, soluble in water, alcohol, and polar solvents
Formulating Considerations: Any ingredients with reactive groups (e.g., polquaterniums) should be added after polymer is neutralized
Form Supplied: Fine white powder
Regulatory Status: Benzene-free
Special Comments: Instantly water-dispersible. Polymer is hydrolyzed to diacid before neutralization
Supplier: ISP

PVP

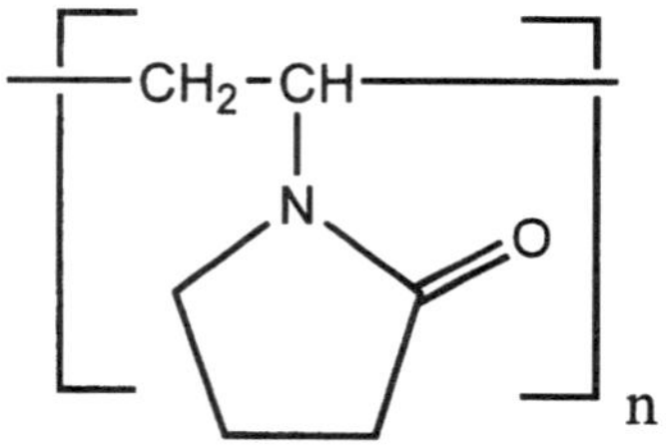

Chemical Name: Poly(vinylpyrrolidone)
Trade Names: PVP K-30, PVP K-90, K-120(ISP), Luviskol K (BASF)
Function in Formula: Film former, hair fixative resin, thickener, dispersant, lubricant skin protectant, adhesion promoter, gel
Use Concentration: <1% in skin care products; 2–5% in hair-setting products; 1–4% in hairsprays (aerosol), <1% in shampoos; 1% in adhesives
Solubility Characteristics: Soluble in water, lower aliphatic alcohols, glycols
Formulating Considerations: Insoluble in hydrocarbons. Incompatible with unneutralized carbomers—becomes compatible above pH 5.0. Compatible with a wide range of hairspray ingredients including propellants and solvents. Add to water or alcohol phase
Form Supplied: Powders and aqueous solutions
Special Comments: Also available as pharmaceutical grade; K values from 12 to 120 available. Fixative hold increases with increase in K value
Suppliers: ISP, BASF

PVP (and) Dimethicone

Chemical Name: Polyvinylpyrrolidone-encapsulated dimethicone dispersed in an aqueous solution of polyvinylpyrrolidone
Trade Name: Polymer ACP-1006
Function in Formula: Conditioning and moisturizing agent
Use Concentration: 2–8% in conditioning shampoos and conditioners, 2–8% in styling aids; <2% in creams and lotions
Solubility Characteristics: Encapsulates not soluble in oil or water
Formulating Considerations: Add at end of batching before preservative and fragrance
Form Supplied: Aqueous solutions
Supplier: ISP

PVP/Acrylates Copolymer

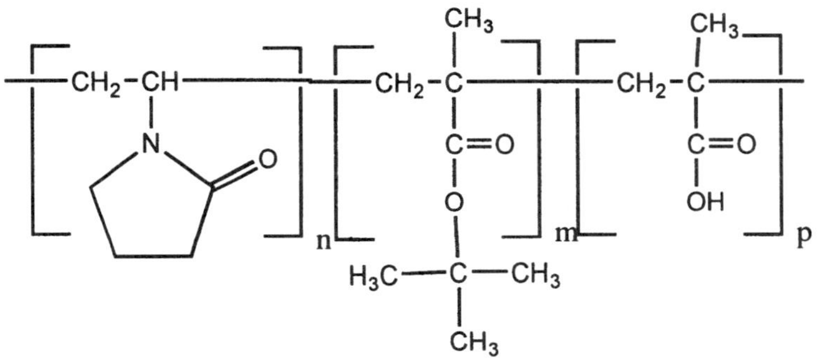

Chemical Description: Terpolymer based on vinyl pyrrolidone and acrylic acid compounds
Trade Name: Luviflex VBM 35
Function in Formula: Film former, hair fixative
Use Concentration: 5–8% in hair fixative
Solubility Characteristics: Alcohol- and alkaline-soluble
Formulating Considerations: Luviflex VBM 35 must be neutralized, neutralize 20–100% for best results. Neutralization is necessary for water solubility
Form Supplied: Alcoholic solutions
Supplier: BASF

PVP/Dimethylaminoethyl Methacrylate Copolymer

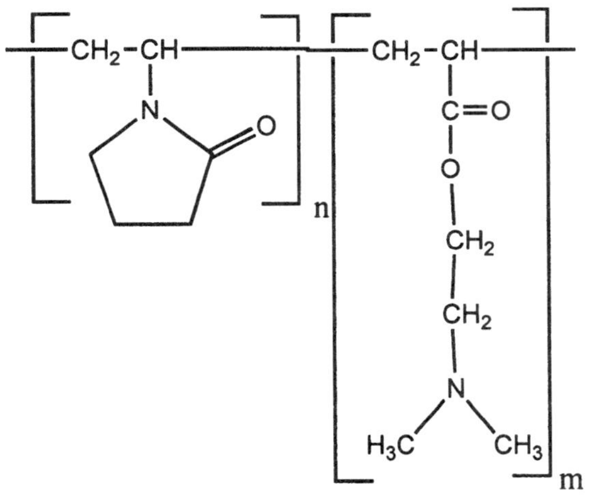

Chemical Name: Poly(vinylpyrrolidone-co-dimethylaminoethyl methacrylate)
Trade Name: Copolymer 845, 937, 958
Function in Formula: Conditioner/hair-fixative resin
Use Concentration: 2–10% in mousse/gel; 2–5% in conditioner/shampoo
Solubility Characteristics: Water- and alcohol-soluble
Form Supplied: Water and alcohol solution
Supplier: ISP

PVP/Dimethylaminoethylmethacrylate Polycarbamyl Polyglycol Ester

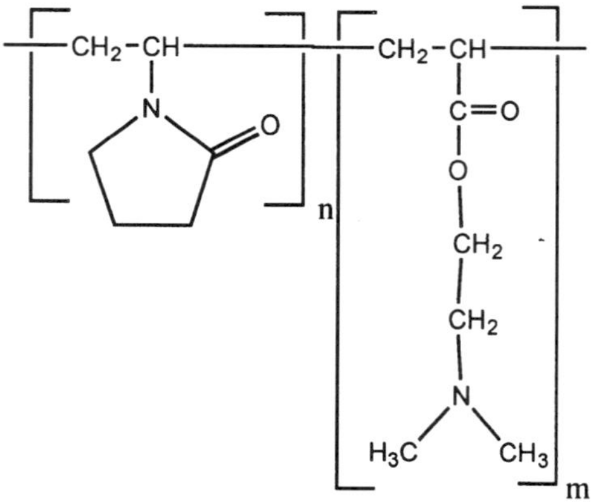

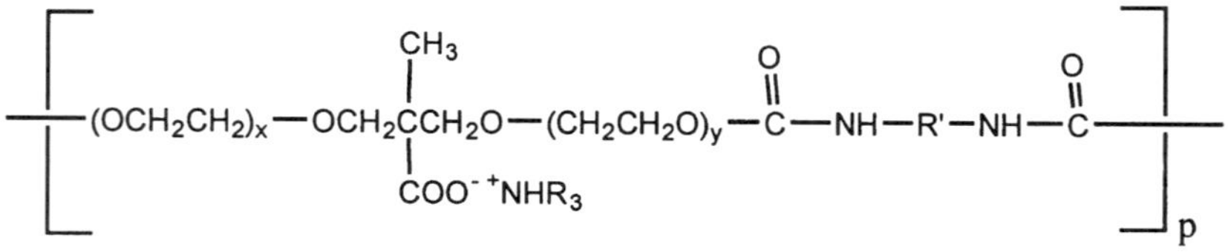

Chemical Name: Poly(vinyl pyrrolidone-co-dimethylaminoethyl-methacrylate)/polyurethane interpolymer
Trade Name: PECOGEL GC-310, GC-1110
Function in Formula: Film former/conditioner
Use Concentration: 3% in conditioner; 2% in shampoo; 5% in mascara
Solubility Characteristics: Water- and alcohol-soluble
Form Supplied: 10% aqueous solution
Regulatory Status: Benzene-free
Special Comments: GC-310: 3 parts PVP/dimethylaminoethylmethacrylate to 1 part polyurethane; GC-1110: 1 part PVP/dimethylaminoethylmethacrylate to 1 part polyurethane
Supplier: Phoenix

PVP/Dimethiconylacrylate/Polycarbamyl Polyglycol Ester

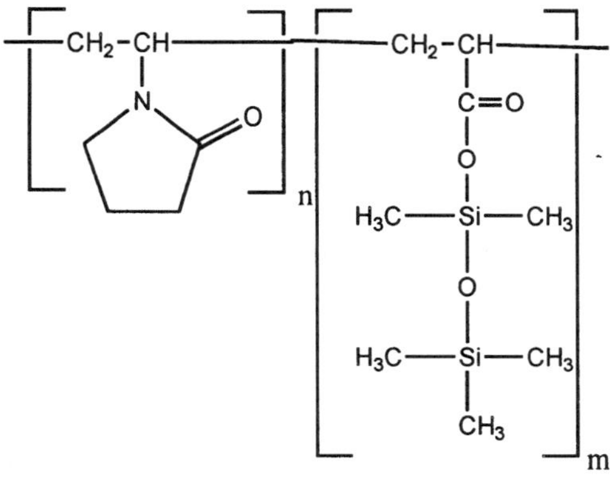

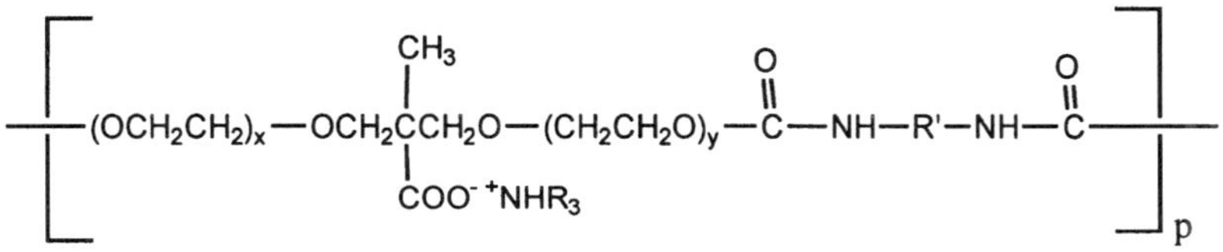

Trade Name: PECOGEL S-1120
Function in Formula: Film former
Use Concentration: 5% in mascara; 10% in sunscreens; 2% in conditioner
Solubility Characteristics: Water- and alcohol-soluble
Form Supplied: 20% aqueous solutions
Supplier: Phoenix

PVP/Eicosene Copolymer

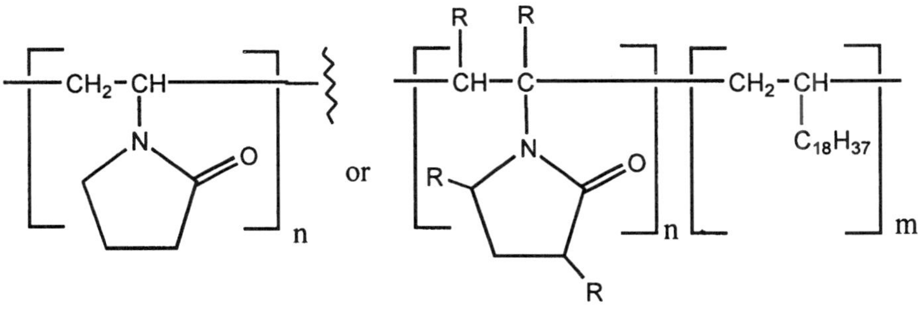

Trade Names: Ganex V-220 (ISP), Unimer V-15 (Induchem)
Function in Formula: Waterproofing film former, pigment dispersant, wear-proofing film former
Use Concentration: 1–6% in sunscreens; 3–10% in makeup; 2–5% in creams/lotions; 2–10% in lipsticks (waterproof, film forming), up to 30% in color cosmetics (pigment dispersion)
Solubility Characteristics: Oil-soluble, water-insoluble
Form Supplied: 100% waxy solid
Suppliers: ISP, Induchem

PVP/Ethyl Methacrylate/Methacrylic Acid Terpolymer

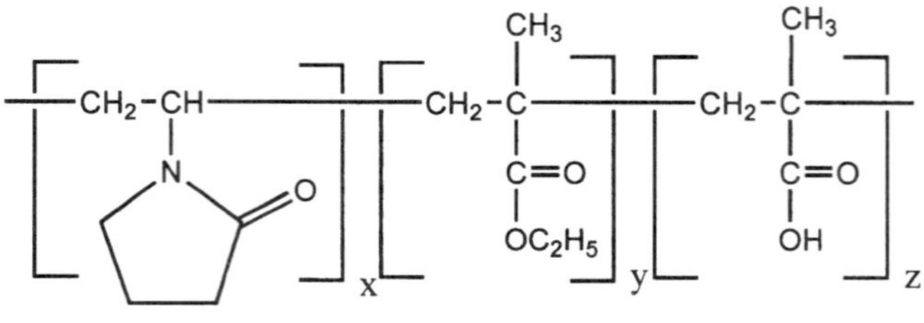

Chemical Name: Poly(*N*-vinyl-2-pyrrolidone-ethyl methacrylate-methacrylic acid)
Trade Name: Stepanhold R-1
Function in Formula: Hair-fixative resin
Use Concentration: 9–10% in hairspray and setting aids
Solubility Characteristics: Soluble in water and alcohol
Formulating Considerations: Complete alcohol solubility gives greater formula stability and more uniform neutralization in production. Clear films result from low levels of neutralization
Supplier: Stepan

PVP/Hexadecane Copolymer

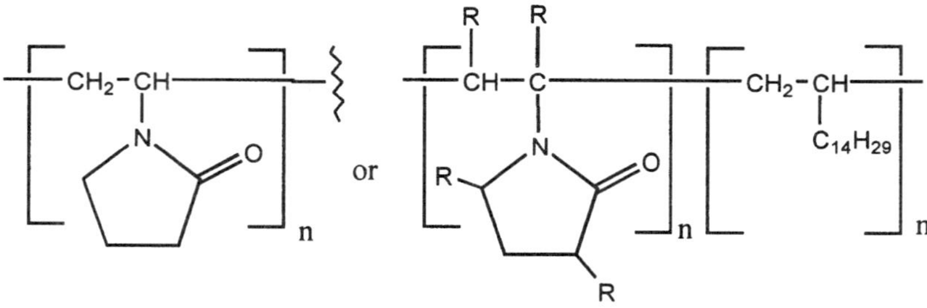

Chemical Name: Poly(vinylpyrrolidone-co-hexadecene)
Trade Names: Ganex V-216 (ISP), Unimer U-151 (Induchem)
Function in Formula: Waterproofing film former, dispersant
Use Concentration: 1–6% in sunscreens; 3–10% in makeup; 2–6% in creams/lotions; 3–10% in makeup; 2–6% in lipsticks/gloss
Solubility Characteristics: Oil-soluble, water-insoluble
Form Supplied: 100% liquid
Suppliers: ISP, Induchem

PVP/Polycarbamyl Polyglycol Ester

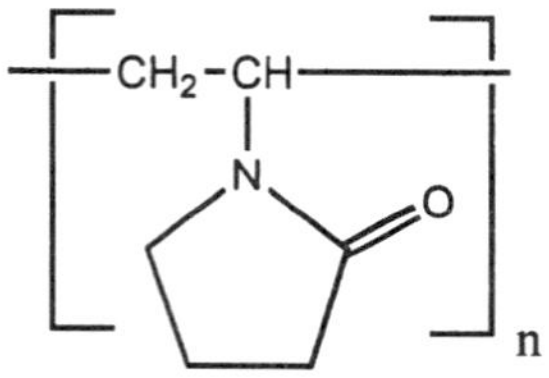

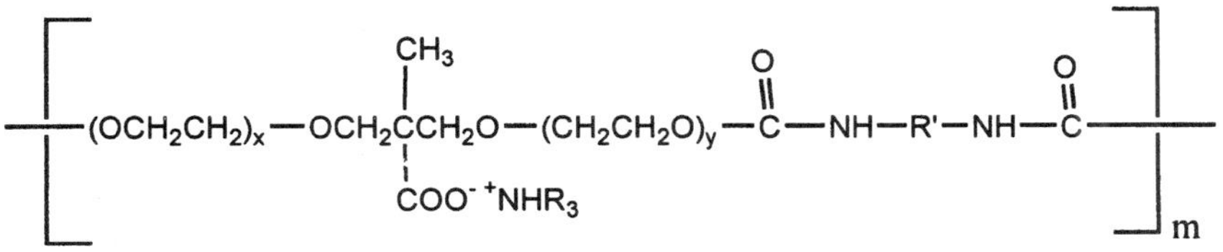

Chemical Name: PVP/polyurethane Interpolymer
Trade Names: PECOGEL H-12, H-115, H-1220
Function in Formula: Film former
Use Concentration: 5% in mascara; 2% in shampoo; 3% in conditioner
Solubility Characteristics: Soluble in water and alcohol
Form Supplied: H-12 is 12% aqueous solution, H-115 is 15% aqueous solution, H-1220 is 20% aqueous solution
Regulatory Status: Benzene-free
Special Comments: H-12 is 3 parts PVP to 1 part polyurethane; H-115 is 1 part PVP to 1 part polyurethane; H-1220 is 1 part PVP to 2 parts polyurethane
Supplier: Phoenix

PVP/VA Copolymer

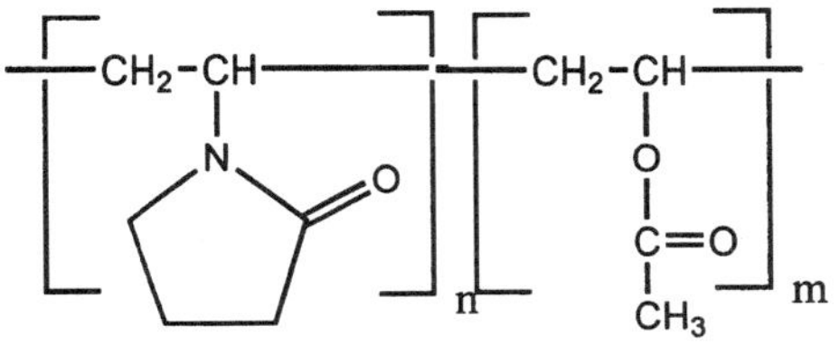

Chemical Name: Poly(vinylpyrrolidone-co-vinyl acetate)
Trade Names: PVP/VA E-735, PVP/VA E-635, PVP/VA S-630, PVP/VA W-735, (ISP); Luviskol VA Grades (BASF)
Function in Formula: Film former, hair fixative
Use Concentration: 2–6% in gel, setting lotions; 4–8% in hair fixatives; 2% in coatings
Solubility Characteristics: Varying water and alcohol solubilities depending on grade
Formulating considerations: Depends on grade. Those with high vinyl acetate content are relatively insoluble in water. All are soluble in ethanol. Not soluble in hydrocarbon alone. Compatible with a wide range of hair spray ingredients including propellants and solvents
Form Supplied: PVP/VA S-630 supplied as white powder; all others are supplied as alcoholic solutions, in which the solvent is either ethanol or isopropanol or water
Special Comments: Available in varying PVP:PVA ratios of 70:30, 60:40, 50:50, 30:70, 20:80
Suppliers: ISP, BASF

PVP/VA/Vinyl Propionate Copolymer

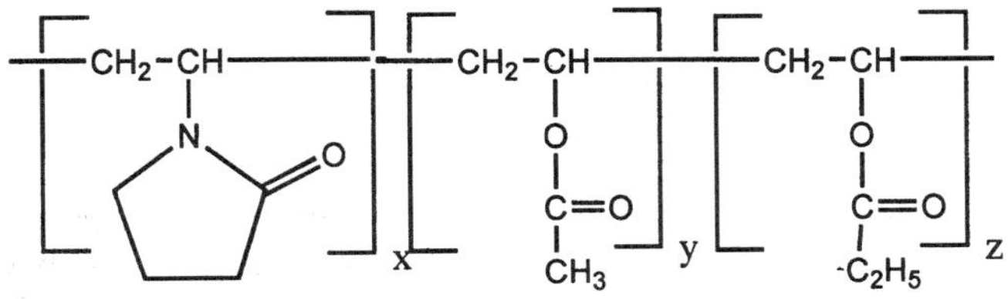

Chemical Description: Terpolymer of vinyl pyrrolidone, vinyl acetate, and vinyl propionate
Trade Names: Luviskol VAP343E, Luviskol VAP343I
Function in Formula: Hair setting resin
Use Concentration: 1–3% in hairsprays; 3–6% in pump sprays, setting lotions
Solubility Characteristics: Soluble in ethanol and isopropanol
Formulating Considerations: >35% ethanol required for hydroalcoholic systems containing 5% solids. Product has hydrocarbon compatibility in hairspray formulations
Form Supplied: 50% solution in ethanol or isopropanol
Special Comments: K value ~ 30
Supplier: BASF

Quaternium-80

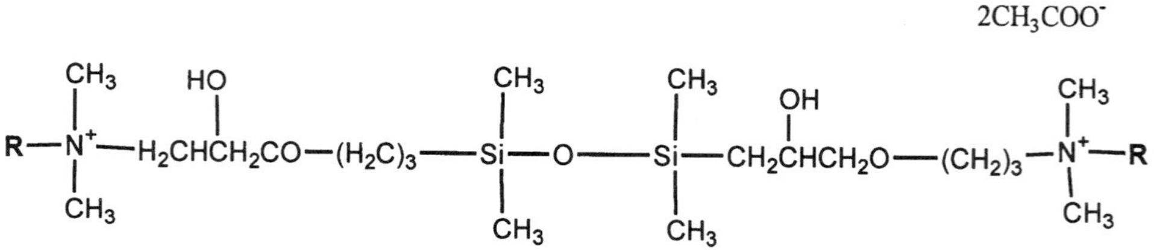

where **R** = long-chainalkyl group

Chemical Name: Diquaternary polydimethylsiloxane
Trade Names: Abil-Quat 3270, 3272
Function in Formula: Substantive to hair, conditioning agent
Use Concentration: 0.5–1.5% in shower and foam baths, shampoos, and conditioners
Solubility Characteristics: Soluble in polar media
Form Supplied: Liquid
Supplier: Goldschmidt

Quaternized Hydrolyzed Wheat Protein/Dimethicone Phosphocopolyol Copolymer

Chemical Description: Polymer hydrolysate of wheat protein reacted with dimethicone copolyol phosphate via an alkyl chloride bridge to form a copolymer, which is then quaternized with monochlorohydrin
Trade Name: PECOSIL SWPQ-40
Function in Formula: Conditioner/film former
Use Concentration: 5% in hair-styling gels, conditioners, and shampoos
Solubility Characteristics: Soluble in water
Form Supplied: 35–38% aqueous solution
Regulatory Status: Benzene-free
Supplier: Phoenix

Silica

Si0$_2$

Chemical Name: Amorphous silicon dioxide
Trade Name: CAB-O-SIL Fumed Silica
Function in Formula: Thickening and gelling of fluids and free flow of powders, antisetting
Use Concentration: 2–4% in gels; 0.5–2% in thickening; 0.2-0.5% in antisettling and free flow
Solubility Characteristics: Soluble in strong alkalies—pH 10.5. Not soluble in water or organics

Formulating Considerations: Must be properly dispersed to achieve good efficiency. Seek advice from technical service for specific recommendations
Form Supplied: Dry powder
Microbial Considerations: None
Regulatory Status: FDA approved
Supplier: Cabot

Chemical Name: Silicon dioxide, fumed amorphous
Trade Name: TC25 Silica, TC10 Silica (Crosfield), Aerosil 200 (Degussa)
Function in Formula: Thickener
Use Concentration: 2–20% in toothpaste; <10% in oil
Solubility Characteristics: Insoluble in water
Formulating Considerations: Compatible with all known active ingredients in toothpaste. Dispersed into liquid phase of product. Use a high-speed mixer to disperse
Form Supplied: Fine white powder, spray-dried powder
Microbial Considerations: <300/g molds and yeasts: <10/g negative: <10/g-using standard plate counts
Regulatory Status: Meet FCC food grade specs
Suppliers: Crosfield, Degussa, Kraft Chemical Company

Sodium Polymethacrylate

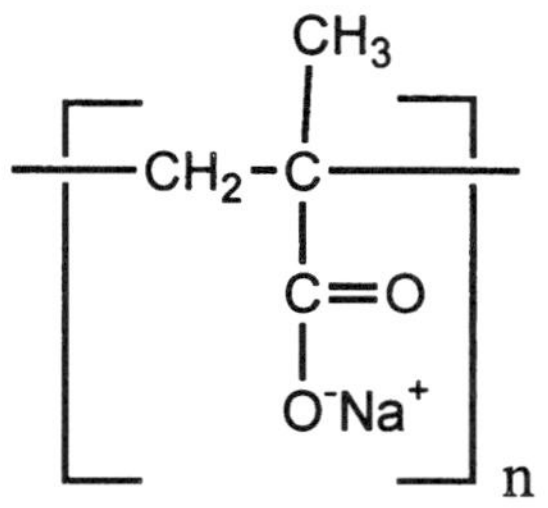

Trade Name: DARVAN No.7
Function in Formula: Dispersing agent
Use Concentration: 0.5–4% of the weight of solids to be dispersed
Solubility Characteristics: Soluble in water
Formulating Considerations: Compatible with anionic and nonionic species. Incompatible with cationics
Form Supplied: Clear colorless liquid—25% active
Supplier: Vanderbilt

Sodium Polynaphthalenesulfonate

Chemical Structure: This product is a mixture of polymeric species. No distinct chemical structure can be drawn
Chemical Description: Sodium salt of polymerized alkyl naphthalene sulfonic acid
Trade Name: DARVAN No.1
Function in Formula: Dispersing agent
Use concentration: 0.5–4% based on weight of solids to be dispersed
Solubility Characteristics: Soluble in water
Form Supplied: Buff-colored powder, 87% min. active
Microbial Considerations: Susceptible to microbial attack, requires preservation
Supplier: Vanderbilt

Sodiumpolystyrene Sulfonate

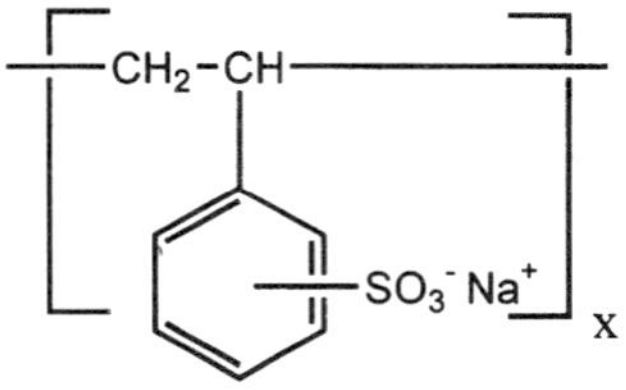

Trade Name: Flexan 130
Function in Formula: Hair fixative/conditioning agent
Use Concentration: 1–3% in mousses and fixative lotions
Solubility Characteristics: Soluble in water
Form Supplied: 30% solution in water
Supplier: National Starch

Stearoxy Dimethicone

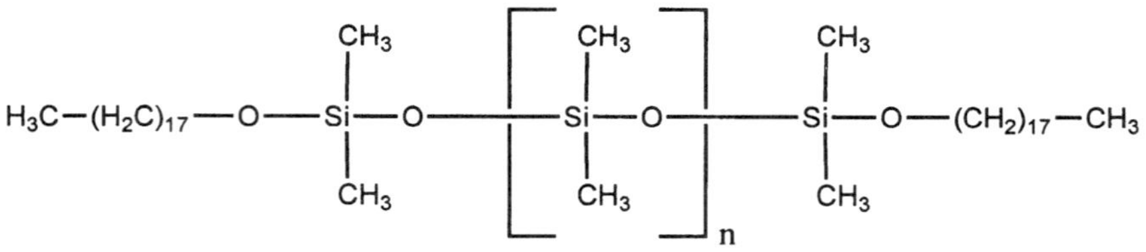

Chemical Name: Dialkoxy dimethyl polysiloxane
Trade Name: Abil Wax 2434 (Goldschmidt); Silicone Fluid Q5-0158A (Dow Corning)
Function in Formula: Emollient, pigment disperser, barrier protection, lubricant
Use Concentration: 1–5% in creams and lotions; 1–5% in pigmented products; 0.1–0.5% in antiperspirants; 1–5% in deodorant sticks, roll-ons
Solubility Characteristics: Soluble in mineral oil, cosmetic esters, cyclomethicone. Insoluble in polar media
Formulating Considerations: Melting point 20–30°C. Add to oil/wax phase
Form Supplied: Waxy semisolid—100% active
Special Comments: Nonionic, improves pigment adhesion, spreading and penetrating properties in lotions and antiperspirants
Suppliers: Goldschmidt, Dow Corning

Stearyl Dimethicone

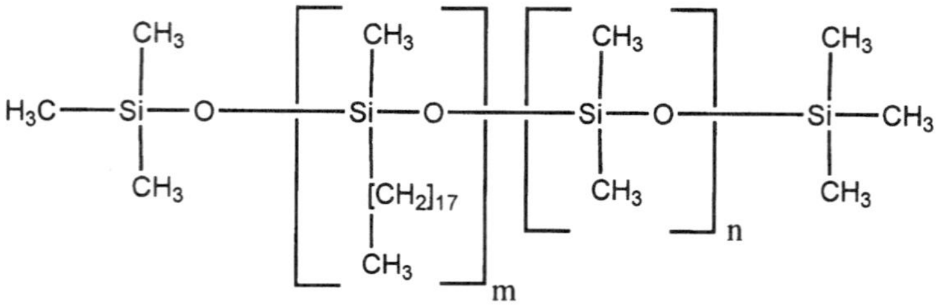

Chemical Name: Polysiloxane polyalkylene copolymer
Trade Name: Abil Wax 9800D
Function in Formula: Emollient
Use Concentration: 1–5% in deodorant sticks; 1–5% in lipsticks
Solubility Characteristics: Soluble in oils. Insoluble in water
Formulating Considerations: Melting point 20–30°C. Add to oil phase of emulsions. Disperse in oils/waxes of pigmented products
Form Supplied: Semisolid wax
Regulatory Status: Nonhazardous
Special Comments: Improves the color of decorative cosmetics
Supplier: Goldschmidt

Stearyl Methicone

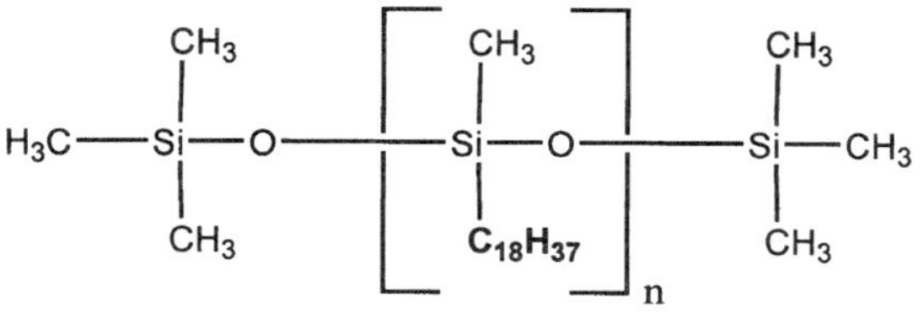

Chemical Name: Polymethylalkyl siloxane
Trade Name: Abil Wax 9809
Function in Formula: Emollient and barrier properties, nonionic
Use Concentration: 0.1–0.5% in antiperspirants; 1–3% in creams and lotions; 2–8% in eye-makeup removers
Solubility Characteristics: Soluble in mineral oil, emollient oils and esters
Formulating Considerations: Add with oil or wax phase. Requires heating to 50°C to liquefy
Form Supplied: Solid wax
Regulatory Status: Nonhazardous
Special Comments: Reduces greasiness of oils, soft emollient after feel, gels mineral oil
Supplier: Goldschmidt

Styrene/PVP Copolymer

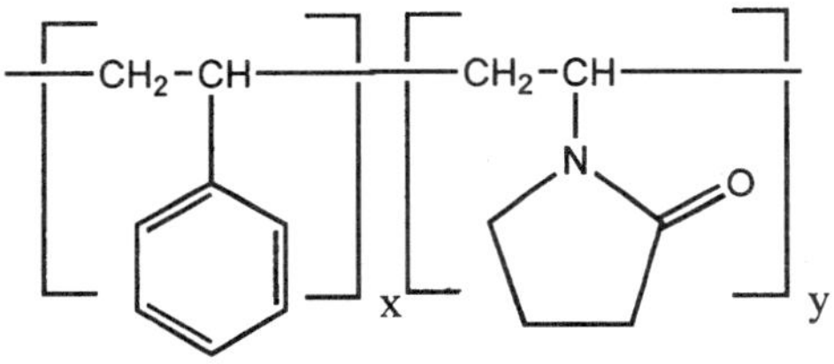

Chemical Description: Vinylpyrrolidone styrene copolymer emulsion
Trade Name: Polectron 430
Function in Formula: Opacifier
Use Concentration: 0.5–2% in shampoos/conditioners; 1-2% in permanent wave solutions
Solubility Characteristics: Dispersions in water
Form Supplied: Water emulsion, 40% solids
Supplier: ISP

Tricontanyl PVP

Chemical Description: Copolymer of PVP and tricontene
Trade Name: Ganex WP-660
Function in Formula: Water- and wear-proofing film former
Use Concentration: 1–5% in sunscreens; 3-10% in makeup products; 2–5% in creams and lotions
Solubility Characteristics: Oil-soluble, water-insoluble
Formulating Considerations: Polymer has an HLB requirement of 6. Fatty esters are recommended as emulsifiers. Add polymer to oil phase at 80–85°C
Form Supplied: Off-white flakes
Supplier: ISP

Trihydroxystearin

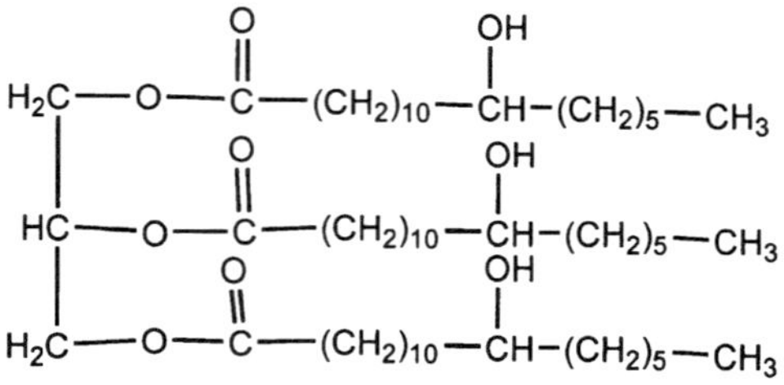

Chemical Name: Glyceryl tri (12-hydroxystearate)
Trade Names: Thixcin; Flowtone (Southern Clay)
Function in Formula: Thickener, suspending agent
Use Concentration: 2% in eye products; 2% in ointments and lipsticks
Solubility Characteristics: Disperses in oils
Formulating Considerations: Needs heat and shear activation. Pregel in binder and solvent preferred, compatible with most ingredients
Form Supplied: White powder
Regulatory Status: On priority list of CIR as of 1987
Suppliers: Rheox, Southern Clay

Trimethyl Silyl Amodimethicone

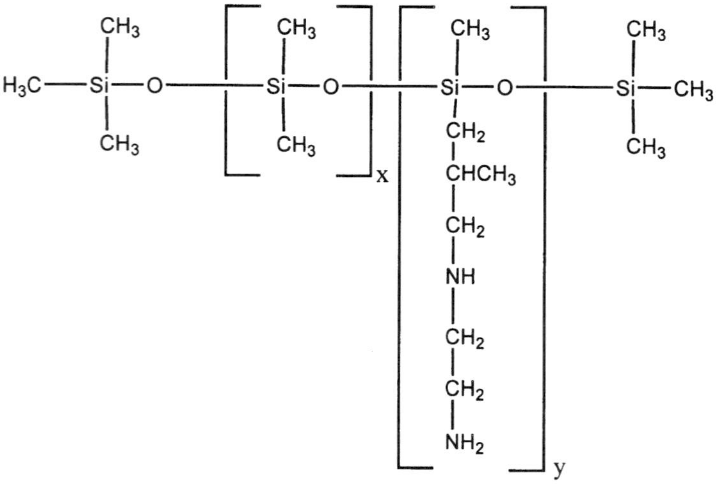

Trade Name: Silicone Fluid Q2-8220
Function in Formula: Substantive conditioner. Adds gloss in hair products
Use Concentration: 2% in hair conditioner
Solubility Characteristics: Insoluble in water, ethanol propylene glycol, and mineral oil; soluble in isopropanol, cyclomethicone, dimethicone
Formulating Considerations: Compatible with typical hair-conditioning agents, including quaternary ammonium salts
Form Supplied: Liquid
Special Comments: Avoid eye and skin contact with the undiluted raw material
Supplier: Dow Corning

VA/Butyl Maleate/Isobornyl Acrylate Copolymer

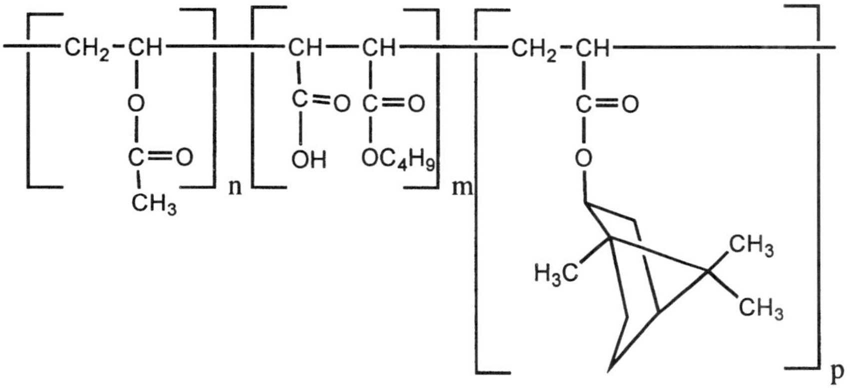

Chemical Description: Terpolymer of vinyl acetate, butyl maleate, and isobornyl acrylate
Trade Names: Advantage CP, Advantage V
Function in Formula: Hair-fixative resin
Use Concentration: 4–12% in hairsprays
Solubility Characteristics: Soluble in alcohol and hydroalcohollic solutions
Formulating Considerations: Compatible with a wide range of hairspray ingredients including propellants and solvents. V polymer is for 80% VOC
Form Supplied: Alcoholic solution
Special Comments: Stiff-holding hair fixative, excellent spray characteristics
Supplier: ISP

VA/Crotonates Copolymer

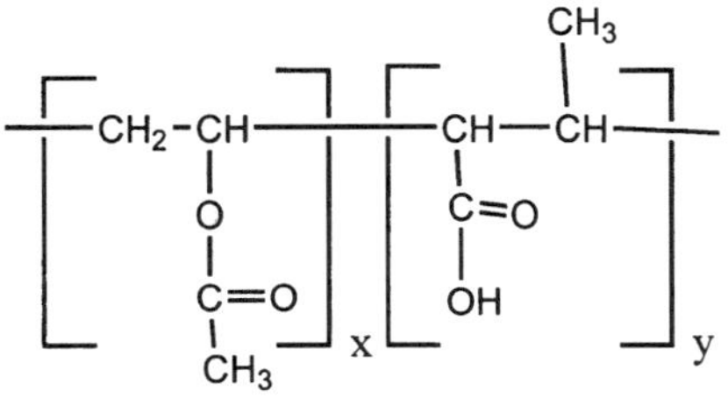

Chemical Name: Poly(vinyl acetate-co-crotonic acid)
Trade Names: Resyn 28-1310 (National Starch), Luviset CA 66 (BASF)

Function in Formula: Binder/hair-fixative resin, film former
Use Concentration: 3–5% in hairsprays, 5% in styling lotions
Solubility Characteristics: Soluble in ethanol and hydroalcoholic systems when neutralized. Alkaline soluble
Formulating Considerations: Generally neutralized 60–90% with AMP when formulated. Becomes water-soluble when 100% neutralized. Neutralizer should be added to alcohol solution first, then resin can be added
Form Supplied: Fine, white beads
Regulatory Status: Benzene-free
Special Comments: Acidity = 1.16 ml/g. Solubility can be controlled by pH adjustment
Suppliers: National Starch, BASF

VA/Crotonates/Vinyl Neodecanoate Copolymer

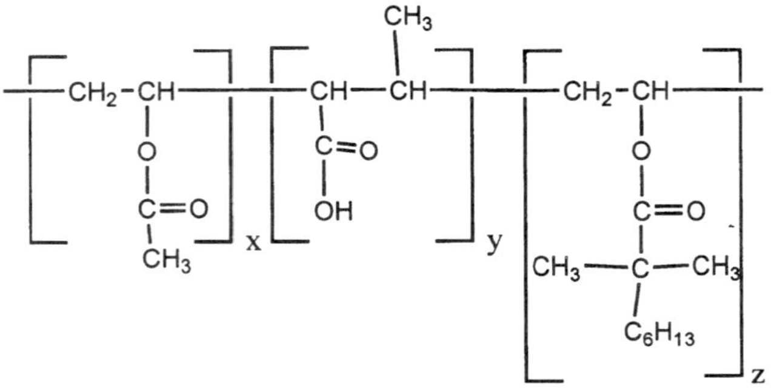

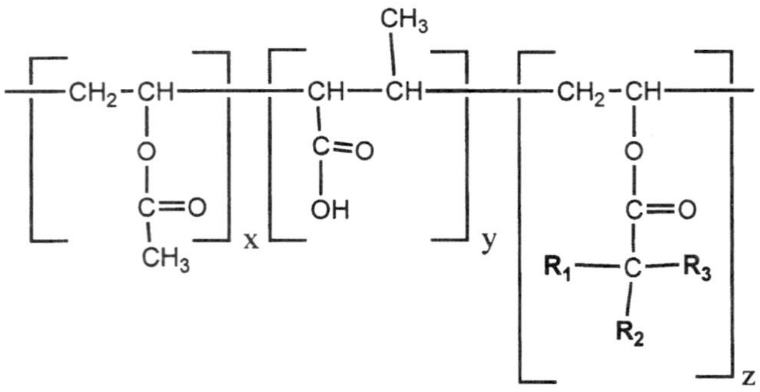

$\mathbf{R}_1$, $\mathbf{R}_2$, and $\mathbf{R}_3$ are saturated alkyl groups

Chemical Description: Copolymer of vinyl acetate, crotonic acid, and vinyl neodecanoate
Trade Names: Resyn 28-2913; Resyn 28-2930
Function in Formula: Hair fixative
Use Concentration: 3–5% in hairsprays; 5% in styling lotions
Solubility Characteristics: Soluble in ethanol and isopropanol
Formulating Considerations: Generally neutralized 80–90% for use in hairspray. Becomes water-soluble when 100% neutralized. AMP is most common neutralizer
Form Supplied: 29-2913: dry beads; 28-2930: fine, translucent beads
Regulatory Status: Benzene-free
Special Comments: 29-2913: acidity = 1.24 mEq/g; 28-2930: Acidity = 1.16 mEq/g
Supplier: National Starch

VA Acetate/Crotonates Acid/Vinyl Propionate Copolymer

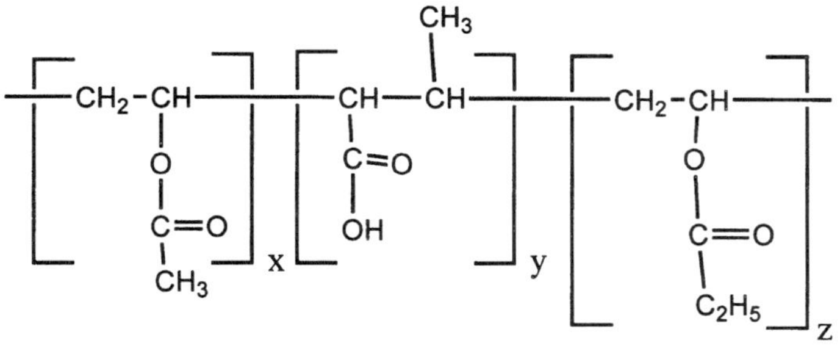

Chemical Description: Terpolymer formed from vinyl acetate, crotonic acid, and vinyl propionate
Trade Name: Luviset CAP
Function in Formula: Hair fixative, film former
Use Concentration: 2–4% in hairsprays and setting lotions
Solubility Characteristics: Soluble in ethanol and isopropanol and alkalies
Formulating Considerations: Has to be neutralized to approximately 75% for best results. 100% neutralization confers water solubility
Form Supplied: Fine beads
Special Comments: Good hydrocarbon compatibility. Solubility can be controlled by pH adjustment
Supplier: BASF

Vinylcaprolactam/PVP/Dimethylaminoethylmethacrylate Copolymer

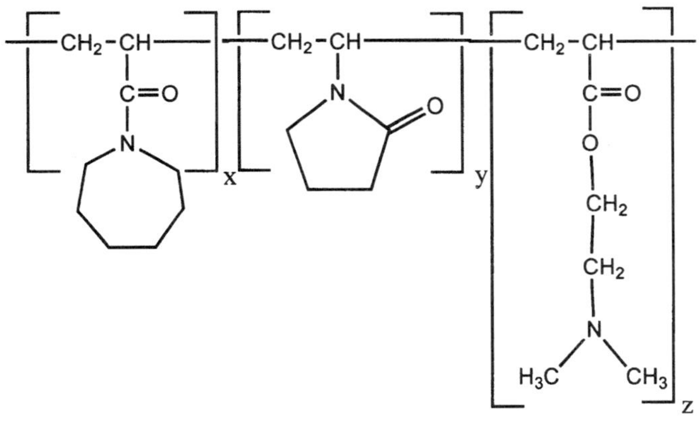

Chemical Description: Terpolymer formed from vinylpyrrolidone, dimethylaminoethyl methacrylate, and vinylcaprolactam
Trade Names: Gaffix VC-713, H20LD
Function in Formula: Film former/hair-fixative resin
Use Concentration: 3–6% in gels; 5–8% in mousses; 3–6% in hairsprays
Solubility Characteristics: Soluble in water and alcohol
Form Supplied: 37% in ethanol or fine white powder
Supplier: ISP

Index

Polymer terminology Appendix appears after Chapter 1
Encyclopedia of common cosmetic polymers appears as primary Appendix after Chapter 12
Bold numbers indicate the start of chapters